Disorders of the Knee

DISORDERS OF THE KNEE

ARTHUR J. HELFET

B.Sc. (Cape Town), M.D., M.Ch. Orth. (Liverpool), F.R.C.S. (England), F.A.C.S.

Emeritus Professor, formerly Chairman, Department of Orthopaedic Surgery, Albert Einstein College of Medicine, New York; Consulting Orthopaedic Surgeon, Hospital for Joint Diseases, New York; Formerly Senior Visiting Orthopaedic Surgeon and Senior Lecturer in Orthopaedic Surgery, University of Cape Town and Groote Schuur Hospital; Hunterian Professor, Royal College of Surgeons

With 27 Guest Authors

Second Edition

J. B. Lippincott Company : Philadelphia : Toronto

SECOND EDITION

For information address J. B. Lippincott Company, East
Washington Square, Philadelphia, Pennsylvania 19105.

1 3 5 6 4 2

Library of Congress Cataloging in Publication Data
Main entry under title:

Disorders of the knee.

Bibliography
Includes index.
1. Knee—Diseases. 2. Knee—Wounds and injuries.
I. Helfet, Arthur J. [DNLM: 1. Knee. 2. Knee in-
juries. WE 870 H474m]
RC951.D57 1982   617′.582   81-8466
ISBN 0-397-50484-5   AACR2

Printed in the United States of America

To Nathalie, Anthony, David, Tim, Tessa, Vanessa, and Marje

CONTENTS

GUEST AUTHORS

ENDRE A. BALAZS, M.D

Boston Biomedical Research Institute
Harvard Medical School
Boston, Massachusetts

ANDREW F. BROOKER, JR., M.D.

Chief of Orthopaedic Surgery
Baltimore City Hospital
Assistant Professor of Orthopaedic Surgery
The Johns Hopkins Hospital
Baltimore, Maryland

VICTOR H. FRANKEL, M.D., Dr.Sci.

Director of Orthopaedic Surgery
Hospital for Joint Diseases
New York, New York, and
Professor of Orthopaedic Surgery
Mount Sinai
School of Medicine
New York, New York

ROBERT H. FREIBERGER, M.D.

Professor of Radiology
Cornell University Medical College
Director, Department of Radiology
Hospital for Special Surgery
New York, New York

RONALD J. FURLONG, M.B., B.S., F.R.C.S.

Hon. Consultant Orthopaedic Surgeon
to St. Thomas' Hospital, London
Hon. Consulting Orthopaedic Surgeon
to the British Army

JERRY GOLDSMITH, M.D.

Staff Physician
Baptist Memorial Hospital
LeBanheur Children's Hospital
St. Joseph Hospital
Memphis, Tennessee

EDWARD T. HABERMANN, M.D.

Professor and Chairman
Department of Orthopaedic Surgery
Albert Einstein College of Medicine
Chief of Orthopaedic Surgery
Montefiore Hospital and Medical Center
Albert Einstein College of Medicine
Bronx, New York

JOHN ELLIS HANDELSMAN, M.B., B. Ch., M. Ch. Orth.
Professor of Orthopaedic Surgery
Brown University
Chief of Pediatric and Orthopaedic Surgery
Rhode Island Hospital
Providence, Rhode Island

DAVID L. HELFET, M.D.
Assistant Professor in Orthopaedic Surgery
The Johns Hopkins Hospital
Baltimore, Maryland

A. W. BROOKES HEYWOOD, M. Ch. Orth., F.R.C.S.
Principal Orthopaedic Surgeon
Princess Alice Hospital
University of Cape Town
Republic of South Africa

DANIEL N. KULUND, M.D.
Assistant Professor
Orthopaedic Surgery and Health and Physical Education
University of Virginia Medical Center
Charlottesville, Virginia

DAVID G. MENDES, M.D.
Chairman of the Orthopaedic Department
Rothschild University Hospital, Faculty of Medicine, Technion
Haifa, Israel

JOSEPH E. MILGRAM, M.D., M.S.
Emeritus Director of Orthopaedic Surgery
Hospital for Joint Diseases
Clinical Professor of Orthopaedic Surgery
Albert Einstein College of Medicine
New York, New York

WALID MNAYMNEH, M.D.
Associate Professor
Department of Orthopaedics and Rehabilitation
Chief, Musculoskeletal Oncology
School of Medicine
University of Miami
Miami, Florida

MAURICE E. MÜLLER, M.D.
Professor of Orthopaedics
University of Berne
Director, Clinic for Orthopaedics and Traumatology, Inselspital
Berne, Switzerland

JAMES A. NICHOLAS, M.D.
Director, Department of Orthopaedic Surgery
Founding Director, Institute of Sports Medicine and Athletic Trauma
Lenox-Hill Hospital
Associate Professor of Clinical Orthopaedics
Cornell University Medical College
Attending Orthopaedic Surgeon
New York Hospital and The Hospital for Special Surgery
New York, New York

MARGARETA NORDIN, LEG. SJUKGYMNAST (R.P.T.)
Associate, Department of Orthopaedic Surgery
Sahlgren Hospital
University of Göteborg
Göteborg, Sweden
Associate, Department of Orthopaedics
University of Washington
Seattle, Washington

RICHARD L. O'CONNOR, M.D.*
Formerly Founding President, International Arthroscopy Association
and Consultant in Orthopaedic Surgery
West Covena Hospital
Los Angeles, California

ANTHONY J. SARANITI, R.P.T.
Institute of Sports Medicine and Athletic Trauma
Lenox-Hill Hospital
New York, New York

JOSEPH SCHATZKER, M.D., B.Sc. (Med.)
Associate, Department of Surgery
University of Toronto
Active Staff, Division of Orthopaedic Surgery
Wellesley and Sunnybrook Hospitals
Toronto, Ontario

W. NORMAN SCOTT, M.D.
Associate, Implant Service and Adjunct Orthopaedic Attending
Lenox-Hill Hospital
New York, New York

LOUIS SOLOMON, M.D., F.R.C.S.
Professor of Orthopaedic Surgery
University of the Witwatersrand Medical School
Chief Orthopaedic Surgeon
Johannesburg General Hospital
Johannesburg, Republic of South Africa

* Deceased

SAKAE TAKEDA, M.D.

Department of Orthopaedic Surgery
Tokyo Teishin Hospital
Tokyo, Japan

E. L. TRICKEY, M.B., B.S., F.R.C.S.

Consultant Orthopaedic Surgeon
The Royal National Orthopaedic Hospital
London, United Kingdom

PETER S. WALKER, Ph.D.

Director of Bioengineering and Associate Scientist
Hospital for Special Surgery
Affiliated with New York Hospital
Cornell University Medical College
New York, New York

MASAKI WATANABE, M.D.

Director, Department of Orthopaedic Surgery
Tokyo Teishin Hospital
Tokyo, Japan

CHARLES WEISS, M.D., B.S.

Chairman, Department of Orthopaedics
and Rehabilitation
Mount Sinai Medical Center
Miami Beach;
Clinical Professor of Orthopaedics
University of Miami
School of Medicine
Miami, Florida

PREFACE

The lyf so short, the craft so long to lerne.
Geoffrey Chaucer, 1340?–1400
"The Parlement of Foules"

Who would looke dangerously up at Planets that
might safely look down at Plants?
John Gerard
"The Herball," 1599

The publisher's request for a revised edition is a reflection of the remarkable progress in the understanding and management of disorders of the knee in the past swift five years; consequently, it has not been difficult to add, alter, and sometimes rewrite chapters.

The additions include the description of a helicoid knee prosthesis and a helicoid knee brace, which give practical expression to the concept enunciated previously that the action of the knee joint is that of a helix and not a hinge. The muscles acting on the knee demand synchronous rotation of the tibia on the femur during flexion and extension. These new devices are designed to comply with muscle demands and so provide for fluid, tensionless movements.

To balance, to run, to carry, or to propel, the knee is a mainspring of athletic performance, and I am grateful that James Nicholas has updated his authoritative contribution, this time with the help of Norman Scott, on the management and rehabilitation of "Major Injuries of the Knee in Contact Sports." A welcome addition is a contemporary chapter on the new and necessary discipline of sports medicine, "The Knee in Athletics," in which Dan Kulund discusses a wide range of interesting features of training for running (from jogging to marathoning), cycling, and other popular sports.

Also new to this volume is a chapter by Walid Mnaymneh on "Common Tumors of the Knee." He presents difficult and sometimes confusing problems in a straightforward and easily understood fashion. The coverage of dislocations of the patella

has been augmented by A. W. Brookes Heywood, and the chapter has been recast to include old and introduce fresh material. The acute and the various forms of repeated dislocation are discussed.

I am convinced that a major cause of mechanical pain in the knee, as in other joints, is instabilities and irregularities in the patterns of movement, whether due to ligamentous weakness or arthritic change. E. L. Trickey's "Pathologic Anatomy of Knee Joint Ligament Injuries" is an illuminating and appropriate introduction to the discussion of these injuries and to the disabilities they produce in work and sport. After meticulous studies of dissections of cadaveric knees, he describes and elucidates the complicated patterns of clinical instability.

Major technological advances in our knowledge of the normal and abnormal in joints are discussed in the chapters on arthritic disorders of the knee.

Etiology, pathogenesis, clinical manifestations, conservative treatment, and intra-articular surgery are discussed by myself in collaboration with Louis Solomon, who devotes a separate chapter to his most recent work on "The Rheumatoid Knee."

Surgical management is divided into a number of specialized sectors: When to carry out total replacement and which type of osteotomy calls for careful decision. Ronald Furlong has extensive experience with osteotomy, in particular, with procedures described by Pauwels and Maquet, whose monographs he has translated.

My discussion of "Clinical Biomechanics of the Helicoid Endoprosthesis" is followed by Peter Walker's erudite illustrated thesis on "The Biomechanics of Knee Prostheses," in which he discusses the evolution and principles of design.

I am indebted to David Mendes who, after his experience with total condylar and other knee implants, has given valuable counsel for the final modifications in the development of helicoid total knee replacement. He describes the indications and techniques, while Edward Habermann adds the benefit of his studies in the "Complications and Malfunctions of Total Knee Replacement."

I am grateful to the contributors who unhesitatingly revised or rewrote their splendid chapters. They illustrate the advantages of combining basic technical and clinical research. Charles Weiss writes on "Microstructure and Biochemistry of Joints," Endre Balazs on "The Physical Properties of Synovial Fluid and the Special Role of Hyaluronic Acid," and Victor Frankel on "Biomechanics of the Knee." Robert Freiberger and Masaki Watanabe, joined by Sakae Takeda, discuss their respective precise techniques of intra-articular diagnosis by arthrography and arthroscopy, to which Richard O'Connor adds his contribution on the

techniques and scope of intra-articular surgery. Jack Handelsman reports on his and other recent work on "The Hemophiliac Knee." Maurice Müller writes on stable internal fixation for articular fractures, complemented by "Management of Juxta-articular Disorders of the Knee Joint" by A. F. Brooker and David Helfet. Joseph Milgram repeats his invaluable report on the interpretation of osteochondral fractures.

As always, I am indebted to *Lydia Gruebel Lee* for her editing and to Stuart Freeman of J. B. Lippincott Company for his ever-ready help and understanding.

Arthur J. Helfet, M.D.

PREFACE TO THE FIRST EDITION

I must believe in order that I may understand.
St. Anselm, 11th century

I must understand in order that I may believe.
Peter Abelard, 12th century

Orthopaedic surgery has benefited from the century's tremendous progress in scientific understanding and technology; this is manifest even on the limited canvas of a specialised treatise. *The Management of Internal Derangements of the Knee,* published in 1963, had as its theme the clinical implications of the helical character of the mechanics of the knee. The new edition reports progress in the management of traumatic and arthritic derangements. But since knowledge of basic structure, joint biomechanics, and biochemistry has advanced considerably over the past decade, additional chapters by clinical scientists who are among the most distinguished pioneers in these fields are included.

Victor Frankel describes the modern concepts of the kinematics which underlie the importance of helicoid motion of the knee joint in a form simple to understand and, in lucid biomechanical terms, explains their relation to derangements of the meniscus.

Charles Weiss who familiarised himself with the first "patterns of erosion" in the operating rooms and laboratories of the Albert Einstein College of Medicine illuminates the origin and nature of joint tissues in terms of his ultramicroscopic and histochemical studies.

Endre Balazs has unravelled a chain of molecular action in the lubrication of joints and has introduced with his extract of hyaluronic acid a variant of treatment by transplant or replacement of normal tissue.

In osteoarthritis of the hip joint, replacement by prosthetic implant has yielded considerable success. The knee is a more complex joint and the results are not as successful. Although patients with advanced osteoarthritis may be relieved of pain, restoration of function is limited. Nevertheless, though it would be premature to commend a particular device, Peter Walker's critical and constructive review of engineering principles presages promising developments.

Robert Freiberger demonstrates that expert arthrography adds to the precision of clinical diagnosis, as does Masaki Watanabe's brilliant arthroscope and camera, which, without injuring tissues, display the nooks and crannies of the joint and its disorders. Both techniques should aid in obviating the widely practiced and unnecessarily traumatic "house cleaning," when simple meniscectomy and limited removal of osteophytes are all that is basically necessary in early osteoarthritis.

Major knee injuries are a frequent sequel to the gladiatorial collisions which are a feature of modern professional football and other sports. James Nicholas relates a thoughtful and most valuable report of his considerable experience in the surgical management and rehabilitation of these athletes. These injuries are a grosser version of the more usual derangements of the knee and result in wider disruption of tissues.

Maurice Müller is a leader among the Swiss surgeons who have united to promote the principle that internal fixation with compression fosters synthesis of bone. With his colleagues, J. Goldsmith and Joseph Schatzker, he describes the elegant techniques that have streamlined treatment and improved results in fractures and especially in joints where accurate stable reduction permits early movement and return of function.

In elaborating his previous contributions, Joseph Milgram has continued his original and thought provoking interpretation of the mechanism and character of osteochondral fractures. He emphasizes anew the warning that articular cartilage is vulnerable to corticosteroid therapy and that ill may follow its use. To his contribution he adds the gift of a most valued friendship and his unsurpassed command of orthopaedic literature.

The knee is not a hinge joint. The realization that the tibia navigates a helical course on the condyles of the femur, gives clarity to certain features in the diagnosis and treatment of injuries of the knee joint, and as the concept is developed, leads to new physical signs in the diagnosis of derangements of the knee joint and then to the inescapable conviction that *most traumatic arthritis of the knee in middle-aged and elderly people is due to minor derangements of the soft tissues especially the menisci, and that the pain and the discomfort of the condition are usually cured by simple operation.*

No longer is the outlook hopeless for the osteoarthritic, rheumatoid or hemophiliac knee. We know that in early osteoarthritis the process may be arrested with relief of symptoms and restoration of function. In due course radiographs may show reversal of the degenerative process.

A new Chapter is included on the surgery of the rheumatoid knee; and, Jack Handelsman contributes an erudite report on the considerable progress that has altered the management and improved dramatically the prognosis for the hemophiliac.

Precise diagnosis, gentle nontraumatic surgery, and adequate rehabilitation, however, remain the requisites for successful surgery of the knee.

The knee is used to carry and to propel, to comfort and to supplicate, and merits care on every count.

I am deeply indebted to the valued contributors and in writing and editing this volume, am most grateful to Eli Sedlin, who worked with me in the department of Orthopaedic Surgery of the Albert Einstein College of Medicine; to George Sacks, whose use of words is a constant delight; to Alan Apley who combines friendship with apt counsel; and to Stuart Freeman of J. B. Lippincott Company, who has blended understanding and helpfulness.

Arthur J. Helfet, M.D.

CHAPTER 1
ANATOMY AND MECHANICS OF MOVEMENT OF THE KNEE JOINT

Arthur J. Helfet

The key to understanding the knee joint is the realization that its movement is helicoid* or spiral in character.[4] The knee is not a simple hinge joint. The opening and the shutting of the front of the joint in the acts of flexion and extension involve the tibia in a winding course set by the configuration of the medial condyle of the femur (Fig. 1-1). As the tibia glides on the femur from the fully flexed to the fully extended position, it descends and then ascends the curves of the medial femoral condyle and at the same time slowly rotates outward. These movements are reversed as the tibia passes back to the fully flexed position. This screw-action gives to any position of the knee joint a stability that would be denied a straight up-and-down hinge joint.

Movement of the tibial tubercle, which is easily observed, demonstrates this spiral action (Fig. 1-2). Moreover, it shows that rotation occurs not only in the last few degrees of flexion and extension, as was thought pre-

* Helicoid—"having the form of a helix; screw-shaped; spiral."—Shorter Oxford Dictionary.

viously, but throughout the whole range of movement (Figs. 1-3, 5-3E—G). The extent of the rotary movement is roughly equivalent to half the width of the patella. When the knee is fully flexed, the tubercle points to the inner half (Fig. 1-4, *left*) of the patella; in the extended knee it is in line with the outer half (Fig. 1-4, *right*).

The anatomy of the knee joint facilitates this pattern of movement and at the same time maintains stability in the lower limb during movement while bearing weight.

THE THIGH MUSCLES— THE CONTROL MECHANISM OF THE KNEE JOINT

QUADRICEPS

The quadriceps group of muscles, of which the medial vastus is the most prominent, runs from without inward, is inserted into the tibia

(text continued on p. 4)

1

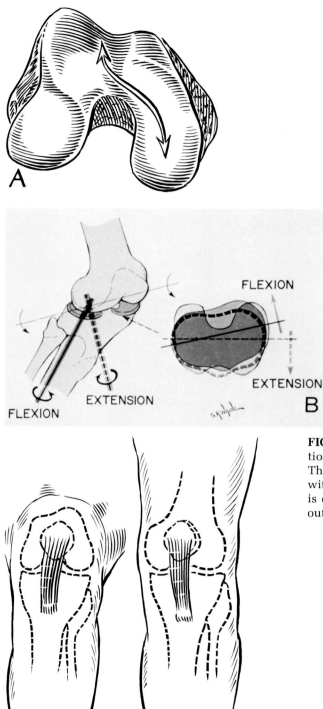

FIG. 1-1. **(A)** The articular surface of the medial condyle of the femur, showing the helicoid track followed by the tibia in flexion and extension of the knee. The tibia descends and then ascends the curves of the medial femoral condyle and at the same time slowly rotates outwards. **(B)** Diagrammatic illustration of rotation of the tibia on the femur during flexion and extension of the knee joint. (Helfet AJ: AAOS Instructional Course Lectures, vol 19. St. Louis, CV Mosby, 1970)

FIG. 1-2. Movement of the tibial tubercle in relation to the patella demonstrates this spiral action. The tibial tubercle of the flexed knee (*left*) is in line with the medial half of the patella. When the knee is extended (*right*) the tubercle rotates toward the outer half of the patella.

FIG. 1-3. The tibial tubercle is in line with the anterior tibial spine and the anterior cruciate ligament, which spiral synchronously.

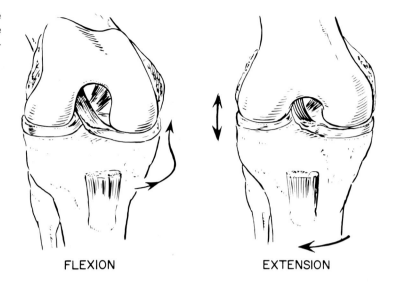

FLEXION   EXTENSION

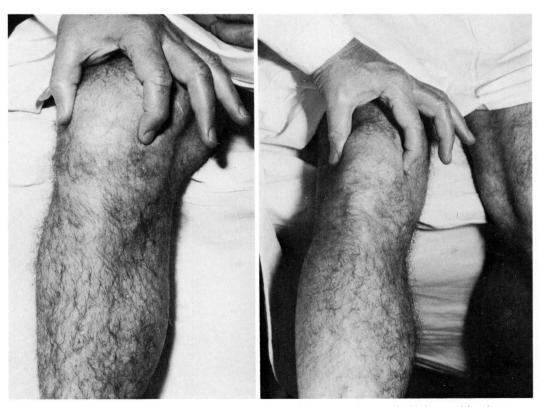

FIG. 1-4. The extent of the rotary movement is roughly equivalent to half the width of the patella. When the knee is fully flexed (*left*) the tubercle points to the inner half of the patella; (*right*) in the extended knee it is in line with the outer half.

through the patella and the patellar ligament, and has a broad fibrous expansion stronger on the medial side (Fig. 1-5). From the direction of their pull and the preponderance of attachment to the medial side of the tibia, their purpose is to rotate the tibia outward while extending the knee. Special fibers from the medial vastus to the quadriceps tendon and the patella control synchronous spiral movement of the patella and prevent lateral dislocation.

MEDIAL HAMSTRINGS

The medial hamstrings are directed from the ischial tuberosity downward and, if anything, slightly inward to be inserted into the upper tibia on its anteromedial and posterior surfaces (Fig. 1-6). Their action is to rotate the tibia inwardly while flexing the knee. In addition, the semimembranosus is inserted into the posteromedial aspect of the capsule of the knee joint, which has firm connections with

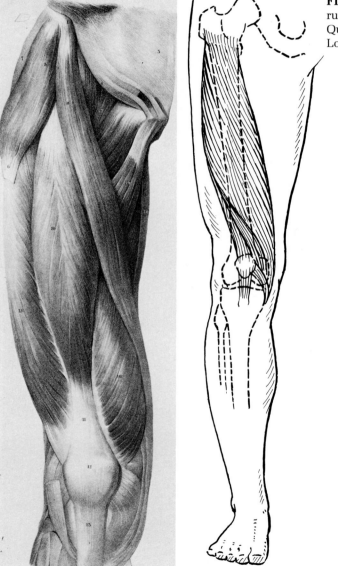

FIG. 1-5. The quadriceps group of muscles runs from without inward. (*Left* drawing from Quain J [ed]: The Muscles of the Human Body. London, Taylor and Walton, 1836)

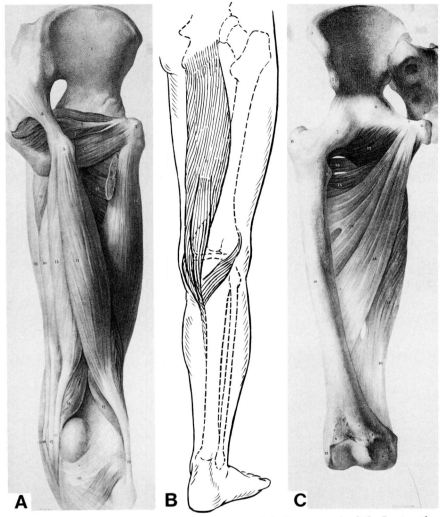

FIG. 1-6. (A, B) The medial hamstrings rotate the tibia inward while flexing the knee. The popliteus anchors the femur and the posterior capsule of the knee joint and so acts as a stabilizer while the medial hamstrings rotate the tibia inward. **(C)** The adductor muscles stabilize the thigh from the inner side. (A, C from Quain J [ed]: The Muscles of the Human Body. London, Taylor and Walton, 1836)

the posterior end of the medial meniscus in this area. When in action, the semimembranosus anchors the posterior end of the meniscus.

POPLITEUS

The popliteus, which originates from the upper end of the posterior surface of the tibia as a fleshy triangular muscle, narrows to a ten-

don which, synovial-sheathed, winds upward and forward around the posterolateral segment of the knee joint to be inserted in a groove on the lateral femoral epicondyle above the joint line. The tendon crosses and grooves the lateral semilunar cartilage, though separated by a fold of synovium. In turn, it is separated from the fibular collateral ligament by its own sheath and sometimes by a small bursa as well (see Fig. 1-16). The popliteus flexes the knee joint and at the same time anchors the femur, while the medial hamstrings rotate the tibia inward. Last points out that en route posterior fibers from the tendon enter the lateral meniscus and so drag the meniscus backward and downward during lateral rotation of the femur.[7] In other words, the posterior end of the lateral meniscus is anchored during flexion of the knee. The muscle also has clinical significance, for synovitis of its tendon sheath causes pain and disability independently of a lesion of the knee joint itself.

THE BICEPS AND THE ILIOTIBIAL BAND

Both the biceps and the iliotibial band are active in stabilizing the fully extended knee. It is suggested also that contraction of these muscles is a preliminary, and sometimes a necessary preliminary, to strong action by the extensors of the knee. In the initial stages of contraction until the quadriceps group of

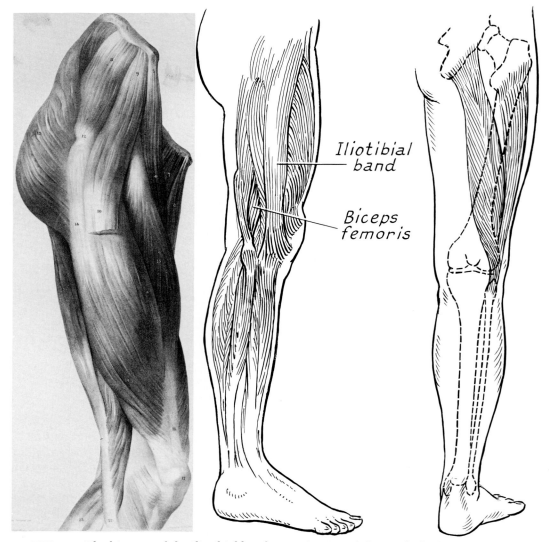

FIG. 1-7. The biceps and the iliotibial band are active in stabilizing the leg on the thigh.

muscles has shortened sufficiently to exert full power, the position and the stability of the knee must be controlled by the action of the biceps and the iliotibial band. The biceps tendon is inserted into the head of the fibula with the fibular collateral ligament, while the iliotibial band finds insertion into the tibia through the lateral capsule and into the fibula through the lateral ligament. The biceps is also a flexor of the knee, and both play a part in external rotation of the tibia. Indeed, in paralytic contracture of the knee, the iliotibial band may be the main contributor to the flexion-external-rotation deformity (Fig. 1-7).[10]

However, their most important function is probably to stabilize the fibular component of the leg in weight-bearing. Through their attachments, they exert control on the superior tibiofibular joint. When the knee is fully extended, rotation of the tibia on the femur is not possible. Also the weight-bearing knee cannot indulge in any change of its exact ratio of flexion-extension to rotation, but the movements of flexion and extension of the ankle

and inversion and eversion of the foot do not take place in isolation in the ankle and the subtaloid and the midtarsal joints. They require a component of rotation in the leg. This necessary movement must take place in the inferior and the superior tibiofibular joints (Fig. 1-8), a factor more easily appreciated when it is realized that the increasing width of the articular surface of the talus posteriorly needs changing accommodation in the ankle mortise. Indeed, one might generalize by saying that most actions of the weight-bearing leg are accomplished by sinuous adaptatory movements of all the joints of the leg from the hip downward. "The coordination of joints, whether stationary or in motion, is a fundamental part of bodily posture and movement."[1]

The movement of the fibula on the tibia may be confirmed quite simply. With the muscles relaxed and the knee bent, the tibia with the fibula can be rotated quite freely on the femur. With weight taken on the leg, independent rotation of the tibia on the femur is no longer

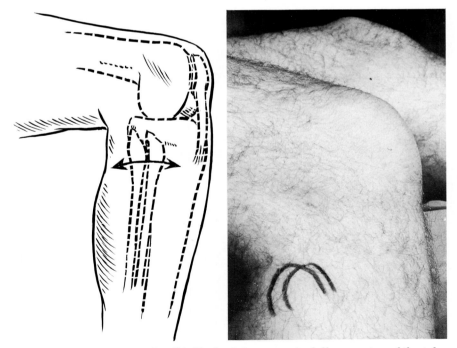

FIG. 1-8. Movement in the tibiofibular joints permits full excursion of the talus in the ankle mortise (see text for description).

possible. The tibia does not rotate on the femur unless the knee flexes and extends. Different widths of the talus occupy the ankle mortise in flexion and extension. The change in space is accommodated by movement of the fibula on the tibia at the inferior and the superior tibiofibular joints. When weight is taken on the leg as the ankle flexes and extends, the head of the fibula can be felt to move backward and forward on the tibia independently and without rotation of the tibia (Figs. 1-8, 1-9).

The experiment may be repeated while taking weight on the bent knee. Invert and evert the foot or flex and extend the ankle, and so long as the angle of flexion of the knee does not alter, rotation of the tibia on the femur does not take place. The adjustment is made by independent movement of the superior tibiofibular joint. This is further proof that the helicoid, or spiral, action of the knee joint when controlled by the thigh muscles, as in weight-bearing, demands that flexion and extension be synchronous with inward and outward rotation of the tibia, respectively, and

that the stable weight-bearing position for each component is definite and cannot be altered.

In other words, the normal movement of the knee joint when bearing weight and under control of the thigh muscles is a synchrony of extension with lateral rotation of the tibia and of flexion with medial rotation. Only when the thigh muscles are relaxed is it possible to rotate the tibia on the femur freely in both directions, and even in relaxation it is not possible to achieve full extension or full flexion without full lateral or medial rotation, as the case may be. When the slack tibia moves from full extension to flexion, the range of free rotation increases. But it should be emphasized again that when the quadriceps and the hamstrings are active, only synchronous movement in each direction is normally possible: when the knee straightens, the tibia must rotate laterally; as it flexes, the tibia must rotate medially.

The superior tibiofibular joint, in the past, has not been accorded proper clinical respect; injury, as will be shown later, may result in

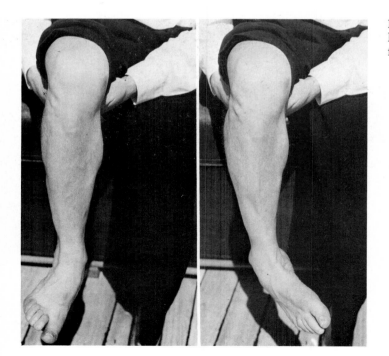

FIG. 1-9. The changing position of the head of the fibula when the ankle or the foot is moved is obvious.

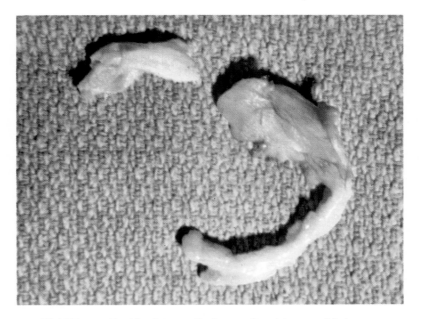

PLATE 1-1. Residual posterior horn of meniscus with (anteriorly) a fibrous shape—the attempt at regeneration of the anterior two-thirds.

appreciable disability. It is important to recognize the symptoms of this disorder, which must be differentiated from those of injury to the lateral semilunar cartilage.

FUNCTIONS OF MUSCLES ACTING ON THE KNEE

A rough classification of the actions of the muscles acting on the knee joint follows:

Quadriceps group—mainly extensors and outward rotators of tibia

Medial hamstrings—mainly flexors and inward rotators of tibia

Stabilizers—popliteus, biceps, tensor fascia femoris, and iliotibial band

CRUCIATE LIGAMENTS AND SEMILUNAR CARTILAGES— THE GUIDE MECHANISM OF THE KNEE JOINT

The spiral movement of the knee is guided by a mechanism of cruciate ligaments and semilunar cartilages (Fig. 1-10). The cruciates do not act as stays to prevent anteroposterior displacement of the tibia on the femur but as guide ropes to keep the tibia on its winding path when the knee extends and flexes. It

would be reasonable to expect that the cruciates develop in support of such normal action rather than as potential obstructions to unnatural anteroposterior displacement.

The anatomic arrangement and continuity of the cruciates with the semilunar cartilages suggests that the function of guiding rotation of the tibia on the femur is shared in the manner presented diagrammatically in Figure 1-11. It is also probable that both the cruciate ligaments and the semilunar cartilages are of similar origin because the cartilages are differentiated from the same embryologic layer in continuity with the cruciate ligaments and are not truly cartilaginous.[5]

The continuity of the ligamentous and cartilaginous structures, in what Sir Harry Platt aptly termed *figure-of-eight anatomy*, was described accurately by Galeazzi in 1927.[3] Three of his illustrations, reproduced here, emphasize this characteristic. Figure 1-12 shows the strong fibrous band, sometimes a centimeter wide, connecting the posterior horn of the lateral cartilage to the femoral attachment of the anterior cruciate ligament. Figure 1-13 (*left*) shows the fibrous bands which connect the anterior cruciate ligament with the anterior horn of the medial and with the anterior horn of the lateral cartilage.

Figure 1-13 (*right*) shows Barkow's ligament connecting the posterior horn of the lateral cartilage and the anterior horn of the me-

FIG. 1-10. The cruciate ligaments and the semilunar cartilages act as guide ropes to keep the tibia on its helical path as the knee extends and flexes.

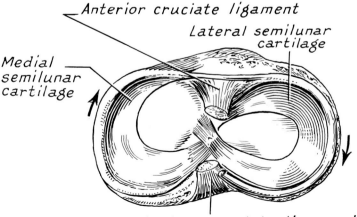

Anterior cruciate ligament

Lateral semilunar cartilage

Medial semilunar cartilage

Posterior cruciate ligament

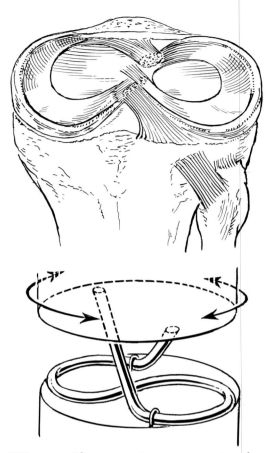

FIG. 1-11. The anatomic arrangement and continuity of the cruciates with the semilunar cartilages suggest that the function of guiding rotation is shared in this figure eight manner.

dial cartilage. Galeazzi also referred to the transverse ligament of the knee (Winslow) which joins the anterior horns of the two cartilages, and he emphasized particularly the firm attachments between the anterior cruciate ligament and medial cartilage.

In addition to their links with the cruciates, the menisci have attachment to the tibia and move with it. There is play between them and the tibia, especially in the anterior half of the medial and the anterior two thirds of the lateral meniscus, where the attachments through a coronary ligament are lax. The posterior half of the medial meniscus is firmly attached to the deep part of the tibial collateral ligament

and the posteromedial capsule. The lateral meniscus is attached equally firmly to the posterior capsule where the popliteus muscle takes part of its insertion.

These arrangements are significant. The medial part of the capsule which is concerned with the quadriceps expansion, in outward rotation of the tibia has, as one would expect, intimate attachments to its pilot, the medial semilunar cartilage. But the lateral ligament, which is designed to stabilize the tibiofibular joint, does not take part in rotating the tibia and therefore is independent of the lateral meniscus, from which it is separated by the tendon of the popliteus and a fold of synovium. Should it become adherent, rotation of the tibia is affected, and flexion of the knee is hampered—a feature to consider in the stiff knee after injury or infection.

The insertion of the popliteus into the posterior capsule and the back end of the lateral meniscus means that as the muscle contracts to flex the knee and to act as anchor for the femur, it also holds the cartilage to the posterior edge of the tibia, thus providing a stable axis of pivot while the tibia rotates inwardly on the femur.

An effect of the firm attachment of the posterior ends of both menisci, compared with the loose capsular attachments of both anterior halves, suggests the explanation for another clinical finding. The "retracted" or detached anterior horn occurs frequently (see Fig. 6-10). The main injury is a rupture of the bands binding the anterior horn to the cruciate ligaments and to each other. The loose posterior horn is usually associated with rupture of the cartilage itself, implying that the meniscus is more vulnerable than the extensive and firm capsular attachments.

Watson-Jones drew attention to the part played by the semilunar cartilages in the rotator mechanism when he described what might be called the *retreating cartilage.*[9]

Place one finger over the joint line on the knee in front of the medial ligament where the curved margin of the medial femoral condyle approaches the tibial tuberosity. Now rotate the foot and leg laterally. It is easy to feel the medial semilunar cartilage disappearing from the surface, leaving a sulcus between the bones.

This sign is present only when the knee is bent and the muscles relaxed; it is an expression of the independence of the figure-of-eight mechanism, of which the cartilage is only a part, when rotation is not accompanied by synchronous extension of the knee. The cartilage maintains its relationship to the margin of the tibia in all normal movements and therefore does so when the leg is bearing weight.

On the other hand, as will be shown, when rupture of the cartilage blocks lateral rotation of the tibia, *absence* of the retreating cartilage sign in the flexed knee may be used diagnostically.

In the young the semilunar cartilages, which are not true cartilage, are smooth and firm but yet resilient. With age the cartilage becomes yellowish in color, firmer and fibrotic in consistency, and less resilient. In the aged the free edge retracts, and the cartilage as a whole is harder and narrower and triangular on section.

The substance of the cartilage is avascular. Blood vessels course only in capsular and ligamentous attachments. Consequently, repair will occur in peripheral lesions, but no tear of the substance of the cartilage will heal.

On the other hand, with this in mind, surgery of the semilunar cartilages may be relatively bloodless both during and after operation. The vascular synovium should be sutured hemostatically, and the meniscus excised by incision into the substance only and not through the peripheral attachments.

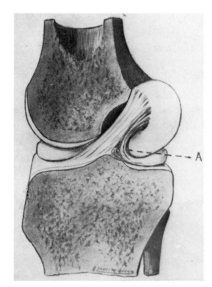

FIG. 1-12. A strong, fibrous band, sometimes 1 cm wide, connects the posterior horn of the lateral cartilage to the femoral attachment of the anterior cruciate ligament. (Galeazzi R: J Bone Joint Surg 9:515, 1927)

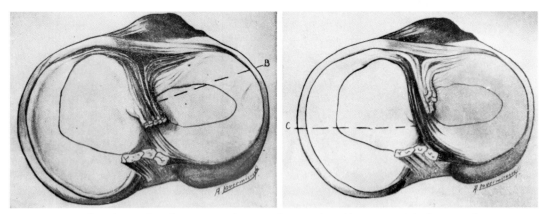

FIG. 1-13. (*Left*) Fibrous bands connect the anterior cruciate ligament with the anterior horn of the medial cartilage and (B) with the anterior horn of the lateral cartilage. (*Right*) Barkow's ligament connects the posterior horn of the lateral cartilage to the anterior horn of the medial cartilage. (Galeazzi R: J Bone Joint Surg 9:515, 1927)

REGENERATED CARTILAGES

I do not propose to enter the controversial speculation on the manner and frequency of regeneration of semilunar cartilages. One may open a knee in which previously a meniscus had been excised and find practically no evidence of regeneration. In most instances, one does find a shape resembling most or part of the meniscus, but it is not of pristine smooth shiny cartilage. Microscopically fibrous tissue in various stages of maturity, but without true cartilage cells, may be demonstrated (see Plate 1-1). In some instances at least, the regenerated shape is no more than organized and fibrosed blood clot, duly shaped and nourished by the joint—in the same way as an erosion of articular cartilage fills, smooths, and shines without apparent vascular nourishment. These regenerated cartilages seem to occur more frequently when special meniscectomy knives, used blindly to free the back end of the meniscus, take their toll on vascular synovial membrane with consequent postoperative hemarthrosis. In the early days of the Middle East campaign during World War II, when a large number of relatively inexperienced surgeons were operating on knees, the incidence of postoperative hemarthrosis in some units was as high as 60% to 80%. At operation each incision should be visualized properly and made into the cartilage itself.

CAPSULAR LIGAMENTS

MEDIAL LIGAMENT

The medial ligament is the main strut of the capular tissues of the knee. The deep portion is a thickened part of the capsule itself and is adherent to the medial meniscus. The superficial part forms a strong, broad strap of triangular shape. Originating just distal to the adductor tubercle, the ligament keeps free of the meniscus and the joint margins and has an extensive insertion into the medial surface of the tibia, at least 1½ inches below joint level. But the posterior border has continuity with the strong posterior capsule of the knee joint, and anteriorly there are fibrous connections with the quadriceps expansion and the patellar ligament. Therefore, the whole medial capsule with its ligament is adequately designed to take strong control of the tibia in all movements of the knee, both by its structure and its intimate connections with the anterior and the posterior muscles of the thigh (Fig. 1-14).

LATERAL LIGAMENT

The lateral ligament extends in two layers from the lateral epicondyle of the femur to the head of the fibula, where it finds insertion in

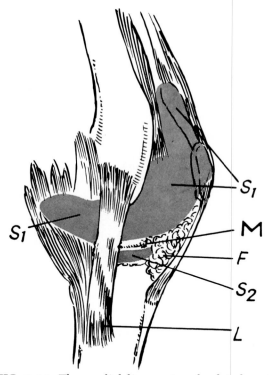

FIG. 1-14. The medial ligament and related anatomy of the knee joint. (L) medial ligament; (F) infrapatellar pad of fat embracing the anterior horn of the meniscus; (M) medial meniscus; (S_1, S_2) synovial cavities; (S_2) fold of synovium between meniscus and articular cartilage of tibia. The meniscus is extrasynovial, as is the fat pad.

intimate relationship with the biceps tendon. The tendon of the popliteus and frequently a bursa separate it from the knee joint and the lateral meniscus (Fig. 1-15). The only connection with the fibrous capsule is at its posterior border, which is continuous with the fascia covering the popliteus and therefore with that muscle's attachments to the posterior horn of the lateral meniscus. Through the superior tibiofibular joint it plays its part in stability of the leg on the thigh and is independent of rotary movements of the tibia. As observed previously, if it were attached to the lateral meniscus, rotation would be prevented, and flexion of the knee curbed. Understandably, because it plays a minor role in the stability of the knee joint, the whole lateral capsule is thinner and weaker than the medial side (Fig. 1-16).

THE PATELLA

The patella is a pulley, and its excursion is controlled by the direction of action of the quadriceps group of muscles and the position of the tibial tubercle which carries the patellar ligament (see Fig. 1-2).

The articular surface of the patella is divided into a large lateral and a smaller medial area. These areas are separated by a vertical rounded ridge (Fig. 1-17). In full extension, its shape fits comfortably and evenly into the trochlear surface of the femur (Fig. 1-18). The ridge then lies in the hollow or trough of the trochlear surface. When the knee is bent, the patella is carried downward and backward on the under aspect of the femur where the trochlear surface is prolonged onto the inner condyle (Fig. 1-19). In flexion the patella tilts away from the lateral condyle so that only the inner part of its articular surface rests against the medial condyle.[2]

As long as the tibial tubercle rotates smoothly, the patella travels its short course smoothly and under even tension. However, any derangement of the joint which prevents lateral rotation of the tibia during extension of

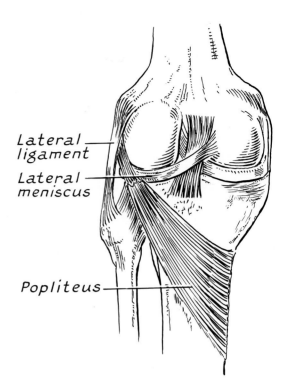

FIG. 1-15. The lateral ligament does not take part in rotating the tibia and therefore is independent of the lateral meniscus, from which it is separated by the popliteus tendon and a fold of synovium.

the knee affects normal tension because contraction of the quadriceps forces the inner border of the patella against the medial condyle of the femur (Fig. 1-20, see Fig. 6-28). This explains the patellar symptoms and signs produced by certain cartilage injuries, such as retropatellar pain on climbing and descending stairs, tenderness of the medial border of the patella, and the pattern of cartilage erosion that develops only on the medial surfaces of the patella and the femur. This pattern differs from that produced by retropatellar arthritis, complicating recurring dislocation when it is the lateral surface of the patellar cartilage that undergoes fibrillation.[6] Later, the medial surface is damaged from repeated drag over the lateral condyle of the femur during reduction, with consequent erosion of articular cartilage. By this time both sides of the patella are tender (Fig. 1-20).

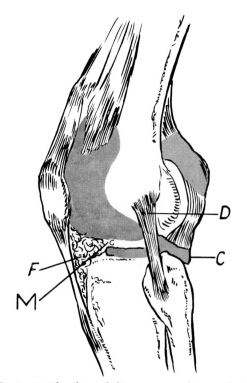

FIG. 1-16. The lateral ligament and its relationships to the knee joint. (*F*) infrapatellar pad of fat; (*M*) lateral meniscus separated by fold of synovium from articular cartilage of tibia; (*C*) popliteus tendon in synovial sheath; (*D*) lateral ligament separated from meniscus by tendon and fold of synovium.

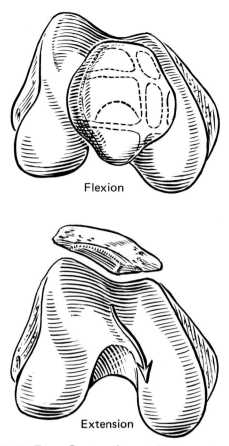

Flexion

Extension

FIG. 1-18. From flexion, the patella ascends a sinuous course from the under-surface of the medial condyle to the trochlear surface of the femur. In full extension, its shape fits comfortably and evenly into the trochlear groove.

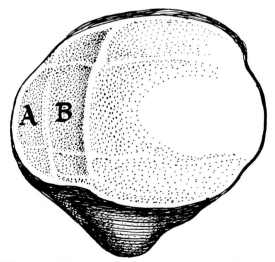

FIG. 1-17. The articular surface of the patella is divided into a large lateral and a smaller medial slope, with vertical division into two planes (*A* and *B*). (Frazer JB: Anatomy of the Human Skeleton. London, Churchill, 1933)

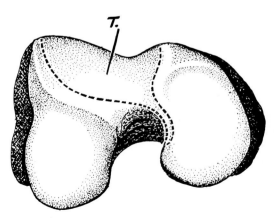

FIG. 1-19. Lower end of right femur, showing trochlear surface (*T*) for patella, extending along inner condyle as an area with which patella articulates in flexion. (Frazer JB: Anatomy of the Human Skeleton. London, Churchill, 1933)

FIG. 1-20. Pattern of erosion expected after recurrent dislocation of the patella, associated in this specimen with genu valgum. The condyles of the femur are relatively unscarred, but the trochlear groove and the patellar articular surfaces are extensively abraded—more on the lateral than on the medial side (*arrows*).

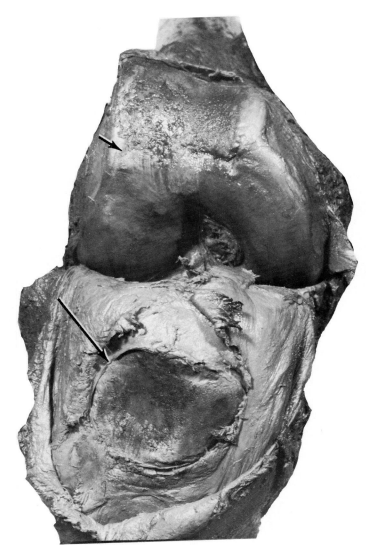

ANATOMY OF DISLOCATION

Dislocation of the patella is encouraged by the angle between the line of action of the quadriceps and the patellar ligament (see Fig. 1-5). The muscles act from without inward, whereas the ligament is vertical. As the late Arthur Steindler pointed out, this introduces a lateral-directed horizontal component which tends to force the patella out of its groove.[8] Stability is maintained by the transverse strength of the medial capsule, by the attachments of the medial vastus to the quadriceps tendon and the patella, and by the depth of the lateral trochlear surface of the femur. The propensity to subluxation is greater if the latter is shallow or short, if the angle is increased—as in genu valgum or external rotation deformity from any cause—or if the attachments of the medial vastus are divided by injury or ill-repaired parapatellar incision. Acute traumatic dislocation occurs at the expense of the medial capsule (see Chap. 22).

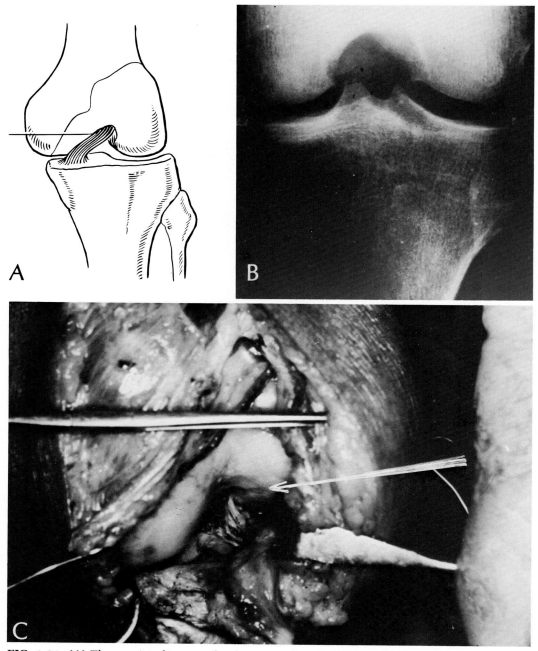

FIG. 1-21. (A) The cruciate ligament hooks across the edge of the medial femoral condyle. **(B)** Rare x-ray film of groove eroded in edge of medial condyle by cruciate ligament. **(C)** Photograph at operation. Arrow points to cruciate ligament and eroded groove.

INFRAPATELLAR PAD OF FAT

The infrapatellar pad of fat extends from the lower pole of the patella to the level of the tibia, behind and on each side of the patellar ligament (see Figs. 1-14, 1-16). The pliable fat is a mobile structure and acts as a true cushion as the front of the joint is closed in straightening the knee. Alar folds of the synovium, which cover the joint surface, are so disposed as to maneuver vulnerable lobes of fat away from injury. The fat pad also contains a high proportion of adipose elastic tissue, which helps it to regain its shape. The pad has connections with the front ends of the semilunar cartilages, which are attached and which it overlaps.

It is important to note that the fat pad is a mobile structure in the knee joint and that interference with its free movement results in pain and disability. Care must be taken not to injure the fat pad when operating on the knee because many discomforts after contusions or rough surgery are due to fibrous scars or adherence to surrounding structures, which affect its mobility. A swollen fat pad, from any cause, may also result in pain as the pad is compressed when straightening the knee. A vicious circle is created because the impingement increases the swelling, which aggravates the pain.

TENSION IN CAPSULE AND LIGAMENTS

The tension in the capsule and the ligaments of the knee joint during all normal movements, that is, with proper synchrony of rotation with flexion and extension, remains unchanged. This may be confirmed by observing the anterior cruciate ligament during operation on the knee. Bend and straighten the leg. The cruciate keeps the tibia on its spiral path gently and without tension. Now straighten the knee while preventing synchronous external rotation of the tibia. The cruciate is tightened and then hooks over the medial condylar edge of the femoral notch (Fig. 1-21). The

same effect is produced by rupture or displacement of the anterior part of a meniscus. The full arc of movement into extension is blocked. In the attempt to force it, the anterior cruciate is tensed over the edge of the medial femoral condyle.

It would seem that any crowding of the anteromedial joint space blocks outward rotation of the tibia. Through the usual medial incision, with the knee bent over the table, the free rotation of the tibia shows very well. Place a sterile rubber catheter across the joint toward the cruciate notch. The tibia can no longer rotate outward. The result is a so-called locked knee.

Experiments on cadaver knees that purport to show changes in ligamentous tension are misleading.[3] The forces applied produce abnormal straight up-and-down movements without the requisite degree of rotation. Such movements would be expected to produce abnormal tensions.

REFERENCES

1. **Barnett CH, Davies DV, MacConaill MA:** Synovial Joints: Their Structure and Mechanics. New York, Longmans Green, 1961
2. **Frazer JB:** Anatomy of the Human Skeleton, 5th ed. Breathnach AS (ed): London, Churchill, 1958
3. **Galeazzi R:** Clinical and experimental study of lesions of the semilunar cartilages of the knee joint. J Bone Joint Surg 9:515, 1927
4. **Helfet AJ:** Mechanism of derangements of the medial semilunar cartilage and their management. J Bone Joint Surg 41-B:319, 1959
5. **Kaplan EB:** The embryology of the menisci of the knee joint. Bull Hosp Joint Dis 16:3, 1955
6. **Langston HH:** Dislocation of the patella and its relation to chondromalacia patellae. Brit Med J 1:155, 1958
7. **Last RJ:** The popliteus muscle and the lateral meniscus. J Bone Joint Surg 32-B:93, 1950
8. **Steindler A:** Mechanics of Normal and Pathological Locomotion in Man. Springfield, Charles C Thomas, 1935
9. **Watson-Jones R:** Fractures and Joint Injuries, 4th ed. Vol 2. Baltimore, Williams & Wilkins, 1955
10. **Yount CC:** The role of the tensor fasciae femoris in certain deformities of the lower extremities. J Bone Joint Surg 8:171, 1926

CHAPTER 2
BIOMECHANICS OF THE KNEE*

Victor H. Frankel
Margareta Nordin

The knee joint transmits loads, participates in kinematic functions, aids in momentum conservation, and provides a force couple for purposeful activities involving the foot. The surgeon is frequently called upon to diagnose and treat knee disorders arising from a pathomechanical state. The assessment of altered function is classically performed by collecting subjective patient data and making a clinical evaluation. Biomechanics provides the tools for a precise scientific evaluation of the disorders of function.

The science of biomechanics as applied to the musculoskeletal system relates force and motion. Kinetics, which includes statics and dynamics, is the engineering science that describes the forces acting on a body. In a static situation, such as standing, there is a state of equilibrium; that is, there are no accelerations acting on the part. In a dynamic situation,

such as walking, jumping, or running, there are accelerations acting on the part. Solid mechanics is the engineering science that describes the internal effects of forces acting on a body. These internal effects cause a state of strain, which results in deformation in the body. This state of strain is associated with an internal force system or a stress, which is a force per unit area in a plane. Kinematics is the engineering science that describes the relative motion of two segments of a body and the velocities of the contacting surface particles. How these engineering disciplines are used to solve problems in human biomechanics is the subject of this chapter.

Although much fine work has been done in the past in the area of knee biomechanics, it has been only lately, during the past generation and through the use of more sophisticated engineering techniques, that it has been possible to perform work on the mechanics of the knee joint that has direct clinical application. Our purpose here is to present several examples of general interest so that readers

* This report was supported by the Social Rehabilitation Service, Grant Number RD–2516–M. The authors wish to thank Laurie Glass for editorial assistance.

will have some orientation in examining from a biomechanical standpoint clinical situations that come to their attention. (Basic engineering material that applies to the musculoskeletal system is presented in publications by Frankel and Burstein,[5] Williams and Lissner,[27] and Frankel and Nordin.[6])

In analyzing physical dysfunctions that have as their etiology pathomechanics of some segment of the locomotor system, one must constantly keep in mind the relationship between force and motion. Abnormal motion is usually perceived and measured either with the protractor or, in dynamic situations, with cinematography or stroboscopic photography, television scanning, or electrogoniometric methods. The forces associated with this motion are more difficult to determine because they must be measured by indirect means until such time as a force transducer is built that can be inserted into a knee joint to measure force directly. The techniques of statics and dynamics are used to determine the forces. The distribution of the force over the joint surface is even more difficult to determine because for this analysis one must know the size and location of, and the distribution of force over, the contact area. The joint pressure has not been determined for any joint, and only approximations have been attempted.

The relationship of force and motion is expressed by two well-known equations:

$$\text{force} = \text{mass} \times \text{acceleration}$$
$$\text{torque} = \text{area moment of inertia} \times$$
$$\text{angular acceleration}$$

The first equation refers to linear motion, the second to angular motion. In the case of the first equation, the force can be determined if one knows the mass of the limb, which can be obtained from tables, and the acceleration, which can be obtained through the use of any of the foregoing kinematic methods. In the case of the second equation, the torque about a joint can be determined if the angular acceleration is found by using kinematic methods

and the mass moment of inertia of the limb is known. The latter can be obtained from tables or from direct calculation. It is important because it represents not only how much mass is present but also the distribution of the mass in the limb. For instance, putting on a heavy shoe may increase the mass of the lower limb by 5% while increasing the mass moment of inertia by 30%.

The relationship between torque, mass moment of inertia, and acceleration can be intuitively grasped if one considers an ice skater spinning on one skate. It is obvious that as she moves at a certain angular velocity, she accelerates by folding her arms tightly across her chest. This in effect decreases her mass moment of inertia, so that for the same torque applied originally to the skate there is now an acceleration.

The forces due to gravitational effects or to accelerations that exist on the joint will have internal effects on the joint structure. A study of the stresses and strains in the joint tissues is complicated by the fact that the material composing the tissues is anisotropic, viscoelastic (time-dependent), and heterogeneous. This means that a simple analysis of the material, such as one would apply to a piece of stainless steel, is inadequate. If a small piece of material is removed from the joint and then subjected to a loading test to generate a stress-strain curve, two things must be specified to obtain meaningful data: the direction in which the specimen has been taken for the test must be noted because the material is anisotopic, and the rate at which the specimen is loaded must be specified because the material is viscoelastic.

All biologic tissues made up of collagenous tissue exhibit viscoelastic behavior. This is demonstrated to a marked degree in taffy or "silly putty." If the material is pulled slowly, it does not take much stress for a great deal of strain to develop. If the material is pulled rapidly, however, a large amount of stress develops with only a small strain.

The viscoelasticity of joint materials was first demonstrated by Hirsch in studies wherein small loads were placed on articular

FIG. 2-1. Deformation-time diagram for articular cartilage of the patella. At zero time, a probe 10.57 mm² was placed on the articular cartilage. There was an immediate deformation to 0.46 mm. When the weight was left on, continued deformation of the cartilage occurred. At the end of 1 min, the deformation was 0.50 mm. The weight was removed, and the compressed cartilage expanded back toward its original position but did not reach its total original position until an additional minute had passed. When the weight was left on for longer periods, continued compression of the cartilage was noted. The recovery period was also lengthened, and after the weight had been on for 2 min, the original geometry was not attained during the experiment. (After Hirsch C: The pathogenesis of chondromalacia of the patella. Acta Chir Scand 90 [Suppl 83], 1944)

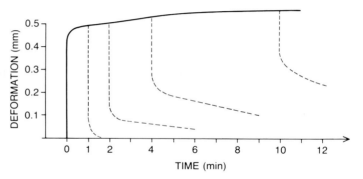

cartilage and then removed (Fig. 2-1).[10] When the load was placed on the cartilage, there was an immediate deformation. As the load remained, the material continued to deform. When the load was released, the material snapped back toward its original shape but did not regain this original shape until a period of time had passed. Cartilage exhibits an elastic deformation that occurs immediately and an inelastic deformation that occurs as the load remains.

The physical properties of the joint structures exhibit regional differences. In the tibial plateau of the dog, Moskowitz* demonstrated differences in histologic structure between the medial and the lateral condyles. Kempson and co-workers demonstrated regional differences in elasticity of the cartilage in the femoral head.[11]

The physical properties of the bony tissue have been summarized by Currey[2] and by Hayes and Carter.[8] The mechanical properties of cartilage have been summarized by Mow and associates.[17] Data on the soft collagenous tissues involved in joint structure have been

* Personal communication.

summarized by Viidik[26] and by Noyes and co-workers.[20]

KINETICS

STATICS

Static analysis can be used to estimate the loads acting at one time on a joint in any position and under any loading configuration. Because a complete static analysis involving all forces imposed on a joint is extremely complicated, a simplified technique is often used that allows the minimum magnitudes of the main forces acting on the joint to be estimated. The technique uses a free body diagram and limits the analysis to the three principal coplanar forces acting on the body.

An example will illustrate the application of the free body technique to the knee. In this case, the technique is used to estimate the minimum magnitude of the joint reaction force acting on the tibiofemoral joint of the weight-bearing leg when the other leg is lifted during stair climbing. The lower leg is considered as a free body, distinct from the rest of the body, and a diagram of this free body in

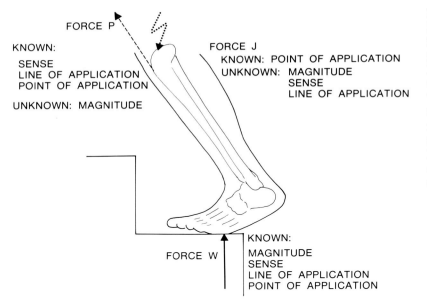

FORCE P

KNOWN:

SENSE
LINE OF APPLICATION
POINT OF APPLICATION

UNKNOWN: MAGNITUDE

FORCE J
KNOWN: POINT OF APPLICATION
UNKNOWN: MAGNITUDE
SENSE
LINE OF APPLICATION

FORCE W

KNOWN:
MAGNITUDE
SENSE
LINE OF APPLICATION
POINT OF APPLICATION

FIG. 2-2. Static analysis of the knee joint during stair climbing. The three principal coplanar forces acting on the lower leg are designated on the free body diagram. Force W is the ground reaction force, force P is the patellar tendon force, and force J is the joint reaction force. (Frankel VH, Nordin M: Basic Biomechanics of the Skeletal System. Philadelphia, Lea & Febiger, 1980)

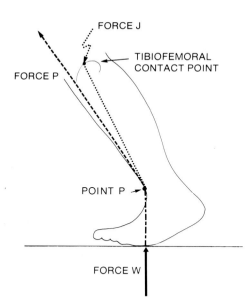

FORCE J

TIBIOFEMORAL
CONTACT POINT

FORCE P

POINT P

FORCE W

FIG. 2-3. On the free body diagram, the lines of application for forces W and P are extended until they intersect (point P). The line of application for force J (the joint reaction force) can now be determined by connecting its point of application (tibiofemoral contact point) wih point P. (After Frankel VH, Nordin M: Basic Biomechanics of the Skeletal System. Philadelphia, Lea & Febiger, 1980)

the stair-climbing situation is drawn (Fig. 2-2). The three main coplanar forces are identified. The ground reaction force (W) has a known magnitude (equal to body weight*), sense, line of application, and point of application (the point of contact between the foot and the ground). The patellar tendon force (P) has a known sense (away from the knee joint), line of application (along the patellar tendon), and point of application (the point of insertion of the patellar tendon on the tibial tuberosity), but an unknown magnitude. The joint reaction force (J) has a known point of application on the surface of the tibia (the contact point of the joint surfaces between the tibial and the femoral condyles, estimated from a roentgenogram of the joint in the proper loading configuration), but an unknown magnitude, sense, and line of application. These three forces are designated on the free body diagram.

In the static situation, advantage can be taken of the fact that for equilibrium to exist, the forces acting on the free body must be concurrent (there must be an absence of couples);

---

* In this case, the ground reaction force is actually equal to body weight minus the weight of the lower leg. Because the weight of the lower leg is minimal—that is, less than 1/10 body weight—it can be disregarded, and the figure for total body weight can be used in the calculation.

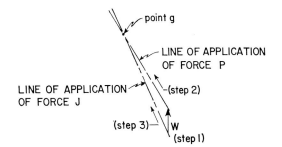

FIG. 2-4. Vector solution of problem of unknown force. A triangle of forces is constructed. Step 1: Vector W is drawn; the magnitude is equal to 1 W. Step 2: Force P is drawn from the head of vector W. Step 3: From the origin of force W, a line is drawn parallel to the line of application of force J. This line intersects vector P at point g, closing the triangle. The lengths of vectors P and J are now known and can be measured in terms of W. (Frankel VH, Burstein AH: Orthopaedic Biomechanics. Philadelphia, Lea & Febiger, 1970)

that is, all forces acting on the surface of the free body will intersect at a point if continued. Thus when force lines P and W are continued, they will intersect (Fig. 2-3, point P). Any other force acting on this free body will also meet at this point. Therefore, the line of application of force J can be found by connecting its point of application on the surface of the upper tibia to the intersection point of forces W and P (point P).

With the line of application for force J determined, it is now possible to construct a triangle of forces (Fig. 2-4). First, a vector representing force W is drawn with the proper line of application and sense. Next, force P is drawn from the head of vector W. The line of application and sense of P are known, but its length cannot be determined because the magnitude is unknown. Since the lower limb is in equilibrium, however, it is known that when force J is added the triangle must close (that is, the head of force P must touch the origin of force J), and the vector sum of the forces will be zero. Therefore, starting at the origin of W, a line is drawn parallel to the line of application of force J. This line intersects vector P at point g. Point g must be the head of vector P and the origin of force J. The magnitude of forces P and J can now be scaled from the

drawings (Fig. 2-5). This technique can be applied to any static equilibrium situation using available anatomic landmarks and geometry.

DYNAMICS

To find the loads occurring during more usual activities, it is necessary to apply a dynamic analysis instead of a static one. Newton's second law of motion, used to find the loads during nonequilibrium situations, is given by

$$F = MA$$

where F is force expressed in newtons,
M is mass expressed in kg, and
A is acceleration expressed in $(m/sec)^2$.

The second law, expressed for angular motion, is given by

$$T = I\alpha$$

where T is the torque, or moment, expressed in newton meters,
I is the mass moment of inertia expressed in newton meters $\times sec^2$, and
α is the angular acceleration expressed in radians/sec^2.

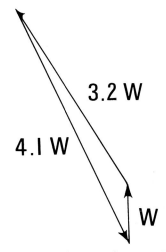

FIG. 2-5. Solution of vector diagram. The patellar tendon force is equal to 3.2 times body weight, and the joint reaction force is equal to 4.1 times body weight.

Kicking a football will illustrate the use of dynamic analysis to calculate the joint reaction force on the tibiofemoral joint at a particular instant during a dynamic activity (Fig. 2-6).[5] The maximal angular acceleration that occurred during the act of kicking the football was measured from stroboscopic photographs at 453 radians/sec² in an athletic male. This acceleration occurred when the lower leg was almost vertical. From anthropomorphic data presented by Drillis and co-workers,[4] the mass moment of inertia about the knee joint center in this subject was found to be 0.35 newton meters × sec². The torque necessary to produce this angular acceleration was calculated from the equation $T = I\alpha$:

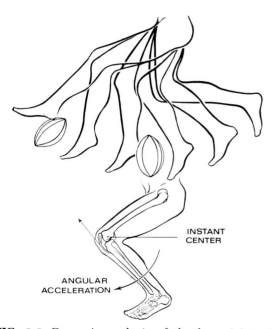

FIG. 2-6. Dynamic analysis of the knee joint. A football is propelled through the air by the foot because of the pull of the quadriceps tendon, which produces an angular acceleration about the knee joint. The angular acceleration can be measured from stroboscopic photographs. The length of the lever arm is the perpendicular distance between the line of the patellar tendon force and the instant center. (Frankel VH, Burstein AH: Orthopaedic Biomechanics. Philadelphia, Lea & Febiger, 1970)

torque = (0.35 newton meters × sec² × (435 radians/sec²) or 158.5 newton meters

The only force that can exert a torque about the center of rotation (instant center) in the knee joint is the tensile force in the patellar tendon. Since the perpendicular distance from this force vector to the instant center was 5.0 cm (0.05 m) in the subject measured, the force on the patellar tendon could be found from this relationship: force × distance = moment, or torque. Thus,

$$\text{force} = \frac{\text{moment}}{\text{distance}} \text{ or}$$

$$\frac{158.5 \text{ newton meters}}{0.05 \text{ m}} \text{ or}$$

$$3170 \text{ newtons}$$

This amount of force was necessary to produce the acceleration needed to kick the football at a particular instant. The force on the knee joint during this instant was found to be 3120 newtons by subtracting the weight of the lower leg, 50 newtons, from the tendon force of 3170 newtons. This weight was subtracted because the radial acceleration was almost zero at the instant when the leg was vertical. This simple example, as well as the static example of stair climbing, gives the reader an idea of the magnitude of forces that can result in a knee joint from common activities.

Walking is perhaps the most common activity in which the knee joint participates. Morrison described the forces acting on the knee joint during walking.[16] His studies first found the accelerations about the knee joint and the external forces acting on the joint for a gait cycle and then identified by means of electromyography the muscles that were contracting. This permitted a determination of the total muscle force associated with the gait.

The dynamic analysis just described demonstrates that of all the forces that produce a load on the knee joint, the muscle forces are by far the largest component. In Figure 2-7, after Morrison, the joint forces in the vertical direction during level walking are shown.[16] The peak force during the stance phase ranged from two to four times the body weight, depending on the individual tested. This peak force occurred in the late stance phase and was associated with gastrocnemius contraction. A force equal to body weight was present in the late swing phase as the hamstrings acted to decelerate the knee. Morrison noticed that during the stance phase of the gait cycle, the joint load was shifted to the medial tibial condyle, and in the swing phase the load acted mainly on the lateral condyle. The forces acting in the medial-lateral direction were generally small, approximately one-fourth the body weight. The peak muscle forces, which occurred in the hamstrings and the gastrocnemius during stance phase, were calculated to be two to four times the body weight. There was no significant difference between the joint forces calculated for male and female subjects when the forces were normalized by dividing by the body weight.

Close pointed out that not only is the magnitude of the force produced by the muscles important, but also the phase of gait in which the muscle activity takes place.[1] Tendon transplantations are not always successful because the tendon may not be pulling during the proper phase of gait. An attempt to control motion about the knee joint by tendon transplantation must take into account the large forces that will act on the tendon if the normal gait cycle is restored.

During the gait cycle, the joint forces are sustained not only by the joint cartilage, bone, and surrounding soft tissues, but also by the menisci. In a normal knee, stresses are distributed over a wide area of the tibial plateau. If the menisci are removed, the stresses are no longer distributed over such a wide area but are limited to a contact area in the center of the plateau. Therefore, removal of the menisci not only increases the magnitude of the stresses on the cartilage at the center of the tibial plateau; it also diminishes the size and changes the location of the contact area. Over the long term, the high stress placed on this smaller contact area may be harmful to the exposed cartilage, which is usually soft and fibrillated in that area.[15,24,25]

The joint force may be greatly modified dur-

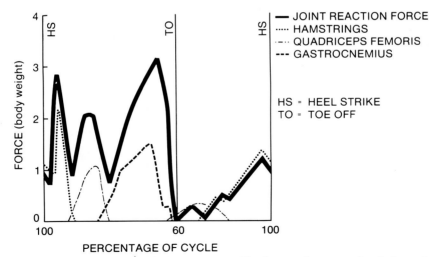

FIG. 2-7. Joint reaction force in terms of body weight transmitted through the tibial plateau during level walking, one gait cycle (12 subjects). The muscle forces producing the peak magnitudes of this force are also designated. (Frankel VH, Nordin M: Basic Biomechanics of the Skeletal System. Philadelphia, Lea & Febiger, 1980)

ing exercise. For any weight-lifting exercise involving flexion and extension, the minimal force multiplier will be 10. For example, if a 100-newton weight is placed in a weight boot and the leg raised from a position of 90° of flexion to full extension of the knee, the quadriceps force required to raise the weight will be approximately 1000 newtons. If this activity is done quickly, an additional force will be required to produce the acceleration needed.

Figures 2-8 through 2-10, after Reilly and Martens, show the quadriceps muscle (QF) force and the patellofemoral joint reaction (PFJR) force plotted against the angle of knee flexion for the various activities investigated.[21] The ranges shown for the forces represent the influence that the errors in measurement (made from the stroboscopic photographs) have on the calculated values. No range is shown in Figure 3-10 for the leg-raising exercise because these results were obtained from a mathematical analysis.

The lowest values for the QF force and the PFJR forces were obtained for level walking (Fig. 2-8). This result is to be expected because an efficient mechanism for walking would be developed to minimize both energy

expenditure and the forces that the skeletal structure would have to bear.

The PFJR force during level walking had a different pattern and different values from those of the tibiofemoral joint reaction force. The highest calculated value for the PFJR force during this activity was 350 newtons, or 0.5 body weight. The magnitude of the PFJR force is not only dependent upon the magnitude of the QF force but also upon the angle of knee flexion. Since the angles of flexion are kept quite low during level walking, the PFJR force is always smaller than the QF force.

The opposite is true for an activity during which the knee is flexed to larger angles, such as knee bends (Fig. 2-9). Here, the larger angles of flexion yield a higher value for the vector sum of the QF force and the patellar tendon force, which the PFJR force must equilibrate. The value calculated for the PFJR force at 90° of flexion was approximately 2500 newtons. Since the subject's body weight was 850 newtons, this joint reaction force is equivalent to about three times the body weight.

For the stair-climbing and descending activities, the PFJR force attained a level of 3.3 times the body weight. This value is almost

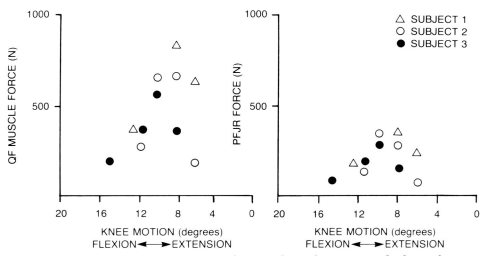

FIG. 2-8. Patellofemoral joint reaction force and quadriceps muscle force during level walking (three subjects). (After Reilly DT, Martens M: Experimental analysis of the quadriceps muscle force and patellofemoral joint reaction force for various activities. Acta Orthop Scand 43:126, 1972)

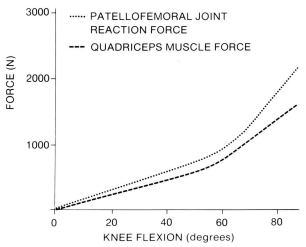

FIG. 2-9. Patellofemoral joint reaction force and quadriceps muscle force during knee bend to 90 degrees (three subjects). (Frankel VH, Nordin M: Basic Biomechanics of the Skeletal System. Philadelphia, Lea & Febiger, 1980)

seven times the PFJR force obtained during level walking. This figure explains why patients with patellofemoral joint derangements experience more pain while climbing and descending stairs. Such patients adapt their gait pattern in stair walking by assisting with the uninvolved side in order to decrease the muscle force. The push-off with the unaffected leg helps considerably in decreasing the muscle force during stair climbing.

Patients with derangements of the patellofemoral joint have the greatest difficulty while descending stairs because the only effective adaptation to prevent high PFJR forces is a lowering of the body with controlled knee flexion at the unaffected side while the involved knee is kept straight. When these patients are treated conservatively with quadriceps exercises against resistance, which require extending the knee from 90° to full extension with a lead boot, most are unable to accomplish the exercise because of retropatellar pain. They are able, however, to do straight-leg raising against the same resistance. The explanation is given in Figure 2-10, in which a maximum PFJR force of 1.4 times the body weight is found at 36° of knee flexion when a 90-newton boot is used. If a heavier

boot is worn, the general shape of the curve obtained remains the same while the force dimension is proportionally scaled upwards.

Figure 2-10 also illustrates that the PFJR force can be kept at a significantly lower level when the straight-leg raising exercise is performed. When the knee is extended, the lines of action of the patellar ligament and the QF forces are almost parallel, and because the angle between those two forces is smaller, their vector sum represents a lower value.

KINEMATICS

RANGE OF MOTION

The kinematic data used to describe normal gait and useful in determining the forces acting in the knee joint have been summarized by Murray.[18] Figure 2-11, after Murray and associates, illustrates the range of motion of the tibiofemoral joint in the sagittal plane during level, free-speed walking in normal men.[19]

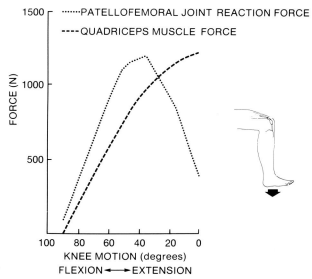

FIG. 2-10. Patellofemoral joint reaction force and quadriceps muscle force during knee extension against resistance provided by a 90-newton weight boot with the subject sitting and the lower leg free-hanging (three subjects). (Frankel VH, Nordin M: Basic Biomechanics of the Skeletal System. Philadelphia, Lea & Febiger, 1980)

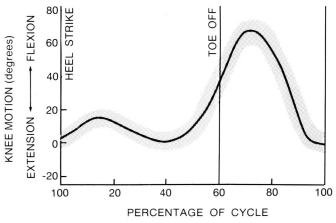

FIG. 2-11. Motion of the tibiofemoral joint in the sagittal plane during level walking, one gait cycle. Shaded area indicates variation among 60 men (age range: 20 years to 65 years). (Frankel V H, Nordin M: Basic Biomechanics of the Skeletal System. Philadelphia, Lee & Febiger, 1980)

Maximal flexion in the stance phase was approximately 18°, and in the swing phase, 75°. The knee joint that does not have this degree of mobility will produce a visible limp during gait. The knee requires full extension both in the beginning of the stance phase at heel strike and at the end of stance phase during toe off. Kettelkamp and co-workers found that the knee reached maximal extension just before heel strike in over 60% of the knees studied, at heel strike in 34%, and between heel off and toe off in 2%.[12]

The range of motion of the knee joint in the transverse plane has been described by Saunders and associates[23] and Kettelkamp and co-workers.[12] This transverse rotation of the tibia on the femur is difficult to measure. Most authors have based their data on passive motion. Levens and associates studied transverse rotation with skeletal pins and photographs.[14] Rotation ranged from 4.1° to 13.3° in 12 subjects, with a mean of 8.6°. Kettelkamp and co-workers, using an electrogoniometer in their studies, found a range of 5.7° to 25.2° in 22 subjects, with a mean of approximately 13°. External rotation of the tibia occurred during extension of the knee and reached a peak value just before heel strike. This external rotation of the tibia is called the *screw home mechanism*, which indicates that as the knee goes into extension the tibia rotates externally on the femur. Helfet has demonstrated the clinical importance of this mecha-

nism.[9] Kettelkamp and co-workers found that maximal abduction of the tibia was associated with the initiation of the stance phase and that maximal adduction occurred as the knee flexed during the swing phase.

The electrogoniographic method of analyzing knee function has been extended by Laubenthal and associates to an examination of the range of knee motion required during activities of daily living.[13] They found that in the sagittal plane the average knee motion was 83° for climbing stairs in a normal manner, 93° for sitting, 106° for tying a shoe, 71° for lifting an object without instructions, and 117° for lifting an object with instructions. The average motion in the coronal and the transverse planes was less than 25° during these activities. They noted a significant relationship between the tibial-foot segment length and the range of knee motion for most of the activities.

SURFACE JOINT MOTION

Kinematics also describes the motion of particles that are attached to the moving limbs. It is the study of the relative motion that can exist between rigid bodies, called *links*. In the case of human joints, the bones are the links. As one link rotates about another, there exists at an instant a point that has a zero velocity; this point constitutes the instantaneous center of motion, or instant center. By means of the

FIG. 2-12. (A, B) Lateral roentgenograms of the knee joint in different positions used to locate the instant center. The femoral shaft is bisected. The intersection of the femoral shaft bisector with the medial femoral condyle defines one point. The second point is found by measuring 7.5 cm upward. (C) Superimposition of roentgenograms A and B. Note displacement of the two points. The instant center is found by connecting the perpendicular bisectors of the displacement lines. (Frankel VH, Burstein AH, Brooks D: J Bone Joint Surg 53-A:945, 1971)

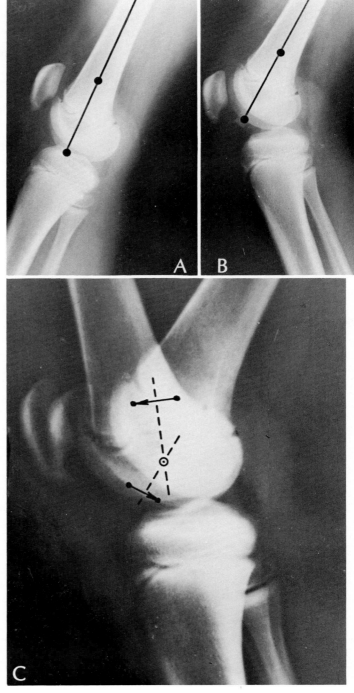

method of Reuleaux, the instant center for knee motion can be located by identifying the displacement of two points on the link as the link moves from one position to another (Fig. 2-12).[22] Lines are drawn connecting each pair of points, and the perpendicular bisectors of these displacement lines are drawn. The intersection of the perpendicular bisectors locates the instant center. This technique has been used by Dempster to identify the hinge point of the knee joint.[3]

Studies identifying the instant center in the knee joint may be performed by using multiple x-ray film exposures, or cineradiography, or by attaching mechanical devices to the bone. The procedure involves exposing six or eight lateral roentgenograms of the knee taken at increments of motion from full extension to 90° of flexion. The patient is positioned with the leg resting on the table and the opposite leg in front of or behind the body. The ankle is supported by a small foam rubber pad so that the tibia is horizontal. An attempt is made to take a lateral film of the knee joint at full extension; the joint is then moved approximately 10° to the next position, care being taken to keep the tibia parallel to the table and to disallow any rotation about the femur. A film is exposed and the leg again moved. In the case of a patient with limited flexion and extension, the knee joint is placed in the maximal tolerated position and actively held in this position.

The films are then superimposed in pairs, with the image of one tibia placed over the other. Points can be identified on these films that will move in space as the joint moves. Films with marked differences in tibial position are not used. A line is drawn on each film, bisecting the femoral shaft and crossing one of the femoral condyles, as illustrated in Figure 2-12A. The point at which the line crosses the condyle is one point used in the analysis; the second is found by measuring 7.5 cm up from the first point along the femoral axis. The displacements of the points are found when the films are superimposed. Perpendicular bisectors of the displacement lines are constructed, and the instant center is located at the intersection of these bisectors (Fig. 2-12C).

An examination of the pathway of the instant centers throughout a range of motion leads to a more complete understanding of the mechanics of joint motion. In Figure 2-13 the instant center is shown together with the relative position of a femur and a tibia. Superimposed on the figure are the directions of the velocities of three points on the femur, obtained by constructing perpendiculars to lines drawn from the instant center to the points in question. Each of these velocities is tangential to the contact surface. In a normal knee, the velocities are tangential to the surface of the tibia for each interval of motion from full extension to full flexion, demonstrating that the femur is sliding on the tibial condyles (Fig. 2-14). If the instant center were to be found on the surface, the joint would have a rolling motion and there would be no sliding friction. In 25 normal knees analyzed in our laboratory, the instant center was located in all positions

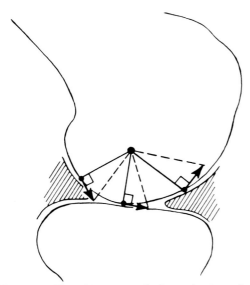

FIG. 2-13. The direction of the velocity of any point on the femoral link may be found by connecting that point to the instant center (*solid lines*) and constructing a perpendicular (*arrowed lines*) to the connecting line at the point in question. (Frankel VH, Burstein AH, Brooks D: J Bone Joint Surg, 53-A:945, 1971)

FIG. 2-14. Instant center study for a normal knee joint. The velocities of the surface particles are tangential to the joint surface as the joint moves from flexion to extension.

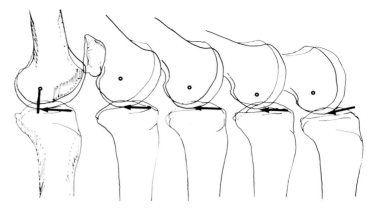

of the knee from 90° of flexion to full extension. In all cases tangential sliding was noted.

Studies of surface joint motion have been performed on knees having internal derangements.[7] The kinematic technique described above was used, and multiple films were exposed with the knee in successive positions from 90° of flexion to as much extension as could be obtained. Because most pathologic changes in the joint surfaces are located in the extension-contact areas, roentgenograms made with the knee in more than 90° of flexion were not included. In many cases, it was found that for some range of extension-flexion the instant center was displaced from the normal position. If the joint is extended and flexed about this position, the joint surface particles do not slide tangentially to the surface but are forced into or away from the surface (Fig. 2-15). This situation is analogous to bending a door hinge, then opening and closing the door and finding that it no longer fits into the jamb. If the direction of the velocity at the joint surface tends to compress the two joint surfaces, further extension or flexion may be blocked.

If structures between the femoral condyles and tibial plateaus are displaced, causing motion to occur about abnormally placed instant centers, the moving structures are forced together and local lesions in the articular cartilage are produced at the sites of compression. Under these circumstances, the joint may accommodate localized high pressures by capsular or ligamentous stretching, which relieves the pressure. This articular wear may occur at a distance from the primary joint lesion. For example, a medial meniscal rupture may be present with wear of the lateral femoral condyle. Cases such as this demonstrate that when there are kinematic disturbances of the type under consideration here, contact with the displaced structure is not the only mechanism by which wear is produced. Abnormal surface velocities may cause high local surface stresses at a distance from the primary pathologic lesion.

It was possible to correlate the site of wear of

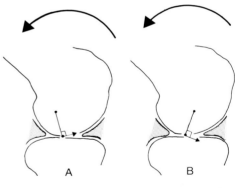

A
DISTRACTION

B
COMPRESSION

FIG. 2-15. Surface motion in two tibiofemoral joints with displaced instant centers. **(A)** The direction of the velocity indicates that with further flexion, the tibiofemoral joint will be distracted. **(B)** The direction of the velocity indicates that with further flexion, the joint will be compressed. (Frankel VH, Nordin M: Basic Biomechanics of the Skeletal System. Philadelphia, Lea & Febiger, 1980)

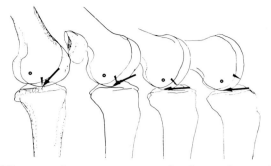

FIG. 2-16. Instant center study from abnormal joint. In the extension range, the instant center was displaced. As the knee joint flexed and extended in this range, the surfaces were either pulling apart or grinding together. In the flexion range, the instant center was normally located. The small triangle indicates the center of a compressed lesion.

the joint surface cartilage with the findings in the instant center study of knees having internal derangements.[7] When the direction of the velocity tended to drive the joint surfaces together, wear could be identified on the joint surface in the range of joint motion where this abnormal compression occurred. The longer that motion about an abnormally located instant center had been present, the greater was the chance of finding wear at arthrotomy. The cartilage lesions were similar to those produced in compression studies of animal joints.

The instant center technique may be used to determine whether or not the surface velocities of the femoral and the tibial articulating surfaces produce efficient sliding. The technique does not help to localize articular changes to either the medial or the lateral side of the joint, nor does it identify prior to surgery the structure responsible for the abnormally located instant center. A kinematic study does allow assessment of the mechanics of the articular surfaces at any degree of flexion.

The instant center technique elucidates a mechanism for the development of traumatic degenerative joint disease secondary to some remote trauma producing an internal derangement of the knee joint. The technique demonstrates the interrelationship between mechanical alterations and biologic response. The scheme presented at the bottom of the page, based on the observations made in our case material, is proposed to explain this relationship.

Figure 2-16 shows the instant centers for an abnormal knee joint. In the extension range, the instant center is displaced in such a manner that the joint is compressed as the knee joint is extended. Figure 2-17 is a photograph of the case in which an area in the medial femoral condyle was compressed in a 12-year-old boy who had been walking for 1½ years with the knee joint forced to rotate about an ab-

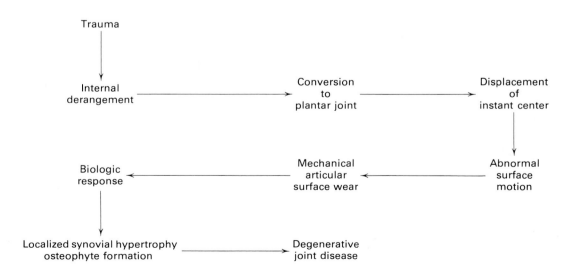

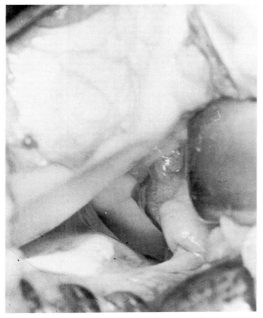

FIG. 2-17. Operative photograph of the knee joint of a 12-year-old boy. The joint had been extending around an abnormally located instant center. There is a compressed faceted area on both the medial and the lateral femoral condyles. An area of synovial hyperplasia is growing toward the center of this compressed area in the margin of the joint.

normally located instant center. Other cases demonstrated wear and early degenerative arthritis in the knee joint; the joint surfaces were sliding together in an abnormal manner, which caused surface damage.

REFERENCES

1. **Close JR:** Motor Function in the Lower Extremity. Springfield, Charles C Thomas, 1964
2. **Currey JD:** The mechanical properties of bone. Clin Orthop 73:210, 1970
3. **Dempster WT:** Study of Hinge Points of Human Body. Wright Air Development Center, USAF Contract No. AF 18(600)-43, 1953
4. **Drillis R, Contini R, Bluestein M:** Body segment parameters; a survey of measurement techniques. Artif Limbs 8:44, 1964
5. **Frankel VH, Burstein AH:** Orthopaedic Biomechanics. Philadelphia, Lea & Febiger, 1970
6. **Frankel VH, Nordin M:** Basic Biomechanics of the Skeletal System. Philadelphia, Lea & Febiger (in press)
7. **Frankel VH, Burstein AH, Brooks DB:** Biomechanics of internal derangement of the knee. Pathomechanics as determined by analysis of the instant centers of motion. J Bone Joint Surg 53-A:945, 1971
8. **Hayes WC, Carter DR:** Biomechanics of the bone. In Simmons DJ, Kunin AS (eds): Skeletal Research—An Experimental Approach. New York, Academic Press, 1979
9. **Helfet AJ:** The Management of Internal Derangements of the Knee. Philadelphia, JB Lippincott, 1963
10. **Hirsch C:** A contribution to the pathogenesis of chondromalacia of the patella: A physical, histologic and chemical study. Acta Chir Scand (Suppl. 83), 90 1944
11. **Kempson G, Spivey C, Freeman M et al:** Indentation stiffness in articular cartilage in normal and osteoarthrosic femoral heads. In Wright V (ed): Lubrication and Wear in Joints. Philadelphia, JB Lippincott, 1969
12. **Kettelkamp DB, Johnson RJ, Smidt GL et al:** An electrogoniometric study of knee motion in normal gait. J Bone Joint Surg 52-A:775, 1970
13. **Laubenthal KN, Smidt GL, and Kettelkamp DB:** A quantitative analysis of knee motion during activities of daily living. Phys Ther 52:34, 1972
14. **Levens AS, Inman VT, and Blosser JA:** Transverse rotation of the segments of the lower extremity in locomotion. J Bone Joint Surg 30-A:859, 1948
15. **Lutfi AM:** Morphological changes in articular cartilage after meniscectomy: An experimental study in the monkey. J Bone Joint Surg 57-B:525, 1975
16. **Morrison JB:** The mechanics of the knee joint in relation to normal walking. J Biomech 3:51, 1970
17. **Mow VC, Roth V, Armstrong CG:** Biomechanics of joint cartilage. In Frankel VH, Nordin M: Basic Biomechanics of the Skeletal System. Philadelphia, Lea & Febiger (in press)
18. **Murray MP:** Gait as a total pattern of movement. Including bibliography on gait. Am J Phys Med 46:290, 1967
19. **Murray MP, Drought AB, Mory RC:** Walking patterns of normal men. J Bone Joint Surg 46-A:335, 1964
20. **Noyes FR, DeLucas JL, Torvik PJ:** Biomechanics of anterior cruciate ligament failure: An analysis of strain-rate sensitivity and mechanisms of failure in primates. J Bone Joint Surg 56-A:236, 1974
21. **Reilly DT, Martens M:** Experimental analysis of the quadriceps muscle force and patello-femoral joint reaction force for various activities. Acta Orthop Scand 43:126, 1972
22. **Reuleaux F:** The Kinematics of Machinery: Outline of a Theory of Machines. London, Macmillan, 1876
23. **Saunders JB DeC M, Inman V, Eberhart HD:** The major determinants in normal and pathological gait. J Bone Joint Surg 35-A:543, 1953
24. **Seedhom BB, Dowson D, Wright V:** The load-bearing function of the menisci: A preliminary study. In Ingwersen OS et al (eds): The Knee Joint. Recent Advances in Basic Research and Clinical Aspects. Amsterdam, Excerpta Medica, 1974
25. **Shrive NG, O'Connor JJ, and Goodfellow JW:** Load-

bearing in the knee joint. Clin Orthop 131:279, 1978
26. **Viidik A:** Biomechanics and functional adaptation of tendons and joint ligaments. In Evans FG (ed): Studies on the Anatomy and Function of Bone and Joints. New York, Springer-Verlag, 1966
27. **Williams M, Lissner HR:** In LeVeau B (ed): Biomechanics of Human Motion, 2nd ed. Philadelphia, WB Saunders, 1977

BIBLIOGRAPHY

TIBIOFEMORAL JOINT

Brantigan OC, Voshell AF: The mechanics of the ligaments and menisci of the knee joint. J Bone Joint Surg 23-A:44, 1941

Brattström HH, Junerfält I, Moritz U: Behandlingen av sträckdefekter i leder: Kontraktur eller fraktur? Läkartidningen 68:304, 1971

Cailliet R: Knee Pain and Disability. Philadelphia FA Davis, 1968

Collopy MC, Murray MP, Gardner GM et al: Kinesiologic measurements of functional performance before and after geometric total knee replacement. One-year follow-up of twenty cases. Clin Orthop 126:196, 1977

Cox JS, Nye CE, Schaefer WW, et al: The degenerative effects of partial and total resection of the medial meniscus in dogs' knees. Clin Orthop 109:178, 1975

Detenbeck LC: Function of the cruciate ligaments in knee stability. J Sports Med 2:217, 1974

Drillis R, Contini R, Bluestein M: Body segment parameters. A survey of measurement techniques. Artif Limbs 8:44, 1964

Ducroquet R., Ducroquet J, Ducroquet P: Walking and Limping. A Study of Normal and Pathological Walking. Philadelphia, JB Lippincott, 1968

Edholm P, Lindahl O, Lindholm B et al: Knee instability. An orthoradiographic study. Acta Orthop Scand 47:658, 1976

Fairbank TJ: Knee joint changes after meniscectomy. J Bone Joint Surg 30-B:664, 1948

Frankel VH, Burstein AH: Orthopaedic Biomechanics. Philadelphia, Lea & Febiger, 1970

Frankel VH, Burstein AH, Brooks DB: Biomechanics of internal derangement of the knee. Pathomechanics as determined by analysis of the instant centers of motion. J Bone Joint Surg 53-A:945, 1971

Hainaut K: Introduction à la biomecanique. Brussels, Presses Universitaires de Bruxelles, 1971

Hallen LG, Lindahl O: The "screw-home" movement in the knee-joint. Acta Orthop Scand 37:97, 1966

Hsieh H-H, Walker PS: Stabilizing mechanisms of the loaded and unloaded knee joint. J Bone Joint Surg 58-A:87, 1976

Ingwersen OS, Van Linge B, Van Rhens ThJG et al:

(eds): The Knee Joint. Recent Advances in Basic Research and Clinical Aspects. Amsterdam, Excerpta Medica, 1974

Johnson RJ, Kettelkamp DB, Clark W et al: Factors affecting late results after meniscectomy. J Bone Joint Surg 56-A:719, 1974

Kapandji IA: The Physiology of the Joints, Vol 2, Lower Limb. London, Churchill Livingstone, 1970

Kettelkamp DB, Jacobs AW: Tibiofemoral contact area—Determination and implications. J Bone Joint Surg 54-A:349, 1972

Kettelkamp DB, Johnson RJ, Smidt GL et al: An electrogoniometric study of knee motion in normal gait. J Bone Joint Surg 52-A:775, 1970

Krause WR, Pope MH, Johnson RJ et al: Mechanical changes in the knee after meniscectomy. J Bone Joint Surg 58-A:599, 1976

Laasonen EM, Wilppula E: Why a meniscectomy fails. Acta Orthop Scand 47:672, 1976

Laubenthal KN, Smidt GL, Kettelkamp DB: A quantitative analysis of knee motion during activities of daily living. Phys Ther 52:34, 1972

Levens AS, Inman VT, Blosser JA: Transverse rotation of the segments of the lower extremity in locomotion. J Bone Joint Surg 30-A:859, 1948

Lindahl O, Movin A: The mechanics of extension of the knee-joint. Acta Orthop Scand 38:226, 1967

Markolf KL, Mensch JS, Amstutz HC: Stiffness and laxity of the knee—The contributions of the supporting structures. J Bone Joint Surg 58-A:583, 1976

Marshall JL, Olsson S-E: Instability of the knee. A long-term experimental study in dogs. J Bone Joint Surg 53-A:1561, 1971

McLeod PC, Kettelkamp DB, Srinivasan V et al: Measurements of repetitive activities of the knee. J Biomech 8:369, 1975

McLeod WD, Moschi A, Andrews JR et al: Tibial plateau topography. Am J Sports Med 5:13, 1977

Moore TM, Meyers MH, Harvey PJ: Collateral ligament laxity of the knee. J Bone Joint Surg 58-A:594, 1976

Morrison JB: Bioengineering analysis of force actions transmitted by the knee joint. Biomed Eng 3:164, 1968

Morrison JB: The mechanics of the knee joint in relation to normal walking. J Biomech 3:51, 1970

Murray MP: Gait as a total pattern of movement. Including a bibliography on gait. Am J Phys Med 46:290, 1967

Murray MP, Drought AB, Kory RC: Walking patterns of normal men. J Bone Joint Surg 46-A:335, 1964

Perry J, Norwood L, Hoise K: Knee posture and biceps and semimembranosis muscle action in running and cutting (an EMG study). Transactions of the 23rd Annual Meeting, Orthopaedic Research Society, Vol 2, p 258, 1977

Pope MH, Crowninshield R, Miller R et al: The static and dynamic behavior of the human knee in vivo. J Biomech 9:449, 1976

Reuleaux F: The Kinematics of Machinery: Outline of a Theory of Machines. London, Macmillan, 1876

Roberts EM, Zernicke RF, Youm Y et al: Kinetic parameters of kicking. *In* Nelson RC, Morehouse CA (eds): Biomechanics IV. Baltimore, University Park Press, 1974

Saunders JB DeC M, Inman VT, Eberhardt HD: The major determinants in normal and pathological gait. J Bone Joint Surg 35-A:543, 1953

Seedhom BB, Dowson D, Wright V: The load-bearing function of the menisci: A preliminary study. *In* Ingwersen OS et al (eds): The Knee Joint. Recent Advances in Basic Research and Clinical Aspects. Amsterdam, Excerpta Medica, 1974

Seireg A, Arvikar RJ: The prediction of muscular load sharing and joint forces in the lower extremities during walking. J Biomech 8:89, 1975

Shrive NG, O'Connor JJ, Goodfellow JW: Load-bearing in the knee joint. Clin Orthop 131:279, 1978

Smidt GL: Biomechanical analysis of knee flexion and extension. J Biomech 6:79, 1973

Smillie T: Injuries of the Knee Joint. Edinburgh, Churchill Livingstone, 1970

Stauffer RN, Chao EYS, Györy AN: Biomechanical gait analysis of the diseased knee joint. Clin Orthop 126: 246, 1977

Townsend MA, Izak M, Jackson RW: Total motion knee goniometry. J Biomech 10:183, 1977

Trent PS, Walker PS, Wolf B: Ligament length patterns, strength, and rotational axes of the knee joint. Clin Orthop 117:263, 1976

Walker PS, Erkman MJ: The role of the menisci in the force transmission across the knee. Clin Orthop 109:184, 1975

Walker PS, Hajek JV: The load-bearing area in the knee joint. J Biomech 5:581, 1972

Wang C-J, Walker PS: Rotatory laxity of the human knee joint. J Bone Joint Surg 56-A:161, 1974

Wang C-J, Walker PS, Wolf B: The effects of flexion and rotation on the length patterns of the ligaments of the knee. J Biomech 6:587, 1973

Warren CG, Lehmann JF, Kirkpatrick GS: Measurement of moments in the knee—ankle orthosis of ambulating paraplegics. *In* Nelson RC, Morehouse CA (eds): Biomechanics IV. Baltimore, University Park Press, 1974

Williams M, Lissner H: LeVeau B (ed): Biomechanics of Human Motion, 2nd ed. Philadelphia, WB Saunders, 1977

PATELLOFEMORAL JOINT

Böstrom A: Fractures of the patella. A study of 422 patellar fractures. Acta Orthop Scand (Suppl) 143, 1972.

Brattström HH, Junerfält I, Moritz U: Behandlingen av sträckdefekter i leder: Kontraktur eller fraktur? Läkartidningen 68:304, 1971

Cailliet R: Knee Pain and Disability. Philadelphia FA Davis, 1968

Drillis R, Contini R, Bluestein M: Body segment param-

eters. A survey of measurement techniques. Artif Limbs 8:44, 1964

Frankel VH, Burstein AH: Orthopaedic Biomechanics. Philadelphia, Lea & Febiger, 1970

Frankel VH, Burstein AH, Brooks DB: Biomechanics of internal derangement of the knee. J Bone Joint Surg 53-A:945, 1971

Goodfellow J, Hungerford DS, Zindel M: Patello-femoral joint mechanics and pathology. I. Functional anatomy of the patello-femoral joint. J Bone Joint Surg 58-B:287, 1976

Hainaut K: Introduction à la biomecanique. Brussels, Presses Universitaires de Bruxelles, 1971

Kapandji IA: The Physiology of the Joints, Vol 2, Lower Limb. Edinburgh, Churchill Livingstone, 1970

Kaufer H: Mechanical function of the patella. J Bone Joint Surg 53-A:1551, 1971

Reilley DT, Martens M: Experimental analysis of the quadriceps muscle force and patello-femoral joint reaction force for various activities. Acta Orthop Scand 43:126, 1972

Seireg A, Arvikar RJ: The prediction of muscular load sharing and joint forces in the lower extremities during walking. J Biochem 8:89, 1975

Smidt GL: Biomechanical analysis of knee flexion and extension. J Biomech 6:79, 1973

Smillie T: Injuries of the Knee Joint. Edinburgh, Churchill Livingstone, 1970

West FE: End results of patellectomy. J Bone Joint Surg, 44-A:1089, 1962

Williams M, Lissner H: LeVeau B (ed): Biomechanics of Human Motion, 2nd ed. Philadelphia, WB Saunders, 1977

QUADRICEPS MUSCLE

Damholt V, Zdravkovic D: Quadriceps function following fractures of the femoral shaft. Acta Orthop Scand 43:148, 1972

Elftman H: Biomechanics of muscle. With particular application to studies of gait. J Bone Joint Surg 48-A:363, 1966

Frankel VH, Burstein AH: Orthopaedic Biomechanics. Philadelphia, Lea & Febiger, 1970

Haffajee D, Moritz U, Svantesson G: Isometric knee extension strength as a function of joint angle, muscle length and motor unit activity. Acta Orthop Scand 43:138, 1972

Helfet A: Disorders of the Knee. Philadelphia, JB Lippincott, 1974

Lieb FJ, Perry J: Quadriceps function. An anatomical and mechanical study using amputated limbs. J Bone Joint Surg 50-A:1535, 1968

Lieb FJ, Perry J: Quadriceps function. An electromyographic study under isometric conditions. J Bone Joint Surg 53-A:749, 1971

Reilly DT, Martens M: Experimental analysis of the

quadriceps muscle force and patello-femoral joint reaction force for various activities. Acta Orthop Scand 43:126, 1972

Smillie IS: Injuries of the Knee Joint. Edinburgh, Churchill Livingstone, 1970

Williams M, Lissner H: LeVeau, B. (ed.): Biomechanics of Human Motion, 2nd ed. Philadelphia, WB Saunders, 1977

Zernicke RF, Garhammer J, Jobe FW: Human patellar–tendon rupture. J Bone Joint Surg 59-A:179, 1977

CHAPTER 3
MICROSTRUCTURE AND BIOCHEMISTRY OF JOINTS

Charles Weiss

Primary functions of the knee joints are to provide for weight bearing and movement. The compressive forces of weight bearing and the shearing forces of movement are brought to bear upon a specialized form of hyalin cartilage that covers the articulating surfaces of those bones that comprise the knee joint. This opalescent covering appears to be homogeneous and inert because it is devoid of both nerves and vessels and contains but a sparse number of cells embedded in a gel-like matrix. Only recently has it been shown to be chemically complex, structurally heterogeneous, and metabolically extremely active. The emphasis in this chapter will be on the structure, physical properties, cellular and chemical composition, metabolism, and nutrition of normal young adult human articular cartilage and how these parameters are altered in osteoarthritis. Developmental and aging processes will be discussed briefly but only as they relate directly to an understanding of normal and osteoarthritic cartilage.

THE ARTICULAR SURFACE

Upon arthrotomy, joint surfaces wet with synovial fluid appear smooth and regular. However, examination under indirect light with only a hand lens shows them to be irregular and undulating. These undulations, which are present in the drawings of the 19th century microscopists,[56] have recently received widespread attention, owing in part to the increasing interest in joint mechanics, particularly lubrication, stimulated by the advent of total joint replacement.

Studies on a wide variety of mammalian species, by incident light microscopy,[55] Linnik interference photomicrography,[54] tally-surf tracings,[186] and scanning electronmicroscopy[30,31,57,185] have described four orders of surface irregularities[87]: the primary joint contours, secondary irregularities (0.4 mm to 0.5 mm in diameter), tertiary hollows (20 μm to 45 μm in diameter and 0.5 μm to 2.0 μm deep with a pitch of 25μm), and quaternary

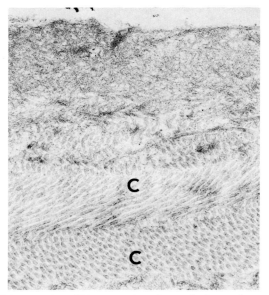

FIG. 3-1. An oblique section through the surface of normal articular cartilage. The surface is covered by a layer of fine fibers 4 nm to 10 nm in diameter, corresponding to the lamina splendens. Collagen fibers (~32 nm in diameter) of the tangential zone are arranged in tightly packed bundles (C) oriented at right angles to each other and running parallel to the articular surface (original magnification × 30,000).

ridges (1 μm to 4 μm in diameter and 0.1 μm to 0.3 μm deep). Under conditions of static loading and presumably during periods of simultaneous weight bearing and movement, the elasticity of cartilage permits flattening of the bearing surface and bulging of the non-bearing surfaces.[54] However, while the primary joint contours are altered, the tertiary hollows remain intact.[54] Quaternary ridges may be due to wearing away of ground substance from the articular surface, thus exposing large fiber bundles.[87]

Under the light microscope, a birefringent line is apparent on the articular surface. McConnaill[91] named this structure the lamina splendens. Scanning[32] and transmission[182] electronmicroscopic studies have demonstrated a layer of fine fibrils (4 to 10 nm in diameter) occurring in random fashion and measuring up to several micra in height, that covers and appears adsorbed to the intact ar-

ticular surfaces (Fig. 3-1, see Fig. 3-8). The composition of these fibrils cannot be determined by their ultrastructural appearance alone. Biochemical analysis suggests that they are probably hyaluronic acid[7] or other proteoglycans[142] derived from the synovial fluid.

JOINT LUBRICATION

Synovial joints, which have a coefficient of friction as low as 0.002, are remarkably efficient in carrying out the dual functions of weight bearing and movement.[93] To date the precise mechanism of this lubrication remains incompletely understood. It is apparent, however, that the special properties of the synovial fluid, the macromolecular covering of the cartilage surface, the primary, secondary, tertiary, and quaternary surface contours, and the physical properties of articular cartilage play significant roles in joint lubrication.

The presence of synovial fluid, slimy to the touch and with the capacity to decrease in viscosity with increasing joint movement and resultant sheer forces,[45,94] led early investigators to postulate a classic hydrodynamic concept of joint lubrication[12]: a wedge of fluid develops between rapidly rotating surfaces, and pressure created in this wedge keeps the surfaces apart. In 1960 Charnley demonstrated that fluid wedges are inconsistent with the reciprocating movement of animal joints.[26] The high rate of shear created by the load that joints support during movement would thin the normally viscous synovial fluid excessively; thus, a hydrodynamic system could function only under low loads and at high speeds. Boundary lubrication, as advanced by Charnley, depends upon the affinity of synovial fluid for the articular surface (the lamina splendens). The low coefficient of friction in this system is due to a molecular film that is physiochemically bound to each of the articulating surfaces and keeps them apart. This system, although effective at low speeds, is ineffective at high loads.

The classic hydrodynamic theory has been modified in two important ways: McCutchen advanced the concept of *weeping* lubrication, a form of hydrostatic lubrication that occurs when, as a result of loading, fluid passes from within the articular cartilage to the joint surface.[92] Second, the elastic deformation of cartilage increases the contact area between surfaces, thereby decreasing the pressure in the lubricating fluid and permitting the film thickness to be independent of load.[42,50,166,167] These two modifications of the hydrodynamic theory have been termed elastohydrodynamic and allow effective lubrication under high loads.[9,42,45,141,142,144] Under lesser loads the concept of boundary lubrication appears valid when the concept of "boosted lubrication" is added to it.[185,187] Synovial fluid subjected to rapid increases in pressure is transformed from a viscous liquid to a gel because water is squeezed out and aggregates of macromole-

cules form a tangled network. This gel can serve as a boundary lubricant and may increase cartilage resiliency. Pools of this *enriched* gel, or concentrate of synovial fluid, have been shown under the scanning electron microscope to be trapped in tertiary undulations when the articular surface is placed under load; in this manner they keep the actual cartilaginous surfaces apart.[42,185,186,187]

THE CELLS

The morphology and disposition of cells in normal adult articular cartilage has allowed microscopists to define four distinct zones (Fig. 3-2). The zone closest to the articular surface is the tangential or gliding zone (often re-

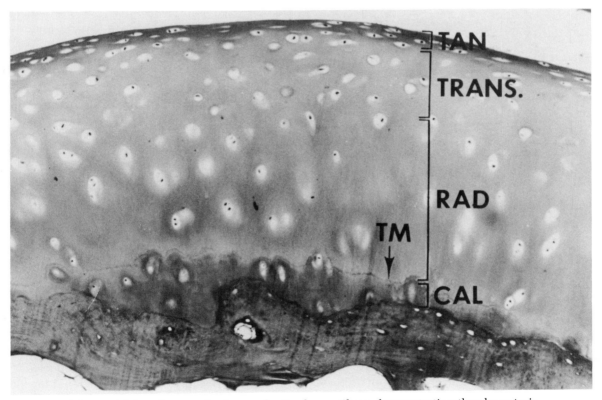

FIG. 3-2. Light micrograph of normal articular cartilage, demonstrating the characteristics of the tangential (*TAN*), transitional (*TRANS*), radial (*RAD*), and calcified (*CAL*) zones and the tidemark (*TM*). The articular cartilage rests upon the subchondral bony plate. (Weiss C: Normal and osteoarthritic articular cartilage. Orthop Clin North Am 10:175, 1979)

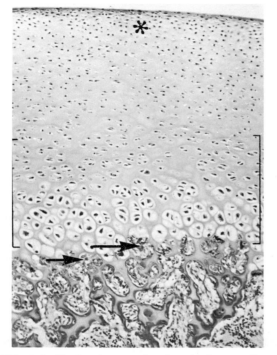

FIG. 3-3. Photomicrograph of articular cartilage from immature animal. The superficial zone consists of flattened cells. Beneath this zone is the growth zone for the articular cartilage (*). The basilar portion of the articular cartilage consists of an epiphyseal plate for the underlying epiphysis (*area in brackets*). A rich vasculature invades the basilar portion of the cartilage (*arrows*). No well defined radial bone or calcified bone is present (H≃E; original magnification ×100).

ferred to as the "skin" of cartilage), which contains several layers of flattened or oval cells whose long axes run parallel to the joint surface. Deep to the tangential zone lies the transitional zone, a much wider area that contains larger, rounded, randomly arranged cells. Below this region, slightly smaller, rounded cells (often in pairs) lie in short irregular columns; this zone is called the radial zone. Beneath the radial zone lies an area that contains few cells (often with pyknotic nuclei) arranged in short columns and surrounded by a calcified matrix; this is called the calcified zone. In material stained with both hematoxylin and eosin, a thin (about

5 mm), basophilic, irregular line separates the radial from the calcified zone. This structure has been designated by Collins as the "tide mark";[33] its significance and composition are still unknown. The calcified zone in turn rests on a dense layer of cortical bone called the bony or subchondral end plate.

Immature articular cartilage differs significantly from that of the adult in being more cellular and having a less distinct zonal pattern (Fig. 3-3). By the eighth embryonic week the developing joint contains cartilage that consists of two separate cell populations, several layers of elongated and tightly packed superficial cells and more loosely arranged, rounded, deeper cells. No radial zone, tide mark, calcified zone, or bony end plate is present. Autoradiographic techniques have demonstrated two zones of cellular proliferation, one immediately below the tangential zone, which presumably accounts for the growth of the articular cartilage, and a second zone in the basilar portion that acts as a microepiphyseal plate for endochondral ossification of the underlying epiphysis.[97,100,102,103,141] With termination of epiphyseal growth and the formation of a well-defined calcified zone and tide mark, mitotic activity ceases.[103,104] This suggests that cartilage is unable to compensate for cell death due to attrition or normal aging, and in fact studies in cattle[151,184] and rabbits[106] have demonstrated a decrease in cell count with aging. Studies of human cartilage indicate that during the period of rapid growth there is a decrease in the number of cells per fixed volume of cartilage. However, at maturity there is little decrease in the cell count despite advancing age.[125,171] It is conceivable that a very low level of mitotic activity is present in aging human articular cartilage because a significant decrease in the number of cells in the tangential zone and a corresponding increase in the number of cells in the transitional and radial zones have been reported.[171] Recent studies have demonstrated that laceration,[100,107] compression,[38,39] enzymatic[196] and arthritic[110,112] insults are capable of initiatin mitotic activity in mature cartilage.

In the past decade, the ultrastructure of cell in articular cartilage has been studied in ma and other species during growth,[41,160] maturation,[10,160,164] and aging,[10,124,131,155,161,164,188] with arthritis,[123,124,126,155,194] and under a variety of experimental conditions.[152,153,160,162] These studies have demonstrated considerable and consistent differences among cells of the various zones and have also shown that these cells are capable of rapid ultrastructural changes in response to environmental alterations. Although early histologic and metabolic studies of chondrocyte activity indicated that cells of the tangential zone were effete,[36,95] recent autoradiographic investigations[192] have shown them to be active in protein and glycoaminoglycan synthesis. Under the electron microscope these elongated cells appear similar in structure to fibrocytes[41,163,195] in that nuclei are elongated and irregular in shape and contain a dense nucleoplasm with chromatin clumping and an intact nuclear membrane. The groundplasm is moderately dense and contains short, dilated cisternae composed of rough endoplasmic reticulum,[135,195] a small Golgi apparatus (consisting of flattened, frequently empty vacuoles),[41,135,160,195] and dense, rounded mitochondria (Fig. 3-4). Large lipid droplets, glycogen deposits, and matrix-containing vacuoles are rare. The cell membrane contains numerous pinocytotic vesicles and forms short cytoplasmic processes on the deep surface.

The rounded cells of the transitional zone are metabolically the most active cells of articular cartilage; this activity is reflected by their ultrastructural appearance (Fig. 3-5).[10,41,123,135,154,161,164,195] They have a large, eccentric, finely granular nucleus that often contains one or more nucleoli and is bounded by well-defined internal and external nuclear membranes with regularly spaced nucleopores.[135] The groundplasm is of moderately low electron density. It contains aggregates of glycogen particles and a small number of intracytoplasmic filaments 7 nm to 10 nm in diameter.[195] Many oval mitochrondria are present, large lipid droplets may be found adjacent to them.[34] An extensive rough endoplasmic reticulum is present.[10,41,135,160,195] The rough surface endoplasmic reticulum, Golgi apparatus, and large secretory vacuoles con-

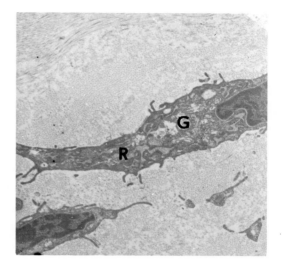

FIG. 3-4. Elongated cell in tangential zone of normal human articular cartilage. Bundles of collagen fibers are arranged at right angles to each other. The elongated cell contains a dense nuclear and cytoplasmic groundplasm. The Golgi apparatus consists of low density lamellae (G), and the rough endoplasmic reticulum (R) is sparse (original magnification × 5,000).

tain fibrillar material similar in electron density to that of the extracellular matrix.[135,195] The juxtanuclear Golgi apparatus is especially well developed and consists of closely packed agranular lamellae with small vesicles and with larger vacuoles (up to 2.5 μm in diameter).[41,131,160,161,195] Ultrastructural autoradiographic studies have shown that these vacuoles migrate from the region of the Golgi apparatus to the periphery of the cytoplasm, where they fuse with the cell membrane and finally rupture to discharge their contents outside the cell.[60] This process occurs all along the cell membrane and results in the formation of large invaginations, or *bays*, that give the cell a scalloped appearance.

In the deeper portions of the radial zone, cells that appear "normal" under the light microscope frequently contain increased numbers of intracytoplasmic filaments (whose function is unknown but is considered degenerative),[10,127,135,154,160,161,195] poorly developed rough endoplasmic reticulum, sparse Golgi apparatus, and small, dense mitochondria.[195]

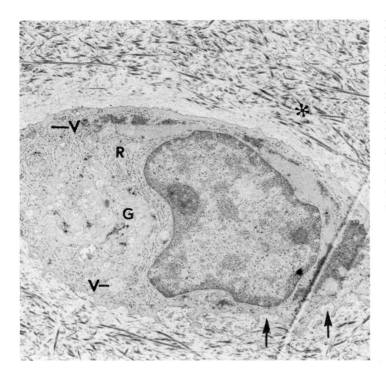

FIG. 3-5. Cell in transitional zone of normal human articular cartilage. The fibrous capsule consists of fibers arranged concentrically around the cell (*). Fine fibers are adjacent to the cell membrane. The cell is rounded, and numerous "bays" give it a scalloped appearance (*arrow*). An extensive rough endoplasmic reticulum (R), large Golgi apparatus (G), and many vacuoles (V) containing material similar in electron density to the extracellular matrix are present (original magnification × 10,000).

Metabolic studies of cells in the calcified portions of articular cartilage have revealed them to be either dead or in an inert phase because they do not take up cytidin³H, an indicator of RNA synthesis.[101]

THE MATRIX

The matrix of articular cartilage consists of a network of collagen fibers embedded in a gel-like ground substance composed of polyanionic proteoglycans (proteinpolysaccharides) and water. For a relatively hard tissue cartilage matrix has an unusually high water content—in the vicinity of 75% to 80%.[6,17,48,82,83,184] This high percentage is relatively unchanged during growth and aging,[15,17,83] but there is a marked increase in patients with osteoarthritis.[98] Although the pericellular areas appear to have an especially high water content,[19] unlike bone, the water of articular cartilage is not highly bound to matrix constituents and may be easily removed by drying or

mild heating.[98] It has been postulated that the ease with which water may be driven from and returned to cartilage explains in part not only the elasticity of cartilage but also the weeping phase of joint lubrication. The concentration of electrolytes in cartilage is the same as that in the extracellular fluid compartment with two exceptions, sodium and sulfate, both of which are elevated.[48,129] Sodium serves as the principal cation for the polyanionic matrix.[62,158] Sulfate concentration is elevated owing to the high content of sulfated glycoaminoglycans.[6,111,165] Small quantities of other organic materials have also been found in the matrix of articular cartilage. Neutral fats, phospholipids, cholesterol, triglycerides, and glycolipids have been seen in articular cartilage matrix with both the light and the electron microscope.[34,58,125,172,173] The concentration of these extracellular lipids increases with aging, possibly secondary to cellular degeneration.[124,172,173] The frequent proximity of these lipids to degenerating cells and membranous cell remnants supports this hypothesis. Sialic acid is also present in small amounts, probably bound to keratin sulfate.[4,67,181]

COLLAGEN

Collagen constitutes the major organic component of articular cartilage, accounting for more than 50% of the dry weight and 90% of the protein content of the tissue.[6,16,24,25,67,112,129,132] The stability of collagen in cartilage is remarkable. The proportion of collagen protein remains constant throughout life; it has a very slow turnover time; it is virtually insoluble in water or dilute acid; and less than 2% can be extracted by solutions of 5M guanidine hydrochloride.[132] To appreciate the contribution of collagen to this complex tissue some idea of its composition, structure, assembly, and properties must be understood (Fig. 3-6).

Collagen is a protein. Its constituent amino acids are assembled on the ribosomes of connective tissue cells to form a protocollagen molecule (Fig. 3-6),[37,139] approximately one-third of its amino acid residues being glycine and one-quarter being proline.[132] This protocollagen molecule has a molecular weight of approximately 100,000 and is arranged in the form of a flexible, left-handed helix. The amino acid composition of all protocollagen molecules is not identical, and these variations have been termed $\alpha 1$, $\alpha 2$, and $\alpha 3$ chains.[132] Enzymatic hydroxylation (a process that requires oxygen, ascorbic acid, ferrous ion, and α-ketoglutarate) of some of the proline and lysine residues results in the formation of hydroxyproline and hydroxylysine, amino acids that are not found to any appreciable extent in animal proteins other than collagen.[75,139] At about the time of hydroxylation two hexoses, glucose and galactose, are attached by an O-glycoside linkage to the hydroxyl group of hydroxylysine as the disaccharide glycosylgalactose.[21] Three protocollagen chains are then assembled intracellularly into a right-handed triple helix held together by easily soluble (salt) hydrogen bonds and forming a stiff macromolecule approximately

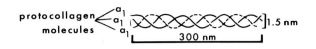

a) Tropocollagen (Triple-helix)

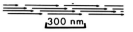

b) Collagen Fibril (Quarter-Stagger)

FIG. 3-6. Schematic representation of the structure of collagen. (Weiss C: Normal and osteoarthritic articular cartilage. Orthop Clin North Ma 10:175, 1979)

300 nm in length and 1.5 nm in diameter called tropocollagen (Fig. 3-6).[139] The intracellular site of hydroxylation, glycolization, tropocollagen assembly, and the mechanism of secretion into the extracellular matrix has not been completely defined, and considerable controversy exists about the role of the Golgi apparatus in tropocollagen synthesis and secretion.[37]

It is in the extracellular matrix that these salt-soluble tropocollagen molecules begin to assume less readily soluble forms resulting from cross linkages between adjacent $\alpha 1$ chains in the same tropocollagen molecule (these chain pairs are called β chains[59]), and from progressive cross linking between chains of adjacent tropocollagen molecules. Very stable cross linkages may result from aldol type condensations; however, it is probable that other cross-linking mechanisms exist as well.[170] The typical collagen fiber with 64-nm periodicity and sub-banding is assembled in the extracellular matrix at a distance from the cell by a linear arrangement of the tropocollagen molecules. These molecules line up in head-to-tail fashion to form long linear polymers. Adjacent polymers are "offset" by approximately 25% of their length, and it is this quarter stagger that produces the characteristic collagen periodicity (Fig. 3-6).[59]

The collagen of articular cartilage differs in

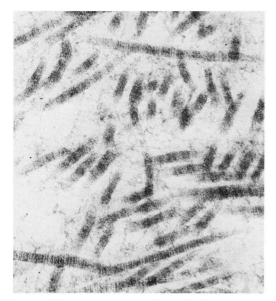

FIG. 3-7. Electronmicrograph of fibrillar matrix in transitional zone. Fibers 4 nm to 10 nm in diameter occupy the spaces between individual collagen fibers and frequently appear attached to adjacent collagen fibers, obscuring the periodicity.

a number of important ways from the collagen of skin and bone. Collagen fibers in articular cartilage do not stain with the usual anionic collagen stains, owing in part to competitive inhibition by the polyanionic matrix in which the fibers are embedded and in part to the specific composition of the collagen fibers. Miller and co-workers have demonstrated that two forms of the $\alpha 1$ protocollagen chain exist—$\alpha 1$ (type I), which is found in skin and bone, and $\alpha 1$ (type II), which accounts for more than 90% of the collagen extracted from cartilage.[130,131,132]

In addition to quantitative differences in several amino acids, the $\alpha 1$ (type II) chain differs from the $\alpha 1$ (type I) chain in that two-thirds of its lysine residues are hydroxylated (a fivefold increase) and it has an unusually high content of protein-bound hexose (containing 16 to 18 hexose residues per chain, or 3% by weight, compared to about 2 residues per chain, or 0.4% by weight, in the $\alpha 1$ (type I) chains.[130] Forty percent of the hydroxylysine

residues are substituted in this fashion. Since more than 90% of extracted collagen consists of $\alpha 1$ (type II) chains, the great majority of tropocollagen molecules in articular cartilage have the structure $\{\alpha 1 \text{ (type II)}\}$.[3] These molecules are less heat-stable than the molecules of skin and bone. It has been postulated that the hexose coat on the collagen molecule hinders the formation of intermolecular cross links, permits sliding required for cartilage elasticity, obscures the distinct periodicity and banding of the individual collagen fibers observed under the electron microscope (Fig. 3-7), repels anionic collagen dyes, and may, by interaction with the glycoaminoglycan side chains of the proteoglycan molecules, play a role in maintaining the structural integrity and properties of cartilage.[118,120,130]

THE FIBROUS ARCHITECTURE OF CARTILAGE

The arrangement of the collagen fibers in adult human articular cartilage has been extensively studied; however, the precise disposition of these fibers remains controversial. Benninghoff concluded that collagen fibers were arranged in arcades that were anchored in the calcified zone, ran vertically in the radial zone, turned obliquely in the transitional zone, and ran tangential or parallel to the articular surface in the superficial or tangential zone.[14] X-ray diffraction studies,[84] on the other hand, demonstrated that collagen fibers in the tangential zone ran tangential to the articular surface and in the deeper zones were arranged in a random fashion except in the calcified zone of old cartilage, where they were arranged perpendicular to the articular surface.

Recent transmission[195] and scanning[32] electron-microscopic-studies have further elucidated the fibrous architecture of cartilage (Figs. 3-1, 3-4, 3-5, 3-6, 3-8). The surface of adult human cartilage is covered by a layer of fine fibers 4 nm to 12 nm in diameter and several micra deep. This layer probably corresponds to the lamina splendens, consisting of either a hyaluronic acid or other protoglycan from the synovial fluid that is absorbed to the articular surface.

The tangential zone of normal young adult human articular cartilage (Figs. 3-1, 3-4, 3-8) consists of tightly packed bundles of collagen fibers (30 nm to 32 nm in diameter with 64 nm periodicity) arranged tangentially or parallel to the articular surface and at right angles to each other (Fig. 3-4).[128,195] Little ground substance separates the individual collagen fibers or fiber bundles. At the summit of the medial femoral condyle this zone is approximately 200 micra deep, and it reaches 600 micra in depth at the periphery of the joint. The tight bundle arrangement of collagen fibers is loosened in the transitional zone, and increased interfibrillar ground substance is present (Fig. 3-7). The individual fibers in this zone are 40 nm to 80 nm in diameter and appear to be randomly arranged (Figs. 13-4–13-8)[22,41,84,160,195] except at the periphery of the lacuna (the perilacunar rim), where they are packed closely together and run concentrically about the cells (Fig. 13-5).[22,41,84,160,195] The space between the perilacunar rim and the cell membrane is filled with fine fibers (4 nm to 10 nm in diameter), which lack typical collagen periodicity.[22,123,160,195] Fibers of similar appearance are found in the interfibrillar matrix and often appear attached to one or more collagen fibers, frequently obscuring their periodicity (Fig. 13-7). These fine fibers, by virtue of their location in areas of high metachromasia and in areas that stain with cationic dyes such as safranine O, are thought to be proteoglycan molecules. Collagen fibers of the deep and calcified zones are large in diameter, and in old cartilage they are frequently arranged perpendicular to the joint surfaces.[84,195]

With aging a number of changes occur in collagen fibers of human articular cartilage.[124,188] Fibers in all zones are increased in diameter, often appear fragmented, and often contain nuclei of calcification in the vicinity of degenerating cells. In the superficial zone, collagen fibers frequently lose their bundle arrangement but remain arranged tangentially to the articular surface. The lamina splendens

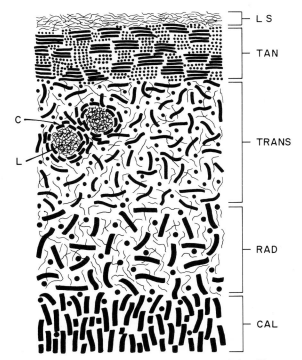

FIG. 3-8. Diagramatic representation of the fibrous architecture of normal, young, human articular cartilage. The lamina splendens (*LS*) is a layer of fine fibrils (4 nm to 10 nm in diameter) several microns thick that covers the articular surface. The tangential zone (*TAN*) consists of tightly packed bundles of collagen fibrils (30 nm to 32 nm in diameter) arranged parallel to the articular surface and often at right angles to each other. The transitional zone (*TRANS*) and radial zone (*RAD*) consist of randomly arranged collagen fibrils (40 nm to 100 nm in diameter) and significant amounts of proteoglycans. The predominant organization of collagen fibrils in the basilar portion of the radial zone is perpendicular to the joint surface. There is an increased concentration of fine fibers and filamentous fibrils (4 nm to 10 nm in diameter) in the lacunae (*L*) and in the interterritorial regions of the transitional and radial zones. Mature collagen fibrils (*C*) appear to encapsulate the lacunae. Collagen fibrils of the calcified zone (*CAL*) are usually more then 100 nm in diameter and are arranged perpendicular to the joint surface. (Lane JM, Weiss C: Review of articular cartilage collagen research. Arth Rheum 18:553, 1975)

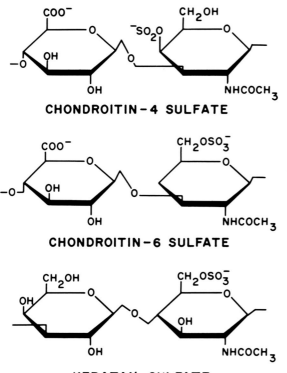

CHONDROITIN-4 SULFATE

CHONDROITIN-6 SULFATE

KERATAN SULFATE

FIG. 3-9. Outline of the chemical structure of the repeating dimeric units that comprise three of the glycoaminoglycans of articular cartilage. Chondroitin-4 sulfate consists of a glucuronic acid molecule linked by a 1-3 ester linkage to N-acetyl galactosamine with a sulfate at the C-4 position. Chondroitin-6 sulfate is similar in structure but with a sulfate at the C-6 position. Keratan sulfate consists of galactose linked by a 1-4 ester linkage to N-acetyl glucosamine with a sulfate at the C-6 position. These dimeric units are 10 Å in length, therefore the negative charges of the Chondroitin sulfates are 5 Å apart, and the negative charges of Keratan sulfate are 10 Å apart.

in older tissue is often replaced by an accumulation of amorphous debris.[188]

THE PROTEOGLYCANS

Proteoglycans are combinations of protein and carbohydrates that form large aggregates within the matrix of articular cartilage and ac-

count for almost 50% of the dry weight of cartilage.[6,12,17,23,25,27,48,62,69,112,118,129,149,165] These proteoglycan aggregates (PGA) may be several hundred million in molecular weight, are highly elastic, expand dramatically in solution, resist compression into a smaller volume, occupy large amounts of water, and form a complex gel entangled with collagen fibrils. These large aggregates are formed by the noncovalent association of proteoglycan subunits (PGS) with hyaluronic acid. The PGS consists of a protein core to which is attached numerous glycosaminoglycan side chains.[8,18,62,73,133,157,158]

Glycosaminoglycans are linear polymers composed of two different sugar residues that alternate regularly. One sugar residue is an amino sugar in which the number two carbon of glucose or galactose is replaced by an amino group that is acetylated.[5,145,159] The other sugar residue is usually glucuronic acid (Fig. 3-9). Four types of glycoaminoglycans have been found in articular cartilage—hyaluronic acid, chondroitin 4-sulfate, chondroitin 6-sulfate, and keratan sulfate. In hyaluronic acid, glucuronic acid alternates regularly with N-acetylglucosamine. This molecule contains negative charges spaced at 10Å intervals. The chondroitin sulfates (Fig. 3-9) are composed of regularly alternating units of N-acetylgalactosamine and glucuronic acid, have a molecular weight of 450 to 500, and are approximately 10Å in length.[17,18,25,62,133,136,149,157,158] The galactosamine carries a sulfate group on the fourth or sixth carbon; thus there are two anionic charges (sulfate and carboxylate groups) spaced at 5Å intervals. Approximately 50 to 70 periods or dimeric units are contained in each chain of chondroitin sulfate. Keratan sulfate (Fig. 3-9) is a smaller molecule composed of 15 to 30 dimeric units and consisting of galactose and N-acetylglucosamine. An ester sulfate is carried on the number six carbon of N-acetylglucosamine. Negative charges are thus spaced at 10Å intervals. The repelling forces of these closely spaced, negatively charged groups cause the glycoaminoglycan chains to assume an extended configuration

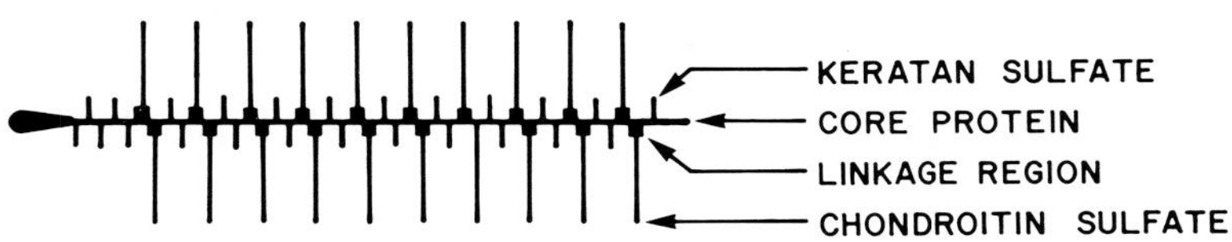

FIG. 3-10. Schematic representation of the proteoglycan subunit. The protein core is about 300 nm in length, 1.5 nm in diameter, and 50 to 100 glycoaminoglycan chains are covalently linked to it. The protein core has three regions: a globular region, a keratan sulfate rich region, and the remainder of the protein core to which chondroitin sulfate and keratan sulfate is attached. (Burleigh PMC, Poole AR [ed.]: Dynamics of Connective Tissue Macromolecules. Amsterdam, North Holland Publishing Co., 1975)

PROTEOGLYCAN SUBUNIT

KERATAN SULFATE
CORE PROTEIN
LINKAGE REGION
CHONDROITIN SULFATE

and to stick out stiffly from the protein core, thus resisting compression into a smaller volume.

In immature cartilage, there is 1:1 ratio of chondroitin 4-sulfate to chondroitin 6-sulfate and almost no keratan sulfate. With aging there is a progressive increase in the amount of chondroitin 6-sulfate, a decrease in chondroitin 4-sulfate, and a marked increase in the amount of keratan sulfate.[62,133,157,159] By middle age, the concentrations of keratan sulfate and chondroitin 6-sulfate are about equal and account for about 90% of the total glycoaminoglycan content of articular cartilage.[12,18,77,85,86,121,174,175]

The concentration and disposition of these polyanions in articular cartilage may be demonstrated by the use of cationic dyes such as toluidine blue, Alican blue, and safranine O, which bind one molecule of dye to each negatively charged group of the glycoaminoglycan. Some of these dyes, such as Alcian blue and toluidine blue, change their absorption spectra maximum in response to their lining up and binding to the glycoaminoglycans.[62,73,140,158,169,176] These are known as metachromatic stains. Other stains such as safranine O bind only to tissue polyanions in a 1:1 ratio and therefore can be used as a quantitative measure of the amount and disposition of glycoaminoglycan in articular cartilage.[146] These studies have confirmed the paucity of glycoaminoglycans in the tangential zone, the

high concentration of chondroitin sulfate in the lacunar space and in the territorial regions surrounding chondrocytes, and the increased amount of keratan sulfate found at greater distances from the cells (the interterritorial regions) and in the lower portions of the radial zone.

The glycoaminoglycans are covalently bound to the protein core of the PGS by attachment to serine and threonine at specialized linkage regions. The PGS, as seen in Figure 3-10, contains three regions—(1) a globular region, 60,000 to 70,000 in molecular weight, rich in aspartic acid, cysteine, and methionine and devoid of glycoaminoglycans for attachment to the hyaluronic acid backbone of the PGA, (2) a keratan sulfate-rich region, and (3) the remainder of the unit, which consists of the protein core to which is attached both chondroitin sulfate and keratan sulfate chains. PGSs are polydisperse, that is, they vary in size and composition.[63,65,66,67,68,147,148] Small molecules consist mainly of the globular and keratan sulfate-rich regions with small amounts of chondroitin sulfate, whereas the larger subunits contain considerably more chondroitin sulfate linkages. The average PGS from articular cartilage has a protein core about 200,000 in molecular weight and 300 nm long. Attached to this protein core are about 100 chondroitin sulfate side chains, each 20,000 to 30,000 in molecular weight and 50 to 60 nm long, and 100 keratan sulfate chains 5,000 to 10,000 in molecular weight and 10 to 20 nm long. The PGS molecule is about 3 million in molecular weight.

Within the matrix of articular cartilage, most of the proteoglycan exists in the form of the aggregate (PGA). The backbone of the aggregate consists of hyaluronic acid with

PROTEOGLYCAN AGGREGATE

FIG. 3-11. Schematic representation of proteoglycan aggregate. (Burleigh PMC, Poole AR [ed.]: Dynamics of Connective Tissue Macromolecules. Amsterdam, North Holland Publishing Co., 1975)

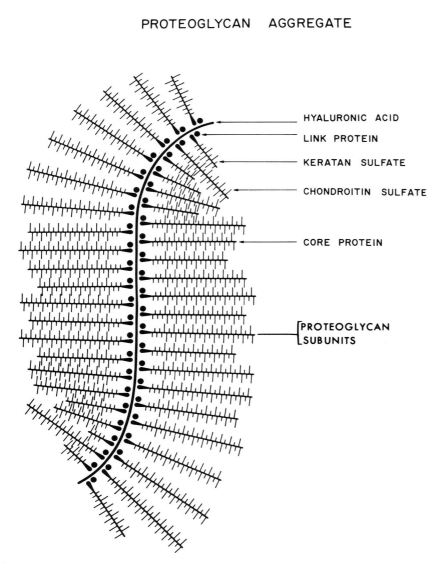

HYALURONIC ACID

LINK PROTEIN

KERATAN SULFATE

CHONDROITIN SULFATE

CORE PROTEIN

PROTEOGLYCAN
SUBUNITS

which many PGSs are noncovalently associated.[63,65,66,67,68,147,148] A low molecular weight protein (link protein) appears to stabilize or strengthen the bond between the PGS and the hyaluronic acid. The typical PGA consists of over 100 PGS molecules (each 2,000,000 to 3,000,000 in molecular weight) bound with link protein to a hyaluronic chain over 4000 nm long, and therefore has an aggregate molecular weight of over 200 million (Fig. 3-11). The repelling force of the thousands of negative charges causes the aggregate to occupy an enormous volume of solution. In articular cartilage the volume occupied by the PGA is constrained by the collagen fibril network. When articular cartilage is subjected to a compressive force, the aggregates are compressed into a smaller volume, and water is released from the cartilage. When the compressive force is removed, water returns into the cartilage, and the volume of the aggregate is restored.

THE METABOLISM OF CARTILAGE

The absence of a vascular supply and the preponderance of extracellular matrix suggests that cartilage is relatively stable and metabolically inert; however, its respiratory rate and energy production on a per-cell basis is quite high.[43,151] Although aerobic, anaerobic, and hexose monophosphate shunts have been demonstrated in cartilage, the tolerance of chondrocytes to potassium cyanide and to oxygen deprivation coupled with their sensitivity to monoiodoacetate, as well as the presence of high lactate concentrations, suggests that the anerobic pathway is used preferentially.[76,90,113]

The synthesis of the protein core of the proteoglycan molecule is similar to the synthesis of the protocollagen molecule described above; however, the synthesis, sulfation, and polymerization of the glycoaminoglycan molecule are a bit more complex and require a number of enzymes including nucleoside diphosphokinase, uridine diphosphate (UDP)-glucose phosphorylase, UDP-glucose dehydrogenase, and a number of transferases and isomerases.[178] In very brief outline, glucose 1-phosphate and N-acetylglucosamine 1-phosphate are converted by uridine triphosphate (UTP) to UDP-glucuronic acid and to UDP-N-acetylglucosamine. These are then united by an ether link to form chondroitin.[47,138,167,185] These steps are probably carried out on or near the ribosome. The addition of sulfate to the glycoaminoglycan unit is rapid,[40] occurs in the region of the Golgi apparatus,[60] and involves the addition of adenosine triphosphate (ATP) to the sulfate to form 3-phosphoadenosine-5-phosphosulfate or *active sulfate*, a high-energy molecule from which sulfate can be added to the C-4 or C-6 position of the N-acetylgalactosamine.[40,137] There is evidence to suggest that the entire glycoaminoglycan molecule is synthesized almost simultaneously by the cell.[1,98,104]

Qualitative and quantitative radioactive tracer techniques (*i.e.*, autoradiography and scintillation counting) using H^3- or C^{14}-labeled amino acids, hexoses, or $S^{35}O_4$ have been utilized to determine the rate and distribution of matrix synthesis and degradation. Studies on the rate of incorporation of glycine-H^3 and $S^{35}O_4$ have shown that glycoaminoglycan synthesis is rapid and linear with time;[113] that it is most rapid in immature animals; that after an initial decline it remains constant despite aging;[106,107] that cortisol,[108,109] antimetabolites,[98] and nitrogen mustard[98] decrease matrix synthesis; and that synthesis is increased following lacerative injury[107] and in certain phases of osteoarthritis.[15,36,110,112] The same isotopic techniques have been used to study matrix degradation and have shown that, although collagen is relatively stable, a large proportion of the proteoglycans are quite labile.[111] More than 23% of the proteoglycans in adult cartilage behave like a "fast fraction," with a half-life of approximately 8 days.[111] This rate of degradation would appear to be far in excess of that necessary to compensate for normal attrition and suggests that this rapid synthetic and degradative activity is part of an extremely active enzyme-dependent internal remodeling system.[104,111]

Several enzymes are capable of breaking down the proteoglycan molecule, including papain,[52,179,180] hyaluronidase,[15,133,158] and a number of intracellular enzymes.[44,51,52,88,179,180] Ali,[2,3] Woessner,[197] and others[28,47,53,61,78,88,164,196] have found a family of lysosomal acid proteases (cathepsin D) that can act to degrade cartilage matrix, and recent studies by Woessner[198] have defined in cartilage a cathepsin D capable of degrading proteoglycans at a neutral pH. This enzyme may be active in osteoarthritis as well as in normal cartilage remodeling.

NUTRITION IN CARTILAGE

Articular cartilage is avascular except embryonically and for a short time postnatally, when vascularized canals extend from the metaphysis and periosteum into the epiphysis and basilar portions of the articular cartilage.[81,89] The source and mechanism by which nutrients reach chondrocytes has fascinated investigators for centuries, beginning with the microscopic and injection studies of Hunter in 1743.[71] During the 19th century, cartilage was thought to be nourished primarily by diffusion from the underlying vasculature,[182] although several authors felt that synovial fluid also played a role.[80,143] More than 50 years ago, Strangeways[177] suggested that nutrition was principally derived by diffusion from the synovial fluid. More recent studies have either supported this view[20,33,117] or suggested that both synovial fluid and the subchondral vasculature provide nutrition to the articular cartilage.[49,72,96] Radioactive tracer studies have confirmed the opinion that in the immature animal with open epiphyseal plates, a significant portion of the articular cartilage derives its nutritional support from the underlying vasculature of the epiphysis. However, with maturation, which is associated with closure of the epiphyseal plate, formation of the subchondral bony end plate, and establishment of the calcified zone and tide mark, almost all the nutrition is derived by diffusion from the synovial fluid.[70]

Early studies revealed that cartilage is completely permeable to cationic dyes, less permeable to neutral, and only slightly permeable to anionic, dyes.[20,74] There are, however, a number of physical and chemical factors that influence the type, size, and rate of diffusion of various substances into this tissue. Maroudas has developed the concept that the articular surface acts as a membrane (with a pore size of 62A as determined by McCutchen[93]) and that Donnan equilibrium and ion exchange theories are applicable in articular cartilage.[114–118] The fixed charge density of the matrix (due to the polyanionic glycoaminoglycans) controls in large measure the diffusion characteristics of cartilage; as the fixed charge density increases with increasing depth of the cartilage, the permeability to fluid flow decreases.[114] The diffusion coefficients for NaCl, K, and SO, have been shown to be approximately 40% of their value in aqueous solution and that for glucose about 30%.[115] Toward smaller molecules the water in cartilage appears to behave like solvent water, but

with large molecules some water becomes inaccessible owing to steric exclusion effects exerted by the proteoglycan molecules. Therefore, the distribution of small molecules such as glucose is only slightly affected, but as the weight of the solute increases, the distribution and diffusion coefficients decrease significantly.[115] Hemoglobin is the largest molecule capable of penetrating cartilage. Solute agitation (joint movement) appears to increase the rate of diffusion of a number of small molecules.[117] Although most investigators have felt that no active cellular transport system exists in articular cartilage (and this view is not unreasonable in view of the high matrix-to-cell ratio), recent studies have demonstrated that the diffusion of nutrients (amino acids, sugars, and sulfate) into articular cartilage is extremely rapid (within seconds) and depends in part upon the presence of viable cells.[193]

To summarize, then, the articular surface acts as a membrane with a pore size of 62A, and the diffusion of molecules into articular cartilage depends upon agitation, molecular size, steric configuration, and the charge of the solute as well as on the pore size tortuosity, fixed charge density, and (possibly) cellular composition of the cartilage matrix.

OSTEOARTHRITIS

The etiology and pathophysiology of osteoarthritis have been the subject of much scientific investigation during the past two centuries.[168] One of the problems inherent in studying this disease is its focal nature. Disease in a single joint may involve the entire histologic and chemical spectrum from normal to far advanced; furthermore, areas of cartilage separated by no more that 100 micra may differ markedly in physical properties, histologic appearance, and metabolic activity (Fig. 3-12). During the 19th and early 20th centuries histologic studies established the anatomic pattern of disease,[13,33,64,168] and recent technological advances have enabled scientists to correlate the anatomic, metabolic,

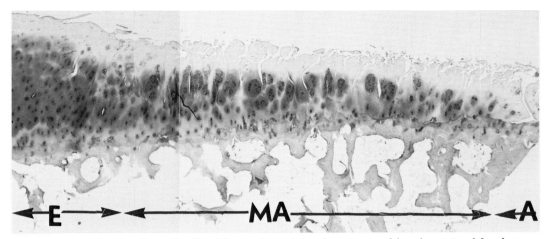

FIG. 3-12. Section from the distal femoral condyle of a 34-year-old male, stained for the presence of mucopolysaccharide with safranin O (*dark stain*) and counterstained with fast green (*light stain*), demonstrating areas of early (*E*), moderately advanced (*NA*), and advanced (*A*) osteoarthritic changes in close juxtaposition. Early osteoarthritis shows superficial fibrillation, slight hypercellularity, and loss of proteoglycan confined to the upper middle or transitional zone. Moderately advanced changes include clefts extending deep into the middle zone and increased numbers of cells in clusters or "clones." Some clones in the superficial and upper middle zones are devoid of proteoglycan halo, whereas those in the middle zone show intense safranin O staining. The loss of proteoglycan extends into the middle zone. Areas of advanced disease contain clefts that extend through the entire thickness of the articular cartilage; the tissue is hypocellular and almost completely devoid of proteoglycan, with safranin O confined to some pericellular areas. The subchondral bone trabeculae are progressively thickened as the cartilage height is diminished. (Weiss C: Fed Proc 32:1459, 1973)

and chemical alterations that occur in osteoarthritic cartilage.[110] Mankin has devised a histologic–histochemical grading system for the osteoarthritic lesion that correlates very closely with the metabolic and chemical analysis of this tissue.[110] For purposes of this discussion we will divide the cartilage changes in osteoarthritis into early, moderately advanced, and advanced stages (Fig. 3-12).[194] The first two stages are characterized by anabolic and catabolic cell function and will be considered together. Advanced disease consists primarily in catabolic cellular function and will be discussed separately.

The changes in early osteoarthritis consist of fibrillation of the articular surface, which extends into but not through the tangential zone, a slight increase of the number of cells per unit volume of tissue, and loss of glyco-aminoglycans (or alteration of the proteoglycan molecule) confined to the transitional zone. Moderately advanced lesions are characterized by a decrease in the overall cartilage height clefts, which extend into the transitional and upper portions of the radial zone, and increased numbers of cells in the form of cell cluster, or *clones*, in the transitional and radial zones. Many clones in the superficial region of the cartilage are devoid of a proteoglycan halo, whereas those in the basilar portion of the transitional zone are surrounded by intense proteoglycan halos. The loss of proteoglycans extends through the transitional zone and into the radial zone.

In early lesions ultrastructural observations of the matrix show minute surface irregularities, loss of lamina splendens, and a decrease in interfibrillar matrix that is most evident

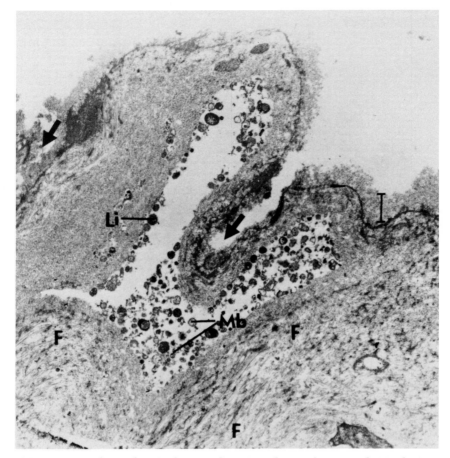

FIG. 3-13. Surface of articular cartilage in advanced osteoarthritic lesion. The surface is thrown into deep folds or clefts. Amorphous debris (*I*) coats the articular surface. Collagen fibrils of small diameter (*F*) are arranged parallel to the surface of the clefts (*arrows*). Lipid (*Li*) and membranous remnants (*Mb*) of a degenerated chondrocyte are present (Weiss C: Fed Proc 32:1459, 1973)

in the transitional zone. With progression to moderately advanced lesions, clefts take the form of progressively deepening infoldings (Fig. 3-13) of the articular surface.[194] Collagen fibers of small diameter are arranged perpendicularly to the joint surface.[84,194] It is probable that the compressive force of weight bearing and the shearing force of movement *in vivo* tend to flatten these clefts, resulting in a functional realignment in which fibers are arranged parallel or tangential to the "true" articular surface.[194] Individual collagen fibers

in moderately advanced lesions appear smaller than those found in age-matched controls.[194] This may indicate either that collagen fibers break down secondary to enzymatic degradation[2,3,28,47,78,197] or that synthesis of new fibers has occurred.[194] In view of recent metabolic studies, the latter explanation seems most plausible.[110,112]

Electron-microscopic studies of early to moderately advanced osteoarthritic cartilage show striking cellular changes.[194] An increase in the number of degenerating cells is found

FIG. 3-14. Cells in the tangential zone of moderately advanced osteoarthritic cartilage. The cells are more rounded than those of normal articular cartilage, and contain a dense groundplasm and well-developed rough endoplasmic reticulum (R), large Golgi apparatus (G), and many vacuoles (V) filled with electron-dense material (original magnification ×6,500).

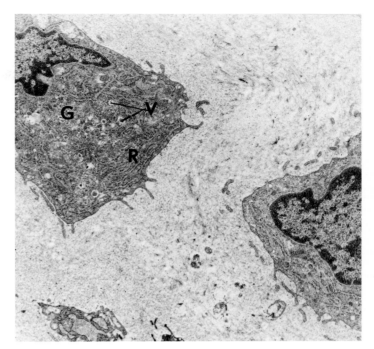

in the superficial and deep zones. These cells are characterized by increased intracellular filaments and a corresponding decrease in other intracellular organelles as well as by dead cells devoid of a nuclear or cell membrane and consisting of aggregates of phospholipid membrane remnants.[124,155,182,194] In the superficial zone viable cells undergo hypertrophy, are surrounded by collagen fibers of small diameter, and appear similar to fibroblasts (Fig. 3-14).[156,182,194] Clones of cells in the deeper zones consist of viable hypertrophied cells that contain well-developed rough endoplasmic reticulum, Golgi apparatus, mitochondria, and numerous secretory vacuoles.[194] These clones are surrounded by halos of fibrillar matrix, probably proteoglycans (Fig. 3-15). Centrioles, possibly indicative of cell division, are present.[194] Cells in various stages of degeneration are commonly found within or adjacent to these clusters (see Fig. 3-15).[194]

Metabolic and biochemical studies have confirmed these histologic, histochemical, and ultrastructural impressions. Despite in-

creased numbers of dead cells in early and moderately advanced osteoarthritis lesions,[194] there is an increase in the number of cells per unit volume of tissue.[97,104,110,112] These lesions are characterized by a progressive increase in thymidine-^{3}H incorporation, which is an indicator of mitotic activity.[110,111] Metabolic activity of the tissue is also increased.[35,36,122,125] Although there is a progressive decrease in hexosamine with increased severity of the disease, there is also a considerable increase in hexosamine synthesis on a per-cell basis, indicating that although the individual cells are producing increased amounts of matrix, it is insufficient to compensate for the progressive degradation of matrix components that occurs with advancing disease.[110] The matrix synthesized by the "blastic"-appearing cells in the osteoarthritic lesion differs from that of normal adult cartilage by having a high content of chondroitin 4-sulfate.[112] Chondroitin 4-sulfate is normally found in large quantities only in immature cartilage. The fact that these cells are again able to divide and to synthesize a more "immature" matrix may indicate that in

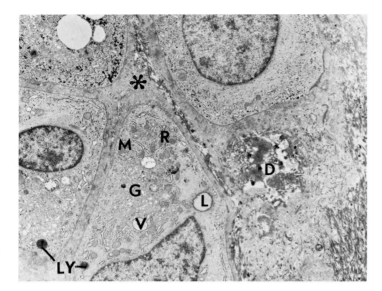

FIG. 3-15. Chondrocyte clone in moderately advanced osteoarthritic lesion. Collagen fibers run perpendicular to the articular surface and have a low interfiber density compared to the pericellular halo (*). Degenerating cells are present within this clone (D). Chondrocytes have well-developed rough endoplasmic reticulum (R), extensive Golgi apparatus (G), numerous vacuoles (V), and mitochondria (M). Large lipid droplets (L) and lysosome-like structures (LY) are also present (original magnification ×6,500).

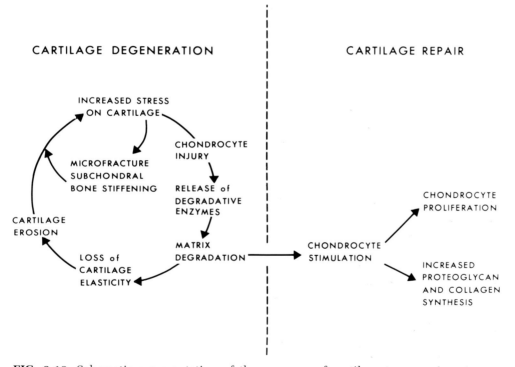

FIG. 3-16. Schematic representation of the response of cartilage to excessive stress. (Weiss C: Normal and osteoarthritic articular cartilage. Ortho Clin North Am 10:175, 1979)

the early and moderately advanced stages of this disease, chondrocytes are stimulated to dedifferentiate in an attempt to reconstitute the altered cartilage.

In the advanced osteoarthritic lesion cartilage height is markedly decreased, clefts extend to subchondral bone, there is a marked depletion of proteoglycans, the tissue is hypocellular, and the tide mark is disrupted (see Fig. 3-12). Ultrastructural studies show a marked decrease in interfibrillar matrix, an increased number of microscars, and extracellular lipids.[194] The cells are often in advanced stages of degeneration.[194] Metabolic studies show a progressive decrease in DNA and hexosamine synthesis and a pronounced decrease in total hexosamine content.[15,16,29,110,112,168] There is a progressive increase in acid hydrolase activity in the advanced stages of the disease.[47,78] The subchondral bony plate increases in thickness.

In summary (Fig. 3-16), increased stress on articular cartilage (physical, chemical, or metabolic) sufficient to injure chondrocytes results in the release of enzymes that degrade the cartilage matrix. The loss of cartilage matrix (proteoglycans and collagen) stimulates both reparative and degenerative reactions. Chondrocytes replicate and increase proteoglycan and collagen synthesis as well as release increased amounts of degradative enzymes. The net result is that the reparative response is inadequate to compensate for the loss of proteoglycan and collagen, thus diminishing the resilient properties of the cartilage. Increased stress is transmitted to the subchondral bony plate, resulting in microfracture, increased trabecular thickness, and stiffness, which in turn result in more force being transmitted back to the overlying articular cartilage. This increased force causes disruption of the articular surface, additional cartilage injury, and cell death. This cycle suggests that treatment aimed at enhancing the reparative response and inhibiting the degenerative processes, both physical and chemical, may be capable of halting and even reversing the arthritic process.

REFERENCES

1. **Adamson L, Gleason S, Anast C:** Sulfate incorporation by embryonic chick bone. Biochem Biophys Acta 83:262, 1964
2. **Ali SY:** The presence of cathepsin-B in cartilage. Biochem J 102:10c, 1967
3. **Ali SY, Evans L, Stainthorpe E et al:** Characterization of cathepsins in cartilage. Biochem J 105:549, 1967
4. **Anderson AJ:** Some studies on the occurrence of sialic acid in human cartilage. Biochem J 78:399, 1961
5. **Anderson B, Hoffman P, Meyer K:** The O-serine linkage in peptides of chondriotin-4 or -6 sulfate. J Biol Chem 240:156, 1965
6. **Anderson CE, Ludowieg J, Harper H et al:** The composition of the organic component of human articular cartilage. J Bone Joint Surg 46A:1176, 1964
7. **Balazs EA, Bloom GD, Swann DA:** Fine structure and Glycosaminoglycan content of the surface layer of articular cartilage. Fed Proc 25:1813, 1966
8. **Barland P, Janis R, Sandson J:** Immunofluorescent studies of human articular cartilage. Ann Rheum Dis 25:156, 1966
9. **Barnett CH, Cobbold AF:** Lubrication within living joints. J Bone Joint Surg 44B:662, 1962
10. **Barnett CH, Cochrane W, Palfrey AJ:** Age changes in articular cartilage of rabbits. Ann Rheum Dis: 22:389, 1963
11. **Barnett CH, Davies DV, MacConnaill MA:** Synovial Joints, Their Structure and Mechanics. Springfield, Charles C Thomas, 1961
12. **Benmaman JD, Ludowieg J, Anderson CE:** Glucosamine and galactosamine in human articular cartilage: Relationship to age and degenerative joint disease. Clin Biochem 2:461, 1969
13. **Bennett GA, Waine H, Bauer W:** Changes in the Knee Joint at Various Ages. With Particular Reference to the Nature and Development of Degenerative Joint Disease. New York, The Commonwealth Fund, 1942
14. **Benninghoff A:** Form and Bau der Gelenk-Knorpel in ihren Beziehungen zur Funktion. S Anat Entwicklungsgesch 76:43, 1925
15. **Bollet AJ:** Connective tissue polysaccharide metabolism and the pathogenesis of arthritis. Adv Intern Med 13:33, 1967
16. **Bollet AJ, Handy JR, Sturgill BC:** Chondroitin sulfate concentration and protein polysaccharide composition of articular cartilage in osteoarthritis. J Clin Invest 42:853, 1963
17. **Bollet AJ, Nance JL:** Biochemical findings in normal and osteoarthritis articular cartilage. II. Chondroitin sulfate concentration and chain length, water and ash content. J Clin Invest 45:1170, 1966
18. **Brandt KD, Muir H:** Characterization of protein-

polysaccharides of articular cartilage from mature
and immature pigs. Biochem J 114:871, 1969

19. **Brower TD:** The localization of chloride in hyaline
cartilage by histochemical techniques. J Bone Joint
Surg 38A:655, 1956
20. **Brower TD, Akohoshi Y, Orlie P:** The diffusion of
dyes through articular cartilage in vivo. J Bone Joint
Surg 44A:456, 1962
21. **Butler WT, Cunningham LW:** Evidence for the linkage of a disaccharide to hydroxylysine in tropocollagen. J Biol Chem 241:3382, 1966
22. **Cameron DA, Robinson RA:** Electromicroscopy of
epiphyseal and articular cartilage matrix in the
femur of the newborn infant. J Bone Joint Surg
40A:163, 1958
23. **Campo RD, Dziewiatkowski DD:** Introcellular
synthese of protein polysaccharides by slices of bovine costal cartilage. J Biol Chem 237:2729, 1962
24. **Campo RD, Tourtelotte CD:** The composition of bovine cartilage and bone. Biochem Biophys Acta
141:614, 1967
25. **Campo RD, Tourtelotte CD, Brelin RJ:** The protein–
polysaccharides of articulars, epiphyseal plate and
costal cartilages. Biochem Biophys Acta 177:501,
1969
26. **Charnley J:** The lubrication of animal joints in relation to surgical reconstruction by arthroplasty. Ann
Rheum Dis 19:10, 1960
27. **Chrisman OD:** The ground substance of connective
tissue. Clin Orthop 36:184, 1964
28. **Chrisman OD, Semonsky C, Bensch KG:** Cathepsins
in articular cartilage. In Workshop on the Healing of
Osseous Tissue, Washington N.A.S.–N.R.C., 1967
29. **Chrisman OD:** Biochemical aspects of degenerative
joint disease. Clin Orthop 64:77, 1969
30. **Clark IC:** Surface characteristics of human articular
cartilage—A scanning electron microscope study. J
Anat (London) 108:23, 1971
31. **Clark IC:** Human articular cartilage surface contours
and related surface depression frequency studies.
Ann Rheum Dis 30:15, 1971
32. **Clark IC:** Articular cartilage: A review and scanning
electron microscope study. J Bone Joint Surg 58:732,
1971
33. **Collins DH:** The Pathology of Articular and Spinal
Disease. London, E. Arnold and Co, 1949
34. **Collins DH, Chadially FN, Meachim G:** Introcellular
lipids of cartilage. Ann Rheum Dis 24:123, 1965
35. **Collins DH, McElligott TF:** Sulphate ($^{35}SO_4$) uptake
by chondrocytes in relation to histological changes
in osteoarthritis human articular cartilage. Ann
Rheum Dis 19:318, 1960
36. **Collins DH, Meachim G:** Sulphate ($^{35}SO_4$) fixation by
human articular cartilage compared in the knee and
shoulder joints. Ann Rheum Dis 20:117, 1961
37. **Cooper GW, Prockop DJ:** Introcellular accumulation
of protocollagen and extrusion of collagen by embryonic cartilage cells. J Cell Biol 38:523, 1968

38. **Crelin ES, Southwick WO:** Mitosis of chondrocytes
induced in the knee joint articular cartilage of adult
rabbits. Yale J Biol Med 33:243, 1960
39. **Crelin ES, Southwick WO:** Changes induced by sustained pressure in the knee joint articular cartilage
of adult rabbits. Anat Rec 149:113, 1964
40. **D'Abramo F, Lipmann F:** The formation of adenosine 3′ phosphate-5′ phosphosulfate in extracts of
chick embryo cartilage and its conversion into chondroitin sulfate. Biochem Biophys Acta 25:211, 1957
41. **Davies DV, Barnett CH, Cochran W et al:** Electron
microscopy of articular cartilage in the young adult
rabbit. Ann Rheum Dis 21:11, 1962
42. **Dawson D, Wright V, Lozfield MD:** Human joint lubrication. Biomed Eng 160, 1969
43. **Dickens F, Weil-Malherbe H:** Metabolism of cartilage. Nature 138:30, 1936
44. **Dingle JT:** Studies on the mode of action of excess
vitamin A 3. Release of a bound protease by the action of vitamin A. Biochem J 79:509, 1961
45. **Dintenfass L:** Lubrication in synovial joints: A theoretical analysis. J Bone Joint Surg 45A:1241, 1963
46. **Dorfman A:** Metabolism of Acid Mucopolysaccharides. In Connective Tissue: Intercellular Macromolecules. Boston, Little, Brown & Co, 1964
47. **Ehrlich MG, Mankin HJ, Treadwell BV:** Acid hydrolases in osteoarthritic and normal cartilage. J
Bone Joint Surg 55A:1068, 1973
48. **Eichelberger L, Akeson WH, Roma M:** Biochemical
studies or articular cartilage. I. Normal values. J
Bone Joint Surg 40A:142, 1958
49. **Ekholm R:** Articular cartilage nutrition. Acta Anat
11:1, 1951
50. **Elmore SM, Sokoloff L, Norris G et al:** The nature of
"imperfect" elasticity of articular cartilage. J Appl
Physiol 18:393, 1963
51. **Fell HB, Dingle JT:** Studies on the mode and action
of excess of vitamin A: G. lysosomal proteases and
the degradation of cartilage matrix. Arthritis Rheum
7:398, 1964
52. **Fell HB, Thomas L:** Comparison of the effects of papain and vitamin A on cartilage. J Exp Med 111:719,
1960
53. **Fessel JM, Chrisman DD:** Enzymatic degradation of
chondromucoprotein by cell free extracts of human
cartilage. Arthritis Rheum 7:398, 1964
54. **Gardner DL:** The influence of microscopic technology on knowledge of cartilage surface structure.
Ann Rheum Dis 31:235, 1972
55. **Gardner DL, McGillivray DC:** Living cartilage is not
smooth. Ann Rheum Dis 30:3, 1971
56. **Gardner DL, McGillivray DC:** Surface structure of
articular cartilage: Historical review. Ann Rheum
Dis 30:10, 1971
57. **Gardner DL, Woodward D:** Scanning electron microscopy and replica studies of articular surfaces of
guinea pig synovial joints. Ann Rheum Dis 28:379,
1969

58. **Ghadially FN, Meachim G, Collins DH:** Extracellular lipid in the matrix of human articular cartilage. Ann Rheum Dis 24:136, 1965

59. **Glimcher MJ, Krane SM:** The organization and structure of bone, and the mechanism of calcification. In Gould BS (ed): Treatise on Collagen, Vol II. New York, Academic Press, 1968

60. **Godman GC, Lane N:** On the site of sulfation in the chondrocyte. J Cell Biol 21:353, 1964

61. **Gregory JD, Laurent TC, Roden L:** Enzymatic degradation of chondromucoprotein. J Biol Chem 239:3312, 1964

62. **Hamerman D, Rosenberg LC, Schubert M:** Diarthrodial joints revised. J Bone Joint Surg 52A:725, 1970

63. **Hardingham TE, Muri H:** Hyaluronic acid in cartilage and proteoglycan aggregation. Biochem J 139:565−581, 1974

64. **Harrison MHM, Schajowicz F, Trueta J:** Osteoarthritis of the hip: A study of the nature and evolution of the disease. J Bone Joint Surg 35B:598, 1953

65. **Hascall VC, Heinegard D:** Aggregation of cartilage proteoglycans I. The role of hyaluronic acid. J Biol Chem 249:4232−4241, 1974

66. **Hascall VC, Heinegard D:** Aggregation of cartilage proteoglycans II. Oligosaccharide competitors of the proteoglycan hyaluronic acid interaction. J Biol Chem 249:4242−4249, 1974

67. **Hascall VC, Sajdera SW:** Protein−polysaccharide from bovine nasal cartilage: The function of glycoprotein in the formation of aggregates. J Biol Chem 224:2384, 1969

68. **Heinegard D, Hascall VC:** Aggregation of cartilage proteoglycans III. Characteristics of the proteins isolated from trypsin digests of aggregates. J Biol Chem 249:4250−4256, 1974

69. **Herring GM:** The chemical structure of tendon, cartilage, dentin and bone matrix. Clin Orthop 60:261, 1968

70. **Honner R, Thompson RC:** The nutritional pathways of articular cartilage. J Bone Joint Surg 53A:742, 1971

71. **Hunter W:** On the structure and diseases of articulating cartilage. Philos Trans R Soc London 42:514, 1743

72. **Inglemark BE, Saaf J:** Ueber die Ernahrung des Gelenkknorpels und die Bildung der Gelenkflussigkeit unter verschiedenen funktionellen Verhaltnissen. Acta Orthop Scand 17:303, 1948

73. **Jeanloz R:** The nomenclature of mucopolysaccharides. Arthritis Rheum 3:233, 1960

74. **Kantor TG, Schubert M:** The difference in permeability of cartilage to cationic and anionic dyes. J Histochem Cytochem 5:28, 1957

75. **Kiurikko KI, Prockop DJ:** Purification and partial characterization of the enzyme for the hydroxylation of proline in protocollagen. Arch Biochem Biophys 118:611, 1967

76. **Krane S, Parson V, Kunin AS:** Studies of the metabolism of epiphyseal cartilage. In Bassett CAL (ed): Cartilage Degradation and Repair. Washington, N.A.S.−N.R.C., 1967

77. **Kuhn R, Leppelmann HJ:** Galaktosamin und Glucosamin im Knorpel in Abhangigkeit vom Lebensalter. Liebig Ann Chem 611:254, 1958

78. **Lack CH, Ali SY:** The degradation of cartilage enzymes. In Bassett CAL (ed): Cartilage Degradation and Repair. Washington, N.A.S.−N.R.C., 1967

79. **Lane JM, Weiss C:** Review of articular cartilage collagen research. Arthritis Rheum 18:553, 1975

80. **Leidy J:** On the intimate structure and history of articular cartilage. Am J Med Sci 17:277, 1849

81. **Levene C:** The patterns of cartilage canals. J Anat 98:515, 1964

82. **Lindahl O:** Ueber den Wassergehalt des Knorpels. Acta Orthop Scand 17:134, 1958

83. **Linn FC, Sokoloff L:** Movement and composition of intrastitial fluid of cartilage. Arthritis Rheum 8:481, 1965

84. **Little K, Pimm LH, Trueta J:** Osteoarthritis of the hip: An electron micrographic study. J Bone Joint Surg 40B:123, 1958

85. **Loewe G:** Localization of chondromucoproteins in cartilage. Ann Rheum Dis 24:528, 1965

86. **Loewe G:** Changes in the ground substance of aging cartilage. J Pathol Bacteriol 65:381, 1963

87. **Longmore RB, Gardner DL:** Development with age of human articular cartilage surface structure. Ann Rheum Dis 34:26, 1975

88. **Lucy JA, Dingle JT, Fell HB:** Studies on the mode of action of excess vitamin A. II. A possible role of introcellular proteases in the degradation of cartilage matrix. Biochem J 79:500, 1961

89. **Lufti AM:** Mode of growth, fate and functions of cartilage canals. J Anat 106:135, 1970

90. **Lutwak-Mann C:** Enzyme systems in articular cartilage. Biochem J 34:517, 1940

91. **McConnaill MA:** The movements of bone and joints. 4. The mechanical structure of articulating cartilage. J Bone Joint Surg 33B:251, 1951

92. **McCutchen CW:** Sponge, hydrostatic and weeping bearings. Nature 184:1284, 1959

93. **McCutchen CW:** The frictional properties of animal joints. Wear 5:1, 1962

94. **McCutchen CW:** Why did nature make synovial fluid slimy? Clin Orthop 64:18, 1969

95. **McElligott TF, Collins DH:** Chondrocyte function of human articular and costal cartilage compared by measuring the in vitro uptake of labelled (^{35}S) sulphate. Ann Rheum Dis 19:31, 1960

96. **McKibben B, Holdsworth FS:** The nutrition of immature joint cartilage in the lamb. J Bone Joint Surg 48B:793, 1966

97. **Mankin HJ:** Biochemical and metabolic aspects of osteoarthritis. Orthop Clin North Am 2:19, 1971

98. **Mankin HJ:** The water of articular cartilage. In

Simon WH (ed): The human joint in health and disease. Philadelphia, University of Pennsylvania. In Press, pp 37–42, 1978

99. **Mankin HJ:** Localization of tritiated thymidine in articular cartilage of rabbits. I. Growth and immature cartilage. J Bone Joint Surg 44A:682, 1962

100. **Mankin HJ:** Localization of tritiated thymidine in articular cartilage of rabbits. II. Repair in immature cartilage. J Bone Joint Surg 44A:688, 1962

101. **Mankin HJ:** Localization of tritiated cytidine in articular cartilage of immature and adult rabbits after intro-articular injection. Lab Invest 12:543, 1963

102. **Mankin HJ:** The calcified zone (basal layer) of articular cartilage of rabbits. Anat Rec 145:73, 1963

103. **Mankin HJ:** Localization of tritiated thymidine in articular cartilage of rabbits. III. Mature articular cartilage. J Bone Joint Surg 45A:529, 1963

104. **Mankin HJ:** The articular cartilages. A review. AAOS Instructional Course Lectures, XIX:204, 1970

105. **Mankin HJ:** Biochemical changes in articular cartilage in osteoarthritis. In Symposium on Osteoarthritis, pp 1–23. St. Louis, CV Mosby, 1976

106. **Mankin HJ, Baron PA:** The effect of aging on protein synthesis in articular cartilage of rabbits. Lab Invest 14:658, 1965

107. **Mankin HJ, Boyle CJ:** The acture effects of lacerative injury on DNA and protein synthesis in articular cartilage. In Bassett CAL (ed): Cartilage Degradation and Repair. Washington, N.A.S.–N.R.C., 1967

108. **Mankin HJ, Conger KA:** The effect of cortisol on articular cartilage of rabbits. Lab Invest 15:794, 1966

109. **Mankin HJ, Conger KA:** The acute effects of intra-articular hydrocortisone on articular cartilage in rabbits. J Bone Joint Surg 48A:1383, 1966

110. **Mankin HJ, Dorfman H, Lippiello L et al:** Biochemical and metabolic abnormalities in articular cartilage from osteoarthritic human hips. II. Correlation of morphology with biochemical and metabolic data. J Bone Joint Surg 53A:523, 1971

111. **Mankin HJ, Lippiello L:** The turnover of the matrix of articular cartilage. J Bone Joint Surg 51A:1591, 1969

112. **Mankin HJ, Lippiello L:** Biochemical and metabolic abnormalities in articular cartilage from osteoarthritic human hips. J Bone Joint Surg, 52A:424, 1970

113. **Mankin HJ, Orlic PA:** A method of estimating the "health" of rabbit articular cartilage by assays of ribonucleic acid and protein synthesis. Lab Invest 13:465, 1964

114. **Maroudas A:** Physiochemical properties of cartilage in the light of ion exchange theory. Biophys J 8:575, 1968

115. **Maroudas A:** Distribution and diffusion of solutes in articular cartilage. Biophys J 10:365, 1970

116. **Maroudas A, Bullough P:** Permeability of articular cartilage. Nature 219:1260, 1968

117. **Maroudas A, Bullough P, Swanson SAV et al:** The permeability of articular cartilage. J Bone Joint Surg 50B:166, 1968

118. **Maroudas A, Muir H, Wingham J:** The correlation of fixed negative charge with glycosaminoglycan content of human articular cartilage. Biochem Biophys Acta 177:492, 1969

119. **Martin GR, Gross J, Piez KA et al:** On the intramolecular cross linking of collagen in lathyretic rats. Biochem Biophys Acta 53:599, 1961

120. **Mathews MB:** The interaction of collagen and acid mucopolysaccharides: A model for connective tissue. Biochem J 96:710, 1965

121. **Mathews MB, Glagov S:** Acid mucopolysaccharide patterns in aging human cartilage. J Clin Invest 45:1103, 1966

122. **Meachim, G:** The effect of scarification on articular cartilage in the rabbit. J Bone Joint Surg 45B:150, 1963

123. **Meachim G:** The histology and ultrastructure of cartilage. In Bassett CAL (ed): Cartilage Degradation and Repair. Washington, N.A.S.–N.R.C., 1967

124. **Meachim G:** Age changes in articular cartilage. Clin Orthop 64:33, 1969

125. **Meachim G, Collins DH:** Cell counts of normal and osteoarthritic articular cartilage in relation to the uptake of sulfate ($^{35}SO_4$) in vitro. Am Rheum Dis 21:45, 1962

126. **Meachim G, Ghadially FN, Collins DH:** Regressive changes in the superficial layer of human articular cartilage. Ann Rheum Dis 24:23, 1965

127. **Meachim G, Roy S:** Intracytoplasmic filaments in the cells of adult human articular cartilage. Ann Rheum Dis 26:50, 1967

128. **Meachim G, Roy S:** Surface ultrastructure of mature adult human articular cartilage. J Bone Joint Surg 51B:529, 1969

129. **Miles JS, Eichelberger L:** Biochemical studies of human cartilage during the aging process. J Am Geriat Soc 12:1, 1964

130. **Miller EJ:** Isolation and characterization of collagen from chick cartilage containing three identical α chains. Biochemistry 10:1652, 1972

131. **Miller EJ, Matukas VJ:** Chick cartilage collagen: A new type of α 1 chain not present in bone or skin of the species. Proc Natl Acad Sci (USA) 64:1264, 1969

132. **Miller EJ, Vanderkorst JK, Sokoloff L:** Collagen of human articular and costal cartilage. Arthritis Rheum 12:21, 1969

133. **Muir H:** Chemistry and metabolism of connective tissue glycosaminoglycans (mucopolysaccharides). In Hall DA (ed): International Review of Connective Tissue Research, Vol 2. New York, Academic Press

134. **Pal S, Doganges PT, Schubert M:** The separation of new forms of the protein polysaccharides of bovine nasal cartilage. J Biol Chem 241:4261, 1966

135. **Palfrey AJ, Davies DV:** The fine structure of chondrocytes. J Anat 100:213, 1966

136. **Partridge SM, Davis HF, Adair GS:** The chemistry of connective tissues. 6. The constitution of the chondroitin sulfate–protein complex in cartilage. Biochem J 79:15, 1961

137. **Pasternak CA:** The synthesis of 3′ phosphoadenosine 5′ phosphosulfate by mouse tissue: Sulfate activation in vitro and in vivo. J Biol Chem 235:438, 1960

138. **Piez KA:** Characterization of a collagen from codfish skin containing three chromatographically different α chains. Biochemistry 4:2590, 1965

139. **Prockop DJ:** The intracellular biosynthesis of collagen. Arch Intern Med 124:563, 1969

140. **Quintarelli G:** Methods for the histochemical identification of acid mucopolysaccharides: A critical evaluation. In Quintarelli G (ed): The Chemical Physiology of Mucopolysaccharides. Boston, Little, Brown & Co, 1968

141. **Raden EL, Paul I:** Joint function. Arthritis Rheum 13:276, 1970

142. **Raden EL, Swann D, Weisser PA:** Separation of a hyaluronate-free lubricating fraction from synovial fluid. Nature, 228:337, 1970

143. **Redfern P:** A Normal Nutrition in the Articular Cartilage. Edinburgh, Sutherland & Knox, 1850

144. **Redler I, Zimny ML:** Scanning electron microscopy of normal and abnormal articular cartilage and synovium. J Bone Joint Surg 52A:1395, 1970

145. **Roden L:** The protein carbohydrate linkages of acid mucopolysaccharides. In Quintarelli G (ed): The Chemical Physiology of Mucopolysaccharides. Boston, Little, Brown & Co, 1968

146. **Rosenberg L:** Chemical basis for the histological use of safranin-O in the study of articular cartilage. J Bone Joint Surg 53A:69, 1971

147. **Rosenberg L:** Structure of cartilage proteoglycans. In Burleigh PMC, Poole AR (eds): Dynamics of Connective Tissue Macromolecules, pp 105–124. New York, American Elsevier, 1975

148. **Rosenberg L, Hellmann W, Kleinschmidt AK:** Electron microscopic studies of proteoglycan aggregates from bovine articular cartilage. J Biol Chem 250:1877–1883, 1975

149. **Rosenberg L, Johnson B, Schubert M:** Protein polysaccharides from human articular and costal cartilages. J Clin Invest 44:1647, 1965

150. **Rosenberg L, Pal S, Beale R et al:** A comparison of protein polysaccharides of bovine nasal cartilage isolated and fractionated by different methods. J Biol Chem 245:4112, 1970

151. **Rosenthal O, Bowie MA, Wagoner G:** Studies on the metabolism of articular cartilage. II. Respiration and glycolysis of cartilage in relation to its age. J. Cell Comp Physiol 17:221, 1941

152. **Roy S:** Ultrastructure of articular cartilage in experimental hemarthrosis. Arch Pathol 86:69, 1968

153. **Roy S:** Ultrastructure of articular cartilage in experimental immobilization. Ann Rheum Dis 29:634, 1970

154. **Roy S, Meachim G:** Chondrocyte ultrastructure in adult human articular cartilage. Ann Rheum Dis 27:544, 1968

155. **Ruttner JR, Spycher MA:** Electron microscopic investigations on aging and osteoarthritic human cartilage. Pathol Microbiol 31:14, 1968

156. **Sajdera S, Hascall VC:** Protein polysaccharide complex from bovine nasal cartilage: A comparison of low and high stream extraction procedures. J Biol Chem 244:79, 1969

157. **Schubert M:** Intercellular macromolecules containing polysaccharides. In Connective Tissue: Intracellular Macromolecules. Boston, Little, Brown & Co, 1964

158. **Schubert M, Hamerman D:** A Primer on Connective Tissue Biochemistry. Philadelphia, Lea & Febiger, 1968

159. **Seno N, Meyer K, Anderson B et al:** Variations in keratosulfates. J Biol Chem 240:1005, 1965

160. **Silberberg R:** Ultrastructure of articular cartilage in health and disease. Clin Orthop 57:233, 1968

161. **Silberberg R, Silberberg M, Feir D:** Life cycle of articular cartilage cells: An electronmicroscopic study of the hip joint of the mouse. Am J Anat 114:17, 1964

162. **Silberberg M, Silberberg R, Hasler M:** Effects of fasting and refeeding on the ultrastructure of articular cartilage. Pathol Microbiol 30:283, 1967

163. **Silberberg R, Silberberg M, Vogel A et al:** Ultrastructure of articular cartilage of mice of various ages. Am J Anat 109:251, 1961

164. **Silberberg R, Stamp WG, Lesker PA et al:** Aging changes in ultrastructure and enzymatic activity of articular cartilage of guinea pigs. J Gerontol 25:184, 1970

165. **Smith JW, Peters TJ, Serafini-Fracassini A:** Observations in the distribution of the protein polysaccharide complex and collagen in bovine articular cartilage. J Cell Comp Physiol 2:129, 1967

166. **Sokoloff L:** Elasticity of aging cartilage: Effect of ions and viscous solutions. Science 141:1055, 1963

167. **Sokoloff L:** Elasticity of aging cartilage. Fed Proc 25:1089, 1966

168. **Sokoloff L:** The biology of degenerative joint disease. Chicago, University, of Chicago Press, 1969

169. **Spicer S, Horn RG, Leppi TJ:** Histochemistry of connective tissue mucopolysaccharides. In Wagner BM, Smith DE (eds): The Connective Tissue. Baltimore, Williams & Wilkins, 1967

170. **Stevens FS:** Multiple stage depolymerization of collagen fibrils. Biochem Biophys Acta 130:202, 1966

171. **Stockwell RA:** The cell density of human articular and costal cartilage. J Anat 101:753, 1967

172. **Stockwell RA:** Lipid content of human costal and articular cartilage Ann Rheum Dis 26:481, 1967

173. **Stockwell RA:** The lipid and glycogen content of rabbit articular hyaline and nonarticular hyaline cartilage. J Anat 102:1, 1967

174. **Stockwell RA:** Changes in the acid glycosaminoglycan contest of the matrix of aging human articular cartilage. Ann Rheum Dis 29:509, 1970

175. **Stockwell RA, Scott JE:** Distribution of acid glycos-

aminoglycans in human articular cartilage. Nature 215:1376, 1967

176. **Stone AL:** Optical rotary dispersion of mucopolysaccharides and mucopolysaccharide-dye complexes. Biopolymers 3:617, 1965

177. **Strangeways TSP:** Observations on the nutrition of articular cartilage. Br Med J 1:661, 1920

178. **Strominger JL:** Nucleotide intermediates in the biosynthese of heteropolymeric polysaccharides. In Connective Tissue: Intercellular Macromolecules. Boston, Little, Brown & Co, 1964

179. **Thomas L:** The effects of papain, vitamin A, and cortisone in cartilage matrix in vivo. In Connective Tissue: Intercellular Macromolecules. Boston, Little, Brown & Co, 1964

180. **Thomas L, McCluskey RT, Potter JL et al:** Comparison of the effects of papain and vitamin A. on cartilage. I. The effects in rabbits. J Exp Med 111:705, 1960

181. **Toda N, Seno N:** Sialic acid in the keratan sulfate fraction from whole cartilage. Biochem Biophys Acta 208:227, 1970

182. **Toynbee J:** In Redfern P: Abnormal Nutrition in the Articular Cartilages. Edinburgh, Sutherland and Knox, 1850

183. **Underfriend S:** Formation of hydroxyproline in collagen. Science, 152:1335, 1966

184. **Wagoner G, Rosenthal O, Bowie MA:** Studies of the cells in normal and arthritic bovine cartilage. Am J Med Sci 201:489, 1941

185. **Walker PS, Dowson D, Longfield MD et al:** Boosted lubrication in synovial joints by fluid enlargement and enrichment. Ann Rheum Dis 27:512, 1968

186. **Walker PS et al:** Behavior of synovial fluid on surfaces of articular cartilage. Ann Rheum Dis 28:1, 1969

187. **Walker PS et al:** Mode of aggregation of hyaluronic acid protein complex in the surface of articular cartilage. Ann Rheum Dis 29:591, 1970

188. **Weiss C:** An ultrastructural study of aging human articular cartilage (abstr). J Bone Joint Surg 53A:803, 1971

189. **Weiss C:** Light and electron microscopic studies of normal articular cartilage. In Simon WH: The Human Joint in Health and Disease, pp 9−21. Philadelphia, University of Pennsylvania Press, 1978

190. **Weiss C:** Light and electron microscopic studies of osteoarthritic articular cartilage. In Simon WH (ed): Human Joint in Health and Disease, pp 112−122. Philadelphia, University of Pennsylvania Press, 1978

191. **Weiss C:** Normal and osteoarthritic articular cartilage. Orthop Clin North Am 10:175, 1979

192. **Weiss C, Mankin HJ:** Unpublished data

193. **Weiss C, Mankin HJ, Treadwell BV:** Diffusion rates in articular cartilage: Evidence for an active transport system (abstr). J Bone Joint Surg 55A:657, 1973

194. **Weiss C, Mirow S:** An ultrastructural study of osteoarthritic changes in the articular cartilage of human knees. J Bone Joint Surg 54A:954, 1972

195. **Weiss C, Rosenberg L, Helfet AJ:** An ultrastructural study of normal young adult human articular cartilage. J Bone Joint Surg 50A:663, 1968

196. **Weissman G, Spilberg IL:** Breakdown of cartilage protein polysaccharide by lysosomes. Arthritis Rheum 11:162, 1968

197. **Woessner JF Jr:** Acid cathepsins of cartilage. In Bassett CAL (ed): Cartilage Degradation and Repair. Washington, N.A.S.−N.R.C., 1967

198. **Woessner JF:** Cartilage cathepsin D and its action on matrix components. Fed Proc 32:1485, 1973

CHAPTER 4
THE PHYSICAL PROPERTIES OF SYNOVIAL FLUID AND THE SPECIAL ROLE OF HYALURONIC ACID

Endre A. Balazs

This chapter was written with two aims in mind: first, to give a brief review of the chemical composition and rheological properties of the synovial fluid in normal and pathologic joints; and second, to present, with critical comments, various current hypotheses on the importance of this fluid in the function of the joint with special emphasis on the biologic role of hyaluronic acid.

There is considerable data available in the literature on the chemical composition and rheological properties of synovial fluid of various species. This review does not intend to be all-inclusive; rather it presents primary data on human joint fluids only. A large number of speculations and hypotheses are recorded in the literature on the lubricating and nutritive functions of the synovial fluid in the joint. This review aims to be selective in this area as well and to present only the most important recent findings and speculations on this subject.

SYNOVIAL FLUID AS AN INTERCELLULAR MATRIX

From a rheological point of view, the natural environment of cells in a tissue can be liquid or solid. The liquid or solid extracellular matter around and between cells is called matrix. In the solid matrix, certain macromolecular components (mostly collagen or elastin, or both) and their aggregates form a continuous solid phase. The rheological qualities of the solid matrix—that is, rigidity, elasticity, and viscosity—vary considerably, as exemplified by the differences between cartilage and the vitreous of the eye.

The solid matrix consists of fixed and fluid

components. The fixed components are made up of such microscopic elements as collagen and elastin fibrils, basal laminae, and the structural network of proteoglycans. The fluid component comprises water and those solutes (salts, small organic molecules, peptides, proteins, and so forth) that, dissolved in water, are distributed between the fixed components of the solid matrix.

The liquid matrix, on the other hand, is water in which molecules of various sizes are dissolved or dispersed. The rheological qualities of liquid matrices also vary considerably, as exemplified by the differences between the aqueous humor of the eye and synovial fluid.

The joint contains both solid and liquid matrices. Of the four tissue elements forming a joint—articular cartilage, synovial tissue, intra-articular ligaments, and synovial fluid—the first three have solid matrices and the last is a liquid matrix.

It is of primary importance to recognize that all three solid matrix compartments of the joint are directly adjacent to the liquid matrix compartment, the synovial fluid. Another important morphological fact is that the solid matrix compartments of the articular cartilage, ligaments, and synovial tissue are not separated from the fluid matrix compartment by a continuous cell layer or basal lamina. Therefore, no visible morphological barrier separates these two types of matrix compartments.

Other adjacent liquid and solid matrices, such as those present in the peritoneal, pericardial, and pleural spaces and in the anterior chamber of the eye, are separated by microscopically recognizable cellular (epithelium) and matrix (basement membrane) barriers. The joint, however, is not the only tissue in which the liquid and solid matrices are not separated by these barriers. Other tissues in the musculoskeletal system are similarly structured, such as the tendons and their sheaths and the space between fasciae and the bursal space.

CHEMICAL COMPOSITION OF THE SYNOVIAL FLUID

PROTEINS

The protein content of normal synovial fluid in all species studied is much lower than that of serum.[49] The general statement can be made that the very large protein molecules of the serum, such as γ-1 macroglobulin, β-lipoprotein, fibrinogen, and α-2 macroglobulin, are absent, and others, such as α-1 antitrypsin and plasminogen, are present in traces in the normal synovial fluid. In addition, some smaller proteins, such as haptoglobulins and prothrombin present in the serum are also absent from normal synovial fluid.[3,20,24,48,55] Because of the absence of fibrinogen and prothrombin, the normal fluid does not clot.

The total protein content of synovial fluid aspirated from normal human knee joints does not change with age of the donor (Table 4-1). In all inflammatory joint diseases, however, the concentration of protein in synovial fluid increases, and the missing plasma proteins appear. Fibrinogen appears, and after aspiration, the fibrin precipitates, or often, the

TABLE 4-1. PROTEINS AND HYALURONIC ACID IN THE SYNOVIAL FLUID OF KNEE JOINTS OF HUMAN SUBJECTS OF VARIOUS AGES

Age Group (yrs)	Knees Investigated	Protein (mg/ml)	Hyaluronic Acid mg/ml	Limiting Viscosity Number (ml/g)
18–20	36	20.5 ± 0.8	3.8 ± 0.1	5200 ± 100
21–23	24	21.0 ± 0.9	3.8 ± 0.2	5300 ± 100
24–27	20	19.4 ± 1.3	3.4 ± 0.1	5000 ± 150
28–35	18	18.5 ± 2.6	2.5 ± 0.04	5800 ± 300
52–78	34	18.5 ± 1.6	2.5 ± 0.2	5400 ± 200

(Data taken from unpublished work of E. A. Balazs, N. W. Rydell, P. O. Seppälä, I. F. Duff, E. W. Merrill and D. A. Gibbs)

fluid clots. From the point of view of protein content, inflammatory synovial fluid is more "plasmalike" than normal synovial fluid.

In most degenerative joint diseases, the protein concentration also increases in the fluid, but it does not necessarily become plasmalike. Although there is no clear proof, there are indications that in these cases, proteins appear in the synovial fluid that originate from the cells and matrix of neighboring tissues.[53]

Proteins with enzymatic activity also appear in the inflammatory synovial fluid. Enzymes present in the lysosomes of leukocytes, such as acid phosphatases, β-glucuronidase, and β-N-acetylglucosaminidase, are released from the destroyed cells. Other enzymes, such as lactic dehydrogenases, collagenase, and muramidase (lysozyme) are also found in pathologic synovial fluids.[1,22,32]

Most importantly, inflammatory synovial fluid contains immune complexes and antibodies that are not present in the normal fluid. In rheumatoid arthritis, the appearance of the so-called rheumatoid factors (primarily antibodies to γG-globulin) and their complexes with immunologically active proteins, as well as activation of components of the complement system, are typical examples of the drastic changes occurring in the protein composition and immunologic characteristics of synovial fluid during inflammation.[44,52,59-61] The extremely complex alteration in the immunologically active proteins of the synovial fluid indicate that the neighboring tissues—first of all, the synovial tissue—are the sites of very intensive protein synthesis during inflammation.

HYALURONIC ACID

The viscoelastic nature of synovial fluid is due to its hyaluronic acid content. This polyanion is present in the synovial fluid of all species investigated. In equine, bovine, and human joints a considerable variation was found in the hyaluronic acid concentration of synovial fluid collected from various joints of the same subject.[56]

Hyaluronic acid concentration also varies with age.[51] In the synovial fluid of human knee joints the hyaluronic acid concentration is highest between 18 and 25 years, after which it decreases. Between the ages of 30 and 80, no change could be observed in normal joints.[7]

The size of the hyaluronic acid molecules in the synovial fluid of human knee joints was determined by various physicochemical methods. The results vary somewhat, depending on the method used for the purification of the hyaluronic acid and for the determination of the molecular weight.

This large molecule occupies an extremely large volume when dissolved in water that contains a physiologic concentration of salts and hydrogen ions. A single molecule of sodium-hyaluronate, with a weight of 5 million, occupies a spheroidal domain with a diameter of 0.5 μm. This means that 1 g dissolved in physiologic saline fills 3 liters of solvent. In other words, the individual molecules, in close contact with one another but without overlapping, occupy the whole volume of solution at a concentration of only 0.33 mg/ml. The concentration of hyaluronic acid in synovial fluid of the human knee joint is 2 to 3 mg/ml. This means that the molecules are "crowded"; they overlap, and therefore, such a solution must be considered as a continuous network of interacting, entangled molecular chains. Any other molecules, large or small, dissolved in the solution are within the domain of this hyaluronic acid network, and any molecule or particle that moves in it must pass through this feltlike molecular network. The chemical activity of the molecules that can penetrate this network may be changed, and other large molecules cannot find space to penetrate the network. In this sense, one speaks about the exclusion effect and the dynamic filtration effect of hyaluronic acid solutions.[38]

Experiments in vitro carried out by many investigators have demonstrated that large protein molecules can be filtered from solution by passage through a filter layer of synovial fluid or hyaluronic acid. Furthermore, due to the exclusion effect, molecules dissolved in hyaluronic acid solutions are altered in their chemical activity (solubility, aggregation, osmotic effect, charge effect, and so on).[34]

Limiting viscosity number (intrinsic viscosity) is a widely used index for characterizing polymers such as hyaluronic acid. The limiting viscosity number of hyaluronic acid in synovial fluid can be measured without separating the polysaccharide from proteins. This measurement gives a meaningful parameter of one hyaluronic acid molecule that expresses the size, volume, and shape of the molecule as well as its interaction with the solvent (water with ions dissolved in it[15,20,51]). The limiting viscosity number of the synovial fluid of normal human knee joint does not change with age (Table 4-1).[7] This indicates that the molecular size of the hyaluronic acid in the joint remains the same during a lifetime, but the concentration of this polymer drops suddenly around 28 to 35 years of age.

THE ELASTOVISCOUS NATURE OF SYNOVIAL FLUID

NORMAL FLUID

Synovial fluid exhibits viscous and elastic properties. Both depend on its size, conformation, interactions, and number of hyaluronic acid molecules present in the fluid.

In recent years, a considerable amount of work has been reported on the elastoviscous nature of human knee synovial fluid obtained from normal and pathologic joints.[6,7,11,20] These studies clearly show that, from a rheological point of view, the synovial fluid and the protein-free ($<1.0\%$) hyaluronic acid prepared from other tissues (umbilical cord and rooster comb) are identical. Up to now, no evidence has been found that would indicate that the presence of proteins in the synovial fluid significantly alters the elastoviscous properties of the pure sodium salt of hyaluronic acid. Of course, this does not eliminate the possibility that some interaction may occur between proteins and sodium-hyaluronate molecules, which could cause minor modifications in the

viscoelastic properties of synovial fluid. The important fact is, however, that sodium hyaluronate without proteins exhibits the same molecular relaxation mechanism as synovial fluid when it is exposed to strain of various frequencies.[29]

To demonstrate the elastoviscous nature of synovial fluid, one has to measure the dynamic shear moduli at various strain frequencies and at various temperatures.[29] The dynamic rigidity of synovial fluid (G^*), which is the ratio of the peak stress to the peak strain in the fluid, can be divided vectorially into two components ($G^* = \sqrt{G'^2 + G''^2}$). One of these components is called the dynamic loss module (G'') or viscous module because it represents the energy that is dissipated as heat when the molecule is submitted to strain. The other component is called the dynamic storage module (G'), or elastic module, because it represents the energy stored when the molecule is submitted to strain. This energy stored in the molecules for a short period of time imparts an elastic nature to the fluid. This elasticity is similar to that described in rubber solutions, and it is based on the interaction between various segments of the molecular chain of hyaluronic acid. It is also called entropy elasticity because it depends on the states of order and disorder in the arrangement of the molecular chains of hyaluronic acid.

A typical set of values of the storage and loss moduli as a function of strain frequency is shown in Figure 4-1. The three sets of curves of dynamic shear moduli are selected as representative samples of synovial fluid obtained from the normal joint of a young (20 yr) and an old (67 yr) donor and from an osteoarthritic joint of an old (63 yr) donor.

In all three fluids, as the strain frequency increases, both the loss and the storage modules increase. The absolute values of these moduli at low frequencies vary considerably. The fluid obtained from the normal young joint has the highest value and that obtained from the osteoarthritic joint the lowest. Most important, as the frequency increases, the curves representing the loss and storage moduli cross each other in the two normal fluids but not in the pathologic fluid. This means that the normal fluids are predominantly viscous at low strain frequency and predominantly elastic at high strain frequency. Since this crossover is not observable in the pathologic fluid, one has to conclude that this fluid behaves in the entire frequency range as a predominantly viscous rather than an elastic fluid. It is important to note that the strain frequencies at which these measurements were made are within the range to which the fluid is exposed in the course of the normal movement of the knee joint (flexing under no load, walking, running).

These observations can be explained on the molecular level by configurational adjustments of the hyaluronic acid chains. At low strain frequencies, the configurational adjustments of the chains, owing to thermal (Brownian) motions are rapid enough to allow the molecule to maintain its original conformation. That is, under imposed strain, the chains slip by each other, which results in a viscous flow. Therefore, the rheological properties of the fluid are predominantly viscous. At high strain frequency, the configurational readjustment of the chains cannot occur between the short periods of the oscillating strain, and the molecules cannot maintain their original con-

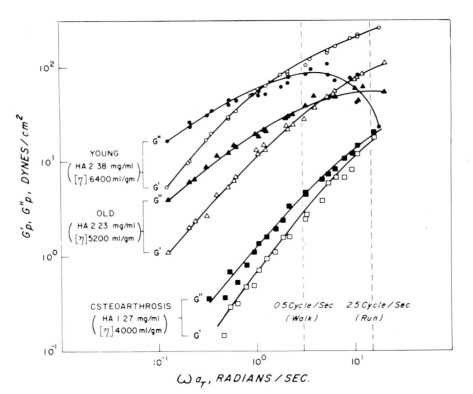

FIG. 4-1. Dynamic elastic modulus, G' (*open symbols*) and dynamic viscous modulus, G" (*filled symbols*) of three human synovial fluid samples aspirated from the normal knee joint of one young (20 years) and one old (67 years) subject and from the osteoarthritic knee joint of an old subject (63 years), plotted against strain frequency. The broken vertical lines indicate the frequencies that correspond approximately to the movement of the knee joint in walking and running. The concentration (*HA*) and limiting viscosity number ([η]) of hyaluronic acid in the aspirated fluid are given in parentheses. (Balazs EA: Univ. of Michigan Med. Ctr. July [Special Arthritis issue]: 255, December, 1968)

formation. That is, under the imposed strain, the molecules deform sinusoidally and alternately store the mechanical energy and then release it elastically. Under these conditions, the fluid's rheological behavior is predominantly that of an elastic body.

The most remarkable behavior of synovial fluid under increasing strain frequency is its rapid transition from viscous fluid to elastic body. This transformation is reversible and has no deteriorating effect on the molecule. Natural rubber and industrial polymers with elastoviscous properties show considerably different behavior in that this transition occurs during a considerably extended frequency range.

What are the biologic implications of this frequency-dependent viscoelastic transformation of synovial fluid? The synovial fluid occupies narrow channels between the soft tissues of the joint, and it is sandwiched between the two cartilage surfaces. The measurements of dynamic shear moduli tell us that the fluid will move like a viscous liquid in these channels when the joint moves at low shear frequency. Under high shear frequency movements, the fluid does not move in the channels; rather, it behaves like an elastic solid, storing the mechanical energy.

But the fluid also impregnates the surface layer of articular cartilage and synovial tissue. Thus, it separates cells (synovial cells) and protein fibrils (collagen), preventing them from direct contact with each other. This means that under slow mechanical loading of the joint, when articular cartilage and synovial tissue are exposed to low frequency strain, hyaluronic acid behaves like a viscous oil. The fluid between the cells and collagen fibrils is displaced (flows) under the mechanical forces, and the tissue itself deforms. On the other hand, at high mechanical loading rates of the joint, when these tissue layers are exposed to high frequency strain, hyaluronic acid transforms into a highly deformable elastic system. Therefore, the fluid, which contains hyaluronic acid, is not displaced, and the tissue itself is not deformed. This means that the hyaluronic acid in the surface layers

of articular cartilage and synovial tissue absorbs mechanical stress, thereby protecting the cells and collagen network from mechanical shock and deformation. In other words, this polysaccharide serves in these tissue layers as a shock absorber.

The cells, which are extremely sensitive to mechanical stress, and the rigid, load-supporting collagen fibrils are surrounded by the elastoviscous hyaluronic acid solution. There is a mechanical coupling between the rigid system of cells and fibrils and the energy-storing and energy-dissipating system of hyaluronic acid. Therefore, a large part of the stress imposed on the entire system is converted to elastic deformation of the hyaluronic acid. By this mechanism, the stress-sensitive elements of the system (cells) are protected, and the structural integrity of the tissue (special organizational pattern of the fibrils) is maintained.

EFFECTS OF AGING*

The rheological properties of synovial fluid change considerably during aging. The elastic (storage) modulus (G') and viscous (loss) modulus (G'') decrease sharply after the age of 27 years. The elastic modulus drops further after the age of 52 years (Table 4-2). As pointed out above, synovial fluids, like solutions of pure hyaluronic acid, show a rapid transition from viscous to elastic behavior when the strain frequency increases. The frequency at which this transition occurs or, more precisely, the point where the curves of the storage and loss moduli cross one another and both moduli have the same numerical value, is specific for a given fluid (Fig. 4-1). This frequency value at the crossover point increases with aging (Table 4-2). The value of the two moduli at the crossover point drops sharply after the 27th year but does not change later. Thus, the rheological properties of synovial fluids in all three age groups stud-

---

* The data reported here are from the work of Balazs, Rydell, Seppälä, Duff, Merrill and Gibbs. While the details of this work are as yet unpublished, a brief review can be found in Balazs, 1969.[7]

TABLE 4-2. RHEOLOGICAL PROPERTIES OF SYNOVIAL FLUIDS ASPIRATED FROM THE KNEES OF HUMAN SUBJECTS OF VARIOUS AGES

Age Group (yr)	Subjects	Elastic Modules G' (dyn/sec^{-2})†	Viscous Modules G" (dyn/sec^{-2})†	Crossover Point of Two Moduli (G', G") (dyn/sec^{-1})	Two Moduli (G', G") at Crossover Point (dyn/sec^{-2})
18–27	16	1170 ± 130	450 ± 82	0.13 ± 0.02	332 ± 41
27–35	18	226 ± 7	72 ± 8	0.21 ± 0.004	59 ± 6
52–78	26	189 ± 33	101 ± 12	0.41 ± 0.12	61 ± 7

† Measured at 2.5 cycle/sec^{-1}.
Data taken from the unpublished work of E. A. Balazs, N. W. Rydell, P. O. Seppälä, I. F. Duff, D. A. Gibbs and E. W. Merrill.

ied are significantly different. The fluid from young subjects is very highly elastic and rigid at relatively low frequencies. The fluid from middle-aged subjects is less rigid but still highly elastic at higher frequencies. The synovial fluid from older subjects is less rigid, less viscous, and less elastic at all frequencies.

The frequencies at which these measurements were carried out were in the same range as the frequencies at which the joints are loaded and flexed during natural movements of the body. Therefore, some conclusions can be drawn about the rheological behavior of the fluid in the joint submitted to various rates of strain. Between the ages of 18 and 39, the synovial fluid undergoes a substantial decrease in rigidity but retains its generally elastic character. With further aging, the elasticity decreases in such a way that under the frequency conditions of normal knee motion the synovial fluid changes from the highly elastic fluid in the young to a nonelastic viscous fluid in the old.

Because the concentration, size, shape, and limiting viscosity number of individual hyaluronic acid molecules does not change in the synovial fluid of the normal human knee joint between the ages of 27 and 78 but the elastoviscous properties of the fluid radically decrease, one has to assume that the interaction between the chains of the neighboring molecules is altered. Recent studies on hyaluronic acid, carried out using x-ray diffraction and optical rotation measurements, indicate that a certain amount of the individual polysaccharide chains form double helical junction points or crosslinks that increase the elastoviscous properties of the polymer. It is possible that during aging the amount of these double helical crosslinks between the chains of neighboring molecules decreases. This in turn would make the molecular chain segments less stiff and the solution less elastic.

PATHOLOGIC FLUIDS*

In the synovial fluids aspirated from joints with osteoarthritis, traumatic arthritis, gout, chondrocalcinosis, and rheumatoid arthritis, the concentration, limiting viscosity number, and molelcular weight of hyaluronic acid is lower than in normal joints.[20,50,56] Consequently, all rheological properties of the fluid, such as the dynamic viscous and elastic moduli and the crossover point of the two moduli are also much below normal values (Table 4-3; Fig. 4-1). Thus, in the pathologic joint, the synovial fluid does not have those rheological properties that protect the synovial tissue and cartilage against mechanical stress.

THE SURFACE OF THE ARTICULAR CARTILAGE

There is some indication that hyaluronic acid is not evenly distributed in the entire joint space. On the surface of the articular cartilage

* Data reported here are from the work of Balazs, Seppälä, Rydell, Gibbs, Duff and Merrill. While the details of this work are not yet published, a brief review of it can be found in Balazs, 1968.[6]

TABLE 4–3. CONCENTRATION AND LIMITING VISCOSITY NUMBER OF HYALURONIC ACID AND THE RHEOLOGICAL PROPERTIES OF SYNOVIAL FLUIDS ASPIRATED FROM HUMAN PATHOLOGICAL KNEES

Pathological Condition	Fluids Analysed	Volume Fluid Collected (ml)	Hyaluronic Acid $[\eta]$		Elastic Modules G' (dyn/sec^{-2})	Viscous Modules G'' (dyn/sec^{-2})	Crossover Point of Two Modules (G', G'') (cycles/sec^{-1})
			mg/ml	ml/g			
Osteoarthritis	11		1.55 ± 0.14	3800 ± 350	85 ± 54	48 ± 28	4.7 ± 1.9
Traumatic Arthritis	3	7–20	0.69–1.76	2100–4200	2–41	2–29	1.3–2.9
Gout	4	3–5	1.28 ± 0.14	3500 ± 690	30 ± 10	15 ± 7	0.9 ± 0.3
Chondrocalcinosis	2	2.5	0.75	3700	5	5	1.7
			1.22	3900	22	13	0.9

Data taken from unpublished work of E. A. Balazs, P. O. Seppälä, N. W. Rydell, I. F. Duff, E. W. Merrill and D. A. Gibbs.

and on the surface of the synovial tissue, a hyaluronic acid layer was observed which cannot be easily washed away from these tissue surfaces. The concentration of the hyaluronic acid in these layers is higher than in the fluid aspirated from the joint. It is not clear what kind of molecular interaction is responsible for the "accumulation" of hyaluronic acid on these tissue surfaces.

Electron microscopic studies showed that a 1- to 2-μm-thick layer of hyaluronic acid−protein complex covers the surface of the articular cartilage. This layer is anchored to the fibrillar collagen matrix of the cartilage and can be removed from it by treatment with proteolytic enzymes or hyaluronidase. With aging, and in osteoarthritic cases, this layer becomes thicker. It is now known, however, how the hyaluronic acid and protein content of the layer change with aging and with various pathologic conditions.[15]

Histochemical and chemical analyses carried out on the cartilage close to the articular surface indicate the presence of hyaluronic acid 50 to 100 μm deep into the cartilage, where it shares the space between the collagen fibrils with sulfated proteoglycans.[8] The deep layers of the cartilage matrix contain only sulfated proteoglycans (proteoglycans of chondroitin 4-sulfate and keratan sulfate) but no hyaluronic acid.

Scanning electron microscopy also shows an accumulation of synovial fluid (hyaluronic acid and proteins) on the surface of articular cartilage[28,35,58] (1970). Under conditions of extreme load, experiments in vitro show, this fluid layer protects the cartilage surface.[58]

One can only speculate about the importance of this layer in the normal function and pathology of the joint. Because it represents the only morphologically visible barrier between the cartilage matrix and the joint space, it is tempting to assume that it is responsible for the protection of the cartilage surface. Because the synovial fluid of the normal joint does not contain appreciable amounts of sulfated proteoglycans, it is possible that the surface layer of the cartilage impregnated with hyaluronic acid forms an effective barrier against diffusion or flow (under pressure caused by compressing the cartilage when the joint is loaded) of the sulfated proteoglycans into the synovial fluid. In various pathological conditions sulfated glycosaminoglycans were found in the synovial fluid,[50] suggesting that the integrity of the surface layer of the articular cartilage impregnated with hyaluronic acid is responsible for the normal maintenance of the cartilage by preventing the leakage of proteoglycans into the synovial space and the subsequent loss of this important component of the cartilage matrix. The missing link in this argument, of course, is the complete lack of knowledge about the chemical composition of the cartilage surface layer in pathological conditions.

THE EFFECT OF HYALURONIC ACID ON CELL ACTIVITIES

Recently, several effects of hyaluronic acid on cells *in vitro* and *in vivo* have been reported. None of these effects have been directly connected to the pathological processes in the joint. Nevertheless, the effect of hyaluronic acid on cell activities is so general that the assumption that it is operative in wound healing and inflammation of the joint is justified.[11]

Sodium-hyaluronate was found to be a cell-immobilizing agent. The movement of cells of the lymphomyeloid system (lymphocytes, granulocytes, macrophages) is inhibited by this biopolymer and by the tissue fluids that contain this molecule (synovial fluid, liquid vitreous). The fast-moving cells of the lymphomyeloid system exhibit different sensitivities to hyaluronic acid. This cell-immobilizing effect is specific for these cells because cells that move slowly *in vitro* (fibroblasts) are not affected. The effect of hyaluronic acid on the motility of cells is not directly related to the bulk viscosity of the solution in which the cells are moving. The effect is dependent on the limiting viscosity number of the hyaluronic acid used. Hyaluronic acid preparations with low limiting viscosity numbers are less effective cell-movement inhibitors than preparations with high limiting viscosity numbers. Pathologic synovial fluids, which have low limiting viscosity numbers, are less effective than normal fluids.[19]

Hyaluronic acid also inhibits the modulation of lymphocytes to lymphoblasts. When blood lymphocytes, stimulated by mitogens (phytohemagglutinin, pokeweed mitogen, streptolysin O, or purified protein derivative of tuberculin) are placed in viscous hyaluronic acid solution, the transformation of lymphocytes to lymphoblasts and the subsequent mitosis is prevented as long as the cells are surrounded and separated from each other by viscous sodium-hyaluronic solutions.[23]

Sodium-hyaluronate can also prevent the target cells from killing sensitized lymphocytes. The cytotoxic effect of lymphocytes is inhibited when the sodium-hyaluronate concentration in the medium separating the target cells from the lymphocytes reaches a certain concentration.[17]

The graft-versus-host reaction could be inhibited with sodium-hyaluronate when the donor cells are injected into the peritoneal cavity. Apparently, the spleen cells injected with sodium-hyaluronate do not find their target organ (spleen, liver), or if they do, their proliferation is inhibited.[19]

Sodium-hyaluronate seems also to influence the wound healing of articular cartilage, tendons, and fasciae. Relatively few experiments have been reported in this area, and therefore one has to regard these results as preliminary. When the dorsal fasciae of rabbits and guinea pigs and the long extensor tendons of the legs of rabbits were traumatized by mechanical damage, and after the trauma, viscous sodium-hyaluronate solution (sterile and pyrogen-free) was applied to the damaged area, the subsequent formation of granulation tissue and fibrous adhesions was considerably suppressed. Sodium-hyaluronate also suppressed formation of granulation tissue around foreign bodies (polyethylene).[23,45,47] All these investigations suggest that hyaluronic acid has a cell regulatory function that specifically affects the lymphomyeloid system during the inflammatory process.

EFFECT ON FRICTIONAL RESISTANCE

It has been generally accepted for a long time that the frictional resistance of those parts of the joint that move adjacent to each other (articular cartilage, synovial tissue, ligaments, tendons within their sheaths, walls of bursae) is decreased by the viscous synovial fluid. The viscosity of the fluid has been regarded as the key to this lubricating effect, and the high-molecular-weight hyaluronic acid as the essential component of the lubricating fluid.[36,40,58]

Recently, this joint lubrication was further defined by separating it into two problem areas—the lubrication of the *soft tissues* (ligaments and synovial tissue) and the lubrication of the cartilage surfaces.[40] The role of hyaluronic acid in diminishing the frictional resistance of soft tissues sliding across each other was confirmed. On the other hand, the same action of hyaluronic acid on cartilage sliding over cartilage was questioned. A glycoprotein fraction was found in the synovial fluid that decreased the coefficient of friction between moving cartilage surfaces.[57] The importance of hyaluronic acid as an agent that reduces the frictional resistance between the moving surfaces inside the joint, and between tendons and their sheaths, is still not fully understood.

ROLE OF THE CARTILAGE SURFACE

As described above, the surface layer of articular cartilage is impregnated with hyaluronic acid. One can visualize the two opposing cartilage surfaces and the thin layer of synovial fluid between as a continuous hyaluronic acid network. The hyaluronic acid network is anchored onto the collagen fibrillar matrix of the surface layer of cartilage of both sides. The space between the two collagen matrices is filled with the same hyaluronic acid molecular network that impregnates the collagen matrix. Therefore, dislocations between the two moving cartilage surfaces occur not between two rheologically different systems (solid cartilage and synovial fluid), but within the hyaluronic acid network. This concept has two important biologic implications. One, there are no asperities or ripples on the sliding surfaces. That is, the beautiful scanning electron micrographs showing the unhydrated cartilage—synovial fluid surface with its many crevices do not picture the real sliding surface. The real sliding surface is not the one that is exposed by breaking the continuity of the hyaluronic acid network, and its dehydrated picture in the electron microscope does not give the proper impression of a highly hydrated hyaluronic acid molecular network. Two, the hyaluronic acid impregnated cartilage surface that serves as a barrier against the movements of macromolecules in

and out of the cartilage is not distributed by the movements in the joint. Therefore, the integrity of this layer and the composition of the cartilage matrix is maintained. According to this hypothesis, the major role of hyaluronic acid on the cartilage surface is to provide the real sliding surfaces and to maintain the integrity of the cartilage matrix.

CONTROL OF CELL INVASION

There is no epithelial barrier on the surface of the synovial tissues that would prevent cell migration from these tissues into the synovial space and on the surface of the soft tissues and the cartilage of the joint. It has been proposed that hyaluronic acid prevents the invasion of cells into joint space.[8,10] This concept is especially important in view of the fact that in all acute or chronic inflammatory processes of the joint, both the concentration and the size of the hyaluronic acid molecules decrease, and at the same time, the cell population in the joint space increases. It is important to note that the pathological fluid is less effective in preventing the migration of the lymphomyeloid cells *in vitro* than normal fluid. These findings, while suggestive, do not present direct proof of the role of hyaluronic acid as a cell movement-controlling factor in the joint.

SODIUM-HYALURONATE AND VISCOSURGERY

In acute and chronic inflammation and in most degenerative processes of the joint, the concentration and molecular size of hyaluronic acid decreases in the synovial fluid. Consequently, the viscosity and elasticity of the fluid also decreases. We suggested that intra-articular application of highly purified (protein content <0.3%) concentrated (10 to 20 mg/ml) sodium-hyaluronate that contains fairly large molecules (molecular weight 1 to 3 million) of this biopolymer can influence the healing and regeneration of the cartilage and soft tissues of the joint. The rationale for this suggestion is that the injected hyaluronic acid will accumulate on the articular and synovial tissue surfaces, thereby "reinforcing" the natural barriers that are most probably deteriorated in the course of the pathologic process. Thus, the injection of hyaluronic acid into a diseased connective tissue compartment in which it is normally present can properly be called a macromolecular implantation. The main objective of the implantation is to increase the hyaluronic acid concentration in the joint well above the pathologic and even the normal level. Because this biopolymer is a natural component of the joint, it metabolizes by diffusion and probably by phagocytic activity of macrophages. Consequently, the elevated concentration in the joint caused by the injection decreases to normal level within days. Nevertheless, one expects that the invasion of the lymphomyeloid cells into the joint space is halted by the temporary increase of hyaluronic acid concentration by the same mechanism as the movement of these cells is inhibited by this biopolymer in vitro. Furthermore, the hyaluronic acid accumulated on the surface of the cartilage and soft tissues may block inflow of proteins (immune complexes) and proteoglycans into the joint space, thereby triggering a healing process in the cartilage and decreasing inflammation in the synovial tissue.

Experiments carried out in dog and rabbit joints indicate that intra-articular cartilage heals better when the sodium-hyaluronate concentration of the synovial space is increased after wounding by implantation of this biopolymer.[47] It was also found that the granulation reaction in subcutaneous tissue after surgical wounds[45] and in adhesion formation between tendon and tendon sheaths after mechanical damage decreases when sodium-hyaluronate is applied to the wounded surfaces.[47]

Viscous pastes (1% to 2%) of sodium-hyaluronate were applied around the lacerated and repaired profundus tendons of monkey fingers.[54] After 4 to 5 weeks of immobilization of the proximal interphalangeal joint in 90° of flexion, the range of motion showed significantly less flexion deformity in the sodium-hyaluronate-treated fingers than in the saline-treated controls. Sodium-hyaluronate did not interfere with the healing of tendons and decreased post-traumatic adhesion formation.

It must be pointed out that not all high-molecular-weight sodium-hyaluronate preparations can be used in in vivo studies. The conventionally prepared sterile, pyrogen-free sodium-hyaluronate dissolved in physiological buffer in a 1% to 2% solution and applied to various tissue compartments causes inflammation.[13] A highly purified, nonantigenic,[42,43] noninflammatory fraction of sodium-hyaluronate was separated from human umbilical cord and rooster comb specimens.[30] This special fraction showed no inflammatory reaction and was not antigenic when used in the most sensitive inflammatory test system.[25,26] This test system uses the eyes of owl monkeys for the quantitative evaluation of inflammatory agents, and it is more sensitive than any other system. This highly purified, noninflammatory, nonantigenic, high-molecular-weight (1–4 million) special fraction of sodium-hyaluronate was named Healon. The 1% solution of Healon dissolved in physiologic buffer (pH 7.2 ± 0.1) forms a solution that is 10^5 to 10^6 times more viscous than the buffer in which it is dissolved.

The therapeutic effect of high-molecular-weight sodium-hyaluronate is based on the viscoelastic nature of the molecules in solution. The protection of the cartilage and soft tissues surfaces,[47] the inhibition of cell motility[10] and phagocytosis, and the prevention of adhesion formation all depend on viscosity. When the viscoelastic solution of sodium-hyaluronate is used during surgical procedures, it serves as a protector of cell layers sensitive to mechanical damage, breaks up adhesions, maintains tissues, and separates tissue surfaces. Such use of viscous solutions in surgical procedures to protect and separate tissue surfaces during and after surgery is known as viscosurgery.[18]

The first studies of the effect of Healon injections on human arthritis were reported by

Rydell,* Helfet, and Peyron and Balazs.† They described an immediate improvement of joint function with painless motion in knee and hip joints when these joints were injected once or twice with 2 ml of 1% Healon solution. Peyron and Balazs measured the molecular weight of the sodium-hyaluronate in 11 synovial fluid specimens before and several weeks after treatment. These measurements suggested a positive correlation between the clinical improvement and the increased molecular weight of sodium-hyaluronate.

In a controlled study by Weiss and Balazs,† knee joints of osteoarthritic patients were injected twice with 2 ml of Healon solution with a 1-week interval between injections. Sixteen other patients received a sham injection, that is, a needle was introduced into the joint and an attempt was made to withdraw fluid, but nothing was injected. Healon injections significantly decreased the level of pain compared with the sham injections. The intra-articular injection of Healon caused a definite improvement in the clinical manifestations of the osteoarthritic condition in these patients, and this effect lasted 3 months after treatment.

Blikra and Bragstad,‡ in a double-blind experiment involving 60 patients, found that two injections of 2 ml of Healon into the knee joint significantly decreased pain and tenderness and increased the range of motion and walking time. The improvement lasted for 3 months. In another double-blind study§ Healon or control solutions of physiologic sodium chloride were injected in the knee joints of 54 patients with severe acute osteoarthritis (involving exudate and severe pain). The Healon-injected joints showed significantly less pain and an overall improvement of joint function compared with the joints injected with the physiologic salt solution. This improvement was especially pronounced when the effect of physiologic salt solution and Healon was compared in the same joint. The improvement found after Healon injection was greater and of longer duration than that observed after the previous injection of the salt solution.

Using the knee joints of 60 patients with mild chronic osteoarthritis (no exudate, mild pain), Stulberg compared the effect of the intra-articular injection of physiologic sodium chloride solution and Healon in a double-blind study.* Both treatments showed a definite decrease in pain and improvement of joint function after injection. Most of the parameters measured showed no significant difference between the treatment with Healon and that with physiologic salt solution.

All these studies suggest that intra-articular injection of physiologic salt solution improves the symptoms of osteoarthritis, especially in patients in whom the level of pain is not high and the inflammation, judged from exudate formation, is not great. One or two intra-articular injections of Healon, on the other hand, causes significant improvement of clinical symptoms in osteoarthritic joints with acute inflammation and severe pain.

Intra-articular injection of Healon in race horses with post-traumatic arthritis improved joint function and relieved lameness in 80% to 85% of the cases studied. This treatment was suggested and first demonstrated by Rydell, Butler, and Balazs.[46] Later, several investigations confirmed their findings.[4,†] It was also shown that the low-molecular-weight sodium-hyaluronate in the synovial fluid of the diseased joint is replaced by molecules of normal size after clinically successful Healon treatment.[14]

The viscoelastic nature of highly purified sodium-hyaluronate (Healon) makes it ideally suitable for viscosurgical procedures in ophthalmology. Healon has been used in retinal detachment surgery for the replacement of vittreus.[2,12,21,33,41] In anterior segment surgery it is used to protect the corneal endothelium and iris during cataract surgery, intraocular lens implantation, and corneal transplantation. Viscosurgical use of Healon also helps to

---

* Rydell N: Personal communication
† Weiss C, Balazs EA: Unpublished data
‡ Blikra G, Bragstad A: Personal communication
§ St. Onge R, Balazs EA, Weiss C: Unpublished data

* Stulberg D: Personal communication
† Swanstrom O, Lee W, Phillips M et al: Personal communication

maintain a deep anterior chamber during and after surgery.[37,31,39]

REFERENCES

1. **Alexandersson R, Nettelbladt E, Sundblad L:** Lactic dehydrogenase isoenzymes in arthritic synovial fluid: Effect of cortisol. Acta Rheumatol Scand 14:243, 1968
2. **Algvere P:** Intravitreal injection of high-molecular-weight hyaluronic acid in retinal detachment surgery. Acta Ophthalmol 49:975, 1971
3. **Andersen RB, Gormsen J:** Fibrin dissolution in synovial fluid. Acta Rheumatol Scand 16:319, 1970
4. **Asheim A, Lindblad G:** Intra-articular treatment of arthritis in race-horses with sodium hyaluronate. Acta Vet Scand 17:379−394, 1976
5. **Balazs EA:** Physical chemistry of hyaluronic acid. Fed Proc 17:1086, 1958
6. **Balazs EA:** Viscoelastic Properties of Hyaluronic Acid and Biological Lubrication. Univ. Michigan Med. Ctr. J. [Special Issue]:255−259, December, 1968
7. **Balazs EA:** Some aspects of the aging and radiation sensitivity of the intercellular matrix with special regard to hyaluronic acid in synovial fluid and vitreous. In Engel A, Larsson T (eds): Thule International Symposium: Aging of Connective and Skeletal Tissue. Stockholm, Nordiska Bokhandelns Forlag, 1969
8. **Balazs EA:** Structure and metabolism of connective tissue under physiological and pathological conditions. In Rüttner J, et al (eds).: Arthritis and Osteoarthrosis. Bern, Stuttgart, Verlag Hans Huber, Wien, 1971
9. **Balazs EA:** Ultrapure hyaluronic acid and the use thereof. United States Patent, 4,141,973, 1973.
10. **Balazs EA, Darzynkiewicz Z:** The effect of hyaluronic acid on fibroblasts, mononuclear phagocytes and lymphocytes. In Kulonen E, Pikkarainen J (eds): Biology of the Fibroblasts. London, Academic Press, 1973
11. **Balazs EA, Gibbs DA:** The rheological properties and biological function of hyaluronic acid. In Balazs EA (ed): Chemistry and Molecular Biology of the Intercellular Matrix III. New York, Academic Press, 1970
12. **Balazs EA, Hultsch E:** Replacement of the vitreous with hyaluronic acid, collagen and other polymers. In Irvine AR, O'Malley C (eds): Advances in Vitreous Surgery. Springfield, Charles C Thomas, 1976
13. **Balazs EA, Sweeney DB:** The use of hyaluronic acid and collagen preparations in eye surgery. In Schepens CL, Regan CDJ (eds): Controversial Aspects of the Management of Retinal Detachment, pp 200−202. Boston, Little, Brown & Co, 1965
14. **Balazs EA, Briller SO, Denlinger JL:** Na-hyaluronate molecular size variations in equine and human arthritic synovial fluids and the effect on phagocytic cells (in press)
15. **Balazs EA, Bloom G, Swann DA:** Fine structure and glycosaminoglycan content of the surface layer of articular cartilage. Fed Proc 25: 1817, 1966
16. **Balazs EA, Friberg S, Freeman MI** (unpublished data)
17. **Balazs EA, Friberg S, Darzynkiewicz Z** (unpublished data)
18. **Balazs EA, Miller D, Stegmann R:** Viscosurgery and the Use of Na-Hyaluronate in Intraocular Lens Implanation. Paper presented at the International Congress and First Film Festival on Intraocular Implanation, Cannes, France, 1979
19. **Balazs EA, Skopinska E, Darzynkiewicz Z** (unpublished data)
20. **Balazs EA, Watson D, Duff IF et al.** Hyaluronic acid in synovial fluid. I. Molecular parameters of hyaluronic acid in normal and arthritic human fluids. Arthritis Rheum 10:357, 1967
21. **Balazs EA et al.** Hyaluronic acid and the replacement of the vitreous and aqueous humor. In Modern Problems in Ophthalmology, 10:1, 1972
22. **Bartholomew BA, Perry AL:** Alpha-mannosidase activity in synovial fluid. Acta Rheumatol Scand 16:304, 1970
23. **Darzynkiewicz Z, Balazs EA:** Effect of connective tissue intercellular matrix on lymphocyte stimulation. I. Suppression of lymphocyte stimulation by hyaluronic acid. Exp Cell Res 66:113, 1971
24. **Decker B, McKenzie BF, McGuckin WF:** Zone electrophoretic studies of proteins and glycoproteins of bovine serum and synovial fluid. Proc Soc Exp Biol Med 102:616, 1959
25. **Denlinger JL, Balazs EA:** Replacement of the liquid vitreus with sodium hyaluronate in monkeys. I. Short term evaluation. Exp Eye Res 30:81−99, 1980
26. **Denlinger JL, El-Mofty Aly AM, Balazs EA:** Replacement of the liquid vitreus with sodium hyaluronate in monkeys. II. Long-term evaluation. Exp Eye Res 31:101−117, 1980
27. **Forrester JV, Balazs EA:** Inhibition of phagocytosis by high molecular weight hyaluronate. Immunology 40:435−446, 1980
28. **Gardner DL, Woodward D:** Scanning electron microscopy and replica studies of articular surfaces of guinea pig synovial joints. Ann Rheum Dis 28:379, 1969
29. **Gibbs DA, Merrill EW, Smith KA et al:** Rheology of hyaluronic acid. Biopolymers 6:777, 1968
30. **Gingerich DA:** The use of force plate in the measurement of equine joint function. In Powers YD, Powers TE (eds): Proceedings of Second Equine Pharmacology Symposium, pp 259−269. Colorado, American Association of Equine Practitioners, 1978
31. **Graue EL, Polack FM, Balazs EA:** The protective effect of Na-hyaluronate to corneal endothelium. Exp Eye Res 31:119−127, 1979
32. **Jasani MK, Katori M, Lewis GP:** Intracellular en-

zymes in synovial fluid joint diseases. Origin and relation to disease category. Ann Rheum Dis 28:497, 1969

33. **Klöti R:** Hyaluronsäure als Glasköpersubstituent. Ophthalmologica 165:351, 1971
34. **Laurent T:** Structure of hyaluronic acid. In Balazs EA (ed): Chemistry and Molecular Biology of the Intercellular Matrix II. New York, Academic Press, 1970
35. **McCall JG:** Scanning Electron Microscopy of Articular Surfaces. The Lancet 1194, 1968
36. **McCutchen CW:** Boundary lubrication by synovial fluid: Demonstration and possible osmotic explanation. Fed Proc 25:1061, 1966
37. **Miller D, Stegmann R:** Use of sodium hyaluronate in auto-corneal transplantation in rabbits. Ophthalmic Surg 11:19−21, 1980
38. **Ogston AG:** The Biological Functions of the Glycosaminoglycans. In Balazs EA (ed): Chemistry and Molecular Biology of the Intercellular Matrix III. New York, Academic Press, 1970
39. **Pape LG, Balazs EA:** The use of sodium hyaluronate (Healon^R) in human anterior segment surgery. Ophthalmology 87:699−705, 1980
40. **Radin EL, Paul IL:** A Consolidated View of Joint Lubrication. J Bone Joint Surg 54A:607, 1972
41. **Regnault F:** Acide hyaluronique intravitreen et cryocoagulation dans le traitement des formes graves de decollement de la retine. Bull Mem Soc F Ophthalmol 84:106, 1971
42. **Richter W:** Non-immunogenicity of purified hyaluronic acid preparations tested by passive cutaneous anaphylaxis. Int Arch Allergy Appl Immunol 47:211−217, 1974
43. **Richter W, Ryde E, Zetterstrom EO:** Non-immunogenicity of purified sodium hyaluronate preparations in man. Int Arch Allergy Appl Immunol 59:45−48, 1979
44. **Ruddy S, Austen KF:** The complement system in rheumatoid synovitis. I. An analysis of complement component, activities in rheumatoid synovial fluids. Arthritis Rheum 13:713, 1970
45. **Rydell NW:** Decreased granulation tissue formation after installment of hyaluronic acid. Acta Orthop Scand 41:307, 1970
46. **Rydell NW, Butler J, Balazs EA:** Hyaluronic acid in synovial fluid. VI. Effect of intra-articular injection of hyaluronic acid on clinical symptoms of arthritis in track horses. Acta Vet Scand 11:139, 1970

47. **Rydell NW, Balazs EA:** Effect of intra-articular injection of hyaluronic acid on clinical symptoms of osteoarthritis and on granulation tissue formation. Clin Orthop 80:25, 1971
48. **Schmidt K, MacNair MB:** Characterization of the proteins of certain post mortem human synovial fluids. J Clin Invest 37:708, 1958
49. **Schubert M, Hamerman DA:** A Primer on Connective Tissue Biochemistry. Philadelphia, Lea & Febiger, 1968
50. **Seppälä PO:** Synovial Fluid in Rheumatoid Arthritis. Scand J Clin Lab Invest [Suppl]16:79, 1964
51. **Seppälä PO, Balazs EA:** Hyaluronic acid in synovial fluid III. Effect of maturation and aging on chemical properties of bovine synovial fluid of different joints. J Gerontol 24:309, 1969
52. **Sliwinksi AJ, Zvaifler NJ:** The removal of aggregated and nonaggregated autologous gamma globulin from rheumatoid joints. Arthritis Rheum 12:504, 1969
53. **Sliwinksi AJ, Zvaifler NJ:** In vivo synthesis of IgG by Rheumatoid synovium. J Lab Clin Med 76:304, 1971
54. **St. Onge R, Weiss C, Denlinger JL et al:** A preliminary assessment of Na-hyaluronate injection into "No Man's Land" for primary flexor tendon repair. Clin Orthop 148:351−357, 1980
55. **Sundblad L, Jonsson E, Nettelbladt E:** Permeability of the synovial membrane to glycoprotein. Nature 192:1192, 1961
56. **Sundblad L, Jonsson E, Nettelbladt E:** Glycosaminoglycans and glycoproteins in synovial fluid. In Balazs EA, Jeanloz RW (eds): The Amino Sugars IIA. New York, Academic Press, 1965
57. **Swann DA, Radin EL, Weisser PA:** Separation of a hyaluronate-free lubricating fraction from synovial fluid. Nature 228:377, 1970
58. **Walker PS et al:** Mode of aggregation of hyaluronic acid protein complex on the surface of articular cartilage. Ann Rheum Dis 29:591, 1970
59. **Ward PA, Zvaifler NJ:** Complement-derived leucatactic factors in inflammatory synovial fluids of humans. J Clin Invest 50:606, 1971
60. **Winchester RJ, Agnello V, Kunkel HG:** Gamma globulin complexes in synovial fluids of patients with rheumatoid arthritis. Partial characterization and relationship to covered complement levels. Clin Exp Immunol 6:689, 1970
61. **Zvaifler NJ:** Breakdown products of C3 in human synovial fluids. J Clin Invest 48:1532, 1969

CHAPTER 5
MECHANICAL EFFICIENCY
OF THE KNEE JOINT

Arthur J. Helfet

Muscles acting on a weight-bearing joint such as the knee have three functions. The first is to maintain posture by stabilizing the leg when standing. The second is kinetic—to move the joint to the limits allowed by its configuration. The third is propulsive—to move the leg on the thigh against resistance. The knee, like other joints in the human body, is wonderfully designed to accomplish these functions with a maximum economy of muscle power. Barnett, Davies and Mac Conaill, in their comprehensive review of synovial joints, indicate the considerable achievement in conservation of muscle energy by the evolutionary conversion of multiaxial into biaxial joints.[1] In addition, there are the advantages in economy of effort in maintaining posture, in lifting, and in propulsion provided by a helicoid as compared with a hinge joint.

The postural function of muscles is to act as stabilizers. The newborn infant crumples to the ground. Barnett and co-workers demonstrate through comparative anatomy how the evolutionary trend toward uniaxial joints

makes for economy of muscle energy. The multiaxial joint requires much greater muscle power for stability in standing than does the biaxial joint. This is evidenced in the bulky muscles of the multiaxial shoulder joint compared with the leaner arm muscles, in most animals, for the biaxial elbow joint. In the animal's total economy the energy required for standing is wasteful. Muscle energy should be expended in moving the animal, especially in searching for food, and not dissipated in maintaining posture at rest. They cite the example of the members of the cat family which sit or lie down as soon as a burst of activity has ended. This avoids wasteful contraction of these postural muscles. Incidentally, the observation is made that

the almost complete inactivity of most of the muscles of the human body during standing, is one of the most striking ways in which a man is a more efficient machine than the great majority of mammals.[1]

A case in point is the muscle requirements of the elbow region of the spiny anteater compared with those of a dog. The anteater's elbow is capable of multiaxial movements, and accordingly, its arm and forearm bulge with muscles whose function is largely postural. The shape of the articular surfaces and the tension in the ligaments of the dog's elbow, in which only flexion and extension are possible, permit a more slender upper arm with flexor and extensor muscles only. The configuration of the knee joint in humans and the pattern of the capsular ligaments are perfectly designed to permit stability in standing with a minimum of muscle effort.

However, if the knee joint were a pure hinge joint, the effort to lift or propel the leg on the thigh against gravity would be enormous, many times as much as needed to pull it up

the helicoid planes of the knee joint. The strength and the energy required to pull a fish straight out of the water may be compared with playing it obliquely to the bank—or the strength required to lift the axle of an automobile compared with that required to lift it by pumping the handle of a jack. A child can push the shaft of a waterwheel (Fig. 5-1, *top*), but it takes a strong man to pull a full bucket of water out of the well (Fig. 5-1, *bottom*).

An engineer explains it as follows:* From the engineering point of view, the construction of the knee joint is brilliantly conceived. Muscle action is nothing more than contraction and mechanically can be considered only

* Helfet HT. Personal Communication.

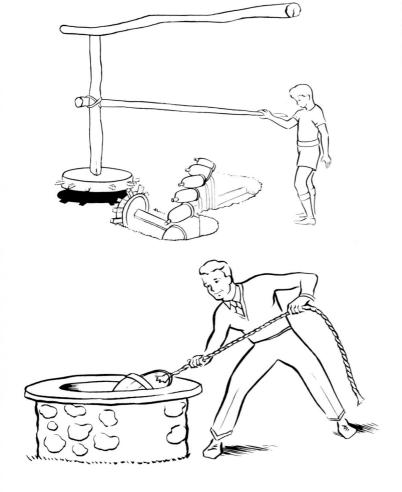

FIG. 5-1. A child can produce a greater volume of water by pushing the shaft of a waterwheel than a strong man can bring up by pulling a full bucket of water out of a well.

as tension—a "pulling force." To illustrate the effect of this, imagine trying to close a door—against a draft—by hooking a finger around the handle and pulling toward the hinge.

In the plan view shown in Figure 5-2, the effective action is a turning movement equal to the force F multiplied by the lever arm A, which is the distance from the point of application of the force to the center line of the hinge. As A is very small, a strong pull is required if there is to be any appreciable effect.

A similar position would apply to the knee —if it were a plain hinge operated by muscular pull—the lever arm being measured from the attachment point of the muscle to a line from the center of the hinge down the middle of the bone (approximately the length of the patellar ligament). An enormous muscular pull would be required to straighten the knee when weight-bearing, for instance, from the position of sitting on the haunches.

However, the actual construction of the joint results in a screw action. The femoral condyles, with the tibia, form a bicondylar joint that can rotate in bending, allowing partial rotation of the calf. The lateral condyle forms a ball joint with the tibia, while the medial tibial tuberosity follows the helical track provided for it on the medial condyle. The quadriceps muscles are attached in such a way that the tension they apply tends to rotate the calf, that is, they produce a torque that forces the tibia to screw itself up, thereby straightening the knee.

The mechanical advantage, or, in other words, the effectiveness of the force applied by the muscles, is increased greatly by this helical action. An illustration of this effect is the ease with which a heavy vehicle can be lifted by means of a screw-jack, whereas it would require a great deal of effort to raise it by a straight pull.

Figure 5-3 shows a model constructed to demonstrate the mechanical action of the knee joint. An eccentric ball-and-socket joint, which represents the action of the tibia on the lateral femoral condyle, is shown. The curved track represents the medial femoral condyle

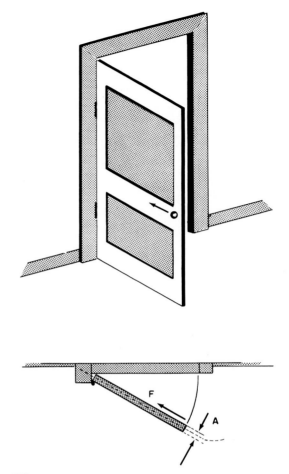

FIG. 5-2.

along which the tibia winds itself in extension and flexion. The rods simulating the femur and the tibia are a dark color on one half and a light color on the opposite half. When the knee is straight, the midlines of both are in continuity, but as the joint is flexed, they rotate on each other, and the proportions change.

EFFICIENCY OF MUSCLES

The efficiency of muscles is linked to training and fitness and is measured by the reaction of muscles to prolonged or increased activity. Should the stamina of the muscles be ex-

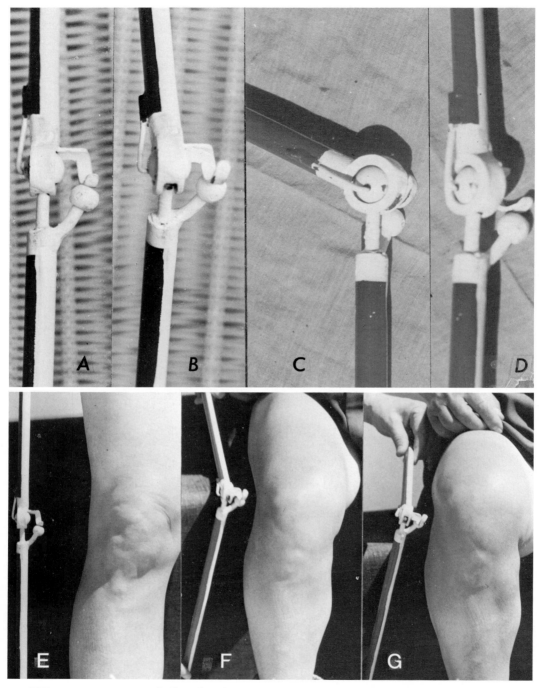

FIG. 5-3. An eccentric ball-and-socket joint represents the action of the tibia on the lateral femoral condyle. The curved part represents the medial femoral condyle along which the tibia winds itself in flexion and extension. **(A,B)** When the joint is extended, the colored strips are in alignment; as it bends and rotates, the proportions change. **C** and **D** are lateral oblique views of the model. The comparable rotation of the tibia on the femur is shown with leg straight **(E)**, with the knee partly flexed **(F)**, and completely flexed **(G).** Note the relationship between the tibial tubercle and the outer border of the patella.

hausted, they protest their willingness or ability to continue functioning. When the muscles controlling the knee tire, a stage of near paralysis is reached when the knee joint loses efficiency and is liable to collapse. I have seen this occur on steep mountain climbs when the legs are too tired to take another step. In ascending, the climber stops, but occasionally on descending the limb gives way altogether. Similarly, when the peronei are exhausted, the ankle may give way.

After extreme or repeated fatigue an effusion develops in the knee joint, accompanied by discomfort or even pain. At the end of a strenuous day the knee aches and, that night or the next day, feels stiff. A laborer or an athlete needs to nurse these symptoms; a hot bath, rest, and gentle exercise afford relief. Repeated or chronic fatigue, however, may result in organization of the effusion with formation of adhesions and stiffness that require more energetic treatment, including stretching by specific exercises or under anesthesia.

An example of such chronic fatigue was seen in a 35-year-old patient. He had not been athletic until 2 or 3 years previously and was without history of injury, when he became addicted to cycling and eventually to long-distance racing. During 3 months of strenuous daily training for a 65-mile road race, he complained of sessions of mild discomfort on the medial side of the right knee.

He completed the race successfully, in tenth place out of hundreds, but subsequently, he was conscious when walking, of weakness, insecurity, and limitation of bending the knee. On examination, no effusion was detected, but the extremes of flexion and extension were uncomfortable, and the joint as a whole was slightly lax. The articular surfaces of the right knee were more tender than those of the left. He could not squat or stand with the knee fully straight without pain. Presumably, the repeated, unwonted stress and fatigue had led to recurrent mild effusion that in time organized into fibrous adhesions and produced these symptoms and signs.

A program of isometric plus knee-stretching exercises was prescribed. As the range of movement improved, the symptoms lessened. When progress slowed, injections of a local anesthetic permitted more forceful stretching. Full recovery took 3 weeks.

This pattern of joint inefficiency develops in athletes who overtrain to exhaustion, especially at the beginning of the season. This should not be confused with the soreness of muscles after unaccustomed use, for which no treatment other than a hot bath and a measure of rest is needed.

The symptoms develop earlier after injury, in the weak and elderly, and when infirmity is due to neuromuscular disease. Other consequences of severe fatigue are muscle spasm, myositis, and ischemia, the extent of the symptom being related to the severity of the strain.

Deformities such as knock-knee, genu recurvatum, and leg-length disparity put muscles at a disadvantage and affect their performance.

Muscle inhibition occurs also as a reaction to pain. A sudden strain, a blow on the thigh, or the movement of a loose body in the knee may cause a sudden stab of pain, muscle inhibition, and giving way of the knee. Accurate diagnosis points the way to correct treatment. Training, designed to build up the muscles to withstand increasingly heavy loads, also increases strength and endurance and engenders the ability to avoid further strain. An adequate joint means well-trained, efficient muscles.

THE KNEE BRACE

The biomechanical design of the knee joint has evolved to conform to the requirements for strength, stability, and movement. This development occurred in response to the functional demands of the muscles of the thigh, which control the knee and which have achieved maximum strength and inherent stability with minimum muscle bulk. Not hinged but helical movement of the knee joint has evolved, and therefore the tibia rotates outward when the knee straightens and inward when the knee flexes. During movement in this normal flexural pathway under control of the muscles, the knee is stable, and tension in the muscles or ligaments does not occur at any point of flexion and extension.

As noted earlier, the muscles of the thigh are so disposed that when they are actively moving the knee joint while weight-bearing, only this helical pattern of movement occurs. That is, femur and tibia in concert follow a definite track, and while on this track the knee is stable and strong.

If the helical movement is blocked, for example, by a ruptured meniscus, the knee locks—that is, rotation is limited, and it is not possible to straighten or flex the joint completely. On the other hand, a torn ligament or capsular or muscle weakness may allow the tibia to go off the track, at which moment the knee becomes unstable and gives way, usually with pain and often with an audible click.

Various braces have been designed to support the knee and restore stability. Invariably, they consist of strong lateral supports with heavy firm fixation joined by straight-path hinges. When in use a conflict ensues between the muscle attempting to extend and flex the knee in its helical track and the constraining hinge action of the brace. This leads to excessive energy expenditure and causes limitation of movement at the point of ultimate conflict between muscle action and hinge design.

The helicoid knee brace is designed to insist on a helical pattern of movement, and so ensures stability without heavy lateral pillars or fixation. It is light, is applied firmly, and is strong enough in ordinary circumstances (i.e., in running and dodging and so on in football, tennis, and other games) to keep the tibia in its track on the femur. The brace acts only as a brake or guide to prevent deviation from the normal pattern of movement and to provide stability when the tibia threatens to run off its helicoid track. For example, if a runner, unprotected by the brace, stumbles or catches his toe, the tibia would be prevented from rotating inward on the femur during flexion or outward during extension, and would thus be at risk of running off its femoral track. The brace gives the damaged knee enough support to

prevent such a dislocation, and the wearer feels secure and free, and is usually able to run and play with the facility and agility of an individual with a normal knee.

The brace is robust enough to counter the usual adduction and abduction strains encountered in contact sports. It is not expected to withstand a heavy lateral tackle by an opposing football player coming at speed, but then, a suit of armor might be necessary to protect the knee from all such forces.

The forms of instability that follow ligamentous injury or muscle weakness are understood and well documented. But in osteoarthritis, in addition to the loss of surface by erosion, the urgent reactions of repair of damaged cartilage lead to changes of shape and depth in the articular surface that cause instability, often minimal, which is not always appreciated.

I am convinced that the resultant minor disorders of movements of one bone or another are a potent and frequent cause of pain and disability in the arthritic knee. These symptoms are usually dramatically relieved by wearing a brace: many patients who have been forced into inactivity and who limp with canes or crutches, are once again able to walk, climb stairs, and play games.

CHARACTERISTICS OF THE KNEE BRACE

The brace consists of a pair of thermoplastic, U-shaped shells connected to one another by stainless steel joints (Fig. 5-4). The shells embrace snugly the front of the thigh above, and the shin below the patella. Firm fixation is provided by two or four straps of elastic limb webbing with Velcro tapes. The locating shells are made of polycarbonate (Lexan), 3 mm thick and 25 mm wide. Each is padded on the inner surface with a 3-mm layer of close-cell polyethylene foam. The joints are riveted to the shells both proximally and distally, provision being made for flexion and extension. The lateral joint allows universal motion, and the medial is a simple pin-in-slot joint (Fig. 5-5), the pin being free to run along the slot as flexion and extension occur (Figs. 5-6, 5-7, 5-8).

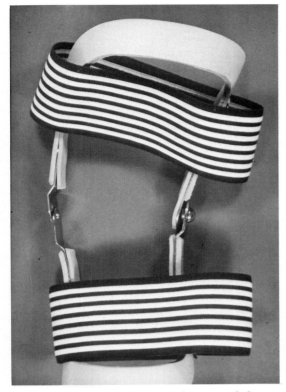

FIG. 5-4. The brace consists of a pair of thermoplastic U-shaped shells connected by stainless steel joints.

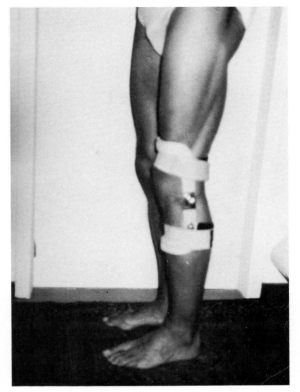

FIG. 5-5. The lateral joint is a hemisphere.

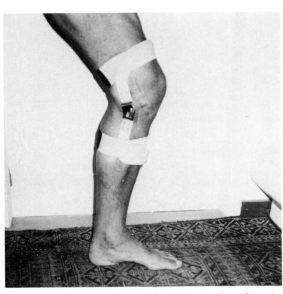

FIG. 5-6. The medial joint is a pin-in-slot, the pin being free to run along the slot as flexion and extension occur.

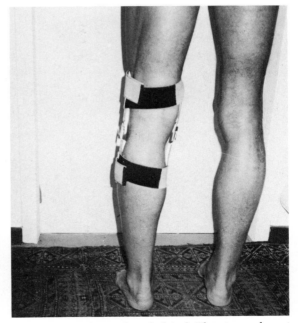

FIG. 5-7. The brace from behind. The straps do not hinder flexion.

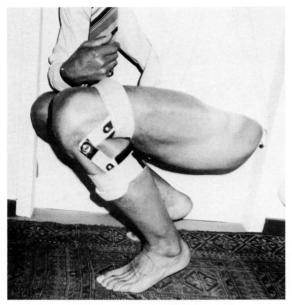

FIG. 5-8. Motion is free and without tension.

Hemispherical motion on the outer side, together with hinge plus sliding motion on the medial side, allows the knee to follow its own helical pattern of movement during flexion and extension without the brace fighting the natural range of movement of the knee. The snug fit of the shells and the rigidity of the stainless steel joints make certain that the tibia remains in its track on the femur, ensuring stability.

A brace weighing approximately 300 g (10¾ oz) is usually efficient in atheletics and football, tennis, squash, and other games in which stability and agility are essential. It has been worn by men weighing between 180 and 200 pounds in the rigorous contact sport of rugby football. In such strenuous sports the additional support of two short lengths of elastic bandage is recommended to prevent the brace from slipping and to insulate the frame.

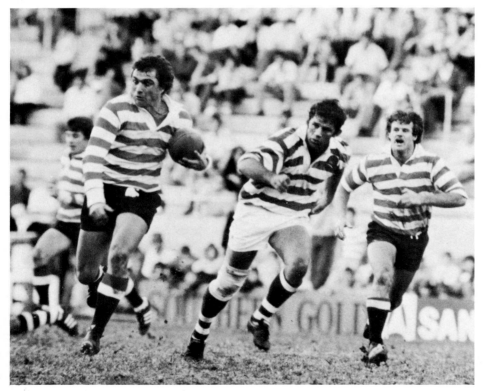

FIG. 5-9. (*Continued on facing page*)

FIG. 5-9. (*Continued*) The player with the brace on his right knee weighs nearly 200 lb (*bottom, facing page*). He had ruptured the posterior lateral capsule and ligaments and felt too insecure to contemplate playing. In the brace, he was always in the thick of the play in an 80 min game. (Newspaper photographs reproduced by kind permission of the Cape Town daily newspapers: the Cape Times and The Argus.)

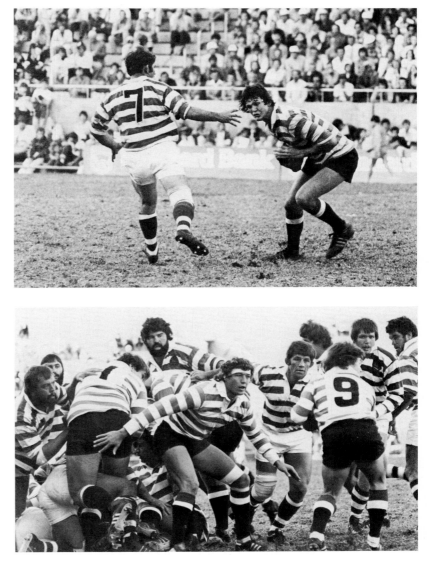

Of the first 100 braces, approximately 50% have been used for sports injuries, 25% have been used for post-traumatic arthritis in middle-aged sportsmen and in other osteoarthritics, 10% have been used for rehabilitation after operation for repair of torn ligaments or menisci, and 5% have been used as a pain-relieving measure for patients with mild rheumatoid or other forms of arthritis.

The brace has proved remarkably rewarding in all these cases. Most of the sportsmen and women have been able to return to their sporting activities (Fig. 5-9). After surgery the brace has relieved discomfort, and swelling has rapidly subsided. Osteoarthritics find that pain is relieved; fine muscle power recovers and often the normal range of movement is regained. Of the small number of rheumatoid patients, most stated that the brace helped to relieve pain.

Indications for using the brace are as follows:

1. Instabilities due to sports and athletic injuries.
2. Convalescence after injury or surgery.
3. Pain in the middle-aged arthritic knee in which instability is also a problem.

Contraindications include the following:

1. Significant destruction of the joint surfaces
2. Distortion of the limb by malunion or juxta-articular fractures
3. Distortion of the limb by muscle wasting or inefficiency after such diseases as poliomyelitis

On one very stout patient with a conical thigh shape and thin calves, the brace continued to slip, and its use was discontinued. It was not possible to provide adequate fixation.

For the arthritic patient it is preferable to allow a fair range of movement, even if the joint is unstable, painful, and swollen.

The brace is not indicated for locked knees with limited movement for those with instability due to severe erosion of cartilage or bone.

In summary, the brace is designed to restore stability and function by facilitating and maintaining helical movement as demanded by the controlling muscles of the knee.

REFERENCE

1. **Barnett CH, Davies DV, MacConaill MA:** Synovial Joints; Their Structure and Mechanics. New York, Longmans Green, 1961

CHAPTER 6

COMMON DERANGEMENTS OF THE KNEE JOINT AND THE MANNER OF THEIR PRODUCTION

Arthur J. Helfet

SEMILUNAR CARTILAGES

When bearing weight, the tibia rotates laterally as the knee joint straightens. It rotates medially when the knee bends. If this synchrony is prevented forcibly, as by the weight of the falling body, the rotator mechanism of the knee is injured. Certain cartilage tears are caused by nothing more than this disruption of the rotator mechanism of the knee. As far as I can determine, only the transverse fracture of the fibrotic medial meniscus of the elderly, which takes place at the junction of the anterior two-thirds and the posterior one-third, may be due to pressure or grinding between the femur and the tibia. All others can be explained by the violent stretching which must occur if medial rotation of the tibia in flexing the knee, or lateral rotation in extending it, is prevented. Similar forces are brought into play if while weight is borne when squatting or kneeling, a sudden twist occurs without ex-

tension or further flexion, or if the tibia twists outwardly while the body lurches backward and increases flexion of the knee.

These are the common causes of injury described by patients. The soccer player catches his toe, trips, and falls while the foot and the leg are rotated outward—flexion occurs without medial rotation (Fig. 6-1). The miner squats with knees fully flexed. An uncontrolled twist—rotation without synchronous extension—is followed by a searing pain, the signal of a tear in the cartilage (Fig. 6-2). One patient, a carpenter, was working in front of a chest of drawers in this attitude. A drawer had jammed. He wrenched vigorously to open it, and the drawer gave suddenly. He twisted on his right knee, and immediately he felt a searing pain over the medial cartilage. To relieve the agony he threw himself onto his left knee with identical consequences to that joint. At operation "bowstring" tears of both medial cartilages were found (Fig. 6-3).

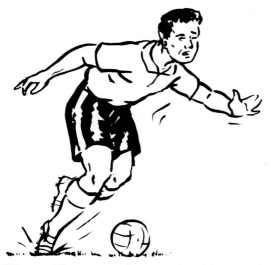

FIG. 6-1. The soccer player catches his toe, trips, and falls. The foot and the tibia are rotated outwardly while the knee flexes. Flexion occurs without medial rotation.

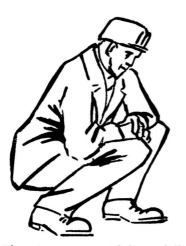

FIG. 6-2. The miner squats with knees fully flexed; an uncontrolled twist causes rotation without synchronous extension.

In another instance, a housewife knelt on her kitchen sink to open the cupboard above it (Fig. 6-4). The door opened suddenly. She lurched backward, increasing the flexion of the knee, but the thigh twisted inwardly instead of outwardly on the leg. A stab of pain signaled detachment of the anterior end of the

medial cartilage. When synchronous rotation is prevented, the knee will flex completely only if the rotator mechanism is stretched the full distance that the tibia normally rotates—in the adult, approximately ½ inch.

At first, presumably, the meniscus straightens out. To allow it to do so, a transverse or oblique split forms in the shorter or free edge (Fig. 6-5). This minor split is the most frequent finding and, as expected and observed also by Smillie,[6] is usually deeper in the lateral than in the medial meniscus because of the longer curve in the latter (Fig. 6-6). If no more than this occurs, the knee might well be symptomless after recovery from the acute injury, although the split itself would not heal. Occasionally, however, the split extends obliquely to form a mobile tag, which causes an irritating and recurring painful catch in the knee (Fig. 6-7).

It is interesting to note that the split usually occurs at the apex of the curve or in the anterior portion of the meniscus. This is to be expected, for the straightening out under tension would take place first in the more mobile portion. The posterior segments are more firmly fixed to the capsule.

A newspaper photographer, who often squatted and knelt in awkward positions to photograph dramatic moments in football matches, suffered this lesion. During clinical examination a twist would occasion a minor click which would "lock" the knee. The signs due to blocking of outward rotation of the tibia, which will be described later, were all present. Another twist and a further click unlocked the knee, which then moved freely and painlessly. He could perform these maneuvers himself with facility. At operation, no more than a pedicled tag on the free border of the medial meniscus was found. The cartilage was removed, and he has had no symptoms since.

If the range of unaccommodated movement is greater, it is achieved either by pulling the cartilage away from its attachments to the anterior cruciate (Figs. 6-8 and 6-9) or away from its capsular moorings at the back (Fig. 6-10) or by splitting the cartilage longitudinally to

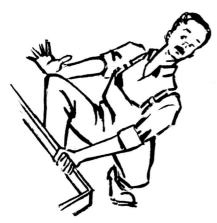

FIG. 6-3. The carpenter twists violently on his flexed right knee when the drawer gives suddenly. He feels a searing pain over the medial cartilage. To relieve the agony, he throws himself onto his left knee, with identical consequences to that joint.

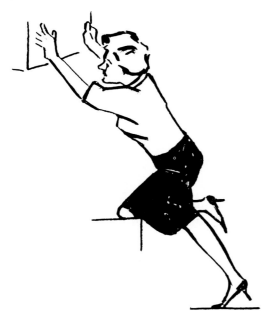

FIG. 6-4. The housewife kneels on her kitchen sink to open the cupboard above. The door opens suddenly. She lurches backward, increasing flexion of knee, but the thigh twists inwardly instead of outwardly on the leg.

allow the free border to form a bowstring across the joint (Figs. 6-11 and 6-12). Occasionally, instead of a longitudinal split, nearly the whole cartilage or the anterior half is wrenched from its peripheral attachments and is bowstrung across the intercondylar space (Fig. 6-13).

As the complete range of rotation is on the order of ½ in or a little more than 1 cm, the displacement need not be great. Allowing for the elasticity of the cartilage, it is always within this measurement.

Whatever the case, the figure-of-eight rotator mechanism is interrupted. As the anterior end of the cartilage is detached, the whole cartilage retracts, and a gap forms between the attachment of the cruciate ligament and the

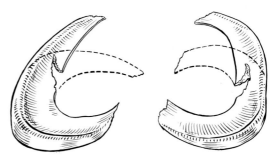

FIG. 6-5. The meniscus straightens out. To allow it to do so, a transverse or oblique split forms in the shorter or free edge.

Split or parrot beak tear of
free edge of meniscus

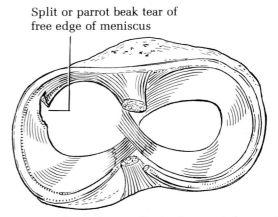

FIG. 6-6. This minor split is the most frequent finding.

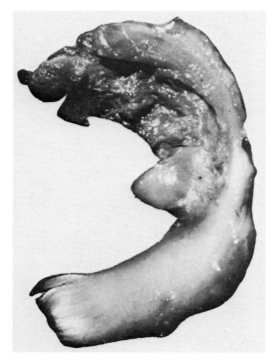

FIG. 6-7. Split posterior horn and a mobile tag, which causes an irritating and recurring painful catch in the knee.

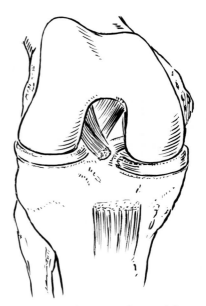

FIG. 6-9. Retracted anterior horn of the medial meniscus.

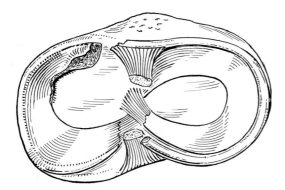

FIG. 6-8. After detachment from the cruciate ligament and the tibial spine, the anterior horn retracts; the gap which forms between the attachment of the cruciate ligament and the torn edge may be recognized at operation. Note the ruffled inner edge of the retracted meniscus.

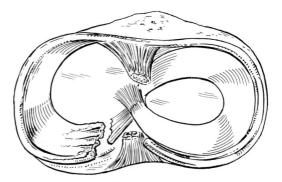

FIG. 6-10. Rupture of its firm attachments to the cruciate ligament and the posterior capsule produces the ragged retracted posterior horn.

torn edge. At operation the gap may be recognized; in a young patient, the free edge of the cartilage will present a ruffle which raises it from the surface of the tibia (Fig. 6-8). The front half of the cartilage is slack and looks too long, and the inexperienced may consider it a "lax cartilage." Sometimes the torn tip of cartilage is coiled up on itself and, as Sir Robert Jones[7] aptly described, "had undergone changes in the loose anterior extremity of the semilunar of the nodular type, some being as

PLATE 6-1. Lesions of semilunar cartilage.

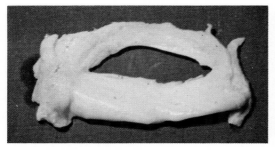

(A) Bowstring meniscus.

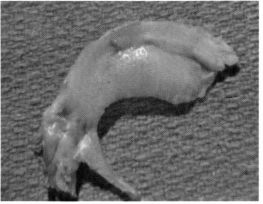

(B) Tear of posterior horn.

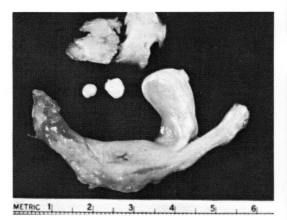

(C) Pedicled tear of posterior horn with loose bodies, fragments of abraded articular cartilage.

(D) Peripheral tear of a discoid meniscus.

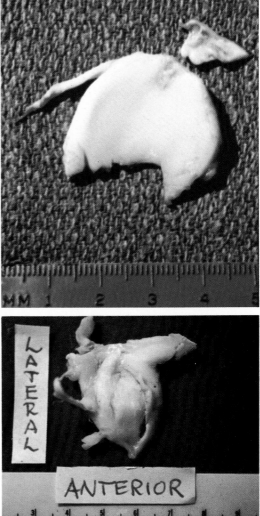

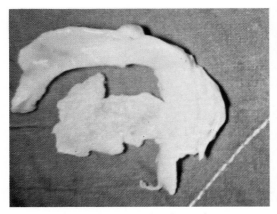

(E) Bowstring tear of a discoid meniscus.

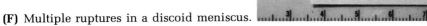

(F) Multiple ruptures in a discoid meniscus.

PLATE 6-1. Lesions of semilunar cartilage. (Continued)

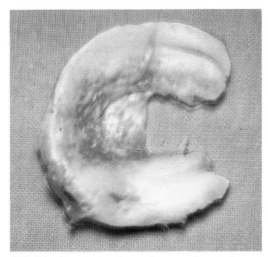

(G) Displaced horizontal tear in a lateral meniscus.

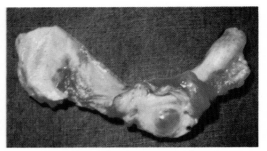

(H) Cyst of a medial meniscus.

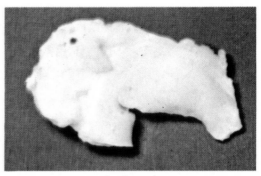

(I) Cyst of a lateral meniscus.

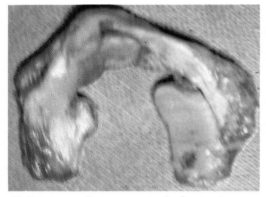

(J) Long-standing rupture of a bowstring meniscus with retraction.

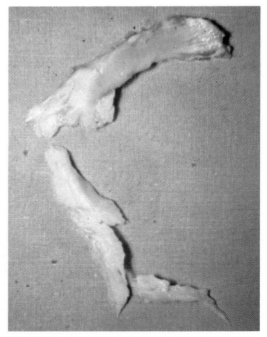

(L) Residual posterior horn of a medial meniscus and a regenerated anterior horn.

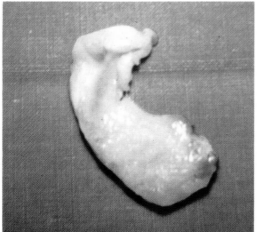

(K) Separated retracted meniscus.

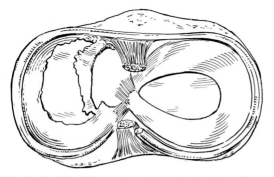

FIG. 6-11. The "bowstring," or bucket-handle, results from splitting of the cartilage longitudinally to allow the free border to bowstring across the joint. The separation is roughly equivalent to the distance the tibia normally rotates.

Complete peripheral
detachment of meniscus

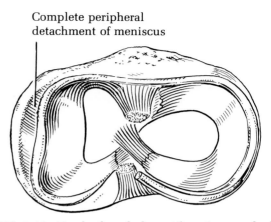

FIG. 6-13. Nearly the whole cartilage is wrenched from its peripheral attachments and bowstrings across the joint.

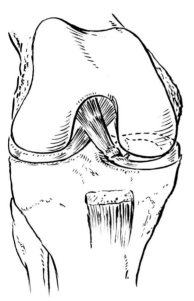

FIG. 6-12. Diagram of bowstring tear from the front.

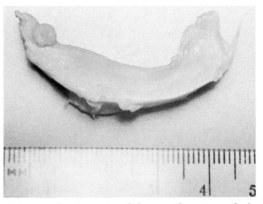

FIG. 6-14. The torn tip of the cartilage is coiled up on itself and "had undergone changes in the loose anterior extremity of the semilunar of the nodular type, some being as lumpy and large as a pea."

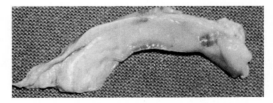

FIG. 6-15. In an older patient, retraction causes a thickening of the anterior half of the cartilage, and a heaped-up mass is formed in the anterior compartment of the joint.

lumpy and large as a pea" (Fig. 6-14). In an older patient with fibrotic and less resilient cartilages, retraction causes a thickening of the anterior half of the cartilage, which is yellowish, hard, and triangular in section, and a heaped-up mass is formed in the anterior compartment of the joint (Fig. 6-15). The lump so formed produces a pattern of erosion over the corresponding area of articular carti-

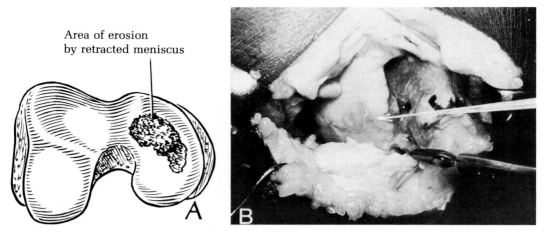

FIG. 6-16. (**A**) Arrow points to the pattern of erosion created by heaped-up retracted anterior horn of medial meniscus. (**B**) Erosion by detached anterior horn.

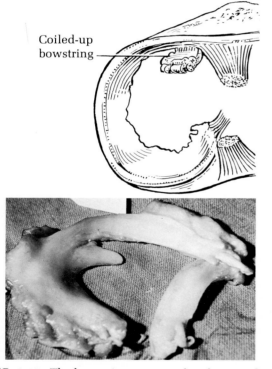

FIG. 6-17. The bowstring snaps and coils up at the fixed end in the anterior compartment.

lage on the anteromedial part of the weight-bearing surface of the medial femoral condyle. After the joint is opened at operation, the observation of this mark or depression or erosion immediately confirms the diagnosis (Fig. 6-16). As this type of cartilage tear presents its own clinical features and sequelae, it should be known as the "retracted" cartilage to distinguish it from the "bucket-handle" cartilage, which itself should be more aptly named the bowstring cartilage. In the latter type of injury the whole or part of the cartilage is bowstrung across the joint, and the symptoms are more severe than in the case of the retracted cartilage. But if in the first attack or subsequently, the bowstring snaps and coils up at the fixed end in the anterior compartment, the clinical picture resembles that of the retracted variety (Fig. 6-17). The first reaction to the snapping of the bowstring is a measure of relief, for the retracted cartilage is so much more comfortable to the patient than is the bowstring. Only later do the sequelae cause symptoms. Manipulation for reduction of the displaced bowstring frequently results in snapping of the bowstring again, bringing relief although temporary. Eventually meniscectomy is necessary. The bowstring injury produces a pattern of erosion on the articular cartilage covering the intercondylar border of the condyle of the femur (Fig. 6-18).

Less frequently, the posterior end of the cartilage is torn (Fig. 6-19). Because the anterior half of the meniscus is mobile with a defined coronary ligament, injury results in a different type of rupture from that in the posterior horn, which is integrated with the capsule in that

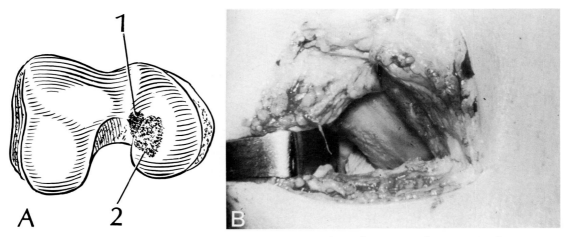

FIG. 6-18. (**A**) Drawing shows the pattern of erosion from the cruciate ligament in the bowstring meniscus (1) and the approximate pattern from the bowstring meniscus itself (2). (**B**) An operative photograph of the same area is included for comparison.

FIG. 6-19. (**A**) Tears of the posterior end of the meniscus. (**B**) Squashed pedunculated tags in triangular fibrotic cartilage of older patient, the "fish tail" meniscus.

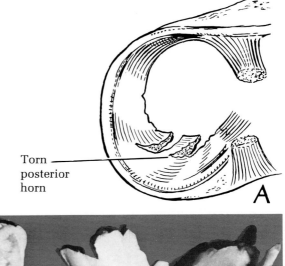

Torn posterior horn

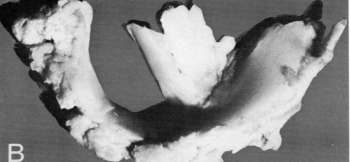

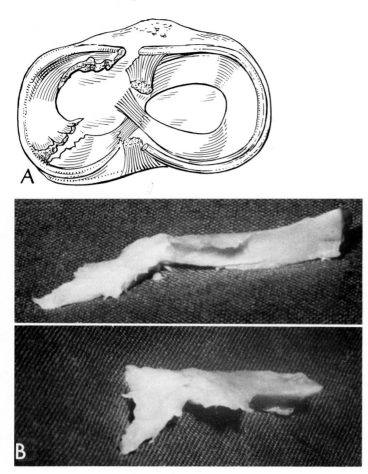

FIG. 6-20. In older people, the anterior half or two thirds of the retracted cartilage thickens. Later, another traumatic incident causes a transverse tear in the posterior half of the cartilage. The torn back end of the front part has a splayed, squashed, and scalloped edge (**A, B**). (**C**) Two fragments which have obviously been separated for some time by a complete transverse tear.

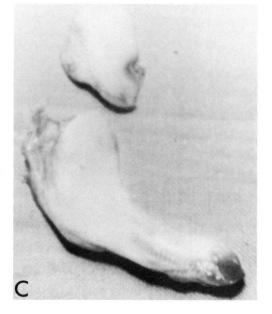

area. The meniscus does not retract but splits in its substance. Only twice have I found the whole back end of the cartilage wrenched from its attachments and the entire cartilage coiled in the anterior compartment. The first of these injuries was sustained during an amateur wrestling match and the second during a soccer scrimmage. We were unable to reconstruct the exact mechanism, except to establish that the injury in each case took place while the knee was well flexed. It is significant that these were the only cartilage injuries in which limitation of extension of the knee was more than 20°, and the block had the elastic consistency mentioned by Sir Robert Jones.

Occasionally violent distraction of the cartilage causes a horizontal split, but rarely does it occur over the whole length of the meniscus. A tear of the inferior layer may pedicle toward the center of the joint, and in two instances it was found insinuated peripherally between the meniscus and the capsule, locking the joint in a particularly painful manner (see Plate 6-1).

When distracted, the hard, fibrotic meniscus in an elderly person tends to pull off from its anterior attachments to the cruciate ligaments and then retracts backward. The anterior half or two-thirds of the cartilage, as described earlier, thickens and forms a heaped-up mass which causes grumbling and increasingly severe symptoms.

Often another and minor traumatic incident causes an acute exacerbation of symptoms that necessitates surgery. At operation a complete transverse tear in the posterior half of the cartilage is found (Fig. 6-20). The torn back end of the front part has a splayed, squashed, and scalloped edge, the fish-tail meniscus. The remaining fragment of the meniscus is relatively normal for the age of the patient. The condition of the fractured end does suggest that it has been nipped off by pressure between the femur and the tibia. It seems that the heaping up or thickening caused by the anterior retraction is all taken up in the front portion and that the weight-bearing surfaces eventually grind through the junction between the thickened and the normal portions of the cartilage.

Alternatively, the second traumatic incident distracts the cartilage, but, as the anterior portion is too thick to glide between the weight-bearing surfaces, the posterior end is wrenched off at the line of the obstruction. Detachment of the anterior horn with retraction occurs frequently, whereas detachment of the posterior horn is uncommon. On the other hand, multiple longitudinal splits of the posterior horn with or without anterior extensions to form a bowstring are comparatively frequent, but these splits are rare in the anterior horn. This is understandable. The more mobile and loosely bound anterior horn tears more easily from its attachments, and the more firmly held posterior horn tears in its substance. In the young, in whom the meniscus is stretchable, the splits are longitudinal. In the aged fibrotic cartilage, the split is transverse.

PATTERNS OF ARTICULAR EROSION

Lesions of the semilunar cartilages result in specific patterns of articular erosion. Each has its own clinical features, though they do tend to merge. Some indication has been given already of the effects of undue tension on the cruciates and the patella by the displaced bowstring tear and by the heaped-up retracted cartilage. They are repeated here for completeness.[4,5]

When rotation of the tibia is prevented during extension of the knee, the cruciate is tensed. It impinges on the lateral side of the medial femoral condyle and in time erodes the surface of the articular cartilage in this area. In turn, the cruciate ligament suffers from the continuous or recurring tension and is slowly stretched, with consequent laxity of the joint; at operation it may show a raw area of granulation on its otherwise shining surface.

The string of the bowstring cartilage etches its pattern medially and posteromedially to that of the cruciate ligaments (see Fig. 6-18).

The effect of the retracted cartilage differs with age. The youthful soft semilunar cartilage is heaped up or ruffled. The anteromedial part of the weight-bearing surface of the medial femoral condyle comes into contact with the thickened anterior part of the retracted cartilage when the knee is extended and thus is slowly worn away (see Fig. 6-16). But because of the protrusion of the femoral condyle, the area of erosion never reaches the edge (see Fig. 7-4). Consequently, after the torn cartilage is removed and full extension and rotational alignment of the femur and the tibia are regained, normal articular cartilage is brought back to the weight-bearing area; this is one reason why, however long its history and whatever the age of the patient, it is worthwhile removing the retracted cartilage.

At operation on older patients the semilunar cartilage may be yellowish and hard. It forms a shorter triangle on section because the free edge has contracted. The narrow hard cartilage tends to erode a more linear groove on the femoral condyle, and the area of erosion seems to extend further backward (Fig. 6-21). At this age, too, transverse tears in the middle third of the cartilage are more common (see Fig. 6-20). The torn end of the front part has a splayed, squashed, and scalloped edge. It seems that the heaping up or thickening caused by the anterior retraction is all taken up in this front portion and that eventually the weight-bearing surfaces nip it off at this junction between the thickened and the normal portions of the cartilage. Therefore, the anterior erosion extends and broadens out further back (Fig. 6-22). Tears of the posterior horn of the cartilage produce a rather broad pattern, but these have not been observed as often as the anterior patterns—probably because this series includes very few patients, such as miners, who normally work in a squatting position.

In time, the posterior horn tear etches its pattern of erosion, as is to be expected, further back on the medial condyle (see Figs. 6-21 and 6-22).

The lateral condyle has a smaller, rounder articular surface (Figs. 6-23 to 6-25).

The third pattern of erosion concerns the medial border of the patella and the surface of the femur with which it is in contact (Fig. 6-26). Attention has been drawn to the effect produced by inadequate excursion of the tibial tubercle on the relationships of the patella and the femur. Normally, in full extension, the line of action of the quadriceps on the patellar ligament settles the patella comfortably on the trochlear surface of the femur. When the tibial tubercle halts short of this line, the patella will deviate medially as the knee extends, particularly when the quadriceps contracts against increased resistance, as in climbing and descending stairs.

It is tensed against the medial slope of the trochlear surface of the femur, and the tension is greatest over the areas of the patella labeled A and B in Figure 1-17 and area T (see Fig. 1-19) of the femur. These are the sites of articular cartilage erosion (Fig. 6-27).

During flexion from complete extension, the increased medial pull on the whole mechanism produces increased pressure by the patella as it slips downward and backward on the extension of the trochlear surface on the medial condyle of the femur, and gradually the complete pattern of traumatic arthritis of the knee is etched (Fig. 6-28).

Normally, in the flexed position the patella tilts onto its medial articular surface. This tilt is accentuated in the blocked knee and will be present even in the position of fullest extension (Figs. 6-29 and 6-30).

A review of two personal series of operations for cartilage injuries reveals that retracted and bowstring cartilages are the most frequent consequences of injury (80.6%—see

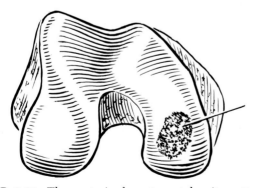

FIG. 6-21. The posterior horn tear etches its pattern (*arrow*) farther back.

FIG. 6-22. The posterior horn tear extends and widens the area of erosion further back. The harder meniscus of the older patient scores the surface more deeply.

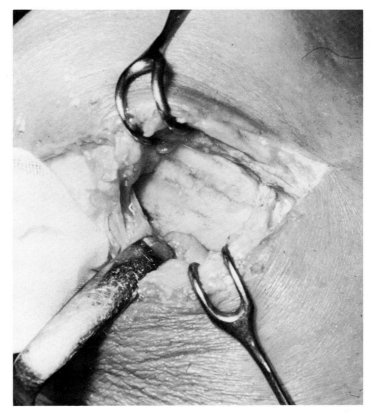

FIG. 6-23. In this cadaveric specimen, note the tear in the cruciate ligament with retraction of the anterior horn of the lateral meniscus and the corresponding patterns of erosion. The medial condyle is unaffected. (Courtesy Royal College of Surgeons, England)

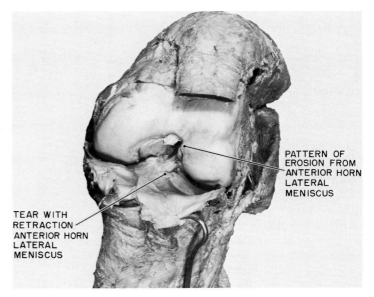

PATTERN OF EROSION FROM ANTERIOR HORN LATERAL MENISCUS

TEAR WITH RETRACTION ANTERIOR HORN LATERAL MENISCUS

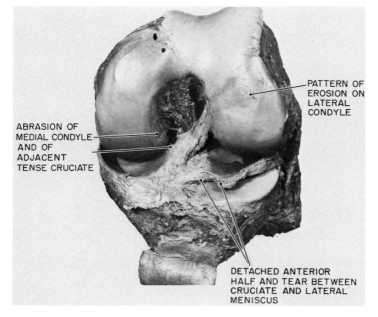

ABRASION OF
MEDIAL CONDYLE
AND OF
ADJACENT
TENSE CRUCIATE

PATTERN OF
EROSION ON
LATERAL
CONDYLE

DETACHED ANTERIOR
HALF AND TEAR BETWEEN
CRUCIATE AND LATERAL
MENISCUS

FIG. 6-24. Cadaveric specimen of displaced anterior half of lateral meniscus. The ligament uniting the anterior horn of the lateral meniscus and the cruciate ligament is partly torn. The infrapatellar pad of fat has been removed to demonstrate the imprint of the scar of the fat pad and the anterior horn of the meniscus on the upper surface of the tibia and the opposing articular surface of the lateral femoral condyle. (Courtesy Royal College of Surgeons, London)

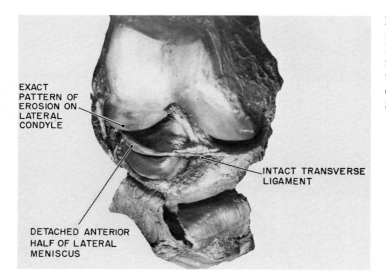

EXACT
PATTERN OF
EROSION ON
LATERAL
CONDYLE

INTACT TRANSVERSE
LIGAMENT

DETACHED ANTERIOR
HALF OF LATERAL
MENISCUS

FIG. 6-25. Cadaveric specimen of bowstring lateral meniscus. Nearly the whole lateral meniscus has been wrenched from its peripheral attachments. Note the pattern of erosion on the lateral condyle. (Courtesy Royal College of Surgeons, London)

Table 6-2). Bowstring tears exceeded the retracted cartilages by 11% in the first series, and by 6.8% in the second series of medial cartilage injuries (Table 6-3), but with increasing age the relative incidence of anterior tears increased (Tables 6-5 and 6-6). This must mean that as the cartilage becomes less resilient and more fibrotic, it is more liable to tear from its ligamentous moorings than to split in its substance.

CYSTS OF THE SEMILUNAR CARTILAGES

Cysts of the cartilages should be mentioned, because most, if not all, are probably traumatic in origin and degenerative in character.

FIG. 6-26. Drawings show areas of erosion due to local compression on the medial trochlear slope of the femur. Operative photograph shows erosions on the medial slope of the trochlear groove.

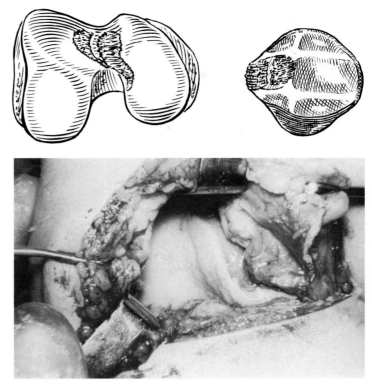

FIG. 6-27. (*Left*) Axial view of right patella, showing erosion of articular cartilage in area B and of corresponding area of trochlear surface of femur. (*Right*) Degenerative changes on medial articular surface of patella.

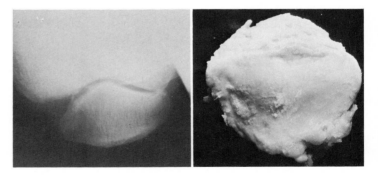

TABLE 6-1. INCIDENCE OF TEARS OF THE SEMILUNAR CARTILAGE—PERCENTAGE OF 627 CASES BY AGE GROUP

Age Group	Percentage
Under 16	3
10 to 20	12
20 to 44	53
45 and over	32

TABLE 6-2. TYPES OF CARTILAGE INJURY (SERIES 1—232 CASES)

	Number	Per Cent
Retracted cartilages	81	34.9
Bowstring or bucket-handle cartilage	106	45.7
Posterior tears	26	11.2
Other tears	19	8.2

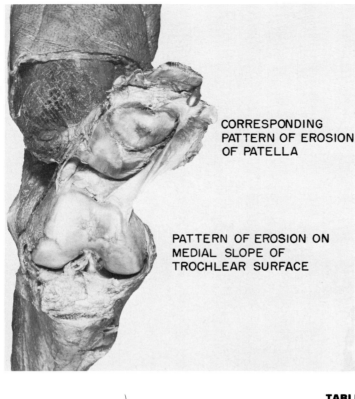

CORRESPONDING
PATTERN OF EROSION
OF PATELLA

PATTERN OF EROSION ON
MEDIAL SLOPE OF
TROCHLEAR SURFACE

FIG. 6-28. This perspective of the retracted anterior horn of the medial meniscus demonstrates the comparable scarring of articular cartilage on the patella and the trochlear surface of the femur. Note the preponderance of damage on the medial surfaces.

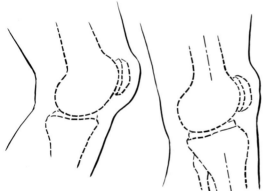

FIG. 6-29. (*Left*) Extension and lateral rotation are limited in traumatic arthritis of the knee. In the fullest extension possible, the patella remains perched on the trochlear extension of the medial femoral condyle. (*Right*) In normal full extension, the patella rests comfortably in the trochlear groove.

I have never seen a cystic cartilage at operation in which there was no evidence of injury. An interesting feature is that the cyst forms in the vascular edges of the cartilages. A cyst in a bowstring cartilage is invariably found in the

TABLE 6-3. TYPES OF MEDIAL CARTILAGE INJURY (SERIES 2—627 CASES)

	Number	Per Cent
Retracted cartilages	191	44.7
Bowstring cartilages	220	51.5
Isolated posterior tears	16	3.8

TABLE 6-4. TYPES OF LATERAL CARTILAGE INJURY (SERIES 2—627 CASES)

	Number	Per Cent
Anterior tears	28	71.8
Posterior tears	11	28.2

TABLE 6-5. TYPES OF INJURY RELATED TO AGE OF PATIENT (SERIES 1—232 CASES)

	Number and Percentage of Cases	
Age	Retracted Cartilage	Bowstring Cartilage
10 to 19	14 (35%)	26 (65%)
20 to 44	53 (43%)	70 (57%)
45 and over	14 (58%)	10 (42%)

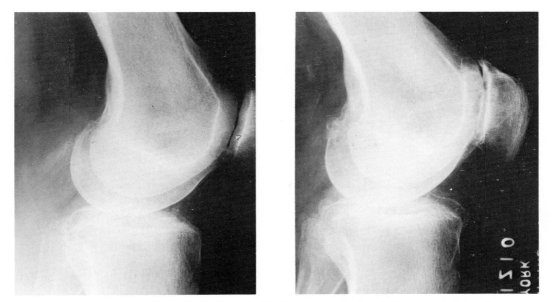

FIG. 6-30. Position of patella in the arthritic knee with flexion deformity. (*Left*) early osteoarthritis; (*Right*) late osteoarthritis.

TABLE 6-6. TYPES OF INJURY RELATED TO AGE OF PATIENT (SERIES 2—627 CASES)

| | Number and Percentage of Cases | |
Age	Retracted Cartilage	Bowstring Cartilage
10 to 19	28 (28%)	72 (72%)
20 to 44	60 (39%)	93 (61%)
45 and over	103 (65.5%)	54 (34.5%)

part attached to the capsule. Although they are sometimes found in the medial meniscus, the majority of cysts form in the middle third of the lateral meniscus, where the meniscus is separated from the capsule by the popliteus tendon and two folds of synovium. Smillie[6] reports an incidence of 2.5% of cystic change in medial and of 22.5% in lateral meniscus tears (Fig. 6-31).

Barrie's recent investigations support these views.[1] He found that 7.1% of surgically excised menisci, by gross and microscopic examination, contained one or more cysts. All were associated with tears, either primarily horizontal or with a horizontal component. Channels leading from the tear to the cysts were often demonstrable, and in some cases of osteoarthritis, detritus of bone was found at

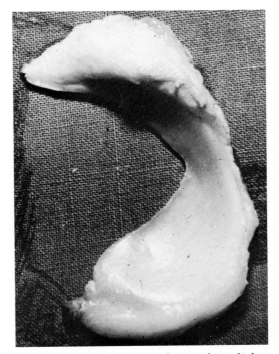

FIG. 6-31. Cyst of anterior horn of medial meniscus.

the periphery of these channels. The fluid resembles synovial fluid histochemically, a factor that discounts the concept of primary myxoid degeneration.

As the cysts arise in its substance, only excision of the meniscus is curative; otherwise, recurrence is common.

Synovial Cysts

Synovial cysts or ganglia arising completely intra-articularly in the intercondylar space are rare. Only four have been found in my experience of over 2500 knee operations. Two developed in the torn attachments between the anterior horn of the medial meniscus and the cruciate ligament (Fig. 6-32), and two arose in the synovium enveloping the cruciate ligaments. One patient in his early fifties suffered for 4 months from unceasing and finally almost constant pain in the knee. At first, swelling and limitation of movement were not remarkable. When, after this time, he sought orthopaedic opinion, an indefinite but tender

swelling could be felt in the posterolateral joint line. Clinically, the posterior horn of the lateral cartilage was tender. Flexion and internal rotation were limited by pain, and on maneuver a click was elicited. At operation for excision of the lateral meniscus, the posterior horn was found to be torn, and during the approach and its detachment, an enormous cyst containing thick yellowish fluid was opened. It stemmed from the attachment and synovial sheath of the cruciates and was tense in the intercondylar and posterolateral space. Removal of the meniscus and most of the wall relieved his pain and other symptoms. Unlike true cartilage cysts, these do not arise from the substance of the meniscus.

DISCOID LATERAL CARTILAGES

Discoid cartilages of all degrees are more liable to injury than normal cartilage. The free edge is shorter and more curved than that of

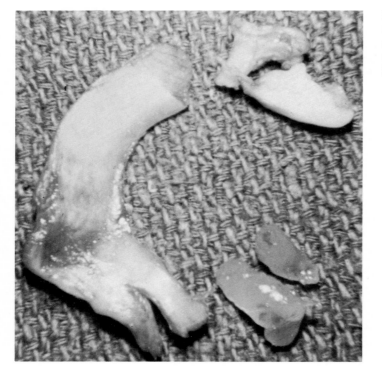

FIG. 6-32. Two synovial cysts developed in the attachments between the anterior horn of the medial meniscus and the cruciate ligament. Note the fractured posterior horn.

the normal lateral meniscus, and transverse and oblique splits are common. Also, the cartilage is thicker in its substance and therefore is vulnerable to lesser strains.

THE CRUCIATE AND THE CAPSULAR LIGAMENTS

Isolated ruptures of the cruciate ligaments are rare and of little clinical significance. Occasionally, when operating for a torn medial cartilage, one finds that the anterior cruciate ligament has been torn from its insertions in the tibia. The injury was violent enough to disrupt the cartilage and the cruciate from their moorings at the same time. But this knee does not demonstrate anteroposterior instability preoperatively or postoperatively, and removal of the cartilage cures all symptoms. Moreover, it is not possible to diagnose the coincidental rupture of the cruciate ligament before operation. Loss of rotation is present because of the injury to the rotator mechanism. No abnormal movement is possible.

By orthopaedic custom, anteroposterior instability of the tibia on the femur is considered pathognomonic of tears of the cruciate ligaments. However, this sign is present only if the capsule is weak and has been injured on one side or the other as well (see Fig. 22-4).

On no occasion has an isolated rupture of the cruciates been detected preoperatively, and it is difficult to imagine a knee in which anteroposterior laxity is possible without weakness in the capsule on one side. So that, whereas a displaced meniscus blocks the rotator mechanism, rupture of the cruciates with its concomitant capsular weakness results in loss of control of helical movement. Normally, the figure-of-eight mechanism keeps the tibia on a well-defined track on the medial condyle of the femur until it has wound itself to stability in full extension. Loss of control due to rupture of the cruciates and the medial capsule results in a type of instability in which the tibia leaves the curved track and slides straight forward from the medial condyle of the femur. This weakness, or anteroposterior

glide, has become the standard test for cruciate ligament injury. However, in any such knee, if the tibia is first rotated outward to its full extent on the femur, (i.e., if it is screwed home), anteroposterior glide can no longer be elicited.

Stabilization by external rotation of the leg may be demonstrated by the patient. Before weight-bearing, the foot is placed on the ground in lateral rotation. This means that the whole limb from the hip downward is turned outward. While the leg is straightened as weight is taken, the knee may be stabilized by turning the femur medially on the tibia (Fig. 6-33). Mitchell (quoted in Helfet[3]) reported one patient who, after 5 months of stumbling and falling, was ready for operation but refused further treatment when he discovered this trick movement. Stabilization by this method may be confirmed clinically in most patients.

Another observation is of clinical interest. When rupture of the cruciates is accompanied by displacement of a semilunar cartilage, anteroposterior glide may be elicited, but complete passive external rotation of the tibia is not possible. In this instance, treatment demands removal of the cartilage as well as extra-articular tendon transposition.

MECHANISM OF INJURY

When the helical element in movement of the knee joint is forcibly prevented, the rotator mechanism is disturbed. When the force is no more than the weight of the body, as in household and most athletic injuries, the semilunar cartilages seem to be able to take the brunt. More violence is needed to disrupt the cruciate ligaments because the capsule must be torn and the tibia must actually be wrenched away from the femur, that is, the disruption is part of a subluxation or dislocation of the knee joint. This has happened to patients in heavy tackles in football, in a motor accident when the foot is caught and the rest of the body is thrown violently (Fig. 6-34), in a fall from a ladder when one foot is impeded or temporarily caught, and in an awkward fall from a

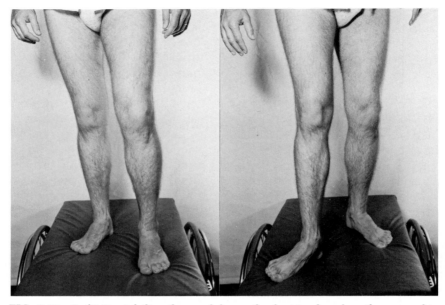

FIG. 6-33. (*Left*) To stabilize the weak knee, the foot is placed on the ground in lateral rotation. As weight is taken, the knee is straightened as the femur is rotated internally on the tibia. Compare this gait with the normal stride (*right*).

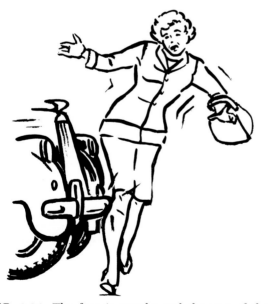

FIG. 6-34. The foot is caught and the rest of the body is thrown violently. This accident caused rupture of the medial and the cruciate ligaments.

height when the patient lands with one leg twisted under the body.

Over a period of time the locked knee may stretch, but cannot rupture, the anterior cruciate ligament. The cruciates, as is proper for guide ropes, are at an even tension in all phases of normal *active* movement of the knee. However, when the synchrony of outward rotation with extension is obstructed by a displaced meniscus, the cruciate ligament is tensed over the intercondylar edge of the medial femoral condyle (see Fig. 1-21). In the course of time, extension is recovered at the expense of stretching the cruciates and the capsule. Mild anteroposterior and general laxity develop. At operation the anterior cruciate shows the localized area of irritation with a corresponding area of erosion of articular cartilage on the affected edge of the femoral condyle (Fig. 6-18). The suggestion sometimes made that this is related to osteochondritis dissecans is unfounded. It is due to superficial traumatic erosion, and the pattern is etched in exactly the same way as are other specific patterns of traumatic arthritis elsewhere in the knee and in other joints.

TEARS OF THE LATERAL LIGAMENTS

The capsular and the cruciate ligaments have been joined under the same heading in this chapter, because rupture of one or the other lateral ligament and adjacent parts of the capsule are components of the same traumatic incident that may cause weakness and profound instability of the knee joint. On the other hand, the lateral ligaments may be injured independently of rupture of the cruciates (Fig. 6-35). Sprains of the medial or the lateral capsule may follow twists of the knee, but ruptures of the ligaments result, in most instances, from violent abduction or adduction forces on the extended leg. Usually the nature of the injury is detachment of the ligament from its insertion to the tibia, the fibula, or the femur, sometimes with a flake of bone. Not infrequently, rupture of the lateral ligament is accompanied by injury to the lateral popliteal nerve.

SPRAINS OF THE CAPSULAR LIGAMENTS

Abnormal strain on the knee joint from any direction may injure the capsular ligaments. As with all tissues that embody elastic elements, damage occurs at the attachments, that is, where the elastic fibers join a less yielding structure. In the knee joint this implies the attachments of the capsule to bone and of the medial meniscus to the medial ligament. The term sprain includes many gradations of partial rupture of ligaments, but the exact distinction between rupture and sprain has not been clearly defined. For the purposes of this chapter the distinction will be clinical, that is, if passive stretching produces pain before or at the normal limit of any angled movement of the joint, the diagnosis will be that of sprain. If the extreme range or more is reached before discomfort is felt, the ligament has ruptured. Difficulties arise when both conditions are present, (e.g., the medial ligament may be avulsed from the tibia while the adjacent cap-

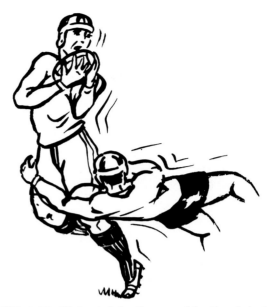

FIG. 6-35. Violent abduction or adduction injuries with the leg straight produce ruptures of the medial or the lateral ligaments.

sular attachments are strained). Passive movement produces pain before instability is detected. When there is doubt, it is necessary to test the stability of the knee joint under local or general anesthetic. Arthrography by x-ray films after the injection of contrast media is helpful in diagnosis. See Chapter 22.

Abduction, adduction, and *hyperextension* sprains occur frequently. Pain, tenderness, and swelling are maximal at, and usually localized to, the affected attachment to bone. Sprains of the fibular attachment of the lateral ligament usually are associated with injury of similar severity to the insertion of the biceps.

Rotation Sprains

A rotational element complicates most sprains, but the most obvious is probably the sprain between the deep portion of the medial ligament and the medial meniscus. Differentiation clinically from the torn meniscus may be difficult unless the semilunar is displaced. Maximal swelling and tenderness is located

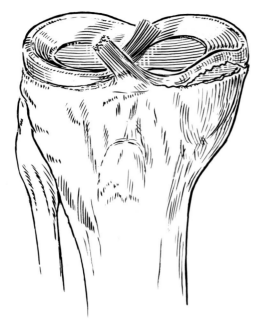

FIG. 6-36. Rupture of the coronary ligaments of the anterior half of the meniscus—a rotation sprain of the medial semilunar cartilage (*see text*).

FIG. 6-37. Prominence of the head of the left fibula.

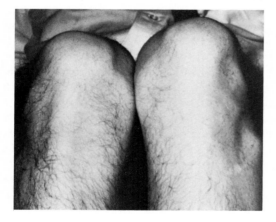

over the midpoint of the meniscus (see Figs. 7-5 and 7-6).

Rotation Sprains of the Medial Semilunar Cartilage

W. Rowley Bristow in the 1930s described certain skiing injuries as "rotation sprain of the medial semilunar cartilage."[1,6] The clini-

cal features are indistinguishable from those of a classic meniscus rupture. Injury is followed by locking and swelling of the knee joint. At operation the only lesion found is hemorrhagic suffusion of the coronary attachments of the medial meniscus to the tibia. It is probable that this is the repair stage after rupture of these vascular structures. The cartilage has been momentarily displaced, but, because of the vascularity of the site of rupture, it is able to heal (Fig. 6-36).

SUPERIOR TIBIOFIBULAR JOINT

As instability and even osteoarthritis of the superior tibiofibular joint do not always incapacitate the patient, it has suffered clinical and literary neglect. Although material disability is rare, three patients suffered much distress, and their symptoms presented problems of diagnosis.

A staff nurse was running on wet sand when someone from behind flicked a towel around her left ankle. She stumbled and fell. Her recollection of the incident was uncertain, but she thought that her ankle had twisted before she fell forward onto her knee, which was almost fully flexed. Later that day she was able to walk and run, but during the evening the anterolateral part of the knee, the calf, and the lower thigh became painful and swollen. She was forced to stay in bed for 3 days, by which time bruising from the superior tibiofibular joint downward had developed in the leg.

She suffered persistent disability. A year later, when examined for the first time, the superior tibiofibular joint was unstable. Although the maneuver was painful, the joint could be subluxated passively.

The violently twisting foot requires increased accommodation for equinovarus movement of the talus in the ankle mortise. When the knee bears weight or is falling, this accommodation is provided by movement of the fibula on the tibia at their two articulations. If torque is excessive, diastasis of the lower tibiofibular or, less frequently, displacement of the superior tibiofibular joint takes place. Operative exploration reveals disruption of the anterior fibers of the capsule.

The second patient was a farmer who had injured his knee falling off a horse 5 years previously. Mistaken diagnosis had led to removal of the meniscus a year later, without relief. After 5 years, the subluxating head of the fibula had eroded the joint surfaces, and cystic degeneration from the torn capsular tissues was present.

In both patients tenderness from strain was present in the tendinous insertion of the biceps, and, among other symptoms, both complained of discomfort in the ankle on walking.

The third patient was a 23-year-old medical student who fractured the lower ends of the right tibia and fibula in 1959. The fractures healed in perfect position, but subsequently she suffered swelling of the ankle after standing. In December, 1961, she assisted at four operations, and increased swelling and discomfort followed. Next morning as she climbed out of bed, she felt sharp pain in the right calf. She had to walk on her toes. Later, pain was referred also up the right thigh. Although no veins were palpable, thrombosis of the deep veins was diagnosed. Anticoagulants and an elastic stocking gave no relief, and any period of standing resulted in intolerable discomfort. She despaired of continuing her interest in surgery.

On examination in April, 1962, the superior tibiofibular joint was tender. Rocking the head of the fibula firmly reproduced her pattern of pain. She could not take weight on the outer border of the right foot without pain, nor could she flex the knee and the ankle while taking full weight on the foot. Injection of procaine into the joint gave immediate though temporary relief. She has since been given three injections of procaine mixed with 25.0 mg of prednisolone into the joint and gentle physiotherapy. Each injection has been followed by 3 or 4 weeks of comfort in spite of full activity before lesser symptoms on prolonged standing reappear. It may be necessary

in due course to excise or arthrodese this joint.

Since publication of these observations in *Management of Internal Derangements of the Knee* in 1963 we have realized that neither *sprain nor frank derangement of the superior tibiofibular joint is uncommon.* Only in blatant dislocations, a rare disorder, is the diagnosis easily made. Often there has been associated major trauma to the foot or leg, and the injury to the small joint is overlooked. Physical impairment from injury is usually not dramatic, but symptoms are grumbling and per-

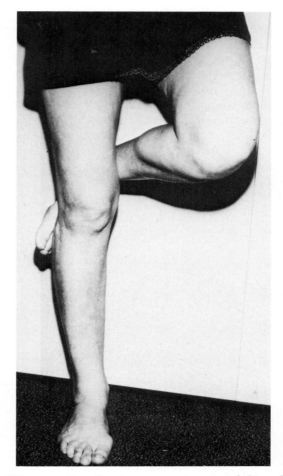

FIG. 6-38. Test for derangement or instability of the superior tibiofibular joint. (Helfet AJ: AAOS Instructional Course Lectures, vol 19. St. Louis, CV Mosby, 1970)

sistent and are often mistaken for injury to the lateral meniscus or for thrombophlebitis. Some of our patients had undergone previous lateral meniscectomy or treatment for thrombophlebitis without benefit.

CLINICAL PICTURE

The presenting symptom is pain in the lateral aspect of the knee, the posterior aspect of the calf, or both. The patient is comfortable at rest. Pain develops with such activities as walking at a brisk pace, running, weight-bearing on a semiflexed knee or in actions which require full dorsiflexion of the ankle.

On examination, tenderness is felt over the superior tibiofibular joint and at the insertion of the biceps femoris to the head of the fibula. Rocking the head of the fibula with the knee flexed, full dorsiflexion of the ankle, and walking with toe-in gait are all painful. Taking weight on the partially flexed knee or forceful contraction of the biceps femoris

against resistance produces the characteristic symptoms. There may be prominence of the head of the fibula (Fig. 6-37). Knee movement itself is full and painless. Involvement of the peroneal nerve may be present when the joint has been dislocated. The lesion may be a simple sprain or a complete luxation. X-ray examination shows no change or occasionally evidence of joint irregularity or deformity of the head of the fibula. Taking an oblique view of the knee is most helpful in displaying the joint.

The importance of the superior tibiofibular joint in bearing body weight while the knee is flexed provides a new diagnostic clinical test.[3]

If the patient with an unstable joint is asked to flex the knee while bearing weight solely on the affected leg it will give way if he or she does not stabilize the leg with the opposite foot (Fig. 6-38). On the other hand, if the joint is arthritic or sprained he will find the test too painful to continue. Injection of a 1% solution

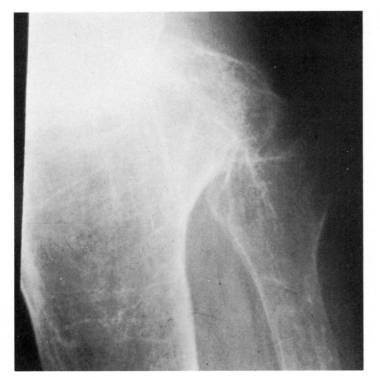

FIG. 6-39. Rheumatoid arthritis of the superior tibiofibular joint.

FIG. 6-40. Anteroposterior and lateral views of exostosis of the head of the fibula distracting the joint.

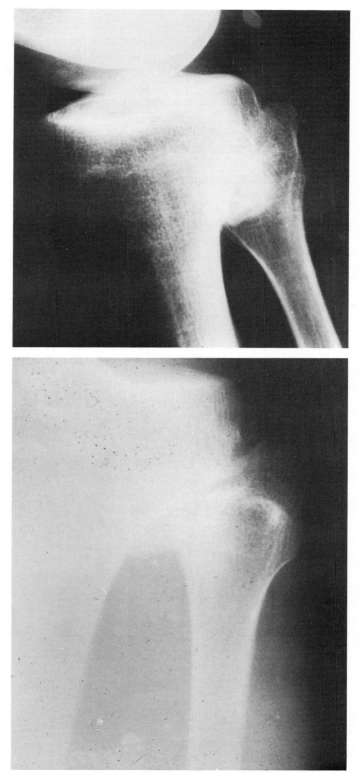

of local anesthetic and 25 mg of hydrocortisone preparation into the joint provides instant relief of the painful symptoms and, because this may last for some time, gives an excellent therapeutic test in all but the unstable joint.

The most frequent cause of derangement is indirect trauma, the ankle being primarily involved. In our series, traumatic arthritis, rheumatoid arthritis, and exostosis of the head of the fibula (Figs. 6-39 and 6-40) have also been noted as causes of the syndrome. Luxation of the joint has been reported among parachute injuries.

It is interesting to note that when the cartilage is damaged, the damage is usually of the retracted and not the bowstring variety, that is, it has been wrenched away from its mooring to the cruciate ligaments and not split in its substance (Fig. 6-34).

4. Violent abduction and medial rotation of the thigh on the fixed tibia while the quadriceps are fully tensed may cause dislocation of the patella.

5. A twist of the ankle which cannot be accommodated by the falling knee may subluxate or strain the superior tibiofibular joint.

SUMMARY

1. Simple abduction or adduction force on the extended knee results in rupture of the medial or the lateral ligament, respectively (Fig. 6-35).

2. Forcible prevention of synchrony of medial rotation of the tibia when flexing and of lateral rotation when extending the knee produces rupture of a semilunar cartilage (Fig. 6-1).

3. The combination of (1) and (2) or either alone, with sufficient additional force to wrench the tibia away from the femur, results in disruption of the cruciate ligaments and capsule with or without concomitant rupture of a semilunar cartilage.

REFERENCES

1. **Barrie HJ:** J Bone Joint Surg, Vol. 61-B (2):184, 1979
2. **Bristow WR:** Internal derangements of the knee joint. J Bone Joint Surg 17:605, 1935
3. **Helfet AJ:** Function of the cruciate ligaments of knee joint. Lancet 1:665, 1948
4. **Helfet AJ:** Diagnosis of internal derangements of the knee. AAOS Instructional Course Lectures, Vol XIX. St. Louis, CV Mosby, 1970
5. **Helfet AJ:** Osteoarthritis of the knee and its early arrest. AAOS Instructional Course Lectures, Vol XX. St. Louis, CV Mosby, 1971
6. **Hertz J:** J Int Coll Surg 24:257−264, 1955
7. **Jones Sir Robert:** Notes on derangements of the knee. Ann Surg 50:969, 1909
8. **Platt Sir Harry:** Report 3rd Congress, Société Internationale de Chirurgie Orthopédique, 1936
9. **Smillie IS:** Injuries of the Knee Joint. Baltimore, Williams & Wilkins, 1970

CHAPTER 7
CLINICAL FEATURES OF INJURIES TO THE SEMILUNAR CARTILAGES

Arthur J. Helfet

INJURY TO SYNOVIUM

After injury to the knee the synovium is irritated and secretes increasing amounts of effusion, mainly muscine. Together with a transudation, the effusion distends the joint. The presence of blood indicates injury to a vascular structure, particularly the anterior cruciates, the periphery of the menisci, or any other attachment of the capsule. When the bone is fractured, the hemorrhage is more extensive, and in this case the blood may clot and may contain globules of fat. After hemorrhage, synovial fluid, normally alkaline, becomes acid. The presence of blood and synovial fluid encourages the formation of fibrous tissue and adhesions.

An injury severe enough to damage the rotator mechanism of the knee joint must cause pain and swelling, but the quality and the severity of both vary considerably. The football player who displaces a meniscus suffers immediate agony. He cannot straighten the knee and adamantly refuses to place weight on the limb. Once the knee is supported and at rest the pain eases. If the cartilage is not displaced or does not remain displaced, or if it is split at the back end only, the acute distress passes in minutes. The player limps but can walk and may even continue in the game. A posterior tear may signify its nature when the knee gives way, not necessarily very painfully, later in the game. This is one explanation of the situation in which a player whose knee is hurt continues after attention, only to leave the field following a second incident. Another explanation is that the cartilage is hurt in the first but displaced only in the second misadventure. In general, injured players who remain on the field either have not displaced the meniscus or have torn only its posterior end.

The retracted cartilage provides a contrast

to this acute onset, especially in middle-aged and older people in whom the trauma may be only minor. A twist while on bended knees or a stumble causes a stab of pain. When the knee is straightened, vague temporary discomfort remains. The whole incident is so brief that 3 weeks or more later the original mild accident is remembered with difficulty or dismissed as "I had a slight sprain only." In these cases the anterior end of the meniscus, usually the medial, is pulled off its mooring to the anterior cruciate. The cartilage retracts and, perhaps because the distraction is gentle, causes little pain. A similar reaction may follow complete rupture of ligaments or tendons. Sprains and partial tears cause much more pain than complete division, which is often relatively painless.

Mention must be made, however, of the acute reaction of the middle-aged knee to a transverse tear at the junction of the anterior two-thirds and the posterior third of the medial meniscus. Often the patient has suffered for some time from recurring effusions, grumbling pain, and limp, which have been diagnosed as osteoarthritis but usually are due to a retracted anterior horn. Suddenly, after another, often minor injury, a transverse fracture occurs, and the knee is acutely painful, swollen, partly flexed, and unable to bear weight. The severe and distressing disablement of the knee is due to displacement of part of the torn meniscus which "locks" the joint.

Synovial effusion, not unduly hemorrhagic if the split is in the avascular substance of the cartilage, will increase slowly and reach its maximum during the night—"when the joint became cold." Then, declares the patient, the knee, even at rest, is stiffer and more painful.

If the vascular structures of the joint are torn, frank hemarthrosis develops rapidly. The knee swells urgently and is much more painful than it is when a slow, simple effusion is present. The usual tests for fluid elicit signs of a tensely distended, very tender joint that is "rubbery" to the touch, in contrast to the softer, much less tender impression given by the simple effusion.

RESTRICTION OF MOVEMENT

Tears and displacements of the semilunar cartilages affect the smooth action of the rotator mechanism of the knee, and the presence of injury is signified in every instance by inability to rotate the tibia to its full extent, and, therefore, to extend or flex the knee completely.

Lesions of the anterior half or more of either meniscus block lateral rotation and extension. To call it "locking" of the joint is inaccurate because only these movements are prevented. Flexion and medial rotation are unaffected and give comfort to the injured knee. The retracted cartilage causes the same limitations of movement but is not so painful. Since the anterior cruciate ligament exerts its guiding action on the tibia in part through the medial cartilage, it seems reasonable to suppose that anterior detachment of the cartilage would impair this function and leave the tibia unable to complete its normal excursion. But this cannot be so, for after excision of the torn cartilage the quadriceps regains full control of the range of rotation of the tibia and, incidentally, of extension as well. The cartilage is an accessory factor in the rotator mechanism. The abnormal cartilage disturbs function, but when it has been excised, the knee can compensate for its absence.*

It appears that any increase in volume of the contents of the anteromedial compartment of the knee prevents full lateral rotation of the tibia. This can be demonstrated experimentally at operation. Through the usual medial incision with the knee bent over the end of the table, the lateral rotation of the tibia during

---

* Sir Robert Jones commented on this point in the appendix to Timbrell Fisher's monograph[7]: "The question, What is the use of the semilunar cartilages? is a fundamental one. Whatever the conclusion to which we arrive, there is no doubt that men can perform the most arduous and expert acts with their joints after removal of the cartilages and without ill effects. I removed the semilunar cartilage in no less than six members of the same International football team. In one case, in which both cartilages were removed, he played through the season without a breakdown."

extension shows very well. If one puts a sterile rubber catheter across the medial joint space, the tibia cannot rotate fully. The reaction to the anterior tear is a blocking of movement by the "heaping-up" of the retracted cartilage.

Similarly, displacement of the posterior horn of the semilunar cartilage blocks full medial rotation of the tibia, and it is impossible to flex the knee completely. Attempts to force these movements cause pain, whereas full lateral rotation and extension of the knee is possible but painless.

The bowstring cartilage blocks extension and lateral rotation, and if the split extends far enough back, flexion and medial rotation also are affected. It is usually the most painful type of cartilage tear, but fortunately is not always complicated by severe hemarthrosis.

The extent of restriction of movement from a displaced or deformed meniscus is, within narrow limits, always the same because only rotation is blocked directly. Limitation of extension is usually some 5° and at most 10°, and the same applies to flexion. This is understandable. If the knee were a hinge joint, the block to movement would be exactly proportional to the size and site of the obstruction, whereas any change in the volume between the articulating surfaces of a helix prevents rotation and converts the joint into a "condyloid" joint, with its own range of movement in one plane. This is one of the reasons for limited movement obtained in the current fashion of knee replacements in which the helix is replaced by condyloid joint action.

ROTATION SIGNS

The blocking of rotation gives us the following clinical signs, which are pathognomonic of injury to the cartilages:

1. When the anterior half of the meniscus is deranged, forced passive extension produces finger-point pain over the site of injury in the anteromedial or the anterolateral compartment of the joint. The patient can pinpoint the pain (Figs. 7-1; 7-4).

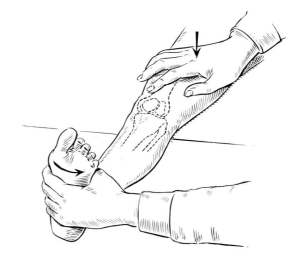

FIG. 7-1. Forced passive extension produces fingerpoint pain over the site of injury in the anteromedial or the anterolateral compartment of the joint.

2. Any attempt to force the final degree of lateral rotation may cause pain localized to the same spot. Flexion and medial rotation of the knee are not affected and, in fact, give the patient comfort. This statement needs a word of qualification: if the effusion in the knee is tense, flexion is limited and painful because of the distention of the capsule as a whole, and if the split in the bowstring cartilage extends to the posterior compartment, the final degrees of flexion and medial rotation may be obstructed also.

3. Forced passive flexion and internal rotation produce finger-point pain in the posteromedial or the posterolateral compartments of the joint when the posterior horn of the meniscus is at fault. If only the posterior end of a cartilage has been injured, extension and lateral rotation are free and painless. The importance of the finger-point pain is readily understandable, as it indicates the site of injury of the cartilage.

4. Two additional signs are associated with anterior lesions. Compared with the normal knee, the outward excursion of the tib-

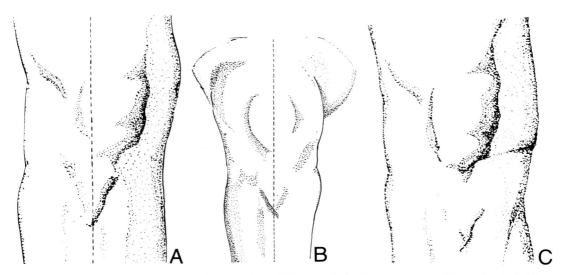

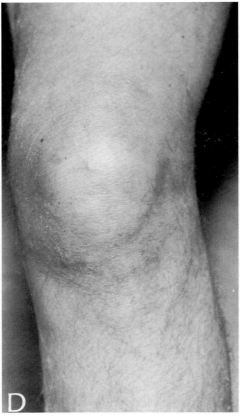

FIG. 7-2. **(A)** When the normal knee is straightened, the tibial tubercle rotates laterally into alignment with the outer half of the patella. **(B)** As the knee flexes, the tubercle rotates medially toward the central axis. **(C)** When blocked by a deranged meniscus, the tibial tubercle of the extending knee cannot rotate beyond the central axis of the patella. The medial femoral condyle protrudes over the margin of the tibia. **(D)** The protrusion of the medial femoral condyle and the blocked rotation of the tibial tubercle are obvious in this knee with a retracted medial cartilage. (Helfet AJ: J Bone Joint Surg 41B:319, 1959)

ial tubercle is limited. When the normal knee is straightened, the tibial tubercle reaches the line of the lateral border of the patella. The tibial tubercle of the injured knee reaches approximately to the central axis of the patella (Fig. 7-2; see also Chap. 2).

5. The final screw-home of the knee in completing extension aligns the borders of the medial femoral condyle and the adjacent tibia exactly. When the screw-home is prevented by an injured cartilage, the femoral condyle is left protruding over the margin of the tibia. Unless the knee is very swollen, this is obvious to the eye (Figs. 7-2 and 7-3). In any case, it can be detected by pal-

FIG. 7-3. (*Left*) The femoral condyle protrudes over the margin of the tibia when the knee is extended. The lower hook grips retracted meniscus. Note the heaping up of articular cartilage on the presenting surface of the femur. The area of erosion is in relation to the meniscus. (*Right*) After removal of the meniscus, the margins of femoral condyle and tibia realign when the knee is extended.

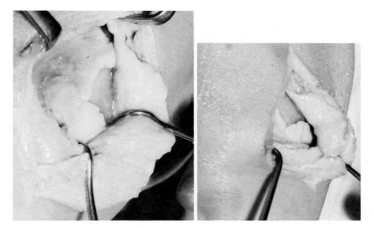

pation. If the examining finger follows the subcutaneous surface of the tibia upward, it will, when it reaches the knee, be obstructed by the protruding medial condyle of the femur, a feature that may be confirmed by comparison with the normal knee. The protrusion is most obvious in the knee in which arthritic changes have become established.

At operation for a torn medial cartilage, these signs may be confirmed. After opening the joint through a medial incision, straighten the knee. The medial femoral condyle overlaps the tibial margin. Remove the cartilage and straighten the knee again. Complete extension is obtained, and the femur and the tibia are in perfect rotational alignment (Fig. 7-3).

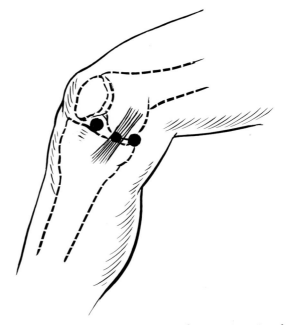

FIG. 7-4. Sites of fingerpoint tenderness associated with injuries to the medial meniscus are (*from left*) the anterior horn, the attachment to the medial ligament, and the posterior horn.

TENDERNESS

Following injury, the whole cartilage may be sensitive, but after a while the retracted cartilage will be tender in the anterior compartment, and the cartilage with a posterior tear will be tender, in the posterior compartment (Figs. 7-4 and 7-5). The complete bowstring cartilage may be tender at both ends. In an untreated tear, tenderness subsequently develops in two other areas. The retracted cartilage, because of its increase in bulk in the anterior compartment, gradually erodes an area of weight-bearing articular cartilage on the medial femoral condyle. The spot is adjacent to the area of condyle that protrudes over the tibia and is most easily located when the knee is flexed. The other site of tenderness is the

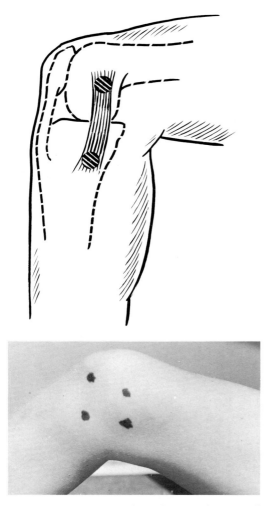

FIG. 7-5. (*Top*) Areas of tenderness from medial ligament sprains or tears are always at the attachment of the ligament to bone. The injured cartilage is tender fore and aft along the joint line. (*Bottom*) The knee is marked to show areas of tenderness from medial ligament or meniscal injuries.

medial border of the patella and the adjacent medial slope of the trochlear surface of the femur (Fig. 7-6); it is caused by injury to the articular cartilage from undue tension between these surfaces of the patella and the femur.

Except in a retracted cartilage, most injuries of the medial meniscus are accompanied by strain of the attachment of the deep fibers of the medial collateral ligament, and therefore there is tenderness over this point in the joint line (Fig. 7-5). Frank strains and rupture of the medial ligament itself occur at the upper or the lower insertion to bone, with corresponding local tenderness (Fig. 7-5).

DIAGNOSTIC CLICKS

Maneuvers that elicit a click from an abnormal or displaced meniscus are useful aids in diagnosis. The well-established tests described by McMurray,[5] Fouche,[2] and Apley[1] use the principle of rotation of the flexed knee with added compression or adduction or abduction to show up instability or displacement of a fragment of the *posterior half* of the cartilage. However, there are two other clicks that may be elicited and have diagnostic significance.

1. There is what may be called the *reducing* click, though sometimes the click signals displacement of the cartilage. The patient has an injured knee with positive rotation signs, limited lateral rotation of the tibial tubercle, prominence of the medial femoral condyle in extension, and finger-point pain on forced extension. Flex the relaxed knee passively, and forcibly rotate it medially and laterally (Fig. 7-7). Suddenly, with a click, lateral rotation is freed. It is possible now to extend the knee fully, and the rotation signs are negative. The reduction often is felt by the patient as well as the surgeon. If rotation alone will not free the cartilage, extension with external rotation or a kick by the patient into full extension may do so (see Fig. 12-3). Sometimes it is possible to displace the cartilage by the opposite maneuver. Flex the knee passively while resisting medial rotation or extend it while resisting lateral rotation of the tibia. Again there is a click, and the rotation signs reappear.

   These reducing and displacing signs are present in *unstable* tears of four kinds—posterior horn, incomplete longitudinal, oblique pedicled tears of the inner margin,

FIG. 7-6. (*Left*) The other site of tenderness is the medial border of the patella and the adjacent medial slope of the trochlear surface of the femur. (*Right*) The knee is marked to show areas of tenderness from the anterior horn of the medial meniscus and the medial border of the patella.

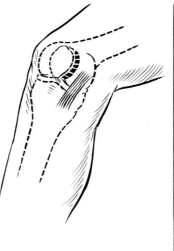

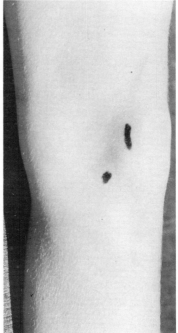

and the retracted medial meniscus in younger people in whom the structure is still reasonably resilient. It forms the basis of the manipulation for reduction of the displaced cartilage.

2. This click is similar to the heavy thud felt over the congenital discoid cartilage. It is like the sensation of a wheel going over a bump and is not felt often. A thickening in the meniscus is the cause, for example, when a tag is folded back on the cartilage, or when the retracted cartilage shortens by becoming thicker fore and aft.

THE McMURRAY CLICKS

The late Professor McMurray described the maneuver to elicit his sign:

In making the examination the patient must be recumbent and relaxed, the surgeon standing at the side of the injured limb; he grasps the foot firmly and the knee is bent completely so that the heel approaches or touches the buttock. The foot is now rotated externally and the leg abducted at the knee

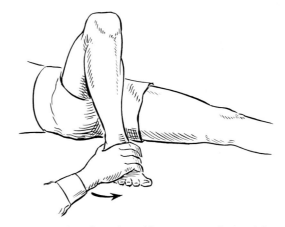

FIG. 7-7. Flex the relaxed knee passively, and forcibly rotate it medially and laterally.

whilst the joint is slowly extended [Fig. 7-8]. With the alteration of the angle of the joint any loose portion of the internal semilunar cartilage is caught between the femur and tibia, and the sliding of the femur over the abnormal portion of cartilage is accompanied by a definite click and pain, which the patient states is similar to the feeling experienced each time the knee gives way. The angle at which this occurs gives the position of the cartilaginous lesion, and, if the maneuver is correctly followed out, the absence of such a click is a definite indication of the absence of any lesion in the posterior or middle portion of the cartilage.

It is difficult to maneuver the leg of a sturdy or heavy patient at the end of the forearm, but the task is facilitated by holding the foot against the examiner's side as shown in Figures 7-8 and 7-9. Movements then are controlled by the examiner's trunk.[3]

Sometimes a positive click is obtained by

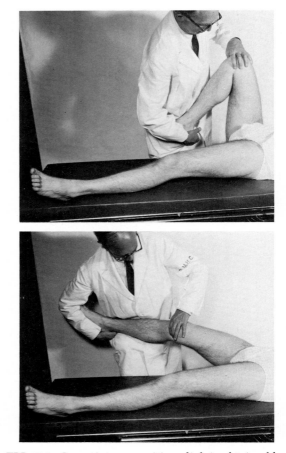

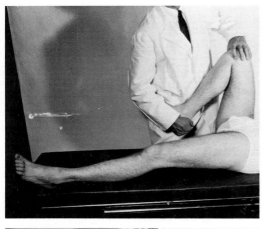

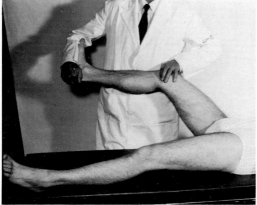

FIG. 7-8. Maneuvers to elicit the "McMurray click." (*Top*) The heel is gripped firmly in the surgeon's hand while the foot is held between the forearm and the side. After complete flexion of the knee, the foot is rotated externally and the leg rotated externally. (*Bottom*) Maintaining external rotation of the foot, the joint is extended slowly.

FIG. 7-9. Sometimes a positive click is obtained by the opposite maneuver. (*Top*) Rotating the foot internally. (*Bottom*) adducting at the knee while slowly extending the joint.

the opposite maneuver—rotating the foot internally and adducting at the knee while the joint is extended slowly (Fig. 7-9).

THE APLEY GRINDING AND DISTRACTION TESTS

With the patient lying on his face, the knee is flexed to 90° and rotated while a compression force is applied; this, the grinding test, reproduces the symptoms of a torn meniscus. Rotation is repeated while the leg is pulled upward with the surgeon's knee holding the thigh down; this, the distraction test, produces increased pain only if there is ligament damage (Fig. 7-10).[1]

These *clicks* all are elicited by the examiner's fingers placed along the joint line and are usually palpable and only occasionally audible as well.

A click (especially if it produces in the patient the sensation of instability) is invaluable in placing the site of the lesion. On the other hand, failure to demonstrate a click does not always exclude a tear, for the sign may not be elicited unless the torn fragment is displaced. Nor will it be elicited in a complete bowstringing of the cartilage nor in the knee in which the displacement (such as the retracted anterior horn) has blocked lateral rotation of the tibia. In these instances the "rotation signs" are sufficient to diagnose the lesion and are pathognomonic.

GIVING WAY OR BUCKLING OF THE KNEE

The mechanics of this phenomenon are uncertain because we must rely on the patient's interpretation of symptoms. *Giving way* is a symptom of instability and may have one or more of six causes, namely:

1. Derangements of the posterior halves of the semilunar cartilages
2. Disruption of the capsular or cruciate ligaments
3. Vertical tears of the posteromedial capsule associated with a torn medial meniscus
4. Recurrent dislocation or subluxation of the patella
5. Instability of the superior tibiofibular joint
6. Weakness of the quadriceps

Any of these may actually cause the knee to give way and the patient to fall and should be distinguished from illusory giving way, which occurs not infrequently as a symptom of *chronic strain of the medial lateral ligament or of adhesion of the fat pad to neighboring fixed structures,* as described in Chapter 8.

The infrapatellar pad of fat is a mobile structure that alters its shape to the changing accommodation in the anterior compartment of the knee joint during flexion and extension. Adhesions limit this movement. Sudden twists of the knee produce a twinge of pain and momentary weakness which the patient may mistake for giving way, and these symptoms may also occur in chronic strains of the ligaments of the knee, especially the medial. The diagnosis is determined by eliciting finger-point tenderness and pain in the same place on reproducing the movement that causes the tension. Occasionally giving way may also be simulated by slipping of a tendon such as the semitendinosis over the cancellous exostosis that forms between the hamstrings on the upper medial tibia.

Unstable tears of the posterior horn of the meniscus are a prime cause of giving way. Tears in or a detached anterior half of the medial meniscus are more liable to produce a painful "catch" than giving way. The following case illustrates the point: A torn cartilage that did not lead to giving way before operation is inadequately removed. A loose posterior fragment remains. Subsequently, the only or the most troublesome symptom is giving way.

Giving way is not necessarily accompanied by pain. More often than not, especially in the lateral cartilage, it is painless. Patients describe a sensation similar to buckling when the unsuspecting straight weight-bearing leg is nudged gently from behind. The knee gives way, as far as we can be certain, during flexion. Presumably, the medially rotating tibia loses control when it reaches the irregularity in its path and is precipitated into further flexion. It may be allied to the "reducing click," which, however, is elicited in the non-weight-bearing relaxed knee.

If the knee buckles after the cruciates and a medial or lateral ligament are torn, it usually gives way during extension. Normally, the intact rotator mechanism keeps the tibia on a well-defined track on the medial condyle of the femur until it has wound itself to stability in full extension. Loss of control by the cruciates and the medial capsule results in a type

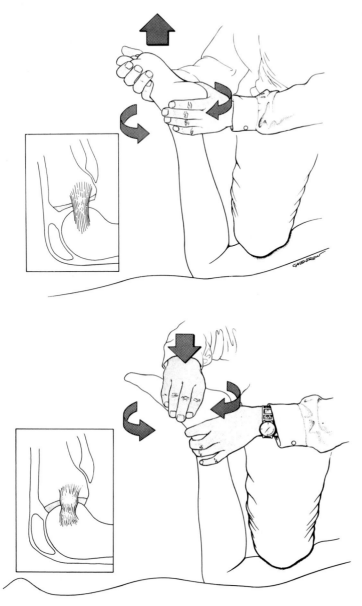

FIG. 7-10. The Apley test.

of instability in which the tibia leaves the curved track and slides straight forward from the medial condyle of the femur. Patients suffering from this injury find their main disability on slopes and ladders where quadriceps contraction and control must be at their maximum. This type of giving way tends to be painful and distressing.

In my experience, buckling of the knee does not occur from isolated detachments or rupture of the anterior cruciate ligament, but only when accompanied by rupture or laxity of capsular ligaments. An isolated detachment of the anterior cruciate is detected when operation is necessary for associated disruption, with retraction of the anterior horn of the medial meniscus.

Both the anterior cruciate ligament and the

anterior horn of the medial meniscus are pulled off the anterior tibial spine by the same twisting force, but the meniscus is responsible for the resulting symptoms. If the integrity of the capsular ligaments is intact, it is not necessary to replace the anterior cruciate. The stump of the ligament may be excised.

Vertical tears of the posteromedial capsule with accompanying rupture of the medial meniscus produce an unusual type of giving way. It seems to occur when the patient is standing and reaches near or full extension of the weight-bearing knee. Apparently, the medial condyle of the femur continues into uncontrolled abnormal internal rotation. The patient describes an odd sensation of weakness, often without pain. Excision of the torn meniscus does not cure, because the peculiar buckling continues until the tear is repaired.

Recurrent dislocation of the patella. Buckling of the knee due to a ruptured semilunar cartilage must also be differentiated from that recorded by the patient suffering from recurring dislocation or subluxation of the patella. The knee is said to give way, but the phenomenon seems to occur, and indeed can only occur, when the weight-bearing leg is straight or nearly straight and while the quadriceps are contracting or contracted. Abnormal internal rotation of the femur or external rotation with flexion of the tibia at this point forces the patella to be dislocated laterally out of the trochlear groove. In my experience, medial dislocation has not been observed.

The leg gives way, or rather collapses, but the knee is locked in slight flexion. The dislocation is reduced by passively straightening the leg while relaxing the quadriceps. In cases of long standing, the quadriceps may be weak, and when the muscles are relaxed, there is gross laxity of the patella.

Instability of the superior tibiofibular joint. Because instability and even osteoarthritis of this joint do not always incapacitate the patient, it has suffered clinical and literary neglect. Although material disability is rare, patients may suffer much distress, and their symptoms present problems in diagnosis.

See Chapters 6 and 16.

Weakness of the quadriceps. The knee gives way when walking, especially down slopes and stairs as the knee flexes beyond a critical angle, this angle depending on the measure of weakness of the quadriceps. It is a common phenomenon in poliomyelitis. To maintain stability, the patient has to lock the knee back in hyperextension. It occurs also after surgery on the knee if the patient walks before the power of the quadriceps has been adequately restored. As soon as the knee fatigues, buckling is experienced. This also troubles mountaineers with adequate quadriceps when they are overfatigued by a long and steep descent. Fixed flexion deformity with inability to extend the knee completely as in osteoarthritis, which is usually accompanied by weak quadriceps, aggravates this type of giving way and leads to the necessity of a knee brace.

DEVELOPMENT OF TRAUMATIC OSTEOARTHRITIS*

Traumatic osteoarthritis should be considered as a repair reaction after injury or wearing or abrasion of the articular surfaces.[4] As a reaction to the traumatic process, or possibly to the constituents of degenerating cartilage, the adjacent bone becomes sclerotic, or patches of aseptic necrosis or small cysts develop. Heaped-up cartilage on the edges of the joint is ossified into osteophytes. The articular cartilage itself first loses its white sheen and tough compressibility or elasticity and becomes yellow, dull, and hard. In the young the cartilage is resilient, but with age it becomes more brittle and less durable, so that an irregularity that might need years to erode the cartilage of youth may do as much in weeks in the elderly.

Articular cartilage is generally considered to be aneural, but after a period of abnormal pressure, whether constant or intermittent, it becomes tender; however, the patient does not apparently suffer *bone pain* until the underlying bone has been reached. Bone pain is of an

---

* See also Chapter 13.

aching, boring character, worse at night when the limb is warm. The patient often finds temporary relief by cooling the limb outside the bed clothes.

The clinical reaction to these changes is a knee that is progressively more susceptible to fatigue and strain. The knee tolerates less and less activity before it aches and swells. The discomfort and swelling is relieved by rest, but as time goes on, the necessary rest periods are longer. Until the latest stages, complete rest in bed or by splinting is usually effective in bringing relief. Progress is aggravated by the tendency of the thigh muscles, which act on the joint, to waste and weaken. Fatigue and strain come on sooner. On the other hand, if the muscles are strengthened, the range of activity is improved, and therefore, building muscle power is an important feature in treatment.

THE MECHANISM OF PAIN

It is interesting to establish a pathologic basis for the various sites and types of pain that follow injury to the medial cartilage. The bowstring tear causes immediate and severe pain. The patient cannot bear weight on the leg. During the next 2 or 3 weeks the symptoms improve, though forcing the knee straight or turning suddenly is still painful. With time, the cruciate ligaments stretch, the patient develops slight anteroposterior laxity, and the knee becomes more comfortable. Each recurrence of the derangement produces less severe symptoms until finally the articular cartilage is eroded and the symptoms of "arthritis" develop—namely, pain and aching during activity referable mainly to the medial compartment of the knee, and aching and swelling after effort, which subside with rest. Later, when the patella is involved, increasing pain on descending or ascending stairs due to pressure between the medial border of the patella and the medial trochlear surface of the femur is the main symptom.

The injury that causes the retracted cartilage produces less pain. The patient may ex-

perience a sharp, momentary stab, which is relieved when the twist is corrected. The joint swells, and there may be recurrent stabs of pain on sudden movements. Later, when the articular cartilage is eroded, the more distressing symptoms of arthritis become manifest—pain in the medial compartment of the knee on walking and aching after effort and, later, at night. The patient may feel that he is "walking with a stone in the knee." The ache is localized to the same area. The patellar symptoms, when they develop, are like those produced by the bowstring cartilage.

Occasionally, the bowstring snaps at one end, usually the anterior (see Fig. 6-17). It coils up in front of the joint and then produces the clinical picture of a retracted cartilage. The first reaction to the snapping of the bowstring is a measure of relief, because the retracted cartilage is so much more comfortable to the patient than the bowstring. Only later do the sequelae cause symptoms. Manipulation for reduction of the displaced bowstring frequently results in snapping of the bowstring, which is the reason for its apparent success.

NONREFERRED PAIN IN THE KNEE WITH OSTEOARTHRITIS OF THE HIP

The patient suffering from osteoarthritis of the hip may feel referred pain in the knee. This referred pain is muscular in origin and is felt in front of or on the sides of the knee, depending on the muscle group that is contracted. A patient with flexion- and abduction- or adduction deformity may feel pain in front of or on the sides of the knee. Because extension contracture, if it ever occurs, is a rarity, pain is not felt behind the knee. It should be noted, too, that it is difficult to walk with a straight knee when there is fixed flexion of the hip. The trunk tends to overbalance forward. The fixed deformities of osteoarthritis of the hip are *always* flexion, *either* adduction or abduction, and *usually* external rotation.

Surprisingly often, with long-established osteoarthritis of the hip, careful examination of the knee reveals fixed limitation of extension and external rotation of the tibia on the femur, prominence of the medial femoral condyle, and tenderness of the medial meniscus and medial border of the patella. Fixed adduction contracture of the hip may also lead to laxity of the medial ligaments of the knee. Referred pain therefore must be distinguished from that is due to changes in the knee joint itself secondary to fixed deformity of the hip.

Although pain in the knee need not necessarily be referred from the hip, the question arises whether the changes in the knee are independent of the hip and part of a generalized osteoarthritis or whether they are secondary to and the consequence of fixed deformity of the hip. The latter is almost certainly the case, because the pattern of disorder in the knee depends on the particular deformity of the hip.

For example, fixed external rotation and flexion of the hip eventually leads to flexion and internal rotation contracture of the tibia on the femur with consequent internal derangement of the knee of the typical pattern. In normal walking, sinuous and synchronous adaptations of movement take place between hip and knee. During flexion the hip rotates outward while the tibia rotates inward, and vice versa during extension. Walking with a fixed flexion–external rotation deformity of the hip demands compensation by flexion of the knee and—in order to point the foot forward—limiting external rotation of the tibia during extension. In time, these factors effect permanent fixed limitation of extension and external rotation of the tibia with retraction of the aging, hardening medial meniscus. This is shown in Figure 1-3 by the limitation of external rotation of the tibia and the prominent medial femoral condyle. These signs persist both while walking and at rest. When present, they represent or portend the typical patterns of erosion of the medial femoral condyle and medial border of the patella and are a frequent cause of pain—pain that may be relieved by simple meniscectomy and, when necessary, debridement of the medial border of the patella.

Adduction deformity adds a valgus strain to the knee and causes medial ligaments and sometimes cruciates to stretch producing instability of the knee. The medial meniscus may be and usually is retracted, as seen in the patient depicted in Figure 1-3. For many years her left hip had been arthritic, flexed, adducted, and externally rotated. Roentgenographs of the knee with valgus stress showed the degree of medial capsule laxity, and the limited external rotation of the tibia and protrusion of the medial femoral condyle denoted a retracted meniscus. These changes plus laxity of the cruciate ligaments were confirmed at operation. All were secondary to the fixed deformity of the hip, and pain felt in the knee was local in origin and not referred.

To stabilize this knee, it was necessary to remove the meniscus and, in addition, to perform an extra-articular tendon transplant of the semitendinosis into a groove in the medial femoral condyle, plus medial transfer of the tibial tubercle. As an advanced example of change secondary to arthritis of the hip joint, this case stresses the importance of examination of the knee joint itself when pain is present with osteoarthritis of the hip.

MUSCLE WASTING

The quadriceps and, to a lesser extent, the hamstrings waste, often rapidly, after injury to the cartilages and the ligaments of the knee. This reaction is due to disturbance of the neurotrophic relationships between the joint and its controlling musculature and varies in degree. Muscle bulk, tone, and control are diminished rapidly, in some instances severely so. It is not due to muscle inactivity alone, though this factor does aggravate both wasting and weakness. In other words, conscientious muscle exercise cannot prevent but does minimize wasting. While effusion remains, wasting is generalized, but the tendency is for the medial vasti to show greater atrophy in sympathy with a medial meniscus injury, while lateral ruptures are associated with atrophy of the lateral vastus.

Although muscle weakness is present, effusion tends to persist and is increased with any activity beyond the power and the endurance of the residual muscle bulk. In turn, the effusion affects the trophic reflexes, and further wasting occurs.

Watson-Jones[8] and Smillie[6] and later in this volume, Nicholas (Chap. 25), very properly stress the urgency in stimulation by controlled muscle exercises in all injuries of the knee, if the period of disability and impairment of function is to be kept to a minimum. The power of the thigh muscles, both quadriceps and hamstrings, must be developed sufficiently to cope with all strains to which the knee will be subjected, and conversely, during convalescence the knee must not be subjected to any strain beyond the power and endurance of the muscles. I stress "endurance," because the commonest form of strain to be countered is fatigue.

As long as displacement of a meniscus remains, muscle bulk and tone cannot recover significantly, despite assiduous exercise. Recovery is impeded further as the patterns of osteoarthritic erosion develop. But if the cartilage is reduced or removed by operation, so that the knee recovers full movement, both the power and the bulk of muscle will increase with exercise. And this happens even if roentgenograms show that preoperative changes in the joint outline persist.

REFERENCES

1. **Apley AG:** A System of Orthopaedics and Fractures. London, Butterworth & Co, 1959
2. **Du Toit GT, Enslin TB:** Analysis of one hundred consecutive arthrotomies for traumatic internal derangement of the knee joint. J Bone Joint Surg 27:412, 1945
3. **Helfet AJ:** Mechanism of derangements of the medial semilunar cartilage and their management. J Bone Joint Surg 41-B:319, 1959
4. **Helfet AJ:** The arrest of osteoarthritis of the hip and knee. In Apley AG (ed): Recent Advances in Orthopaedics. London, J & A Churchill, 1969
5. **McMurray TP:** The Robert Jones Birthday Volume. London, Humphrey Milford, 1928
6. **Smillie IS:** Injuries of the Knee Joint. Baltimore, Williams & Wilkins, 1962
7. **Timbrell-Fischer AG:** Internal Derangements of the Knee Joint, Note 2, p 189. New York, Macmillan, 1933
8. **Watson-Jones Sir Reginald:** Fractures and Joint Injuries, 4th ed. Vol 2. Baltimore, Williams & Wilkins, 1956

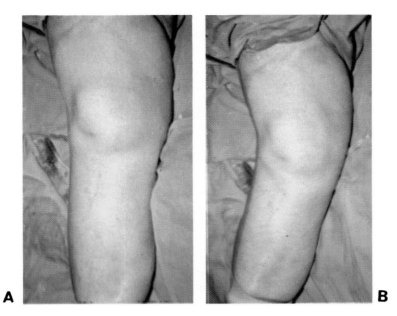

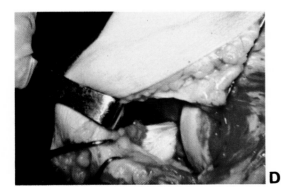

A   B

PLATE 7-1. Knee of a patient who had a long-standing fixed flexion-adduction deformity of the hip. **(A)** Lack of rotation of the tibial tubercle and protrusion of the medial femoral condyle in extension are obvious and denote an intra-articular block to rotation, probably by a meniscus. **(B)** Valgus stress demonstrates the laxity of the medial collateral ligament. A positive "anterior drawer sign" indicated cruciate instability. Roentgenogram in valgus stress showed the extent of medial laxity. **(C)** On opening the anteromedial joint space, the loose medial meniscus with corresponding condylar abrasion are shown. The anterior cruciate ligament is lax. **(D)** The anterior drawer sign demonstrates that the anterior cruciate ligament is stretched and attenuated, not torn. **(E)** The loose medial cartilage is excised. After semitendinosus transfer (see Chap. 22), the patient walked with comfort and stability. The ligaments of this knee had been stretched and the meniscus deranged secondarily to the deformity of the hip.

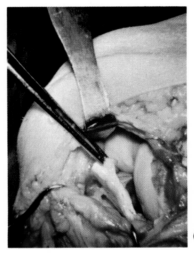

C

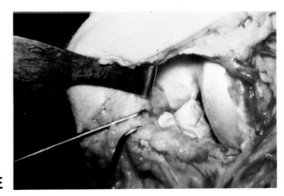

D   E

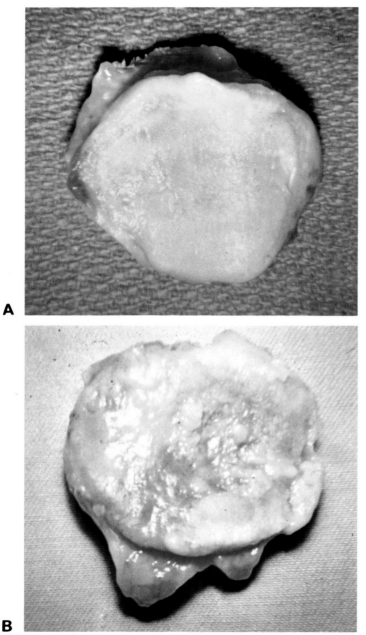

A

B

PLATE 8-1. **(A)** Articular cartilage on both sides of the patella is eroded. **(B)** The cartilage is soft, fissured, and frayed with irregular patterns of disorganization.

CHAPTER 8
DIFFERENTIAL DIAGNOSIS OF TEARS OF THE SEMILUNAR CARTILAGES

Arthur J. Helfet

Accurate diagnosis is essential for successful surgery of the knee. This finely adjusted joint brooks no unplanned or meddlesome surgery. There is little place for opening the joint "to have a look." Indeed, every endeavor should be made to diagnose not only a ruptured cartilage but also the site of rupture.

During the acute stage the knee is grossly swollen and limited in movement, but even then local tenderness and the rotation signs may be elicited. After 3 weeks, if displacement remains, swelling may have disappeared and local tenderness may be faint, but the typical pattern of restriction of movement remains. At a later stage, new areas of tenderness of the articular cartilage, due to continuing tensions, develop on the medial condyle, the trochlear surface of the femur, and the patella.

MEDIAL OR LATERAL CARTILAGE?

The distinction between the medial and lateral cartilage is reasonably straightforward. After reflection most patients can indicate the site of injury and pain, or the side on which something "catches" or "slips." Because the medial cartilage has a longer excursion during flexion and extension of the knee, symptoms on the medial side tend to be more severe. On occasion, a torn posterior end of the lateral cartilage may result in recurrent buckling of the knee, without remarkable "initial" injury, but forced extension or forced flexion usually results in pain that blocks further movement at the site of injury. This is confirmed by finger-point local tenderness and, when present, the palpable click. There is one exception. Very occasionally, pain is felt on one side, usually the medial, when the lesion exists in the opposite meniscus. This may be due to the longer course that the medial meniscus has to travel. The rotary movement pivots on the posterior attachments of the lateral cartilage, whereas the medial side covers the curved tract on the longer medial condyle. If a tear of the lateral cartilage locks rotation, the tension of attempted movement may be felt more sensitively in the longer and more vulnerable medial cartilage and capsule. Although subjective pain may be felt on the opposite side, the site of tenderness and the diagnostic click usually coincide with the main lesion and are sufficient to localize it. If there is doubt, provocative exercise under a skilled physiotherapist will accentuate the signs.

TEARS OF BOTH SEMILUNAR CARTILAGES

Both cartilages are torn more often than one would expect. The presenting features of the injured medial meniscus may obscure those of the lateral side. A careful history may provide a clue in the severity of the accident or an atypical story. Pain may be reported on both sides, or, if the patient is uncertain in localizing the pain, an even more elaborate examination may be necessary. Again, provocative exercises may be helpful. Even so, the symptoms of the second rupture may be obvious only after the first cartilage has been removed. As will be discussed in the chapter on "the dashboard knee," severe contusions of the bent knee tend to injure both cartilages. So does severe wrenching of the extended knee, as in the case of a rider who is dragged by a foot caught in the stirrup after being thrown from a horse.

ANTERIOR TEAR

The anterior tear also has its characteristics. The patient complains of locking or catching in the knee. The rotation signs—limitation of excursion of the tibial tubercle and protrusion of the medial femoral condyle, finger-point pain over the anteromedial or the anterolateral compartment on forced extension, and local tenderness in the same site are all present. A click can be elicited, but not consistently, if the anterior portion of the cartilage has been thickened and, more frequently, if a "pedicled" tag of the free margin can be manipulated in and out of position. In this event the rotation signs are switched on and off synchronously.

This picture includes the *retracted medial cartilage*. In the young, the onset and the course are less severe than they are with the tear with displacement, but the incidence of retracted medial cartilage is greatest in middle and old age, when it is, in my opinion, *the most frequent cause of traumatic osteoarthritis of the knee.*

As with all injuries in older people, the onset may be very distressing, but more often it is mild and sometimes almost unnoticed. At intervals a typical sequence of attacks of discomfort and swelling follow any undue activity, and as the condition deteriorates, it needs less strain to produce the same reaction. The joint swells on each occasion. Decrease in the patient's activity results in increased weight, which in turn adds to the strain on the knee. Eventually, retropatellar pain is caused by going down and later, going up stairs. The patient begins to feel that the bunched-up anterior horn is "like a stone in the knee." The final phase is bone pain at night.

At first, the physical signs are those of any anterior tear. The patient finds relief only by flexing the knee; as time goes on, the range decreases, and the fixed flexion is greater. Finally, the classic osteoarthritic knee with a medially rotated tibial tubercle, a prominent medial femoral condyle, a prominent patella, and a wasted thigh (Fig. 8-1) is established. There are tender spots in the anteromedial compartment just in from the edge of the articular surface of the medial femoral condyle and on the medial border of the patella (see Fig. 7-6, *right*). However, the lateral border of the patella and the lateral side of the joint are not as tender or not tender at all. Painful retropatellar grating may be elicited.

Sometimes a fresh incident, usually a fracture of the posterior third of the medial cartilage, results in grave aggravation of the condition of the knee as a whole. Should this be so, tenderness is felt also over the posterior horn, and a click may be elicited.

POSTERIOR TEAR

The characteristic symptoms of posterior tears of the meniscus are giving way of the knee and pain on full flexion. Sometimes it is difficult for the patient to localize the pain to one side or the other, but tenderness and a diagnostic click usually provide a definite clue. The symptom of giving way is often painless, especially on the lateral side. The torn posterior horn of the medial meniscus is more frequently painful, and a residual tag after inadequate removal of a meniscus causes pain as well as buckling.

THE BOWSTRING CARTILAGE

The type of violence that produces the bowstring (bucket-handle) tear is usually followed by severe pain and swelling. The knee is limited in extension, and the rotation signs are present. If the split extends well aft, the later range of flexion and medial rotations are limited as well and produce pain. While at rest the knee finds comfort anywhere in the intermediate range. Tenderness is felt over the front and the back of the joint line, and, as after all severe incidents, there is another tender spot half way back over the attachment of the deep fibers of the medial ligaments. Even if the knee is not reduced, the swelling and pain subside after a week or 10 days, and the patient can take weight with a limp and with the knee slightly flexed. Eventually, the knee straightens, though at the expense of the capsule, because the rotation signs of limited movement of the tibial tubercle and protrusion of the femoral condyle remain. The stretch in the anterior cruciate ligament and the medial capsule is shown by slight laxity of

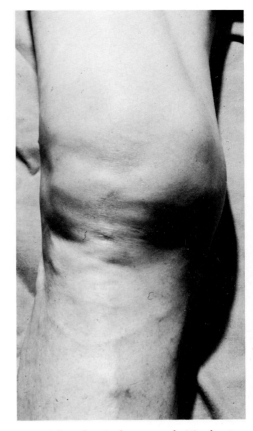

FIG. 8-1. The classical osteoarthritic knee, with medially rotated tibial tubercle, prominent medial femoral condyle, prominent patella, and wasted thigh.

the whole joint. A few degrees of anteroposterior glide and medial ligament laxity are demonstrable. Most often, a diagnostic click is easily palpable.

ROENTGENOGRAPHY AS AN AID TO DIAGNOSIS

In the acute phase and to some extent also in the later stages, roentgenograms have a negative rather than a positive value in diagnosis. Their main purpose is to differentiate internal derangements of the knee from fractures, loose bodies, and diseases that may produce comparable features. Arthrography and ar-

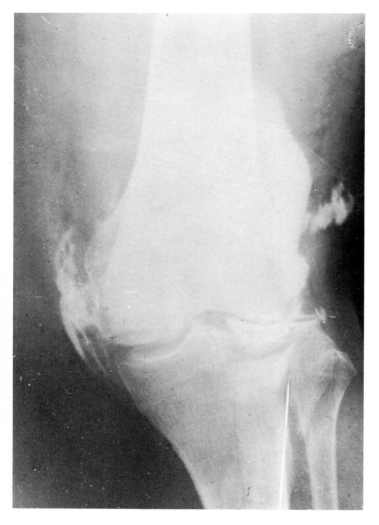

FIG. 8-2. Arthrogram showing ruptured medial ligament and fractured lateral tibial plateau, a combination difficult to diagnose clinically. (Helfet AJ: AAOS Instruction Course Lectures, vol 19. St. Louis, CV Mosby, 1970)

throscopy are valuable in the hands of skilled practitioners. To the experienced clinician such aids are not always necessary, for the clinical patterns described are usually quite clear and are adequate for accurate diagnosis of ruptures of the semilunar cartilages. However, when there is any doubt, and especially in the presence of associated instability due to ligamentous and capsular weakness and tears or other disorders, these aids, as demonstrated by distinguished exponents in Chapters 9 and 10, become invaluable (Fig. 8-2).

Of course, the semilunar cartilages themselves do not show up on x-ray films, except in the rare instances when part of the meniscus is calcified. Even then the picture does not help in the diagnosis of rupture because calcification is not continuous, and the meniscus does not tend to tear through the calcified portion (Fig. 8-3).

After a recent injury the picture is usually negative. When traumatic erosion has occurred, irregularities of joint surface may be seen. Frank osteoarthritic changes, when these have supervened, are also visible. Of note are the tilted posture of the patella below the trochlear groove and the changes in its outline, especially in the skyline view (see Fig. 6-27, *left*). At this stage loose bodies and osteophytes may also be evident. Roentgenographic "loss of joint space" is a misleading description and is often due to an abnormal position of rotation of the femur on the tibia (Fig. 8-4). Hence the sometimes miraculous recovery of roentgenographic joint space after removal of the cartilage and restoration of normal movement and positioning. These features may be more accurately assessed in osteoarthritis by anteroposterior views taken when the patient is at rest and when bearing weight.

INJURIES TO THE INFRAPATELLAR FAT PAD

Contusion, scarring, adhesions, and adherence of the fat pad to the tibia and the meniscus are difficult to distinguish from lesions of the anterior horns of the menisci, with which, of course, they may be associated (Fig. 8-5). The subject is considered in detail in Chapter 18 ("The Dashboard Knee"). The meniscus may be damaged coincidentally with the fat pad, with which it has intimate connections, or the alar flaps of the fat pad may be contused and become adherent to the meniscus. In either case, the anterior horn and the fat pad acquire a point of fixation. This interferes with easy function, and disability ensues. The patient suffers vague aching in front of the knee joint with pain on forced extension and tension or pain in the same area at the extreme of flexion. The swelling and the symptoms are aggravated by activity and relieved by rest, and the history suggests progressive deterioration as time passes.

On examination, tender fullness on both sides of the patellar tendon can be observed. Squeezing the fat pad on both sides of the tendon between the thumb and the forefinger is painful. In an isolated injury of the anterior horn there is tenderness only on direct pressure over the lesion.

If adhesions form that anchor the mobile fat pad and/or the meniscus, the clinical picture

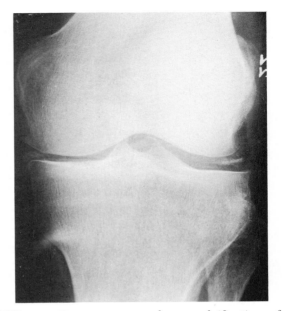

FIG. 8-3. Roentgenogram shows calcification of both the medial and the lateral portions of the meniscus.

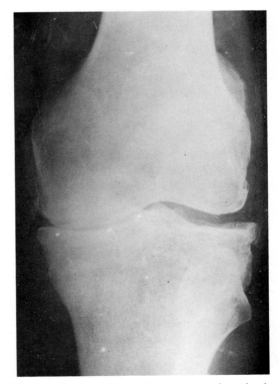

FIG. 8-4. Apparent loss of joint space, largely due to rotation and flexion deformity.

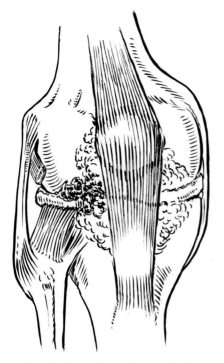

FIG. 8-5. Scar in the infrapatellar pad of fat, involving the anterior horn of the lateral meniscus.

may be complicated by painful limitation of rotation of the tibia and incidents that the patient wrongly interprets as giving way due to acute stabs of pain. The progressive character of the condition and a careful local examination of the extent of swelling and tenderness are the keys to diagnosis. When the anterior horn is obviously damaged, the associated fat pad lesion may be detected only during the operation.

CHONDROMALACIA OF THE PATELLA

In the absence of a meniscal injury chondromalacia of the patella presents a recognizable clinical picture, but when long-standing derangement has established the typical patterns of erosion on the medial surface of the patella and the trochlear slope of the femur,

great difficulties in diagnosis may arise. It is possible that at least some of the early recorded cases of chondromalacia were these sequelae of semilunar cartilage displacement. The pathology and the clinical signs have been clarified by Hirsch and associates,[5] and Soto-Hall,[12] Cave,[8] Wiles and co-workers,[15,16] and Devas.[6] The condition develops in young adults who complain of pain of aching character, worse after sitting, and transient swelling after exercise. Pain is intermittent, may be catching in character, and is worse on slopes and stairs when the contracted quadriceps pulls the tender patella tight against the trochlear surface of the femur (Fig. 8-6). Slight stiffness, persistent swelling, and wasting of the thigh muscles follow. Percussion of the patella against the underlying bone is painful. At a late stage momentary catching with a feeling of sudden insecurity may resemble locking or buckling of the knee joint. Retropatellar crepitation on active movement is characteristic. Soto-Hall[12] elicits this sign by having the patient lie on his back with knee and hip flexed. He is then asked to flex and extend the knee slowly without moving the hip.

Diagnosis is aided by finding that with the muscles relaxed full passive extension is possible without pain, for the patella then rests without tension in the trochlear groove of the femur. The articular surface of the patella is tender. This compares with the meniscal derangement of the knee when the medial border is the only tender part or is significantly more tender than the lateral border. Lateral roentgenograms of the extended knee show the normal patellar excursion, whereas, as shown in Chapter 13, when external rotation of the tibia is limited, the patella remains perched on the lower extension of the medial trochlear slope. Skyline views do not show the unilateral erosion or the osteophytic changes of the patella as seen in Figure 6-27, *left*. They may show thinning of the articular surface (Fig. 8-7).

When examined at operation, the distinction from the arthritic patella is usually obvious, for, instead of a specific pattern of erosion, the articular cartilage is soft, fissured, and frayed, with irregular patterns of disorganization in the late stages (Plate 8-1).

LOOSE BODIES IN THE KNEE

A loose body tends to reveal its presence without subterfuge. Frequently the patient is conscious of "a mouse in the joint" and of the diagnosis. Recurrent attacks of momentary pain and locking, varying in site, followed by an effusion are characteristic. The loose body may be palpable. These incidents differ from those due to the recurrent derangement of a meniscus, in which pain and locking always occur at the same spot. A particularly unstable meniscal tear may also displace momentarily, and the attack then resembles that from the brief intrusion of the loose body between the articulating surfaces; usually derangement of the knee by a torn cartilage is a more protracted experience. When, as is common, the loose body is radiopaque, the roentgenogram is conclusive (Fig. 8-8).

The early stages of osteochondritis dissecans may be misleading clinically. This con-

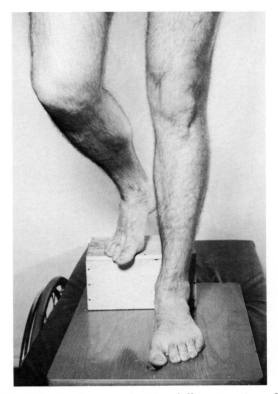

FIG. 8-6. On slopes and stairs, full contraction of the quadriceps pulls the tender patella tight against the trochlear surface of the femur.

FIG. 8-7. Note thinning of the articular surface in these roentgenographic views of chondromalacia of the patella.

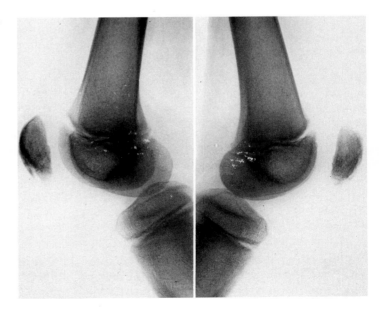

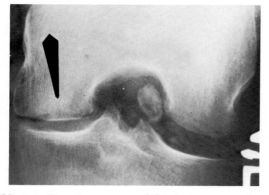

FIG. 8-8. Roentgenogram of third stage osteochondritis dissecans with separated fragment.

dition develops usually between adolescence and completion of growth and presents in three clinical phases. The first is that of a mildly irritable knee and is the reaction to the early products of degeneration of the affected area of articular cartilage. The knee swells and aches after exertion and may be uncomfortable at night. Roentgenograms usually, but not always, reveal the lesion at this stage (Fig. 8-9A). Both knees may be affected, but clinical signs may be more marked or entirely absent on one side.

In 1967 Wilson[17] described the following sign:

The diagnosis of osteochondritis dissecans should be immediately considered in a child who presents a lateral rotation gait and complains of pain, and possibly swelling in the knee. The child may show the following sign which, I consider, is probably diagnostic of the condition. The child is examined in the supine position. The knee on the affected side is flexed through about 90 degrees, and the tibia is medially rotated. The knee is then gradually extended, and at a point about 30 degrees short of full extension, the child will complain of pain over the anterior part of the medial femoral condyle. Lateral rotation of the tibia relieves this pain immediately.

The gradual separation of the fragment introduces the second clinical phase. When one edge is free, the fragment may be pedunculated into the joint and will then simulate the displacement of a semilunar cartilage (Fig. 8-9B,C,D). By this time the roentgenograms are diagnostic.

Once the fragment separates completely, the picture is that of a free loose body (Figs. 8-8, 8-9E,F and see Chap. 28 on osteochondral fractures).

Because a ruptured meniscus may coexist with the separating fragment—both lesions originating from the same injury—careful clinical examination is always essential. Positive rotation signs and finger-point tenderness suggest a second lesion.

The lesions in osteochondritis dissecans differ from the patterns of erosion of articular cartilage seen in osteoarthritis, the latter produced by recurrent pressure or friction of the displaced meniscus, the tensed cruciate ligament, or the friction between the medial facet of the patella and the trochlear groove in the "blocked" joint. In osteochondritis dissecans the surface of the articular cartilage of the separating or separated fragment is not eroded. The fragment of articular cartilage together with a wedge of underlying bone eventually separates from the joint surface.

Paul Aichroth, in a scholarly survey of nearly 200 patients with osteochondritis dissecans of the knee joint at the Royal National Orthopaedic Hospital, has tabulated the common sites of the osteochondritic lesion and implicates injury to the articular surface as the predominant etiologic factor.[1] He adds that many patients had direct injuries and most had taken part in sports or athletics at a high level. In others, mechanical abnormality of the knee joint was found which subjected the joint surface to abnormal stress.

Seventy-five percent of the lesions occurred in the classic site, on the lateral edge of the medial femoral condyle, 10% on the inferocentral surface of the medial, and 13% on the inferocentral surface of the lateral condyle. These are also common sites of erosive lesions. More than 60% of the patients were classified as excellent or good athletes, and the higher the level of their participation the higher the incidence of osteochondritis dissecans. Sixteen of the patients had dislocated or subluxated the patella. Seventeen had a later-

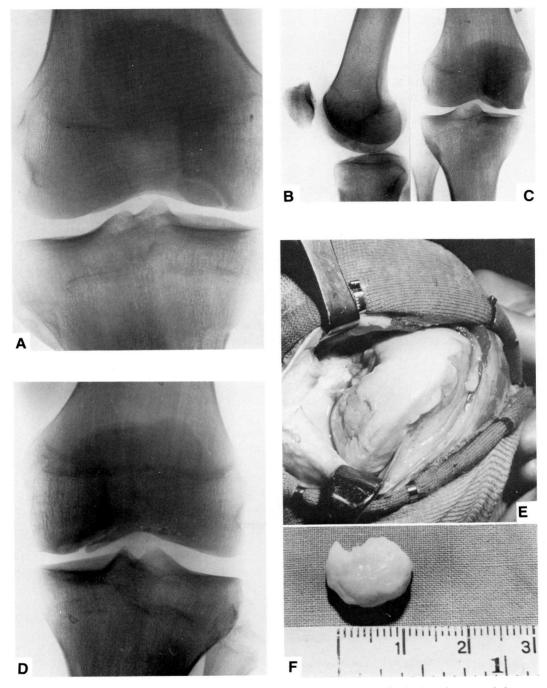

FIG. 8-9. **(A)** The first stage of osteochondritis dissecans, in which detachment of the fragment has not commenced. **(B, C)** The second stage of osteochondritis dissecans; the fragment is separating and forming a mobile pedicle into the joint. **(D)** Another instance in which the fragment has separated. **(E)** The site of separation of an osteochondritic fragment and **(F)** the loose body itself.

ally rotated tibia, and in seven epiphyseal abnormalities were present. On the other hand, 11 patients had osteoarthritic lesions of other joints, and similar lesions have been seen after steroid administration in rheumatic disease and Gaucher's disease. Aichroth concludes that all features point to injury as the main etiologic factor in osteochondritis dissecans of the knee.

In the early stages before separation of the fragment, when aching and swelling are the predominant symptoms, conservative treatment is indicated—an elastic knee guard reinforced with two whalebone struts, to limit the extremes of movement, and limited activity. The only exercise should be isometric muscle drill. The patience of both the young athlete and the surgeon may be tried, but the condition does tend to settle down. Once the fragment pedunculates into the joint or separates to become a loose body, surgery is necessary. It has been my practice to excise the affected piece of cartilage with fragment of bone completely plus any loose bone debris. Often a crescent or disc of dull or yellowish cartilage larger than the attached bone fragment is raised from the underlying bone. This whole disc should be carefully excised. I have seen problems from leaving dead cartilage that subsequently separates and forms another loose body. This is obviated when the whole area is carefully removed. After the operation, the joint should be protected from strain for 6 to 12 weeks until healing is evidenced by comfortable functional recovery.

Replacement of the fragment with internal fixation has not been practiced. On the other hand, for patients referred after fixation but with continued or recurrent symptoms it has been necessary to remove pins and ununited or malunited bone fragments. In any event, it seems unnecessary to undertake an operation, which does not always result in perfection of surface or satisfactory union and which requires prolonged aftercare, to preserve a fragment without which the knee seems to be able to function perfectly well. The area concerned seldom takes part in weight bearing.

Every endeavor should be made to preserve

the patella when it is involved. Prolonged protection by splinting and limited activity after adequate débridement, or after semipatellectomy when indicated, is preferable to removal.[11] However good the initial results of patellectomy may be, in the long run a weak and painful knee ensues, and this is a serious consideration for osteochrondritis dissecans, which is most common in young people.

RECURRING SUBLUXATION AND DISLOCATION OF THE PATELLA

Dislocation of the patella presents little difficulty in diagnosis. Impaction of a meniscus causes acute pain and giving way of the knee, which cannot straighten completely but can flex, often bringing relief by so doing. Acute dislocation locks the knee which can neither straighten nor bend, and the patient falls forward as if tripped.

Recurring subluxation is more deceptive, and many menisci have been erroneously excised. The diagnosis should be suspected in the young and especially in young women, in whom it is more common than meniscal injuries. The patient has a feeling of giving way, of momentary instability with or without a click, and pain on the medial side of the knee. Each incident is followed by an effusion. Tenderness is felt over the medial capsule in line with the border of the patella and chiefly above the joint line, whereas a meniscal tear is tender locally in the joint line. The lateral facet of the articular surface of the patella is tender.

An important sign is that the patient resents and tries to prevent attempts to displace the patella laterally—the apprehension test described by Fairbank[7] and Apley[2] (Fig. 8-10).

SUBLUXATION OF THE SUPERIOR TIBIOFIBULAR JOINT

Subluxation of the superior tibiofibular joint is a rare, or perhaps rarely diagnosed, lesion. A possible explanation of injury was suggested in Chapter 6. When present it must be differentiated from ruptures of the lateral meniscus.[4,9,10,13,17]

In retrospect, the symptoms and signs of three patients are enlightening. During the first week after the accident a nurse suffered severe pain, swelling, and bruising of the anterolateral lower thigh, the knee, and the tibial compartment of the leg. The case notes record a small effusion and stable ligaments, with full extension, but flexion of the knee limited to 110°. She felt cramplike pain on walking, first on the inner and then on the outer side of the calf.

She returned to work after 3 weeks of physiotherapy and limited activity. A normally athletic girl, she gave up all games but still suffered increasing discomfort over the next year, after which she again reported for examination. She complained that although the knee was comfortable when she woke, halfway through the morning pain was felt over the lateral side of the knee and worsened as the day wore on. Examination revealed keen tenderness over the tendon of biceps and the superior tibiofibular joint, but not over the lateral joint line of the knee. The maneuver for the McMurray click resulted in a painful thud which might be confused with the click of a discoid cartilage but was, of course, the slip of the head of the fibula. It was produced by the forced rotation of the leg obtained through the grip on the foot and the ankle.

The diagnosis was confirmed by rocking the head of the fibula anteroposteriorly on the tibia, which produced the pain of which she complained. Comparable roentgenograms showed protrusion of the fibular head behind the posterior border of the tibia.

The second patient also presented with pain over the outer side of the knee, cramps in the calf, and aching in the ankle after walking. Rocking the head of the fibula resulted in the same knee pain. Roentgenograms showed displacement of the head of the fibula and signs of osteoarthritic change.

Pain induced by rocking the head of the fibula, tenderness of the joint, and the distribution of pain also clinched the diagnosis in the

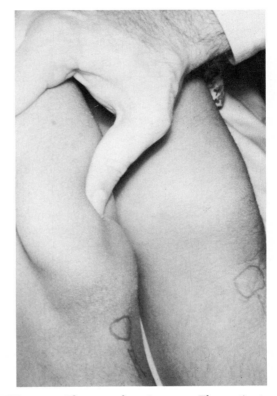

FIG. 8-10. The apprehension test. The patient resents and tries to prevent attempts to displace the patella laterally.

third patient. In all patients, the new test (Fig. 6-38) confirms the diagnosis.

The first joint was repaired and reconstructed. The second was arthrodesed. In both cases the symptoms were completely relieved. Each patient returned to work in approximately 8 weeks. The third girl was kept comfortable for a long time by intra-articular injections of prednisolone. She finally required surgery.

Since 1963 six patients have required arthrodesis of the superior tibiofibular joint for instability and one for intractable osteoarthritis. More recently, equal success has been achieved in three patients by the simpler procedure of subperiosteal excision of the head of the fibula with careful repair of the tibiofibular ligament.

Eleven patients suffering from chronic

sprain, osteoarthritis, or rheumatoid arthritis have been relieved by intra-articular injections of local anaesthetic and corticosteroids. An elastic bandage or strap wound firmly round the upper calf has also given comfort.

TENOSYNOVITIS OF THE POPLITEAL TENDON

Another rare lesion is tenosynovitis of the popliteal tendon. In this series only two cases were diagnosed and treated, but as recorded by Kuland, the condition does develop in running and other sports. Diagnosis was not difficult. The first patient, a radiologist, complained of pain but limited swelling on the outer side of the knee, aggravated by walking but chiefly on bending the knee. At its worst the pain was of a "burning, sharp, stabbing type" that occurred on kneeling when pressure was put on the joint and, to a lesser extent, on passive hyperflexion. Flexion was limited and painful, and this is understandable, because then the tendon is actively engaged. The knee ached at night. Palpation revealed the tender swollen course of the popliteal tendon without effusion in the knee joint. Attempts to rotate the leg laterally against resistance were painful.

Injection of procaine and hydrocortisone acetate into the tendon sheath relieved the condition dramatically.

The second patient suffered from a disabling osteoarthritis of the right hip, which had been treated successfully by cup arthroplasty. Easy comfortable movement of the hip with good muscle control had been achieved.

He related that before the arthroplasty he had complained also of pain on the outer side of his knee which was worse postoperatively. A year later it was decided that the lateral meniscus was at fault, and it was removed. His symptoms were not relieved. He could not exercise the knee, and walking on crutches was accomplished only with discomfort. He could not take pressure on the outer side of the knee and so could not sleep on his right side. He

suffered cramps in his calf from pain radiating to the outer side of the knee.

On examination, tenderness was localized to the popliteus and the insertions of the lateral ligament and the biceps. With the muscles relaxed, movements of the knee, including rotation, were painless, but with the knee flexed, lateral rotation of the leg on the thigh against resistance caused pain. Taking weight when standing was immediately painful, and bending the knee while bearing weight was impossible because of pain.

Procaine injected into the lateral ligament had no effect but injected into the tendon sheath of the popliteus it caused complete and immediate relief. He could move and walk a short while without pain.

ROTATION SPRAINS OF THE MEDIAL SEMILUNAR CARTILAGE

In the acute stage these lesions are often indistinguishable from derangements of the medial meniscus of the knee. The history of injury and locking followed by rapid swelling are typical and properly so, for the lesion is probably a temporary displacement of the anterior half of the meniscus. The effusion is hemorrhagic and painful, because the vascular coronary attachments are strained or torn. The anteromedial compartment of the knee is tender, and forced extension is painful in the same place.

The rotation sprains differ from the ruptured semilunar in that after rest and physiotherapy the knee settles down without recurrence of symptoms. Operation is not necessary because the tear in the vascular coronary ligaments heals.

Occasionally, the healing of the tear occurs by fibrous adhesions between the tibia and the meniscus. In this event, tenderness and pain on rotation in one direction may persist, but the signs of meniscal displacement or instability—locking or giving way—do not recur. This is the single lesion in which manipulation of the knee may "cure" a meniscal lesion, and it is the reason for most successes claimed by manipulators.

Because the differentiation of peripheral detachments from ruptures in the substance of the meniscus is difficult, even with the aid of arthrography or arthroscopy, it is not customary to operate after the first accident. (See Chap. 12.) Initial examination is often negative, and confirmation depends on recurrence of the derangement.

REFERENCES

1. **Aichroth PM:** Osteochondritis dissecans of the knee. J Bone Joint Surg 53-*B*:440, 1971
2. **Apley AG:** The diagnosis of meniscus injuries. J Bone Joint Surg 29:78, 1947
3. **Apley AG:** A System of Orthopaedics and Fractures. London, Butterworth & Co, 1959
4. **Barnett CH, Napier JR:** The axis of rotation at the ankle joint in man. Its influence upon the form of the talus and the mobility of the fibula. J Anat 86:1, 1952
5. **Cave EF, Rowe CR, Yee LB:** Chondromalacia of the patella. Surg Gynecol Obstet 81:446, 1945
6. **Devas MB:** Chondromalacia of the patella. Clin Orthop 18:54, 1960
7. **Fairbank Sir HAT:** Internal derangement of knee in children. Proc R Soc 3:11, 1937
8. **Hirsch C:** A contribution to the pathogenesis of chondromalacia of the patella. Acta Chir Scand [Suppl]90:83, 1944
9. **Lord CD, Coutts JW:** A study of typical parachute injuries occurring in two hundred and fifty thousand jumps at the parachute school. J Bone Joint Surg 26:547, 1944
10. **Lyle HHM:** Traumatic luxation of the head of the fibula. Ann Surg 82:635, 1925
11. **Sacks S:** Semipatellectomy. S Afr Med J 36:518, 1962
12. **Soto-Hall R:** Traumatic degeneration of the articular cartilage of the patella. J Bone Joint Surg 27:426, 1945
13. **Stratford BC:** Simple dislocation of the superior tibio-fibular joint. J Bone Joint Surg 41-*B*:120, 1959
14. **Vitt RJ:** Dislocation of the head of the fibula. J Bone Joint Surg 30-*A*:1012, 1948
15. **Wiles P, Andrews PS, Bremmer RA:** Chondromalacia of the patella. J Bone Joint Surg 42-*B*:65, 1960
16. **Wiles P, Andrews PS, Devas MB:** Chondromalacia of the patella. J Bone Joint Surg 38-*B*:95, 1956
17. **Wilson JN:** A diagnostic sign in osteochondritis dissecans of the knee. J Bone Joint Surg 49-*A*:477, 1967

CHAPTER 9
ARTHROGRAPHY OF THE KNEE

Robert H. Freiberger

Arthrographic examination of the knee joint has been available for many years but has been used only sporadically in spite of the diagnostic accuracy of the procedures.[1,3,4,5] The examination is now becoming more widely used and is gaining acceptance as a routine diagnostic procedure because of the increasing desire to obtain graphic confirmation of clinical diagnosis. The newer, water-soluble contrast media, particularly the meglumine salts, cause practically no irritation to synovial tissues, and inadvertent extra-articular injection causes little or no pain. Fractional millimeter focal-spot x-ray tubes are now generally available, and current flow and x-ray output are sufficient to produce high-quality arthrograms. This is particularly important when fluoroscopic methods are employed, because the usual large focal spot used for spot filming does not provide the sharp radiographs necessary for adequate evaluation.

Arthrography is now used and taught in many medical centers, and it is increasingly possible for the surgeon to request an arthro-gram as he would any other radiographic examination.

The first arthrograms of the knee used air as a contrast medium. The superiority of the water-soluble, radiopaque contrast media now appears clearly established, and at present either a positive contrast substance alone or a combination of air and positive contrast medium is used. Arthrography of the knee is performed best and most easily by a fluoroscopic and spot-film method using a fractional millimeter focal spot for spot filming. Published data on large series of arthrograms show a high degree of accuracy of diagnosis of meniscal tear.

TECHNIQUE

After cleansing the skin and draping the knee, a 20-gauge needle is inserted between the femoral condyle and the patella, from either the medial or the lateral side of the knee. Local anesthesia may be given but is usually unnecessary. Fluid, if present, should be

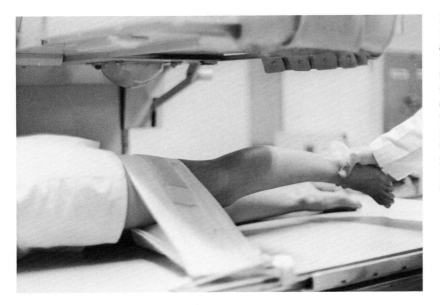

FIG. 9-1. The patient is positioned for examination of the anterior midportion of the lateral meniscus. A sling fastened to the table stabilizes the distal thigh. Pressure exerted on the ankle distracts the area being examined. The protective leaded curtains of the fluoroscope have been raised for the photograph. (Courtesy Appleton-Century-Crofts)

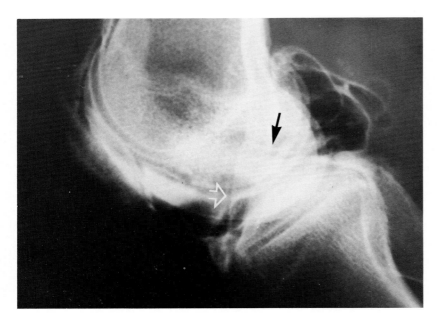

FIG. 9-2. The synovial surfaces of the anterior cruciate ligament (*white arrow*) and the posterior cruciate ligament (*black arrow*) can be seen on this double contrast arthrogram. The exposure was made with the fluoroscopic spot film device.

aspirated as completely as possible; 20 ml of room air is then injected, followed by 5 ml of a meglumine-positive contrast agent. Another 20 ml of room air is injected, and the needle is withdrawn. Unless medically contraindicated, 0.3 ml of 1:1000 epinephrine solution is added to the contrast agent to slow its absorption. In most instances, a horizontal beam lateral film of the knee is made first for depiction of the cruciate ligaments. The patient sits on the edge of the x-ray table; a pillow is placed between the table and the calf, and the patient's foot is pushed backward causing forward stress on the upper tibia, thus simulating the drawer sign. This maneuver stretches the anterior cruciate ligament so that its anterior synovial surface appears as a straight line extending from the femoral condyles to a point approximately 8 mm posterior to the anterior margin of the tibial plateau. The posterior cruciate ligament is seen to extend to the posterior edge of the tibia.

For examination of the menisci, the patient is placed face down and rotated on the x-ray table. The distal part of the thigh is stabilized, either by a sling fastened to the edge of the table or by fixation devices that permit distraction of the side of the knee to be examined (Fig. 9-1). The knee is rotated from a position in which the x-ray beam is tangential to the anterior tibial plateau (an almost lateral projection) to a position in which the x-ray beam is tangential to the posterior tibial plateau, creating the opposite lateral projection. Each meniscus is examined separately. Positioning is monitored with an image-amplified fluoroscope. Two spot films, each with 6 or 9 exposures for a total of 12 to 18 projections, are routinely made of each meniscus. The examination is followed by a second examination of the cruciate ligaments, this time using the vertical x-ray beam and fluoroscopic spot filming (Fig. 9-2). Forward stress on the proxi-

mal tibia is obtained by placing a sling around the patient's calf and pushing the ankle backward against the sling. Then, slightly oblique lateral views of the patella showing its articular cartilages are made with the knee fully extended. Erosion of the cartilage can be demonstrated in severe cases of chondromalacia or osteoarthritis.

ANATOMY PERTINENT TO ARTHROGRAPHY

The medial meniscus is firmly attached to the capsule along its periphery. Because of its complete peripheral attachment, contrast agent cannot normally be seen on the peripheral aspect of the meniscus or within it except through a tear (Fig. 9-3). The arthrogram shows the tightness or laxity of the tibial attachment of the medial meniscus. Occasionally, the recess formed between the capsular attachment and the margin of the tibia is so irregular and so deep that a coronary ligament tear can be assumed. Usually, the clinical significance of the loosely attached medial meniscus remains undetermined.

The lateral meniscus is somewhat more cir-

FIG. 9-3. The contrast agent enhances the free edges of this normal medial meniscus. No contrast agent is seen at the periphery marked by arrows.

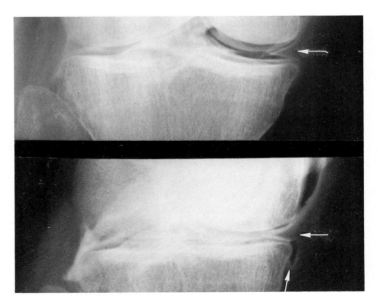

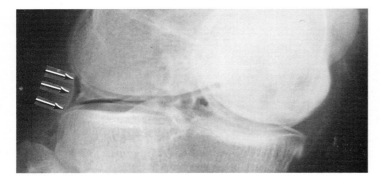

FIG. 9-4. In this roentgenogram of the posterior portion of a normal lateral meniscus, the arrows point to the sleeve of the popliteous tendon, which is filled with air. Its margins are enhanced by positive contrasts, which gives the meniscus a peripherally-detached appearance.

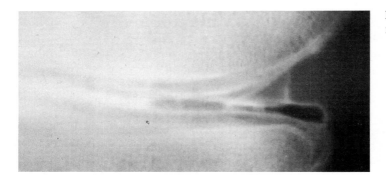

FIG. 9-5. Vertical tear with the fragments in close apposition.

cular than the medial meniscus, and therefore its most anterior and posterior portions at their attachment to the tibial plateau are not depicted on the tangential views of the arthrogram. In general, the lateral meniscus has a much looser tibial attachment normally, allowing a greater degree of mobility. There are no criteria for when the arthrographically demonstrated laxity of the attachment of the lateral meniscus is of clinical significance. In addition, the lateral meniscus is separated from its capsular attachment posterolaterally by the bursa of the popliteal tendon, which communicates with the knee joint. The popliteal tendon bursa is therefore always filled with contrast substance, and this normally gives the posterior portion of the lateral meniscus a peripherally detached appearance (Fig. 9-4). The combination of a more circular configuration, greater mobility, and the presence of the contrast-filled popliteal tendon

sleeve makes arthrographic evaluation of the lateral meniscus more difficult than that of the medial meniscus.

The cruciate ligaments are extra-articular structures with broad, fan-shaped insertions into the tibial plateau and the intercondylar area of the femur. They are covered by synovia that is reflected over both the anterior and posterior cruciate ligaments at their crossing in the center of the knee joint. Contrast agent, therefore, does not envelop each cruciate ligament completely, and arthrographic examination must be meticulous to be accurate. Because tears of the cruciate ligaments can take place without a complete or persistent tear of their synovial surface, they may be evident only by laxity of the ligament when forward stress is applied. By careful technique and by paying attention to detail on the arthrogram, good diagnostic accuracy of cruciate ligament tears can be achieved.

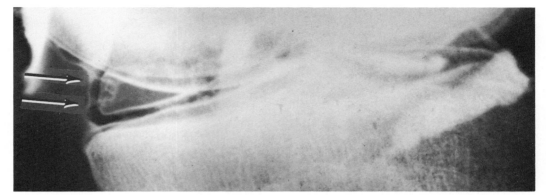

FIG. 9-6. Vertical tear of the medial meniscus with the fragments slightly separated.

FIG. 9-7. Tear of the medial meniscus with the inner fragment displaced into the intercondylar notch.

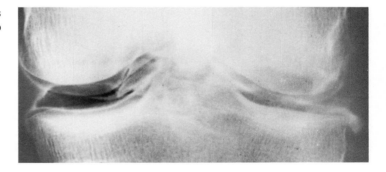

DIAGNOSTIC FEATURES OF MENISCAL TEARS

There are two major types of meniscal tear, vertical and horizontal. The vertical tear splits the meniscus from its superior to its inferior surface; the bucket-handle (bowstring) tear falls into this category. On the arthrogram the two fragments are seen either in close apposition (Fig. 9-5), slightly separated (Fig. 9-6), or with the inner fragment completely displaced and with only the amputated outer fragment remaining (Fig. 9-7).

The horizontal tear indicates a splitting of the meniscus into superior and inferior portions. No major displacement of fragments is usually present (Fig. 9-8). Combinations of these types of tears are frequently found. There is no need to describe the type of tear in great detail, but the extent of the tear and whether it is located predominantly in the anterior middle or posterior portion of the meniscus should be noted. Diagnosis of the discoid or partially discoid lateral meniscus, which can be recognized by its abnormal width, is usually not difficult (Figs. 9-9, 9-10). Difficulties in making a diagnosis of a torn discoid lateral meniscus are encountered occasionally. An oblique tear in a discoid meniscus with displacement of the inner fragment may leave the peripheral portion of normal width, and the tear may thus not be recognized.

Cysts of the lateral meniscus are frequently associated with degenerative horizontal tears, and the contrast agent in such a tear extends irregularly beyond the margin of the tibial plateau, indicating a torn cystic lateral meniscus (Fig. 9-11). When the cystic meniscus is

(text continued on p. 144)

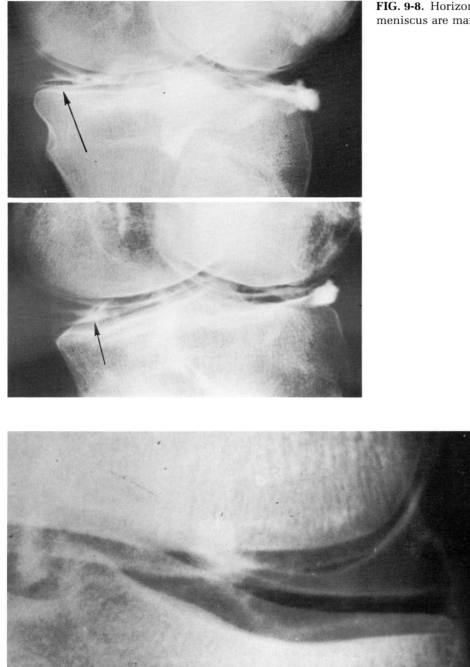

FIG. 9-8. Horizontal tears of the medial meniscus are marked by arrows.

FIG. 9-9. Discoid lateral meniscus. Note the abnormal width.

FIG. 9-10. Torn discoid lateral meniscus in a child.

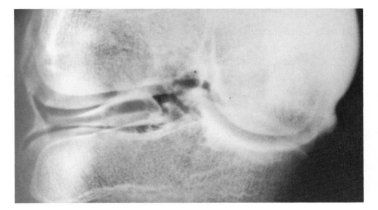

FIG. 9-11. Note the extent to which the contrast agent has dispersed in a soft-tissue bulge at the periphery of the torn cystic lateral meniscus.

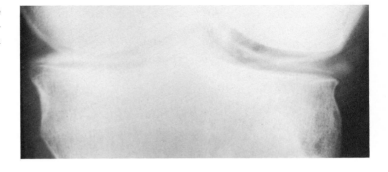

FIG. 9-12. Small chondral fracture of the medial femoral condyle.

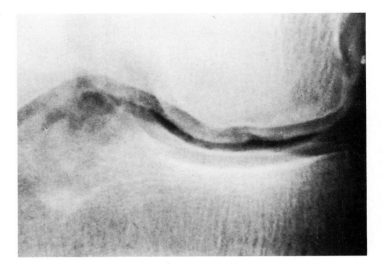

not associated with a tear, the arthrogram will appear essentially normal. However, one may be able to see a soft tissue bulge at the periphery of the meniscus.

The contrast-coated articular cartilages can also be evaluated, the major cartilage erosions, chondral fractures (Fig. 9-12), or loose cartilaginous bodies can be identified. The minor cartilage erosions of chondromalacia are usually not visible. If an arthrogram is requested specifically for the identification of loose cartilaginous bodies or for soft-tissue masses, as for instance in pigmented villonodular synovitis, either an air-only or a contrast-only arthrogram may be preferable in the double contrast study. In such a study, air bubbles that may be confused with loose cartilaginous bodies can form. Capsular ruptures are detected by the extravasation of contrast agent through the ruptured portion of the capsule. Because capsular tears heal to watertight condition rather rapidly, usually within 3 or 4 days, the arthrogram should be performed within 3 days of an acute injury.

COMPLICATIONS

One infection and 10 cases of mild urticaria have occurred in our series of over 25,000 arthrograms.

REFERENCES

1. **Andren L, Wehlin L:** Double contrast arthrography of the knee with horizontal roentgen ray beam. Acta Orthop Scand 29:307, 1960
2. **Butt P, McIntyre J:** Double contrast arthrography of the knee. Radiology 92:487, 1969
3. **Lindblom K:** Arthrography of the knee. Roentgenographic and anatomic study. Acta Radiol (Suppl) 74, 1948
4. **Freiberger RH, Kaye JJ:** *Arthrography*. New York, Appleton-Century-Crofts, 1979
5. **Freiberger RH, Killoran PJ, Cardona G:** Arthrography of the knee by double contrast method. Am J Roentgenol 97:736, 1966
6. **Nicholas JA, Freiberger RH, Killoran PJ:** Double-contrast arthrography of the knee. Its value in the management of two hundred and twenty-five knee derangements. J Bone Joint Surg 52-A:203, 1970
7. **Pavlov H, Freiberger RH:** An easy method to demonstrate the cruciate ligaments by double contrast arthrography. Radiology 126(3):817–818, 1978
8. **Pavlov H, Torg JS:** Double contrast arthrographic evaluation of the anterior cruciate ligament. Radiology 126(3):661–665, 1978

CHAPTER 10
ARTHROSCOPY OF THE KNEE JOINT

Masaki Watanabe
Sakae Takeda

The expression "internal derangement of the knee," coined by William Hey in 1784, describes various lesions and disorders of the meniscus, cruciate ligaments, collateral ligaments, and other structures in the knee joint. It is a condition seen frequently in daily practice, but, owing to the complexity of the structure and the biomechanics of the knee joint, accurate diagnosis is not always easy. With the progress of orthopaedic surgery, however, this condition has been analyzed and classified into an increasing number of clinical components. The classification of internal derangement of the knee, in my estimation at present, is as follows:

1. Lesion or disorder of the meniscus
2. Lesion or disorder of the cruciate ligament
3. Lesion or disorder of the collateral ligament
4. Others
   a. Loose bodies, osteochondral fracture, osteochondritis dissecans, osteochon-

dromatosis, aseptic osteonecrosis, chondromalacia of the patella
   b. Lesion of the infrapatellar fat pads, Hoffa's disease
   c. Lesion or disorder of plica synovialis supra, infra-, or mediopatellaris, chorda cavi articularis genu, chorda obliqua synovialis, popliteal tendon
   d. Tumorous conditions in the joint cavity (pedunculate xanthomatous giant cell tumor, hemangioma, fibroma, ganglion, and so on)

In the diagnosis of internal derangement of the knee, especially of the meniscus lesion, the following are essential:

Knowledge of the normal anatomy and biomechanics of the knee

A correct history, especially details of the manner of the injury

Clinical symptoms

Clinical tests based on the mechanism of knee joint motion

X-ray film, to rule out fracture

Helfet, in this and previous publications, considers that most meniscal lesions can be diagnosed from a careful history and physical examination. Smillie reports the percentage of error reduced from 7.2% to 4.0% with increasing experience. But he adds, "the surgeon who states that he has never excised a normal meniscus is either departing from the truth or is missing more diagnoses than he makes." It is often difficult for a surgeon to diagnose not only the existence of rupture of a meniscus but also the detailed finding of a meniscal tear on which methods of treatment can be based.

In the diagnosis of a lesion of a collateral or cruciate ligament, examination by various maneuvers for stability of the joint, such as valgus or varus stress, drawer sign, and stress radiography, are very important. But dislocation of a piece of the ruptured medial collateral ligament into the joint space or an isolated incomplete rupture of the anterior cruciate ligament is not always easy to confirm by clinical examination.

The knee joint is not a simple hinge joint. Its movement is helicoid or spiral in character and is controlled or guided mainly by a mechanism of collateral ligaments, cruciate ligaments, and menisci. As the normal spiral movement of the knee is a synchrony of extension with external rotation of the tibia and flexion with internal rotation, knee lesions that occasionally are caused by a complex distortion of this pattern may be difficult to diagnose. However, accurate diagnosis is essential for successful surgery and to avoid unnecessary surgery.

More precise diagnosis of meniscal or other lesions is possible by employing three additional methods of visualization: arthrography, arthroscopy, and arthrotomy.

ARTHROTOMY

Arthrotomy for diagnostic purpose should be abandoned because of its associated morbidity and quadriceps inhibition. Further, it is difficult to survey most parts of the menisci by arthrotomy without cutting the extensor apparatus.

ARTHROGRAPHY

Arthrographic diagnosis of meniscal lesions has made great progress during the past two decades, owing mostly to the efforts of Lindblom, Andren and Wehlin, Ricklin, Rüttiman, and more recently, Freiberger (see Chap. 9), Nicholas, and Killoran. It has become a routine examination, and the ratio of errors in the hands of these specialists is less than 5% or 10%. Arthrography has an advantage over arthroscopy in detecting a cleavage in the undersurface of the meniscus or a parameniscal tear without dislocation. However, arthrographic diagnosis is an indirect method, and therefore its interpretation is not easy, especially when the arthrogram is complicated. It is also difficult to confirm a negative arthrogram for a meniscal lesion. Arthrographic diagnosis of the cruciate ligament is still uncertain except in rare cases.

ARTHROSCOPY

Arthroscopic examination of meniscal lesions is a direct observation, and therefore its interpretation is much easier than that needed by indirect methods. The most important problem in arthroscopic diagnosis of a meniscal lesion is how to visualize the entire meniscus. For many years, such visualization was difficult until our No. 21 arthroscope was developed for this purpose in 1959.

The direct viewing telescope of the No. 21 arthroscope has made possible observation of most of the meniscus (with the exception of some small areas) through one puncture, the lateral infrapatellar approach. The posterior segment of the meniscus or an anomalous posterior horn of the lateral meniscus and Wrisberg's or Humphry's ligament are more easily observed by arthroscopy than by surgery. The major advantage of arthroscopy over arthrotomy for diagnostic purposes is the complete absence of quadriceps inhibition and the minimal morbidity following examination.

Arthroscopy also provides additional information from inspection of the synovium and articular surface. For example, we know that in most cases of a torn and degenerated meniscus an erosion or ulcer is found in the cartilaginous surface of the corresponding femoral condyle.

ARTHROSCOPES

Today, the Storz and the Wolf arthroscopes are also used widely. The Storz arthroscope is characterized by its Hopkin's lens system, which provides a very bright image. However, because we have little experience in using these instruments, we shall describe here knee arthroscopy using the No. 21 arthroscope.

The No. 21 direct viewing arthroscope, designed in 1959, was the first arthroscope that allowed inspection of most of the knee joint cavity including the menisci as well as the taking of color photographs. The new model of the No. 21 (1972) consists of a direct viewing and a fore-oblique viewing telescope plus accessories (Fig. 10-1). The size and visibility of the telescopes are presented in Table 10-1. A fore-oblique viewing telescope is also used in turn when necessary.

The direct viewing, or fore-oblique viewing, telescope and a bulb carrier are nested within the same sheath, which has a 6-mm outside diameter. Interestingly enough, the bulb carrier outside the sheath functions as a retractor, which helps in seeing the menisci.

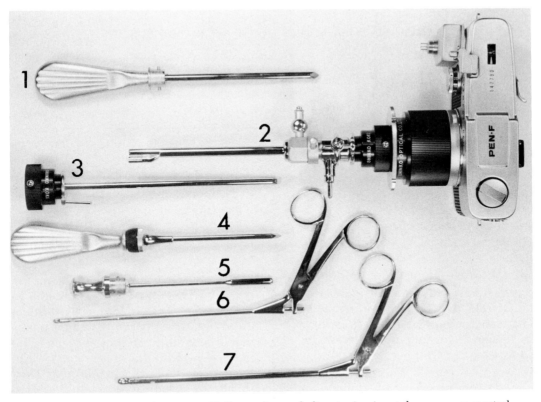

FIG. 10-1. No. 21 arthroscope. Bulb carrier and direct viewing telescope are nested within a single sheath.

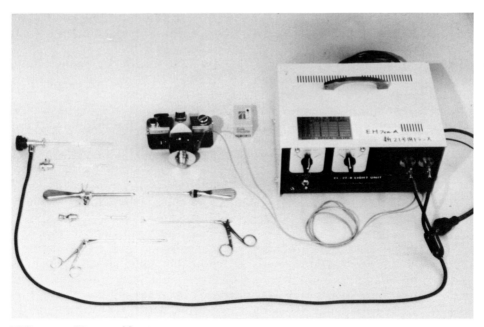

FIG. 10-2. CL-type, No. 21.

TABLE 10-1. TELESCOPES OF THE NO. 21 ARTHROSCOPE

	Length (cm.)		Gauge of	Visibility	
	Total	Tube	tube (mm.)	Axis (°)	Angle (°)
Direct viewing telescope	16.0	9.7	4.9	0	100
Fore-oblique viewing telescope	16.7	10.0	4.9	60	100

The main characteristics of the direct viewing telescope are as follows:

Wide field of vision—visual angle is 100° in air and 88° in water. This is wide enough for normal use.

Depth of focus—from 1 mm to infinity.

Magnification—10 times at a distance of 1 mm, double this at 1 cm, unity at 2 cm, growing smaller at greater distances. Accordingly, image distortion must always be allowed for (see Fig. 10-8).

Light source—small but relatively bright and long-lasting tungsten light source, which is carried alongside the telescope.

Ease of use—both the bulb carrier and the telescope are nested within the same sheath, when in use, as seen in Figure 10-1.

Versatility—with an appropriate transformer, inspection is carried out at 6 V, and photography is performed at 15 V.

The characteristics of the scope are such that when the tip is placed in the joint, it amounts to placing a human eye with extraordinary close vision in the same position, so that is is not difficult for a surgeon to interpret the meniscal findings.

The No. 21 arthroscope with the 6-mm sheath is available for use in children over the age of about 6 years as well as in adults.

Some small areas such as the popliteal cavity, the posteromedial corner of the medial meniscus, and the tibial surface of the meniscus are often difficult to see with the No. 21 scope. For observation of these areas, the No. 24 arthroscope with a 1.7-mm or 2.2-mm diameter should be used in combination with the necessary punctures. Plate 10-1 is a view of the posteromedial corner of the medial meniscus seen from a posteromedial approach with the No. 24.

The No. 21 CL-type of arthroscope, with a glass-fiber light guide (Figs. 10-2, 10-3), was developed in 1975. Plate 10-2 is a view of normal synovial villi photographed with the CL-type at 1/500-sec exposure.

The No. 24 selfoc arthroscope, 1.7 mm in diameter, was developed in 1970 for arthroscopy of smaller joints. It is not a fiberscope but a glass rod lens with an ocular device coupled to it. Selfoc means self-focusing. Selfoc is prepared by ion-exchange treatment of a specially constituted glass rod 1 mm in diameter. As the refractive index of this substance gradually reduces from its central axis to the periphery, the light beam is transmitted through a sine curve configuration with transmission loss lower than that found in optical fiber (Fig. 10-4). Figure 10-5 shows the structure of the selfoc arthroscope.

The No. 24 may be used also as a knee arthroscope. Compared with the No. 21, however, arthroscopic interpretation is much more difficult with the No. 24. The No. 24 is used primarily for viewing very narrow

spaces into which other scopes cannot reach or for special cases such as a stiff knee that precludes manipulation of the No. 21 in the joint, or the knee of an infant.

TECHNIQUE OF ARTHROSCOPY OF THE KNEE JOINT

ANESTHESIA

Anesthesia may be general, spinal, epidural, local, or regional. There are several opinions about the best anesthesia for arthroscopy of the knee joint; each method has its merits and demerits. In Japan, arthroscopy was carried

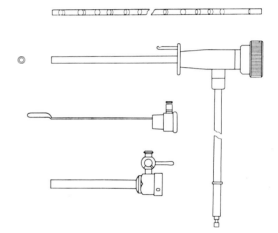

FIG. 10-3. Structure of the CL-type, No. 21.

FIG. 10-4. Light transmission in No. 24 Selfoc arthroscope.

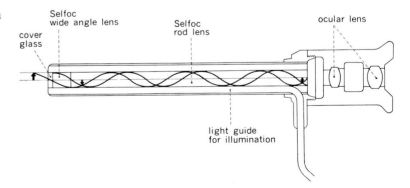

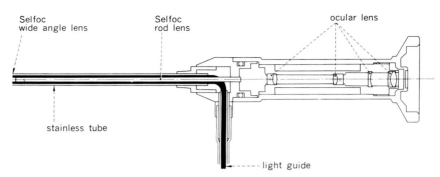

FIG. 10-5. Structure of the new No. 24 with improved ocular.

out under local anesthesia until epidural anesthesia became routine 15 years ago. To view the meniscus in detail, full muscle relaxation is essential. We commonly do arthroscopy of the knee under epidural anesthesia. After examination the patient can return home the same day.

MEDIUM

Normal saline is a physiologic, harmless medium, in which we can observe the natural condition of the synovial villi. It is also useful for lavage of the joint cavity. However, it is inadequate when an electrical instrument is used in the joint because it is an electrolyte.

A gas medium such as N_2 or CO_2 is available for arthroscopy, especially for arthroscopic surgery when an electrical instrument or a laser knife is used. Some arthroscopists use a CO_2 medium, the Pneu-Automatik.

APPROACHES

Many approaches may be used in arthroscopy of the knee joint. The standard method which Watanabe proposed in 1960 is a lateral infrapatellar approach. Occasionally, two or more approaches may be used in combination. Whipple and others have recently described a polypuncture method for more detailed observation. Gillquist's transtendinous approach, using the Storz arthroscope, is useful for viewing the posterior part of the medial meniscus and the distal part of the posterior cruciate ligament.

After mastering the standard method of arthroscopy, one can modify it for special purposes. However, both the standard and special methods should be based on the gross anatomy of the joint. At the same time, the function of each scope to be used should be taken into consideration because each has its own special size, visual axis, visual angle, magnification, depth of the focus, and so on.

STANDARD PROCEDURE WITH THE NO. 21 ARTHROSCOPE

Arthroscopic procedures and the arthroscopic images obtained differ according to the type of arthroscope used. The standard procedure with the No. 21 that I proposed in 1960 uses a lateral infrapatellar approach. In this procedure the following three points are important:

1. Selection of the puncture site
2. First stage of trocar puncture
3. Second stage of trocar puncture

Selection of Puncture Site

The trocar puncture is made at a point on the anterior joint line just lateral to the patellar tendon. This point is in the lateral infrapatellar triangular fossa, which is composed of the lateral side of the patellar tendon, the anterior margin of the lateral tibial plateau, and the antero-inferior ridge of the lateral femoral condyle. After the joint cavity is fully distended by injecting 75 ml to 100 ml of normal saline at room temperature, the knee is bent to 20° and the anterior joint line is palpated with both thumbs of the examiner alongside the patellar tendon. The point depressed with the thumb is the puncture site for either the lateral or the medial infrapatellar approach.

First Stage

The trocar is inserted through a 6 mm to 8 mm skin incision. It is directed obliquely into the infrapatellar fat pad in a posteromedial and proximal direction.

Second Stage

The trocar is then directed parallel to the patellar groove of the femur and introduced through the patellofemoral joint space into the suprapatellar pouch while pressing the suprapatellar region with the free hand to distend the patellofemoral joint space; this is necessary to avoid injury to the cartilaginous surface with the trocar. The trocar should pierce the infrapatellar fat pad at its middle part. If the trocar is directed too far medially and pierces the fat pad at its medial part, observation of the medial compartment will be easier, but it will be difficult to observe the lateral compartment. If the trocar is directed too laterally and pierces the fat pad at its lateral part, observation of the lateral compartment will be easier, but observation of the medial compartment will be difficult.

SYSTEMATIC OBSERVATION

The suprapatellar pouch and bursa are examined with the knee extended. On withdrawing the scope slightly while bending the knee to 20°, the patellofemoral joint can be observed in profile. To observe the patella, it is better to use a fore-oblique viewing scope instead of attempting a direct view. The patellofemoral joint is best observed using a side-viewing scope and a lateral upper approach.

The tip of the arthroscope in the suprapatellar pouch is then directed medially and moved downward, along the medial ridge of the medial femoral condyle while the knee is gently bent to 60° to 90°, imposing a slight valgus strain on the joint. Dropping the patient's foot over the side of the table, thus keeping the knee bent and allowing gravity to assist in opening the medial joint space, provides a better view of the medial meniscus. The joint is extended slowly as the tip of the scope is returned to the suprapatellar pouch.

The knee is then bent with a varus stress while the arthroscope is slightly withdrawn along the patellar groove. The tip of the scope is moved on the medial surface of the lateral femoral condyle into the lateral compartment of the joint. To permit full observation of the lateral meniscus, the knee should be flexed to 60° to 90° in a maximum varus position. This corresponds to the tailor's position. Observation of the lateral meniscus progresses from the posterior segment to the middle and then to the anterior segment.

Observation of the meniscus is made by gently extending and flexing the knee, rotating the tibia externally and internally under valgus or varus stress, and placing pressure with the free hand on the peripheral border of the meniscus. It is very useful to use an instrument introduced into the joint for manipulation of the meniscus. If pathology of the posteromedial corner of the medial meniscus is suspected, the use of the No. 24 arthroscope by the posteromedial approach is essential. Posteromedial puncture is made with the knee in a 60° flexed and maximum varus position.

After observation of the lateral compartment, including the anterior cruciate ligament, the femoral insertion of the posterior cruciate ligament, the plica synovialis infrapatellaris, the popliteal tendon, and other structures, the tip of the scope is reversed again to the suprapatellar pouch.

On conclusion of the examination, including photography and punch biopsy, the joint is irrigated with 500 ml to 1000 ml of normal saline, and the skin incision is closed with a single stitch.

ARTHROSCOPIC DIAGNOSIS

MENISCUS

Because arthroscopy is a direct visualization, the form, size, location, color, glossiness, and flatness of the meniscus can be observed as well as rupture, fibrillation, or tiny cleavages in its surface. In arthroscopy of the meniscus with the No. 21, some areas are difficult to see (Fig. 10-6). Interpretation is thus easy or difficult according to the site and type of the meniscal lesion.

Medial Meniscus

Arthroscopic views of the normal medial meniscus are shown in Plate 10-3*A* to *C*. The middle segment is obscured by the rounded femoral condyle, but when the tip of the arthroscope is pointed closely at it with the knee in a flexed and valgus position, a close-up view of the inner rim of the middle segment can be obtained. The inner rim here makes a few small undulant folds over the tibial plateau owing to normal laxity of the meniscus in the flexed position of the knee (Plate 10-4). The inner rim is concave; it is sharp in the young but becomes irregular and frayed with age. Loss of normal concavity of the inner rim curvature is always an important finding.

If the middle segment is easily found lying under the rounded condyle, a dislocation of that part of the meniscus toward the center of the tibial plateau should be suspected. This finding may be due to a tear localized in the

body of the meniscus, thus making a hole, or to a parameniscal tear in this region; alternatively, it may be due to a medial incomplete discoid meniscus (Fig. 10-7, Plate 10-5).

The insertion of the anterior horn is obscured by fat. Occasionally the anterior part of a normal medial meniscus can be seen lying over the anterior margin of the tibial plateau. An L-shaped tear that makes a pedunculate tag, a transverse tear, or a cross tear can be detected easily (Plates 10-6, 10-7). A bucket-handle (bowstring) tear is also easy to detect—the inner rim curvature of the dislocated part looks convex (on the contrary), and the outer margin is reduced in width (Plate 10-8). However, it is better to confirm the bucket-handle tear with an instrument introduced into the joint. A complete discoid medial meniscus occupies the medial side of the tibial plateau, and its inner rim looks quite thick (Plate 10-9).

The outer margin of the posterolateral part of the medial meniscus is difficult to observe with the No. 21 arthroscope. This part should be observed with a thin No. 24 arthroscope introduced through a medial posterior approach. The undersurface of the meniscus is also difficult to see. By means of the No. 24 fore-oblique viewing arthroscope, some parts of the undersurface can be seen while the inner rim is held up with forceps introduced into the joint. Interpreting what is seen on the undersurface, however, remains a difficult problem.

The space between medial meniscus and tibial plateau is normally very narrow; if it is too wide, rupture of the medial collateral ligament should be suspected (Plate 10-10).

Arthroscopically observed, the posterior part of the medial meniscus enters the tibiofemoral joint space when the tibia is rotated externally in flexion of the knee, and it exits when the tibia is rotated internally. This phenomenon is considered to suggest the mechanism of McMurray's test. When a longitudinal tear is found, it is necessary to trace it in both directions in order to distinguish it from an L-shaped tear (Plate 10-11).

A tear of the meniscus without dislocation is often difficult to find. Observation of the

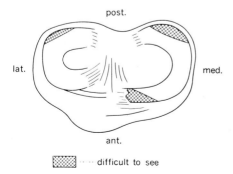

post.

lat.   med.

ant.

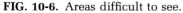 ---- difficult to see

FIG. 10-6. Areas difficult to see.

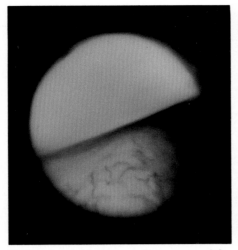

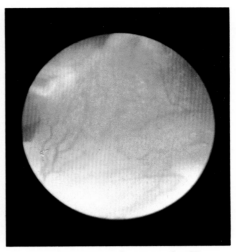

PLATE 10-1. Posteromedial corner of the medial meniscus of the right knee joint.

PLATE 10-2. Normal synovial villi.

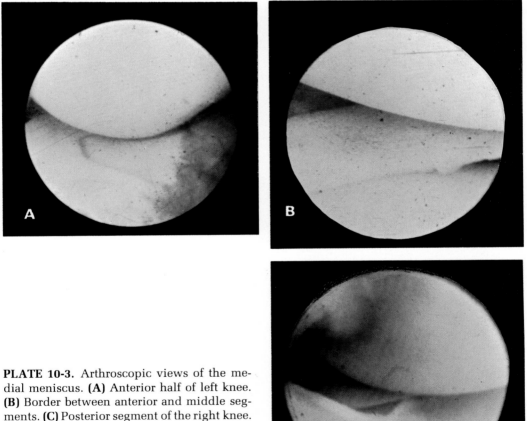

PLATE 10-3. Arthroscopic views of the medial meniscus. **(A)** Anterior half of left knee. **(B)** Border between anterior and middle segments. **(C)** Posterior segment of the right knee.

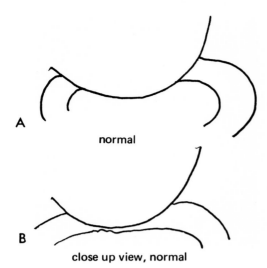

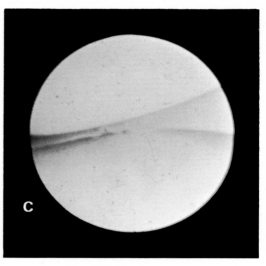

A

normal

B

close up view, normal

PLATE 10-4. Normal medial meniscus. (A) The middle segment is obscured by the rounded condyle. In the close-up views (B, C) of the inner rim of the middle segment, normal wavy folds are visible.

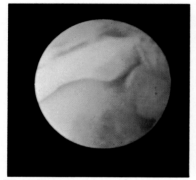

PLATE 10-5. Incomplete medial discoid meniscus in the right knee.

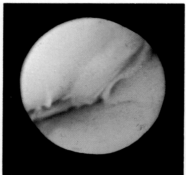

PLATE 10-6. L-shaped tear of the medial meniscus of the right knee.

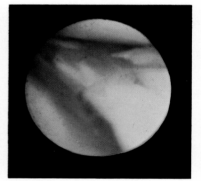

PLATE 10-7. Cross tear of the medial meniscus of the right knee.

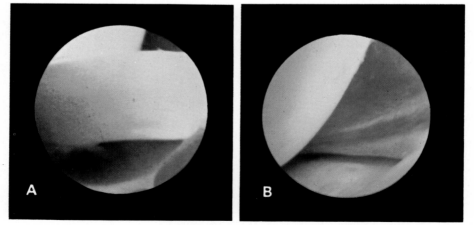

PLATE 10-8. Bucket handle (bowstring) tear of the medial meniscus of the right knee. (A) Bucket handle. (B) Outer ridge.

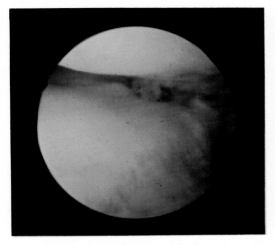

PLATE 10-9. Complete medial discoid meniscus in the left knee.

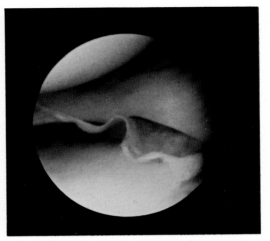

PLATE 10-10. Ruptured medial collateral ligament of the right knee.

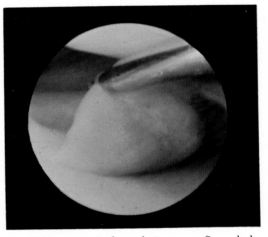

PLATE 10-12. Lateral meniscus of the right knee.

PLATE 10-11. L-shaped tear confirmed by palpation with an instrument.

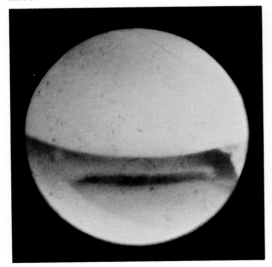

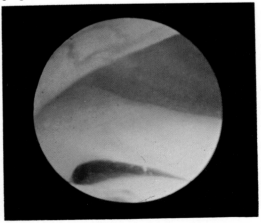

PLATE 10-13. Posterior segment of the left-knee lateral meniscus shows abnormal looseness.

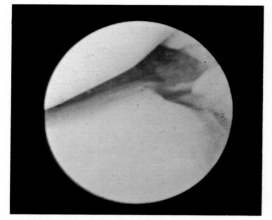

PLATE 10-14. Complete lateral discoid meniscus in the right knee.

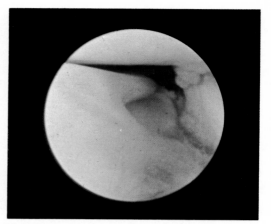

PLATE 10-15. Incomplete lateral discoid meniscus in the right knee.

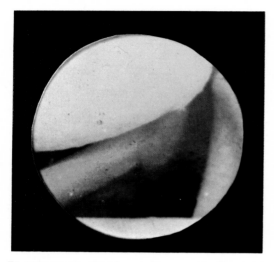

PLATE 10-16. Wrisberg's ligament in the right knee.

PLATE 10-18. Posteromedially dislocated lateral discoid meniscus in the right knee.

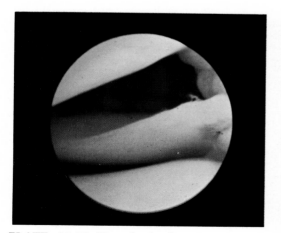

PLATE 10-17. Humphry's ligament in the right knee.

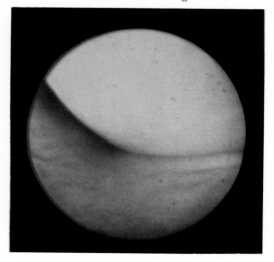

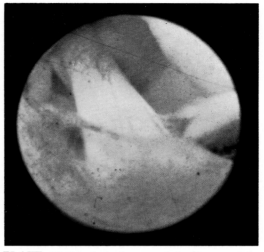

PLATE 10-19. Anterior cruciate ligament in the right knee.

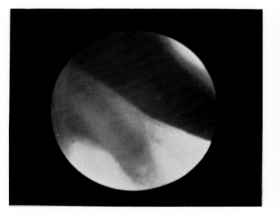

PLATE 10-20. Incomplete rupture of the anterior cruciate ligament in the right knee.

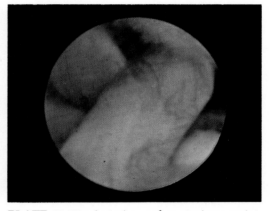

PLATE 10-21. Anterior and posterior cruciate ligaments in the left knee.

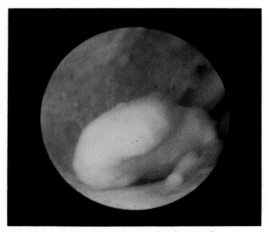

PLATE 10-22. This loose body in the suprapatellar pouch was removed under arthroscopic control.

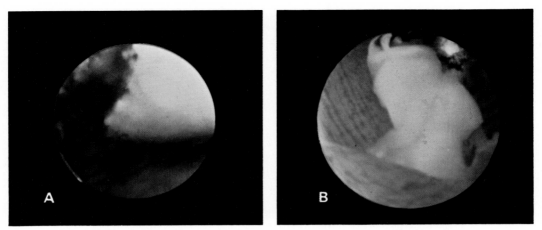

PLATE 10-23. **(A)** Lateral marginal fracture of the patella. **(B)** The fragment in the lateral pouch was taken off without opening the joint.

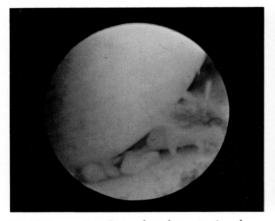

PLATE 10-24. Osteochondromatosis—loose bodies in the knee.

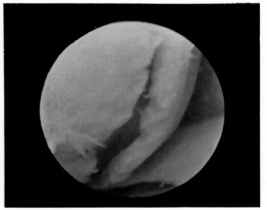

PLATE 10-25. Osteochondronecrosis in the medial femoral condyle of the right knee.

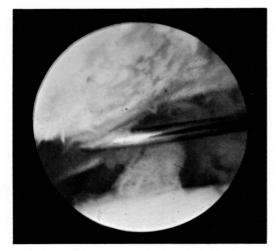

PLATE 10-26. Chondromalacia of the patella, seen from suprapatellar side.

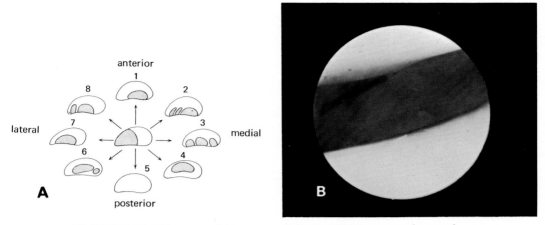

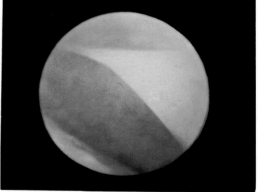

PLATE 10-27. Plica synovialis suprapatellaris. **(A)** Diagrams of normal (*center*) and variations. **(B)** Complete left-knee septum, seen from below.

PLATE 10-28. Plica synovialis mediopatellaris of the right knee.

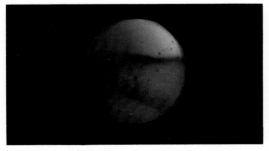

PLATE 10-29. A huge shelf in the right knee of an 8-year-old boy caused some disorder of the joint. The plica was elongated by cutting it partially under arthroscopic control, and the symptoms disappeared.

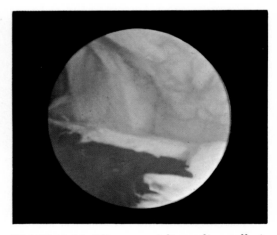

PLATE 10-30. Plica synovialis mediopatellaris caused a disorder of this joint. Biopsy revealed cartilagelike change of the synovium.

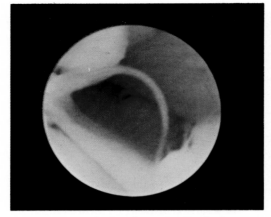

PLATE 10-31. A chorda cavi articularis genus (Mayeda).

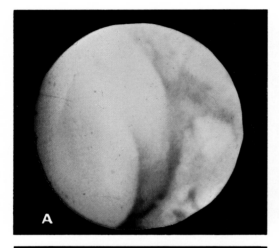

A

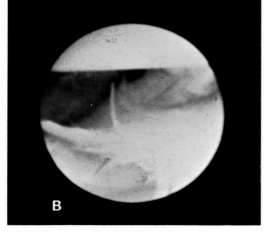

B

PLATE 10-32. Popliteal tendon. (A) Femoral insertion. (B) Running obliquely behind the torn and frayed lateral discoid meniscus of the left knee.

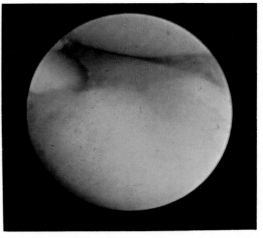

PLATE 10-33. Medial meniscus of the right knee elevated by an underlying ganglion.

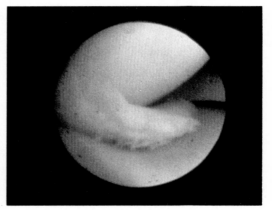

PLATE 10-34. L-shaped tear of the medial meniscus of the right knee joint.

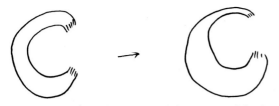

FIG. 10-7. Optical distortion of the image of the lateral meniscus. (*Left*) actual form. (*Right*) image.

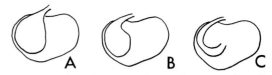

FIG. 10-8. Classification scheme for anomalous lateral meniscus. (**A**) Complete discoid meniscus. (**B**) Incomplete discoid meniscus. (**C**) Wrisberg's ligament type.

meniscus, therefore, should be made carefully, using the various manipulations. In patients with a combined rupture to the medial collateral ligament and the medial meniscus, the anterior cruciate ligament must be carefully observed. On the other hand, there are cases in which the medial collateral ligament is completely ruptured but the arthroscopic view of the medial meniscus and anterior cruciate ligament appears normal. When the unhappy triad is suspected, the lateral meniscus must also be examined carefully.

When a suspected injury of the medial meniscus has been neglected arthroscopically, it is important to observe the lateral meniscus because occasionally pain is felt on the medial side when the lesion exists in the lateral meniscus.

Lateral Meniscus

Observation of the lateral meniscus proceeds from the posterior segment to the middle, and then to the anterior segment. The posterior horn can be traced closely to the point of its insertion, which appears red due to blood vessels lying in its surface. Ofter anterior and posterior segments are seen in one field of vision. Sometimes a whole view of the lateral meniscus can be commanded in one field of vision (Plate 10-12). In judging the form and width of the meniscus, optical distortion of the image must be taken into consideration (Fig. 10-7). Therefore, observation should be done by moving the tip of the arthroscope and changing the distance. The outer margin in the border between the middle and posterior segments is difficult to observe with the No. 21 but can be seen with the No. 24 arthroscope under maximal varus strain. The space be-

tween the posterior segment and the tibial plateau is relatively wide compared with that on the opposite side. However, if this space is too wide due to excessive laxity, a parameniscal tear should be suspected (Plate 10-13).

Lateral Discoid Meniscus

The lateral discoid meniscus is not rare among the Japanese. Smillie classified it into three types—primitive, intermediate, and infantile.[30] Kaplan pointed out that no discoid meniscus was found in any stages of fetal development and that the discoid form develops gradually after birth. It is the result of abnormal motion of the lateral meniscus combined with an anatomic variation in which the posterior horn is not attached to the tibial plateau.[16] It is this type of discoid meniscus that Kaplan failed to find in any fetuses that he examined at Carnegie Institute and in the cases that he personally observed at Columbia University.

In Japan, Nemoto examined knee joints of 70 fetuses in which he found three cases of bilateral lateral discoid meniscus.[24] Matsushita of our clinic investigated the same subject in 16 fetuses and found one case of bilateral lateral discoid meniscus.[18] On the other hand, we also see an anomalous lateral meniscus in which the insertion of the posterior horn is defective but its size is fairly normal; I termed this "Wrisberg's ligament type." I therefore believe that among so-called lateral discoid menisci there are both congenital discoid menisci, as Smillie stated, and secondarily developed discoid menisci, as described by Kaplan.

From the viewpoint of arthroscopy, I have classified the lateral discoid meniscus into the three types shown in Figure 10-8. The complete discoid meniscus occupies the lateral side of the tibial plateau and blocks the view of the tibial plateau completely (Plate 10-14). Such a discoid meniscus appears as if it were the tibial plateau itself, and observation must therefore be done by placing pressure with the free hand on the peripheral border of the meniscus to distinguish it from the true tibial plateau. The incomplete discoid meniscus shows many variations in its size, form, and structure. In arthroscopy of the incomplete discoid meniscus, the close-up view of its concave part of the inner rim often resembles the view of the normal meniscus lying on the tibial plateau (Plate 10-15). The anomalous posterior horn of the lateral meniscus shows variations in size. Wrisberg's ligament is easy to detect (Plate 10-16). Humphry's ligament is rare in Japanese (Plate 10-17). The lateral discoid meniscus often dislocates posteromedially; it is diagnosed from its relationship to the corresponding rounded condyle (Plate 10-18). A ruptured and degenerated discoid meniscus sometimes loses its meniscal appearance.

Clinical Statistics

From 1958 to 1971, 320 knee joints suspected of internal derangement were examined arthroscopically in our clinic. Among them were 208 meniscal lesions or disorders, 18 ruptured ligaments, and 94 other disorders. Among 208 meniscus cases, surgery was performed on 153, and the results are shown in Table 10-2. The ratio of ruptured medial menisci to lateral menisci is approximately 1 : 2 (29 : 54), but when the discoid meniscus is excluded, the ratio should be corrected to 3 : 1 (27 : 9).

CRUCIATE LIGAMENTS

The anterior cruciate ligament is better observed by a lateral infrapatellar approach and with the knee bent to 60° to 90° (Plate 10-19). It looks like a white tendinous band coated by a thin synovial membrane and contains a few blood vessels. The anterior ligament can be traced to its femoral insertion as well as to the divergent inferior part. Complete or incomplete rupture of the anterior ligament can be observed (Plate 10-20).

Behind the anterior ligament, the femoral insertion of the posterior cruciate ligament can be seen (Plate 10-21), bordered by a red, eroded areola in the cartilage in the medial condyle (Plate 10-3C). The posterior ligament is sometimes difficult to see; fat pads in this region hinder its view. When the anterior ligament is torn (or worn out), observation of the posterior ligament is very easy.

COLLATERAL LIGAMENTS

There is not much to be emphasized in arthroscopic examination for injury of the collateral ligaments. The diagnosis is made by clinical examination, and from the viewpoint of arthroscopy, careful observation of any combined injuries is most important. If the medial ligament is ruptured just below the meniscal attachment, a widening of the gap between the medial meniscus and the tibial plateau is evident arthroscopically (Plate 10-10). If a piece of ruptured medial ligament is impacted into the joint space, it can be detected by arthroscopy.

OTHER INJURIES OR DISEASES

Loose bodies, osteochondral fracture, osteochondritis dissecans, osteochondromatosis, aseptic osteonecrosis, and chondromalacia of the patella are included in the last category.

TABLE 10-2. RESULTS OF SURGERY ON 153 MENISCI

Meniscus operated	Medial (torn)	Lateral (torn)	Total
Meniscus excluding discoid meniscus	32 (27)	19 (9)	51 (36)
Discoid meniscus	6 (2)	93 (45)	99 (47)
Meniscus ganglion	2	1	3
Total	40 (29)	113 (54)	153 (83)

Some examples are shown in Plates 10-22 to 10-26.

Hoffa's disease is usually diagnosed by clinical examination. Intra-articular lesions of the infrapatellar fat pads or synovial fringe are sometimes found as a suggillation in the tissue.

Synovial pleats or chordae sometimes cause characteristic disorders of the joint. Plica synovialis supra-, infra-, and mediopatellaris are three main synovial pleats of the knee joint. Plica synovialis suprapatellaris, an incomplete septum between the bursa and the recessus suprapatellaris, separates these structures in the medial half and is a good mark for interpretation of the location of the tip of the arthroscope. However, there are many variations in its extent (Plate 10-27A). Plate 10-27B shows a view of a complete septum. I have never yet encountered a single example of a lesion of this plica. The plica synovialis infrapatellaris can be observed running over the anterior cruciate ligament. As the joint cavity is distended with saline during arthroscopy, this plica becomes somewhat stretched so that it usually looks thinner and the blood vessels running through it become visible. In some cases a membranous septum is found between the plica and the anterior ligament. It is possible to damage this plica by careless arthroscopic procedure, but its clinical significance is not clear. I have encountered only one case in which the plica synovialis infrapatellaris was thickly scarred and caused some disorder of the joint.

The plica synovialis mediopatellaris is a synovial pleat on the medial wall of the knee joint cavity starting from the medial plica alaris and running toward the medial part of the plica synovialis suprapatellaris. It is very often seen in the knee joint of Japanese (nearly half), and Iino called it "the band" in his work on arthroscopy of the knee joint in 1939.[12] It is also called simply "the shelf," because of its shelflike appearance (Plate 10-28), but it shows many variations. The plica synovialis mediopatellaris is considered, as are the preceding two synovial pleats, to be a persistence of the synovial septum of the fetal stage. A considerable number of cases of internal derangement of the knee due to a certain change of the plica synovialis mediopatellaris have been reported in Japan. In my estimation, however, it causes some derangement of the joint only when it is too large (a huge shelf) or becomes rigid (Plates 10-29, 10-30).

The plica synovialis mediopatellaris, the so-called medial shelf, had, in fact, been thought to be peculiar to Japanese; however, this structure seems not to be limited to Japanese. They also reported disorder of the knee due to this structure as "medial shelf syndrome" and pointed out that this syndrome is an important part of the internal derangement of the knee.

The chorda cavi articularis genu[19] is a cord-like or stringlike structure found in various sites of the joint cavity (Plate 10-31). Mayeda considered it to be a retained septum in the synovial cavity and classified it into six types according to the site of its insertion.[19] From the viewpoint of arthroscopy, I classified it into three types according to its relationship to the main synovial pleats. Only when a chorda becomes very thick and hard does it tend to cause derangement of the joint.

The chorda obliqua synovialis refers to a chorda in the synovial membrane that can be palpated in the extended position of the knee either medial or lateral to the patella; it runs obliquely toward the medial or lateral joint line (Fig. 10-9) and is not palpable when the knee is flexed to about 90°. It is a special structure in the synovial membrane, and its clinical significance was investigated by Takahashi of our clinic in 1960.[32]

The lateral outer pouch consists of the lateral wall of the joint cavity and the lateral synovial surface of the lateral femoral condyle. The popliteal tendon can be seen in the depth of the lateral pouch, which runs in a postero-inferior direction and disappears as it curves medially behind the lateral meniscus to its exit in the posterior capsule (Plate 10-32). I have performed arthroscopy in one case of popliteal tendon click, in which a mechanism of the click was investigated.

Pedunculate xanthomatous giant cell tumor,

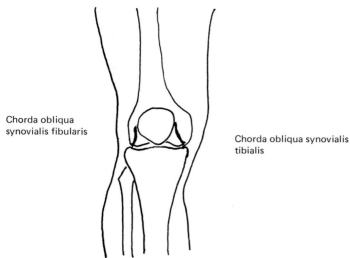

FIG. 10-9. Chorda obliqua synovialis.

Chorda obliqua
synovialis fibularis

Chorda obliqua synovialis
tibialis

Chorda obliqua synovialis.

hemangioma, fibroma, and ganglia have been observed in the knee joint. Plate 10-33 shows a ganglion under the medial meniscus.

ARTHROSCOPIC SURGERY

It is natural and reasonable that a surgeon who has been doing knee arthroscopy for many years should think of using the arthroscope for surgery without opening the joint. An ordinary arthrotomy usually requires hospitalization for a few weeks and extended after-treatment. Arthrotomy also may result in morbidity and quadriceps inhibition. Arthroscopic surgery, on the other hand, avoids surgical opening of the joint with its subsequent ill effects. It requires only one or two days' stay in the hospital. Removal of loose bodies or pedunculate tumors, cutting of adhesions in the joint, and release or removal of a pathologic synovial plica have been performed under arthroscopic control.

The first case of arthroscopic meniscectomy was carried out in 1962. A 17-year-old boy twisted his right knee joint while playing basketball. Arthroscopy revealed an L-shaped tear of the medial meniscus (Plate 10-34). The flap was cut and removed under arthroscopic control. The patient returned home on foot the same day and 6 weeks later was able to play basketball again.

Arthroscopic meniscectomy is a very interesting field of arthroscopy, and the number of cases is rapidly increasing. Until comparatively recently, the indications for arthroscopic meniscectomy had been limited to the L-shaped tear and the bucket-handle tear, but with progress in technique and instrumentation, it is being performed more frequently.

Recently, O'Connor perfected the methodology of arthroscopic meniscectomy and brought most types of meniscectomy within the scope of arthroscopic control.[26] His efforts in this field are worth special mention.

In arthroscopic surgery the instruments to be used should be very small in order to reach the site but also strong enough to serve the purpose. At present, the mode of operating instruments differs according to the individual arthroscopist who designs them. There are dozens of such instruments.

There are three ways of using an operating instrument. It may be introduced into the joint through the same sheath as the scope, that is, an operating arthroscope; through separate 3-mm or 5-mm sheaths, or, directly through a hole pierced by a trocar or formed percutaneously through a small incision (portal). For arthroscopic meniscectomy, general anesthesia is best. The tourniquet is applied to the upper thigh but is not inflated unless bleeding occurs. The most adequate position of the knee and the best approach for the arthroscope and operating instruments should be chosen in each instance (Fig. 10-10).

The instrument to be used is usually introduced into the joint on the side opposite that of the scope's approach. When the scope and instrument are introduced from the same side, it is best to introduce the scope from the upper side and the instrument from below.

In my estimation at present, however, it is unnecessary to carry out all meniscectomies under arthroscopic control, except for those performed on athletes. The best way may be to plan the operation on the basis of the detailed findings obtained by preoperative arthroscopy and to perform it first under direct vision and then, if necessary, in combination with one or two small incisions into the joint, so that the surgery progresses without difficulty and ends in a short time. For instance, if one end of the bowstring of a torn meniscus has been cut under arthroscopy and the other end is difficult to cut, a small incision can be made. This means a half arthroscopic, half open meniscectomy, but it is a practical method. Also, detachment of the posterior horn of the meniscus prior to open meniscectomy may simplify the meniscectomy.

In arthroscopic partial meniscectomy the stability of the retained part of the meniscus should be carefully confirmed by manipulation. A color-TV system is extremely useful in arthroscopic surgery, because assistants can help the surgeon by watching the TV screen (Fig. 10-11). In the near future operating instruments for arthroscopic surgery will be standardized, and the technique for intra-articular manipulation will be discussed in detail. It will also be possible to use a laser knife for arthroscopic meniscectomy. However, it must be realized that good technique in diagnostic arthroscopy is essential for successful arthroscopic surgery.

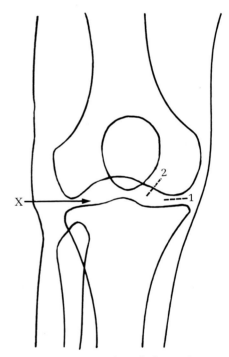

FIG. 10-10. Example of medial meniscus surgery. (**X**) Insertion site of the scope. (*1, 2*) Portals.

FIG. 10-11. Color TV system for endoscopy.

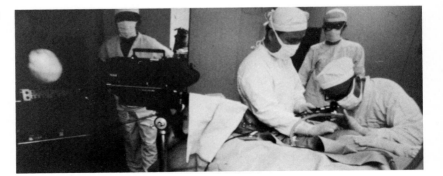

SUMMARY

Through the development of the No. 21 arthroscope, arthroscopy has become a practical means of diagnosing internal derangement of the knee. Since arthroscopy is a direct visualization, its interpretation is easy. The use of arthroscopy has permitted not only diagnosis of rupture of the meniscus but also observation of detailed findings of a meniscal tear on which methods of treatment can be based. In order to improve accuracy of arthroscopic diagnosis of the meniscus, the original technique for knee arthroscopy is essential.

Arthroscopy is a procedure with minimal morbidity. It does not cause quadriceps inhibition and can be performed repeatedly. Further, we are conducting research into the use of the No. 24 arthroscope, employed in tandem with the No. 21, to observe areas of the knee joint, such as the undersurface of the meniscus, the outer ridge of the meniscus in the border between the middle and posterior segments, the tibial half of the posterior cruciate ligament, and the popliteal cavity, at present inaccessible to the No. 21 alone.

Arthroscopic surgery is progressing rapidly, mainly through the efforts of American orthopaedic surgeons; however, successful arthroscopic surgery will be attained only when good diagnostic arthroscopic procedures are followed.

REFERENCES

1. **Andrén L, Wehlin L:** Double-contrast arthrography of knee with horizontal roentgen ray beam. Acta Orthop Scand 29:307, 1960
2. **Aritomi H, Yamamoto M:** A method of arthroscopic surgery: clinical evaluation of synovectomy with the electric resectoscope and removal of loose bodies in the knee joint. Orthop Clin North Am 10:565, 1979
3. **Carson RW:** Arthroscopic meniscectomy. Orthop Clin North Am 10:619, 1979
4. **Casscells WW:** Arthroscopy of the knee joint. J Bone Joint Surg 53A:287, 1971
5. **Freiberger RH, Nicholas JA, Killoran PJ:** The value of double-contrast arthrography in the surgical management of the knee injury. J Bone Joint Surg 49A:1482, 1967
6. **Gillquist J, Hagberg G, Oretorp N:** Arthroscopic visualization of the posteromedial compartment of the knee joint. Orthop Clin North Am 10:545, 1979
7. **Guhl JF:** Arthroscopic treatment of osteochondritis dissecans: Preliminary report. Orthop Clin North Am 10:671, 1979
8. **Helfet AJ:** Mechanism of derangements of the medial semilunar cartilage and their management. J Bone Joint Surg 41B:319, 1959
9. **Helfet AJ:** Management of Internal Derangements of the Knee. Philadelphia, JB Lippincott, 1963
10. **Heller L, Langman L:** The menisco-femoral ligaments of the human knee. J Bone Joint Surg 46B:307, 1964
11. **Humphrey GM:** A treatise on the human skeleton including the joints. Cambridge, Macmillan, 1958
12. **Iino S:** Normal arthroscopic findings of the knee joint in adults. J Jpn Orthop Assoc 14:467, 1939
13. **Ikeuchi H:** Meniscus surgery using the Watanabe Arthroscope. Orthop Clin North Am 10:629, 1979
14. **Jackson RW, Abe I:** The role of arthroscopy in the management of disorders of the knee. J Bone Joint Surg 54A:310, 1972
15. **Kaplan EB:** The lateral meniscofemoral ligament of the knee. Bull Hosp Joint Diseases 17:176, 1956
16. **Kaplan EB:** Discoid lateral meniscus of the knee joint. J Bone Joint Surg 39A:77, 1957
17. **Lindblom K:** Arthrography of the knee. Acta Radiol Scand [Suppl]:74, 1948
18. **Matsushita A, Watanabe M, Takeda S:** Investigation on so-called discoid meniscus. J Jap Orthop Assoc 35:851, 1961
19. **Mayeda T:** Ueber das strangartige Gebilbe in der Kniegelenkhöhle (Chorda cavi articularis genu). Mitt Med. Fak Kaiserl Univ Tokyo 21:507, 1918
20. **McMurray TP:** The semilunar cartilages. Br J Surg 29:407, 1940
21. **Mital MA, Hayden J:** Pain in the knee in children: The medial plica shelf syndrome. Orthop Clin North Am 10:713, 1979
22. **Mizumachi S, Kawashima W, Okamura T:** So-called synovial shelf in the knee joint. J Jpn Orthop Assoc 22:1, 1948
23. **Nemoto H:** Study on discoid meniscus of the knee. Niigata Med J 64:404, 1950
24. **Nicholas JA, Freiberger RH, Killoran PJ:** Double-contrast arthrography of the knee. J Bone Joint Surg 52A:203, 1970
25. **O'Connon RL:** Arthroscopic Surgery of the Knee. A. A. O. S. Symposium on Arthroscopy and Arthrography of the Knee. St Louis, CV Mosby 1978
26. **Okazaki H:** Clinical significance of arthrography and arthroscopy to diagnosis of internal derangement of the knee. Clin Orthop Surg 3:1046, 1968
27. **Ricklin RP, Rüttimann A, Del Buono MS:** Die Meniskusläsion. Stuttgart, Georg Thieme Verlag, 1964
28. **Sakakibara J:** Study on "Iino's band"—a synovial pleat in the knee joint of Japanese. J Jpn Orthop Assoc 46:846, 1972

29. **Smillie IS:** Injuries of the Knee Joint, 4th ed. Edinburgh E & S Livingstone, 1970

30. **Stone RG:** Peripheral detachment of the menisci of the knee: A preliminary report. Orthop Clin North Am 10:643, 1979

31. **Takahashi S:** On the chorda obliqua synovialis of the knee joint. Teishin Igaku 12:1, 1960

32. **Takeda S:** Reconstruction of the anterior cruciate ligament under arthroscopic control. Arthroscopy 2:41, 1977

33. **Watanabe M:** The development and present status of the arthroscope. J Jpn Med Instr 25:11, 1954

34. **Watanabe M:** Arthroscopic diagnosis of internal derangement of the knee. J Jpn Orthop Assoc 42:993, 1968

35. **Watanabe M:** Arthroscopy: The present state. Orthop Clin North Am 10:505, 1979

36. **Watanabe M, Takeda S:** The No. 21 arthroscope. J Jpn Orthop Assoc 34:1041, 1960

37. **Watanabe M, Takeda S, Ikeuchi H** et al: Chorda cavi articularis genu (Mayeda) from the viewpoint of arthroscopy. Clin Orthop Surg 7:986, 1972

38. **Watanabe M:** Arthroscope—present and future. Surgical Therapy 26:73, 1972

39. **Watanabe M, Takeda S, Ikeuchi H:** Atlas of Arthroscopy 3rd ed. Tokyo, Igaku Shoin, 1979

CHAPTER 11
ARTHROSCOPIC SURGERY
OF THE KNEE

Richard L. O'Connor

Operative arthroscopy developed as a natural sequence to the initial work with the arthroscope as a diagnostic instrument. As experience with diagnostic arthroscopy increased, surgeons became aware that because they were able to visualize and understand the pathology present, it might be possible to develop the equipment and the technique that would allow surgical correction. From this perception sprang the early efforts at operative arthroscopy. The original attempts to remove articular obstructive material arthroscopically were made by Dr. Masaki Watanabe's group in Japan. Dr. Watanabe* removed a bucket-handle tear in 1962, and during the ensuing years loose bodies, foreign objects, and selected meniscal flaps were occasionally removed.

My experience with operative arthroscopy began in 1971 with the removal of loose bodies. Subsequently, I excised a meniscal flap in an elderly woman, with complete relief of pain and mechanical obstruction; however, this result was achieved with injury to the already damaged articular cartilage that would be unacceptable in a patient of lesser years who had normal articular surfaces. Encouraged by the work of Dr. Hiroshi Ikeuchi* (one of Dr. Watanabe's associates) in excising meniscal tears and by the intellectual stimulus of Dr. Robert Jackson† of Toronto, who believed a method should be found to preserve as much meniscus as possible, I began to work on developing some surgical instruments that would safely allow excision of meniscal tissue without damage to the adjacent articular cartilage. By the end of 1974, a series of approximately 70 patients treated by arthroscopic partial meniscectomy had been collected. These patients were highly selected, that is, their tears had to conform to certain criteria before a partial meniscectomy was performed. A superficial comparison of the results

---

* Watanabe M: Personal communication, 1971

* Ikeuchi H: Personal communication, 1972
† Jackson RL: Personal communication, 1971

achieved in this group with the results in a group treated by subtotal meniscectomy mandated a change in philosophy: henceforth, all meniscal tears would be excised with arthroscopic equipment to determine which tears could be treated arthroscopically and which required arthrotomy and subtotal meniscectomy. In this second series, which extends to the present time, arthrotomy has been necessary on three occasions, all within the first year and all due to the inexperience of the surgeon. I have found no tear that could not be excised arthroscopically, but some tears are technically much more difficult to excise than others.

PARTIAL MENISCECTOMY

Partial meniscectomy performed through an arthrotomy incision is a surgical procedure whose merit has been debated off and on for years. Its proponents stress the advantage of lowered morbidity, whereas its opponents warn that hidden tears may be missed during the procedure, requiring repeated meniscectomy. Both arguments are valid, but with the new technology offered by the use of arthroscopy, additional tears in the peripheal rim may be detected either prior to or following arthrotomy and partial meniscectomy, because the peripheral rim can be evaluated visually. This may be cumbersome, however, because it necessitates an arthroscopic set-up following arthrotomy and partial meniscectomy. The age and the type of tear may definitely affect the result. Longitudinal tears of recent origin are not often associated with secondary tears. However, flap tears of the meniscus frequently have secondary tears in the peripheral rim on the medial side, which may be undetected owing to the obstruction of the medial femoral condyle. A partial meniscectomy is obviously riskier on a medial meniscus with a flap tear or with a long-standing longitudinal tear.

A major advance in knee surgery has been the ability to perform partial meniscectomy without resorting to arthrotomy, using instead the arthroscope with its limited exposure to perform arthroscopic partial meniscectomy. Successful application of this technique requires the observation and rigid adherence to certain principles:

The peripheral rim must be stable.

All mobile tissue must be completely excised. During the course of investigation into the arthroscopic excision of meniscal tears, the source of meniscal pain became apparent (Plate 11-1). The mobile fragment protruding into the joint line, which is still attached to the capsule by the meniscal capsular fibers, is forced centrally by the compressive effect of the tibia and femur during weight-bearing and rotation toward the intercondylar notch. The stretch on the capsular attachment of the meniscus, resulting from the displacement of the flap, results in pain. No other explanation can explain adequately the amelioration of pain that occurs with predictable regularity when only a small meniscal fragment is excised. What this means is that any fragment of meniscus that may be forced centrally, placing abnormal or unbalanced tension on the capsule, will cause pain. Therefore, any mobile tissue must be excised. If this requires total meniscectomy, it can also be performed using arthroscopic equipment.

CRITICISM OF PARTIAL MENISCECTOMY

Critics of partial meniscectomy have stated three reasons for excising the entire meniscus rather than just the offending fragment.

The argument that a partial meniscectomy will leave a rim capable of inflicting damage on a contiguous articular cartilage may be valid in patients who have had partial meniscectomy through an arthrotomy incision, if additional tears in the peripheral rim were missed. However, in patients treated with arthroscopic partial meniscectomy, observation of the articular cartilage at a later date has not revealed degeneration that was not present at the original arthroscopic examination.

The second and probably most valid criticism is that secondary tears may be missed during partial meniscectomy. As mentioned previously, if partial meniscectomy is done through an arthrotomy incision without the benefit of arthroscopic study, this could be a valid criticism. Using an arthroscope to study the peripheral rim will markedly decrease, but certainly not entirely eliminate, the chance of missing tears in the peripheral rim. Obviously, excision of the entire meniscus will avoid the possibility that tears in the rim will occur later. In our later series of 408 consecutive knees, 2% of the patients treated were thought to have retorn the peripheral rim (at times it is difficult to make a clear-cut distinction between a rupture overlooked and a recent rupture in a retained segment).

The last objection to partial meniscectomy is that excision of the entire meniscus will allow a replica of the meniscus to reform from the capsule. This has not been my observation in a large number of partial meniscectomies that have been reexamined arthroscopically (Plate 11-1A). The rim following meniscectomy is narrow, between 1 mm and 3 mm in width, and is composed of fibrotic synovium; furthermore, the tibial anchorage, anterior and posterior, is absent. In no way can this fibrotic ribbon assume any of the functions of the meniscus.

TYPES OF MENISCAL TEARS

Basically, meniscal tears are of two types:

Longitudinal (Plate 11-2)

Horizontal cleavage tears (Plate 11-3)

The former has a propensity for occurring in younger people. A tear occurs parallel to the longitudinally oriented collagen bundles, which limits its peripheral extent. The horizontal cleavage tear occurs along the middle perforating transverse collagen bundles, dividing the meniscus into roughly a superior femoral layer and an inferior tibial layer. The horizontal cleavage tear is inhibited to some degree in its peripheral extent by the circumferential longitudinal fibers, but this inhibi-

tion is not as decisive as that of the longitudinal tear due to its principal orientation. It allows peripheral dissection between the longitudinal collagen bundles. The arthroscopic appearance of a meniscal tear is predicted on the orientation of the tear as well as on the subsequent action of the femur on the flap originally created. There is a natural tendency for the joint to clear the joint line of any mechanically obstructive tissue, forcing any partially detached tissue to a sanctuary either above or beneath the peripheral meniscal rim in the case of a horizontal cleavage tear (Plates 11-4 and 11-5). A displaced bucket-handle tear, constraining the femoral condyle, is subjected to repeated rotational forces and eventually ruptures, usually at the junction of the middle and posterior thirds but occasionally at its posterior or anterior attachment.

In the presence of a long-standing meniscal tear, tears in a different plane from the original may develop, resulting in a complex tear (Plate 11-6). The importance of classification of the tear to be excised cannot be overemphasized, because the attachment of the mobile fragment to be excised must be distinguished from the normal peripheral rim, and the area of excision must be determined before the original cut in the meniscus to preserve as much meniscus as possible.

ADVANTAGES OF ARTHROSCOPIC PARTIAL MENISCECTOMY

Arthroscopic partial meniscectomy can be performed as an outpatient procedure, but preferably the patient is hospitalized for 2 nights and 1 day. Following surgery, a compression dressing is applied for 24 hours. A range of motion of 100° is usually obtained within 12 hours, and the patient is ambulatory on the night of surgery. Straight leg raising, static quadriceps exercises, and range of motion exercises are instituted in the recovery room. In a particularly fit person, a return to vigorous sports is possible in 5 to 7 days in the absence of an effusion. The average return to preoperative endeavor is between 2 and 3 weeks. Pain is minimal and is most often relieved by Darvon, and no quadriceps inhibition has been recorded.

An abnormal effusion rate, defined as perceptible swelling lasting longer than 10 days, is present in approximately 10% of patients. Another minor problem seen belatedly in the postoperative period is fat pad tenderness, which usually occurs between 3 weeks and 3 months after operation, and if mild will subside spontaneously. If severe, it requires a corticosteroid injection into the fat pad. In approximately 4000 cases of operative arthroscopy, four patients developed a septic process, although in three of these patients it is doubtful that the infection was related to the surgery. Thrombophlebitis occurred in two patients, but there were no cases of thromboembolism. Intra-articular instrument breakage is a major concern, especially to the surgeon just starting to develop his skills. Removal of a small metallic fragment accelerates the surgeon's maturation process greatly.

DISADVANTAGES OF ARTHROSCOPIC PARTIAL MENISCECTOMY

The major disadvantages of arthroscopic partial meniscectomy are the initial cost of the equipment and the time necessary to become proficient in the technique. Stereotactic skills come only with fumbling about within the joint, and until one is comfortable using a probe in one hand and the arthroscope in the other, therapeutic use of the arthroscope should be deferred. At first, an arthroscopic partial meniscectomy is quite a time-consuming venture, but with expertise a meniscal tear can be excised more rapidly than by arthrotomy. Proficiency with this technique, as a rule, is directly proportional to the number of cases performed.

REQUIREMENTS OF ARTHROSCOPIC PARTIAL MENISCECTOMY

The requirements for arthroscopic partial meniscectomy include a full set of arthroscopic equipment with a variety of optical angles, 4 mm to 5 mm diagnostic arthro-

scopes (Plate 11-7), and an operating arthroscope (Plate 11-8), a motorized shaving device (Plate 11-12), and a full set of ancillary mechanical instruments, such as knives (Plate 11-11), scissors (Plate 11-9), and basket forceps (Plate 11-10). Although it is possible occasionally to perform a partial meniscectomy under local anesthesia, it is also very difficult to obtain adequate exposure in some tight knees because the joint line will not open up. Therefore, the use of general anesthesia is the rule; local anesthesia is the exception. The exposure of the meniscus is facilitated by proper positioning—for the lateral meniscus, a position of approximately 20° of flexion, varus, internal tibial rotation (Fig. 11-1), and for the medial meniscus, 10° flexion, moderately severe valgus, and external tibial rotation (Fig. 11-2).

METHODS

Two types of surgical techniques may be used to perform arthroscopic partial meniscectomy. The first is a double puncture triangulation method in which the arthroscope is introduced through one portal and the operative instruments through a second (Fig. 11-3). The meniscal tear is usually removed piecemeal.

The second technique is also a triangulation method, in which the operating arthroscope is inserted through one portal and the meniscal clamp is retracted through another (Fig. 11-4). This has the advantage of placing the surgeon's eye in tandem with the resecting instrument; in this manner, large meniscal fragments can be excised and removed *in toto*. This method is useful in displaced buckethandle and large flap tears.

Reconstitution of the Peripheral Rim

Following arthroscopic partial meniscectomy in a relatively healthy meniscus, the peripheral rim triangulates over a period of several weeks to months, and the ragged surface is smoothed over by increased deposition of ground substance and cartilage cell hypertrophy (Plates 11-13 to 11-15).

FIG. 11-1. Position of the leg in varus, useful for work in the lateral compartment.

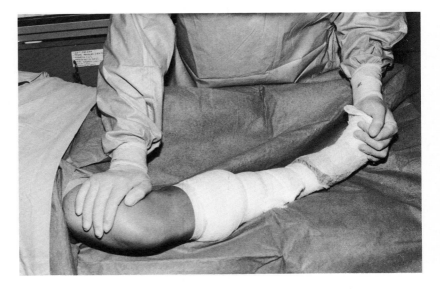

FIG. 11-2. Position of the leg in valgus, useful for work in the medial compartment. Note external tibial torsion applied to the lower extremity.

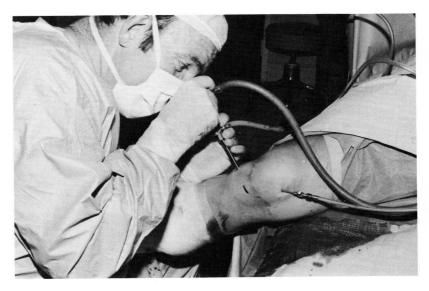

CONDITIONS AMENABLE TO ARTHROSCOPIC SURGERY

Although the arthroscope is uniquely suited to the study and excision of meniscal lesions, it has also been found useful in treating a variety of other conditions, such as:

Loose bodies
Shelf or medial patella plica

Chondromalacia of the patella
Fibrous ankylosis

OSTEOCHONDRAL LOOSE BODY

The osteochondral loose body (Plate 11-16) is commonly found and can generally be treated by arthroscopic removal. Occasionally, the loose body cannot be found, and arthroscopy is repeated when the loose body moves into

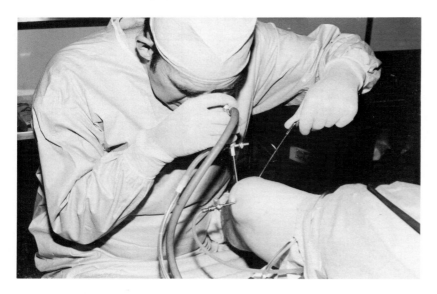

FIG. 11-3. Operating instruments in the joint, using double puncture technique.

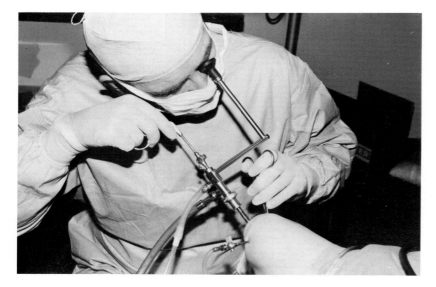

FIG. 11-4. Operating arthroscope in the joint. Retracting instrument to place the meniscal fragment on the stretch through the second portal.

an accessible location. If the ossific nucleus is less than 6 mm, the loose body may not be radiopaque and may not be visible, if x-ray films are obtained in the operating room. The sites in which the loose body resides, in order of frequency, are the quadriceps bursa, the intercondylar notch, the lateral gutter, the posterior medial compartment, and above and below the posterior third of the lateral meniscus.

SHELF OR MEDIAL PATELLA PLICA

The medial patella plica (Plate 11-17) is a synovial duplication running along the medial side wall of the knee. It extends from the upper extent of the superior level of the patella and runs distally to attach to the fat pad. The width, length, thickness, and consistency of this band vary from knee to knee, and observation alone will not enable the surgeon to determine if the band produces symptoms. To confuse the matter further, the duplication is present in approximately 60% of knees. The diagnosis is a clinical one. Usually, the patient gives a history of a blow to the partially flexed knee (such as striking it against the dashboard). The symptoms usually recounted are pain just medial to the patella and one thumb's breadth above the inferior pole of the patella, aching at the end of the day, restriction of the terminal few degrees of flexion because of pain, a sensation that something is catching beneath the patella, and occasional buckling. Physical therapy or exertion tends to exacerbate the patient's discomfort.

On physical examination the maximum point of tenderness is located one thumb's breadth above the inferior pole of the patella and just adjacent to it. A shelf can mimic a tear of the medial meniscus, chondromalacia of the patella, or patellar subluxation. Treatment is simple, consisting of arthroscopic excision of the band.

CHONDROMALACIA OF THE PATELLA

The arthroscopic treatment of chrondromalacia of the patella (Plates 11-18 and 11-19) is usually quite straightforward, and produces a relatively high incidence of good results over a short follow-up period. The surgical attack is directed toward the fibrillated fragment of articular cartilage, using a motorized shaving device. The fibrillated and fragmented articular cartilage is sucked into the aperture, and an inner revolving blade cuts the damaged articular cartilage. Many orthopedists have expressed reservations about the effectiveness of shaving off these areas of degeneration, but my experience, confirming that of Dr. Johnson,* is that the retropatellar discomfort and

* Johnson L: Personal communication, 1978

crepitus are greatly alleviated by this treatment. If patellar malalignment exists, a lateral capsular release is performed in addition.

FIBROUS ANKYLOSIS

The arthroscope is extremely valuable in the treatment of fibrous ankylosis (Plates 11-20 to 11-23), because it allows lysis of adhesions and partial synovectomy to be performed without an arthrotomy incision. The ability to initiate a relatively painless range of motion exercises immediately allows maximum retention of the range of motion secured by surgery. As an example, a 40-year-old operating room nurse was treated by medial meniscectomy, followed 6 months later by lateral meniscectomy for continuing mechanical symptoms. She developed fibrous ankylosis after this, for which she was treated with quadriceps plasty. Nine months later, her range of motion was restricted to 70° of flexion despite vigorous physiotherapy. Under anesthesia the range of motion measured 80° of flexion passively. The joint capacity measured 40 ml of saline solution, as opposed to the normal capacity of 90 ml to 100 ml. The quadriceps bursa was completely obliterated by fibrotic synovial adhesions. Using the arthroscope, the adhesions were divided, and a partial synovectomy was performed with a motorized cartilage planer. Her postoperative range of motion measured 120° of flexion. Active range of motion was instituted in the recovery room.

In conclusion, the use of the arthroscope in the correction of intra-articular abnormalities of the knee is in its infancy. The initial results appear promising in regard to lowered morbidity and rapid return of function, but the original goal of joint preservation cannot be proved or disproved because the follow-up is of short duration.

PLATE 11-1. (A) Diagram of pain production of meniscal tear. With weight-bearing, valgus stress, and external rotation, the mobile fragment is forced centrally into the joint. Traction is placed on the capsule through the intact collagen bundles of the meniscal pedicle, producing pain. **(B)** Rim of reformed meniscus. Note the thin, triangular mass of fibrous tissue. This triangular wedge does not articulate with the articular surfaces in either complete extension or 90° of flexion, and it is useless in providing either stability or weight dissipation.

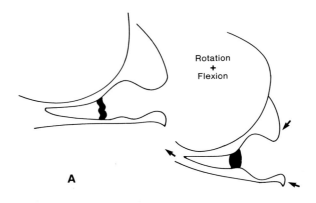

A

B

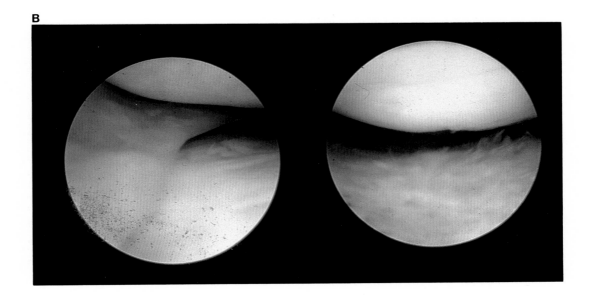

PLATE 11-2. Longitudinal tear of posterior third of medial meniscus.

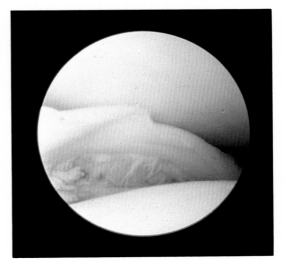

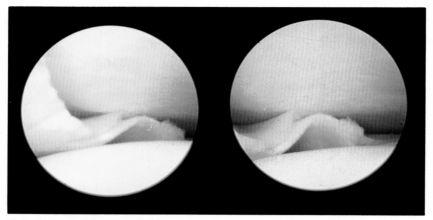

PLATE 11-3. Horizontal cleavage tear of medial meniscus. This is the early appearance of such a tear.

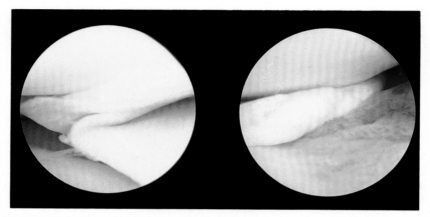

PLATE 11-4. Superior flap tear of medial meniscus. The oblique fragment has been propelled forward by the femoral condyle and lies in a position superior to the main body of the meniscus.

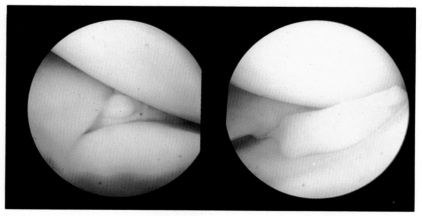

PLATE 11-5. Inferior flap tear of medial meniscus. The femur has propelled the oblique tear anteriorly and lies beneath the main body of the meniscus. This tear may be forced from its sanctuary into the joint line, causing intermittent symptoms of buckling.

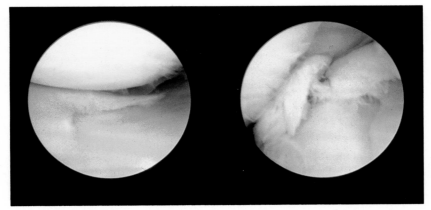

PLATE 11-6. Complex tear of medial meniscus. Continued joint action on a meniscal tear results in tears in various planes to the long axis of the meniscus. Excision of this type of tear is tedious. One flap, usually the most anterior, is excised at a time until a stable rim is achieved.

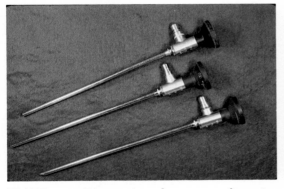

PLATE 11-7. Diagnostic arthroscopes of varying angles: 10° offset, 25° offset, and 70° offset.

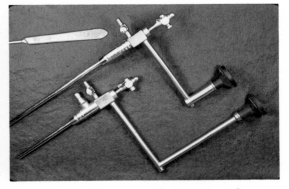

PLATE 11-8. Operating arthroscopes with recent modification.

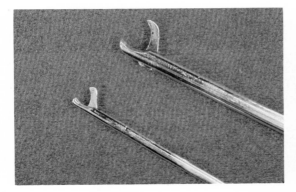

PLATE 11-9. Meniscal scissors. Note that these scissors cut at the tip and can be used to apply gentle traction as the cut is made.

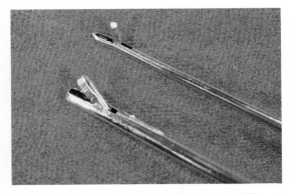

PLATE 11-10. Basket biopsy forceps, in different sizes. These instruments can be used through the operating arthroscope or through a separate stab wound and are useful in trimming the peripheral rim.

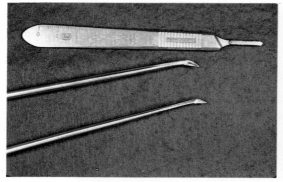

PLATE 11-11. Retrograde knife. This instrument is helpful in excision of flap tears at their base, but it is particularly useful in excision of tears of the anterior third of the lateral meniscus, a previously inaccessible area.

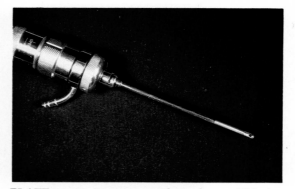

PLATE 11-12. Dyonics cartilage shaver. This instrument is useful for shaving the retropatellar surface, less useful in removing fibrillated articular cartilage from the femoral condyles. It is helpful in synovectomies and most variable in removing small debris from the joint and trimming the peripheral rim following partial meniscectomy.

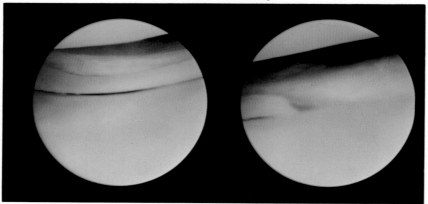

PLATE 11-13. Oblique tear, posterior third of lateral meniscus, associated with a torn anterior cruciate ligament.

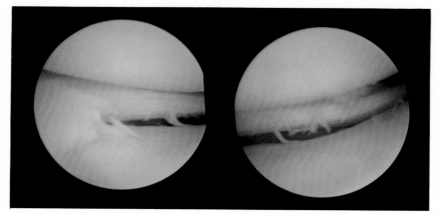

PLATE 11-14. Postoperative excision of tear seen in Plate 11-13.

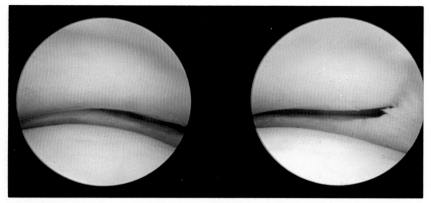

PLATE 11-15. One-year follow-up of excision of tear. The patient was admitted with a tear of the medial meniscus. Note the triangulation of the rim, which has smoothed out, and the healthy articular cartilage of the femoral condyle and the tibia.

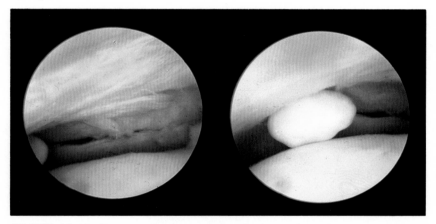

PLATE 11-16. Osteocartilaginous loose body in lateral compartment, 3 years following total lateral meniscectomy.

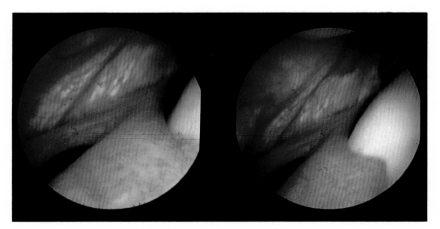

PLATE 11-17. A fenestrated shelf. The shelf arises from the medial sidewall and extends to insert distally into the medial fat pad.

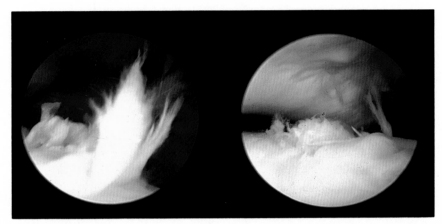

PLATE 11-18. Chondromalacia of the patella, prior to shaving.

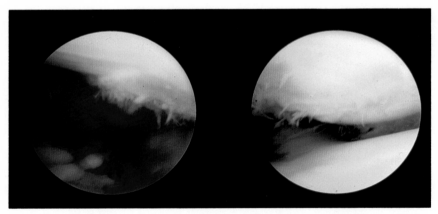

PLATE 11-19. Chondromalacia of the patella, following shaving with the interarticular shaver.

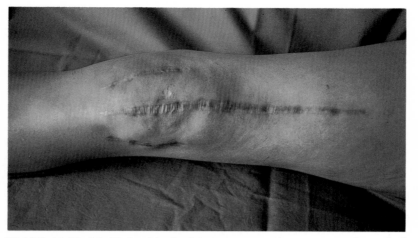

PLATE 11-20. Multiple skin incisions representing 3 years of surgical practice. A total medial meniscectomy was performed first. Because of continuing symptoms, a lateral meniscectomy was then performed. Finally, due to marked restriction of motion, a quadricepsplasty was performed, resulting in only 70° of passive motion 9 months later.

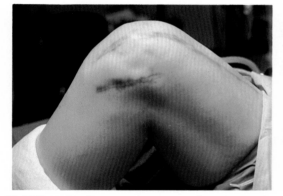

PLATE 11-21. Preoperative range of motion under anesthesia.

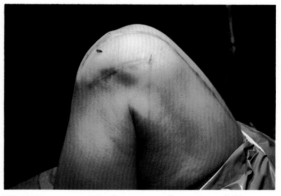

PLATE 11-22. Final range of motion following excision of adhesions in quadriceps bursa under anesthesia.

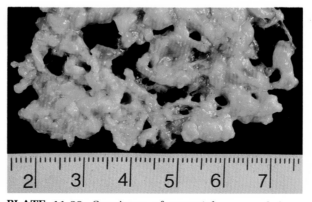

PLATE 11-23. Specimen of material removed from quadriceps bursa using Wolf cartilage shaver, rongeurs, and basket biopsy forceps.

CHAPTER 12
MANAGEMENT OF INJURIES
TO THE SEMILUNAR CARTILAGES

Arthur J. Helfet

Because only peripheral tears of the cartilage are likely to heal, treatment of ruptured semilunar cartilages in most instances includes surgical excision. After the first accident to the knee it is impossible to determine whether the tear is peripheral or not. Therefore, it is reasonable, if successful reduction is possible, to treat the acute injury conservatively. When the cartilage has been deranged twice or more often, healing is most unlikely, and operation should be advised—the sooner the better. Surgery is also necessary and urgent if attempts to reduce the displacement fail. The persistently displaced or retracted cartilage inexorably produces patterns of traumatic erosion and stretching of the capsular structures. These changes are irreversible. Early operation is preventive, but removal of the offending cartilage is also advisable, as will be argued, at any stage of the resultant traumatic arthritis. Surgery should be advised also if the patient's occupation is one in which a potentially unstable knee would be especially hazardous, for instance, work on ladders or at heights. During the war it was not customary to send a soldier back to a fighting unit until the injured meniscus had been removed.

Treatment of the pain and distress of the initial incident includes rest with splinting, management of the resultant effusion, and reduction of any displacements of cartilage. Relief from weight-bearing or a Jones bandage give adequate rest. Complete immobility is not necessary, but movements which would displace the cartilage again should be avoided. Sir Robert Jones[10] described a compression bandage composed of a thick layer of cotton wool, a firm calico, flannel, or crepe bandage, reinforced by a second layer of wool and a firmer bandage (Fig. 12-1). If weight-bearing is urgent, the addition of a plaster-of-paris or other rigid back splint is necessary. The splint should extend from just below the buttock to 6 in above the ankle and should be fixed to the thigh and the leg at least at three, and preferably at four, points.

Acute pain is relieved quite simply by the injection of 5 ml to 10 ml of 1% procaine, made up in normal saline, into the suprapatellar pouch (Fig. 12-2). With proper aseptic precautions, this is a safe office procedure and has value not only for relieving pain but also as a sufficient anesthetic for aspiration of the effusion or reduction of the displaced cartilage.

ASPIRATION OF THE KNEE

Mild effusion requires no more than the compression bandage, but if it is tense or rapidly increasing, it requires aspiration. The easiest

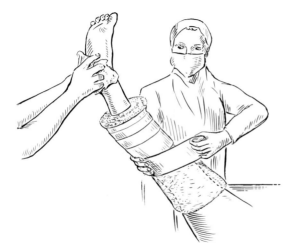

FIG. 12-1. The Jones compression bandage applied from midthigh to midcalf.

route, shown in Figure 12-2, is through the natural notch formed behind the insertion of the quadriceps into the upper pole of the patella. At this point only skin and fibrous capsule cover the synovium, and the route is relatively insensitive. The skin should be cleansed with soap and water, then alcohol, and then painted with iodine or sprayed with a thin layer of one of the self-sterilizing aeroplastic solutions. The latter helps to seal the puncture wound afterward, but all that is required is the firm pressure of an iodine dab for a few seconds after the needle is removed. The skin quickly seals itself. Aspiration always should be followed by firm bandaging with either a Jones' compression bandage or a crepe bandage applied thickly and firmly but not tightly.

Hemarthrosis requires a needle of slightly thicker bore than that used for a simple effusion. The necessity for aspiration is more urgent and invariably should be followed by a compression bandage.

REDUCTION OF THE RUPTURED MENISCUS

The essence of reduction of the displaced meniscus is reversal of the torque of the original injury. If extension and lateral rotation of the tibia are the movements blocked, attempts to overcome the block by manipulating further in these directions will aggravate the rupture

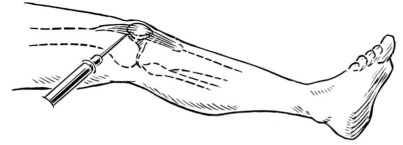

FIG. 12-2. Aspiration of the knee through the suprapatellar pouch. The needle is inserted into the natural notch formed behind the insertion of the quadriceps into the upper pole of the patella.

FIG. 12-3. Reduction of displaced meniscus. (*Top, left*) The patient sits on the edge of the table. The knee is flexed passively. (*Top, center*) Full medial rotation of the leg. (*Top, right*) Lateral rotation is repeated until the full range is obtained. (*Bottom*) The leg is kicked out, as if at a ball, to the limit of extension.

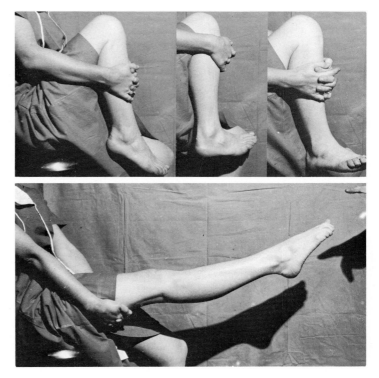

and the displacement. Instead, the tibia must be unwound into flexion and medial rotation. Once the cartilage is slack, a jerk into normal extension will pull the cartilage back into line. The simplest method is to inject local anesthetic into the knee joint and show the patient how to do the maneuver himself. The patient sits on the edge of a table. The knee is flexed passively. Full medial and then lateral rotation is repeated until the full range is obtained, usually suddenly and sometimes with a click. Then the patient kicks the leg out—as if at a ball—to the limit of extension (Fig. 12-3). Sometimes a sticky knee may be helped by rocking the flexed tibia forward and backward on the femur (Fig. 12-4). If unsuccessful, the manipulation may be repeated under Pentothal anesthesia, when abduction or adduction while extending and externally rotating the leg may also be tried. If displacement persists, that is, if the rotation signs remain, there is no alternative to operation.

Prolonged skin traction in bed is not recom-

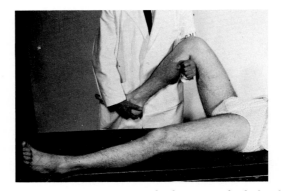

FIG. 12-4. Sometimes a sticky knee may be helped by rocking the flexed tibia forward and backward on the femur.

mended. When accompanied by regular isometric thigh muscle drill (quadriceps and hamstrings), the acute symptoms do settle down and the effusion subsides. But the rotation signs denoting persistence of the displacement of the torn meniscus usually persist. Recurrent effusions in an aching knee, with or without locking and giving way, eventually demand meniscectomy.

CONSERVATIVE TREATMENT

Conservative treatment for the first injury should be continued for 4 weeks, by which time the peripheral tear should heal soundly. (Most ligamentous structures repair in that time.[3,11]) A compression bandage or splint is kept on for 10 days and is followed by a crepe bandage and, most important, limited activity. In other words, the knee requires protection from further injury rather than immobilization.

MUSCLE EXERCISE

As with injury to any joint, rehabilitation of the power and excursion of all muscles acting on the knee is essential. Quadriceps drill should be augmented by hamstrings drill. It is as easy to do static contractions of both together as of either separately. It is of interest that when these two groups are contracted, automatic contraction of the gastrocnemii and the popliteus takes place as well. The whole muscular mechanism of the knee is activated.

Wasting of the muscles associated with an injured joint is more rapid than that occurring through disuse and inactivity alone. A neurotrophic reflex, it would seem, is abolished. The wasted muscles plus inactivity in turn delay the disappearance of joint effusion and swelling. The circulation of the joint and its musculature are complementary and under the same neurotrophic control, and it is probable that muscle activity acts chiefly by increasing the blood supply to the joint and therefore, by increasing absorption of fluid and the products of injury.

The patient should be instructed to contract all the thigh muscles to their full extent, to hold the contraction for a full second, and then relax as fully. The exercise is repeated 12 times per waking hour. No more is required. Overexercising often induces fatigue and a new effusion. As power improves, straight-leg raising exercises may be substituted, but not before the patient realizes that straight leg means *full extension*. The value of much exercise is lost by raising the leg with the knee slightly flexed.

Full extension is even more important postoperatively. Before the cartilage is removed, the final arc of extension and lateral rotation has been absent for some time. After operation it is essential that the patient recover this final stabilizing phase of movement. There is *never* difficulty in recovery of flexion. On the contrary, the knee has the failing of finding comfort in flexion at any time of stress. In older patients whose cartilage lesions have reached a stage of traumatic arthritis, full comfort postoperatively is not attained until the knee can achieve full extension in walking. This is understandable, because only in full extension does the patella lie comfortably, with equal tension on both slopes of the trochlear groove of the femur.

Other forms of physiotherapy may be used if it is understood that their only function is to improve circulation and therefore the absorption of fluid and the metabolites of injury. Heat and massage in any form cannot strengthen muscle. Only exercise can achieve this. Faradization may teach the patient how to contract the muscle and prepare it for exercise, but for restoration of power it cannot compete with active and forceful contraction.

SURGERY OF THE SEMILUNAR CARTILAGES

The requisites for successful and relatively pain-free surgery of the knee are *accurate diagnosis, gentle atraumatic surgery,* and *clear visualization of each step,* associated with controlled preoperative and postoperative rehabilitation. These factors are inherent in the whole technique to be described and apply to assistant as well as to surgeon. Overenthusiastic retraction results in postoperative pain and effusion. So that he can see every step, the assistant should face the side of the knee that bears the incision. The incision must be adequate but not excessive. It is never necessary to use forceful traction to reach the posterior end of the cartilage, and powerful forceps are a temptation to be resisted. Special knives that incite blind incision into the posterior end of the cartilage should not appear on the instrument tables of any but those who devise them, have trained themselves to use them safely, and who presumably require additional reach. I have seen more damage to the synovium and the posterior capsule and more postoperative pain and hemarthrosis from these devices in the hands of the less experienced than from any other cause.

The following technique is based on that of the Liverpool school as used by Sir Robert Jones, Sir Harry Platt, T. P. McMurray, W. R. Bristow, and most of their disciples. During the last 30 years and from the study of over 2500 operations, minor modifications have been made in the incision and in the amount of posterior horn that it is necessary to excise.

SKIN PREPARATION

Forty-eight hours of skin preparation had always been a ritual, but a few hours preparation is now considered safe and sufficient. The limb from groin to toe is shaved, scrubbed with soap and water, painted with 70% alcohol, and wrapped in sterile towels. After the tourniquet has been applied, the skin is painted with two coats of 2% iodine in 70% alcohol or preferably betadyne. Operating through sterile stockinette is not advocated.

HEMOSTASIS

In young patients the limb is exsanguinated by an Esmarch bandage. A tourniquet, preferably pneumatic, is applied well up the thigh. To avoid the use of a tourniquet in old people, the method described to me by Amnon Fried of the Beilenson Hospital in Tel Aviv is recommended. The skin and the capsule in the area of the skin incision are infiltrated with 0.5% procaine or Leostessin in saline with 0.75 ml of 1:1000 Adrenalin per 100 ml. The

rest of the 100 ml is injected into and distends the knee joint. After 5 minutes the joint is anesthetic and the quality of hemostasis is remarkable. A sucker copes with the fluid after the joint is opened. At the end of the operation the patient is able to extend the knee actively. With the technique to be described, postoperative oozing is negligible.

OPERATIVE TECHNIQUE

The leg is placed to hang over the end of the operating table at right angles to the thigh. The leg should be free of the edge by at least an inch. The draped foot is gripped by the gowned knees of the surgeon. This permits easy rotation and abduction and adduction of the bent knee and allows good vision of the intercondylar space or the back end of the cartilage as the need arises—an essential for gentle surgery. A small sandbag along the edge of the table lifts the thigh and facilitates free movement of the leg at the knee (Plate 12-1A).

The Incision

The incision that I prefer is almost horizontal, sloping very slightly downward and backward in line with the upper surface of the meniscus (Plate 12-1B). It does not extend far enough back to injure the medial or the lateral ligament. The whole extent of the incision is over the joint and does not cross the lower border of the femur. Infrapatellar branches of the saphenous nerve (Fig. 12-5) are always cut, and the patient should be warned that there will be a patch of anesthesia in front of the knee after the operation and that it may last for months. It is rarely permanent and causes no disability; when this is realized the patient feels no concern. In no instance have I seen the notorious "neuroma" form in this scar. It happens only in the scar that crosses and becomes adherent to the edge of the femur (Fig. 12-6) and causes pain when the scar is tensed. Excision of the neuroma and freeing of the capsule from the bone relieves the symptoms.

When the articular surface of the patella

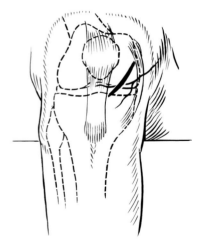

FIG. 12-6. This oblique incision may cut branches of the saphenous nerve where they cross the lower border of the femur and so give rise to a painful neuroma.

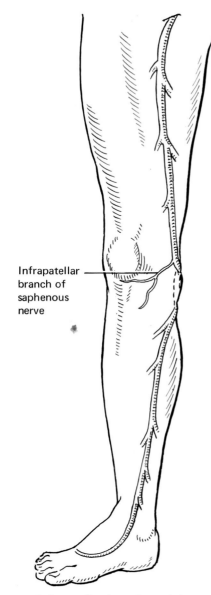

Infrapatellar branch of saphenous nerve

FIG. 12-5. Infrapatellar branches of the saphenous nerve are always cut.

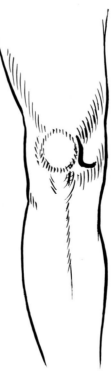

FIG. 12-7. For inspection of the patella, the anterior end of the horizontal incision should be curved upward.

needs inspection, the skin incision for the medial cartilage should be curved upward from the anterior end to run in the gap between the patella and the medial edge of the femoral condyle (Fig. 12-7).

The posterior compartment of the knee is explored through a vertical incision in line with the posterior border of the tibia. With the leg hanging at a right angle, the hamstrings on the medial side are well out of the way, and only the capsule and the synovium need to be traversed (Fig. 12-8). On the lateral side, the incision is above and in line with the head of the fibula. The biceps and the peroneal nerve are below the area of operation (Fig. 12-9). Skin should be sutured gently and without tension. Few minor details in surgical technique cause as much pain as tight skin sutures.

The Operation

The joint is opened in the line of the skin incision. Three layers are traversed, and each must be carefully and separately sutured when closing up. The superficial fascia contains the infrapatellar branches of the saphenous nerve, and a few stitches of fine catgut relieve tension and add to comfort. After the capsule is divided, a sweep of the knife above and below frees it from the underlying synovium. This is a useful practice, especially on the lateral side, as it facilitates sewing up. W. Rowley Bristow taught this maneuver and nominated it as his major contribution to the operative surgery of the knee joint. When opening the synovium, the incision should skirt the fat pad; care should be taken not to cut into it at all, since scars and adhesions of the fat pad are a potential cause of pain (Plate 12-1C).

After the joint is open, the assistant retracts the synovium gently with two blunt hooks, the fat pad is pulled forward by a Langenbeck type right-angled retractor, and the interior is inspected (Plate 12-1D).

Lesions of the anterior two-thirds of the semilunar cartilage are evident—the transverse tear and "parrot beak" of the free edge, the longitudinal bowstring tear in the substance of the cartilage, the peripheral detachment from the capsule, and the retracted anterior end. The last are the most interesting and are relatively common, so much so that in 1909 Sir Robert Jones, reporting on 117 cases, found that 53 cartilages were torn from their

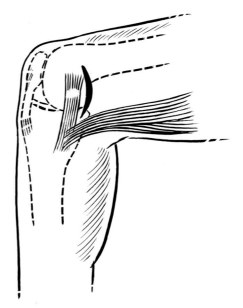

FIG. 12-8. The posterior compartment on the medial side is explored through a vertical incision.

FIG. 12-9. On the lateral side, the incision is above the biceps and the peroneal nerve, in line with the fibula.

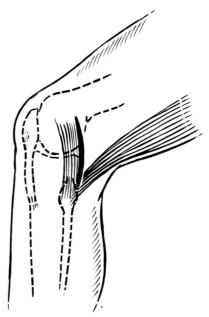

anterior attachment, compared with 16 bow-string tears and 8 complete peripheral detachments. *

Thomas Annandale of Edinburgh described the retracted cartilage for the first time.[1] On November 16, 1883, he performed not the first meniscectomy (which is to the credit of Bradhurst of St. George's Hospital, London in 1866) but the first recorded operation for displaced semilunar cartilage. He found "that the internal semilunar cartilage was completely separated from its anterior attachment to the tibia and was displaced backwards about half an inch."

He did not excise the cartilage but cured his patient by drawing the cartilage forward and stitching it to its former attachment. Ten weeks later the man was back at his work with a normally functioning knee.

Replacement and suture of the retracted anterior horn has proved most suitable for the young and pliable meniscus when it is uncomplicated by tear or detachment elsewhere. In the middle-aged and older patient, when the meniscus has hardened and retracted with thickening longitudinally, its shape and volume have changed, and it is no longer possible to regain anatomical pliability. Full extension is prevented and, as described earlier, causes a patch of local erosion of the opposite femoral surface. At least the misshapen anterior, normally mobile, part of the meniscus should be removed.

If the anterior end is free, it may be picked up with a pair of dissecting forceps. Other-

wise, a blunt hook is passed around the free margin, and the cartilage is dissected off near the edge of the tibia close to the synovial margin (Plate 12-1E).

There would seem to be little purpose in freeing the whole cartilage by dividing the peripheral attachments. If each incision is made into the substance of the cartilage, there is no bleeding postoperatively, whereas dividing the vascular peripheral attachments often results in hemarthrosis. Nothing is lost by leaving a rim of cartilage. It may even minimize the minor radiologic changes described by Fairbank after meniscectomy.[8] Out of hundreds of knees with the residual rim of cartilage, not one has developed a single detrimental symptom. On the other hand, the rim must be meticulously trimmed. No tag or fringe must be left to float frondlike into the joint. These may give rise to continued symptoms due to nipping. On the lateral side, cutting into the meniscus protects the lateral inferior geniculate artery which may be involved if the synovium is damaged (Plate 12-1F).

The freed anterior end of the meniscus is gripped in Kocher's or other forceps. Mild tension is exerted by pulling forward and toward the center of the joint, and a sharp blade splits as much as cuts the meniscus along the edge. The author prefers a fresh Bard-Parker blade, but any keen knife may be used. The strokes are gentle, and care is taken not to scratch the articular cartilage of the tibia.

The pull on the meniscus invaginates the posterior capsule into the joint, and by rotating the foot between his knees the surgeon brings more of the meniscus into view. In the laxer joint still more may be seen if the assistant pulls the whole tibia forward on the femur.

Ultimately, the meniscus is dislocated into the intercondylar space. By rotating the leg in the opposite direction, the posterior attachments to the tibial spine are brought into view and divided (Plate 12-1G, H).

The stage at which the meniscus slips into the center of the joint varies. If the posterior horn is detached, it occurs early, and the oper-

---

* Out of 117 cases operated on (1906, 1907, 1908) for injury to the cartilage in which a lesion was found
  53 were torn from their anterior attachment
  16 were split longitudinally
   8 were attached by the cornua and torn from the capsule
   7 were displacements of the posterior horns
  12 were fractured transversely opposite the internal lateral ligament
   8 were loosely bound circumferentially with no other appreciable abnormality
   8 had undergone changes in the loose anterior extremity of the semilunar of the nodular type, some being as lumpy and large as a pea
   3 exhibited no trace of the cartilage
   2 showed the anterior part doubled and adherent to the posterior part

PLATE 12-1. The technique of medial meniscectomy.

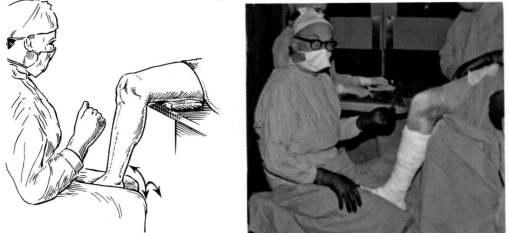

(A) The foot is gripped by the gowned knees of the surgeon. A small sandbag along the edge of the table lifts the thigh and facilitates free movement of the leg at the knee.

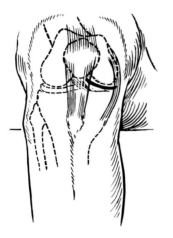

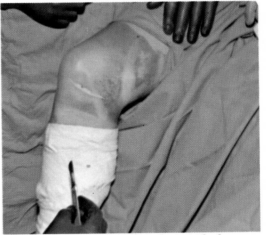

(B) The horizontal incision slopes very slightly downward and backward, in line with the upper surface of the meniscus.

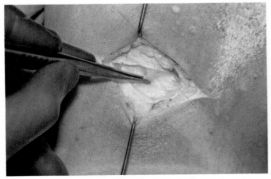

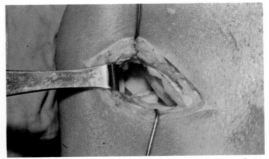

(C) The capsule is divided and the synovium is picked up preparatory to incision.

(D) The anteromedial joint space is opened. A bowstring tear is obvious, as is the erosion on the articular surface of the medial femoral condyle. The cruciate ligament is intact.

PLATE 12-1. The technique of medial meniscectomy. (Continued)

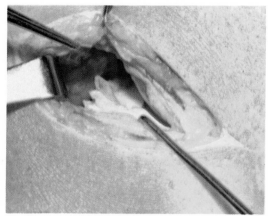

(E) The anterior horn of the meniscus is freed from the tibial spine.

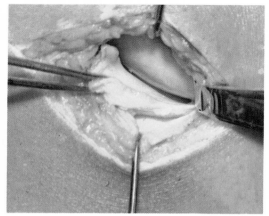

(F) The meniscus is excised by splitting its substance near the peripheral attachment.

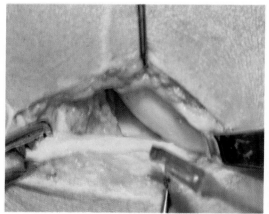

(G) As the posterior border is freed, the meniscus is slipped into the intercondylar space.

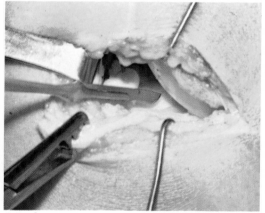

(H) The posterior end is divided from the tibial spines in the intercondylar space.

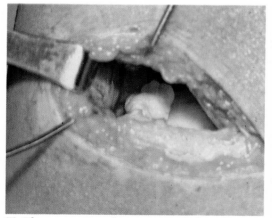

(I) The enormous bowstring of this discoid meniscus is removed as an almost separate body.

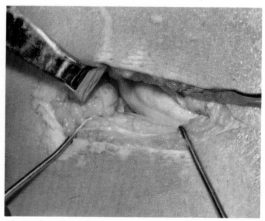

(J) Early chondrophyte formation is seen on the edge of the medial femoral condyle.

PLATE 12-1. The technique of medial meniscectomy. (Continued)

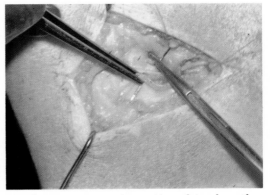

(K) The synovium is closed with a hemostatic lock-switch suture of fine catgut.

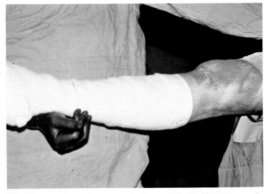

(L) The same suture is continued to close the capsule.

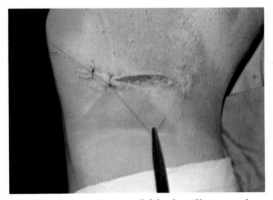

(M) Separate sutures of black silk or nylon are used to close the skin.

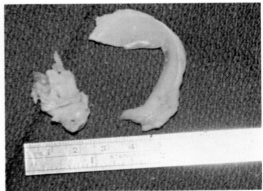

(N) Extension is complete, with full external rotation.

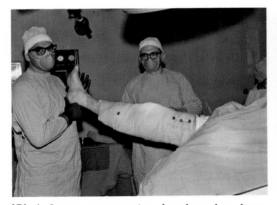

(O) A Jones compression bandage has been applied.

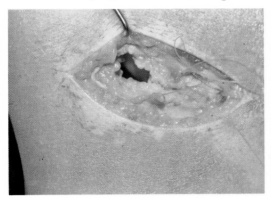

(P) The fragments of the bowstring discoid meniscus.

ation is simple. If the posterior horn is normal and the joint tight, it is more difficult. But usually only a little patience to ensure that each incision is made under direct vision is needed to complete the operation. Charnley's retractor is most suitably angled to expose the curve of the semilunar cartilage.

DIFFICULTIES WITH THE POSTERIOR HORN

Without ill-advised blind dissection it is impossible to remove the whole posterior horn through an anterior incision. A small segment always remains. But as long as the rim is firmly attached to the capsule, and if its substance has not been damaged by accident or during the operation, no harm ensues. In such cases there is no necessity to open the posterior compartment to remove it. The removal of the posterior fragment through a separate incision is essential (1) when a tear or pedicle of the residual fragment is seen from the front, (2) whenever there is a history of giving way of the knee and the loose posterior horn has not been adequately removed, and (3) after accidental fracture of the meniscus during operation.

After repeated derangements of the knee, as most writers have emphasized, there is often more than one split in the posterior horn. Giving way is usually associated with lesions of the posterior halves of the cartilage. Preoperatively, too, the appropriate click over the posterior horn is elicited. If there is no such history or clinical finding, it may be assumed that the back end is intact. The fragment that remains only because of the technical impossibility of removal through an anterior incision in an otherwise tight posterior horn does not merit the additional posterior arthrotomy. The number of times in which judgment based on these criteria has been wrong, and subsequent operation has been necessary, is negligible.

A second operation is usually the result of a subsequent accident to the knee in which the posterior horn has been injured. Accidental fracture of the meniscus during the operation may occur through excessive traction on the cartilage or with an unusually deep transverse or oblique tear, or when the bowstring has left too meager a margin.

Views expressed in this chapter differ from the deeply rooted surgical inclination to remove the meniscus in its entirety. Also, without the indications listed above, it is unnecessary to make a second incision to remove a *stable* posterior fragment.

PARTIAL OR TOTAL MENISCECTOMY

I have long followed the practice of excising the meniscus, leaving the avascular rim. This refinement reduces postoperative pain and hemorrhage.

An increasing number of surgeons now recommend removal of the loose fragment of the bowstring cartilage only as an easier, quicker operation with better recovery and convalescence of the patient. Even the most skillful and gentle surgeon must do more damage to the synovium and capsule if he removes the entire meniscus. A long-standing criticism of the limited operation has been that a tear or multiple tears of the posterior horn might be missed, necessitating a subsequent operation.

In my experience, both the short- and long-term results after partial meniscectomy are an improvement upon the more extensive operation. An editorial in the British Medical Journal of 29th April, 1978, expresses similar views:

> Even in experienced hands, removal of the whole meniscus must mean more extensive injury to the knee with extra hazards to the capsule, ligaments and articular cartilage. Fresh evidence is now reopening this argument.

The initial advantages of partial over total meniscectomy have been confirmed repeatedly. In one prospective trial the early morbidity was "much less." A more detailed retrospective review found that partial meniscectomy was followed by less pain and more rapid recovery of quadriceps power, allowing the patient to be discharged from the hospital, on the average, 1 day earlier. Subsequent recovery of joint function to the point when unprotected use of the leg could be permitted was substantially quicker, with a gain of 5 days. These short-term advantages would be insufficient justification for partial meniscectomy if the more remote results were poor, but this is not the case. Entirely satisfactory results were reported in 40 patients in one series of 46 partial meniscectomies. Another 10-year review of 78 partial, and 125 total, meniscectomies 10 to 30 years later gave a slight advantage in good and excellent results to the smaller operation. In one series, all 20 patients after partial meniscectomy were enthusiastic about the result compared with 30 of 38 who had had the whole meniscus removed. In another group, effusion was four times as common and loss of motion twice as common after total meniscectomy. In both series the bigger operation was followed more frequently by late radiographic evidence of joint deterioration. In a prospective survey of 107 total, and 33 partial, meniscectomies, 31 of the latter had no symptoms compared with only 66 in the total meniscectomy group.

Experience has not, therefore, borne out the fear that recurrent symptoms might be more frequent after partial meniscectomy. In fact, there is both clinical and radiological evidence of less late deterioration in the knee when it has been possible to restrict the operation to removal of the loose fragment only. So we can no longer justify an uncritical policy of total meniscectomy.

The whole cartilage minus the avascular rim must be removed for multiple splits or for a peripheral tear, but for a bowstring (bucket-handle) tear or a tear of the free margin, the loose fragment alone should be excised. The surgeon must then make sure that he has overlooked no further lesion. A considerable advance is that partial meniscectomy may now be performed through an arthroscope, as described by Watanabe in Chapter 10, and by Dandy[4] and Dandy and Jackson.[5] Arthroscopy makes possible accurate preliminary diagnosis and atraumatic partial meniscectomy.

OPERATION TO REMOVE A SEPARATE POSTERIOR HORN

The vertical incision (Fig. 12-8) in line with the posterior border of the tibia crosses the joint line. The synovium of the posterior compartment is entered above the level of the meniscus. The space is well displayed by a right-angled retractor. Straightening the leg a little may show up the residual fragment of meniscus to better advantage. The cartilage is divided anteriorly and posteriorly as necessary. The synovium, the capsule, and the fascia are sutured in separate layers with fine plain catgut.

THE INFRAPATELLAR PAD OF FAT

The anterior end of the meniscus has intimate attachments to the fat pad, which must be meticulously protected from injury. Freeing of the cartilage must be careful and gentle. This applies particularly to the retracted cartilage, the anterior stump of which may be thickened and somewhat fibrous and involved in scar with the fat and the synovium. Presumably, the scarring is the sequel to hemorrhage at the time of the detachment of the meniscus from the cruciate ligament. The thickened stump-plus-scar leaves its mark on the articular cartilage of the condyle of the femur. If the condition has been present for any length of time, straightening the knee will show the indentation or erosion on the anterior articular surface of the condyle. It is produced during weight-bearing when the knee is straight. Both the bulk of the stump and the scar should be trimmed.

THE LATERAL MENISCUS

Lateral meniscectomy does not differ materially from excision of the medial cartilage. The joint space is smaller, but the middle segment is not attached to the capsule, and once the anterior end is free, the meniscus slips more easily into the center of the joint. Care must be taken not to injure the lateral inferior geniculate artery, which runs outside the synovium between the lateral ligament and the posterolateral aspect of the meniscus.

For the last 10 years, the approach described by Bruser[2] has been used. The fibers of the iliotibial band (when the knee is fully flexed) are horizontal and parallel with the joint line. Splitting the fibers in this line provides an easy and atraumatic exposure of the joint. Instead of having the patient supine and flexing the knee on the table as advised by Bruser, the knee is flexed over the end of the table with the foot grasped by the knees of the surgeon as for the medial meniscus. To open the joint, the knee is raised until it is well flexed. Bruser's horizontal incision splits the iliotibial band in line with the joint and is extended as far anteriorly as the patellar tendon. The relaxed fibular collateral ligament is at the posterior end of the incision and must not be injured. The synovium is opened in the joint line, and care is taken not to injure the fat pad, by sloping the anterior end of the incision upward. The foot is then lowered so that the thigh rests on the flexed table. I prefer this because gravity, aided by the weight of the suspended foot and, if necessary, traction by the knees of the surgeon, increase the joint space.

Good exposure of the meniscus is obtained and complete excision is possible. Incision into the meniscus, especially posteriorly, should leave a narrow rim to avoid incising vascular synovium and capsular attachments. A hemostatic lock stitch closes the synovium. The edges of the iliotibial band are opposed by a few intermittent sutures of fine catgut.

INSPECTION OF THE OPPOSITE MENISCUS

Unless the alar folds are exceptionally voluminous, it is possible to inspect the anterior end of the opposite meniscus. A right-angled retractor or flat dissector holds the pad of fat forward, and a light is shone across the joint. Detachments of the anterior end and bowstring tears may be observed. It is also useful to examine the articular cartilage of the lateral condyle, because patterns of erosion give specific information. These and changes in the patella will be discussed in Chapter 13.

The wound is sutured in four layers—synovium, capsule, fascia, and skin. A lock stitch using a small fistula needle with No. 2–0 plain catgut ensures hemostasis in the synovium, and the same stitch is continued to close the capsule. A few sutures to join the

fascia relieves tension in this sensitive layer rich in nerve fibers (Plate 12-1L, M, N).

POSTOPERATIVE CARE

With the knee straight, and before the tourniquet is released, a Jones compression bandage is applied from midthigh to midcalf. It is applied firmly but not tightly. No splint is necessary (Plate 12-1O).

The nursing staff and the physiotherapists must be made to understand that the patient's objective is to recover full extension of the knee. Often this has been impossible for some time before the operation. After an uncomplicated operation, recovery of flexion is never difficult (Plate 12-1P).

The leg must lie flat on the mattress. Pillows behind the knee are forbidden, and flexion must not be attempted. A sandbag along the outer side of the leg and the foot prevents the leg rolling over and adds to comfort, as does a bolster against the sole of the foot.

Static muscle drill for the thigh is instituted as soon as possible, often on the first but usually on the second day. If the patient has learned the procedure preoperatively, there is little difficulty. Once a *complete contraction* is achieved, convalescence is comfortable. This is an interesting phenomenon. Full contraction of the thigh muscles induces a feeling of normality—really, the absence of conscious sensation—and thereafter the exercises are quite comfortable.

If the foot swells, as it does occasionally, denoting that the bandage is too tight, it should be unwound without disturbing the inner layer of wool and reapplied. A dozen full contractions an hour are sufficient. Overexercise is of no value; in fact, it disposes to effusion. After a few days attempts are made to lift the straight leg, and this may be assisted by the surgeon or the physiotherapist.

On the tenth day the Jones bandage is removed, the sutures are taken out, and a crepe bandage is applied firmly and thickly but not tightly. It should extend no more than 1 in above the upper border of the patella and 2 in below the upper surface of the tibia and be applied in figure-of-eight fashion, crossing behind the knee. Gentle, active flexion is permitted and encouraged as soon as the patient can do so comfortably, usually on the second or third day. When contraction of the thigh muscles is strong enough to lift the leg when straight, the patient is permitted to stand and then walk, the distance depending on muscle tone and control. This should be the yardstick in rehabilitation. As long as exertion is within the compass of the thigh muscles, increasing activity rapidly improves power and tone, but overexertion and repeated fatigue result in wasting of muscle and recurrent or persistent effusion. If this occurs, a day's rest in bed, followed by non-weight-bearing exercises is the quickest course.

The prognosis is good. The fit athlete on a guided program of exercises resumes sporting activities including football in 6 weeks. The middle-aged are fit for all normal activities in 6 to 8 weeks. The most resolute and fit patient in my experience was the regimental sergeant major of a Royal Marine Commando unit, who returned to full duty in his unit in 3 weeks. In my unit at Drymen Military Hospital during one year of the war, 120 servicemen operated on for internal derangement of the knee all were transferred to the Convalescent Depot for Scottish Command. Before returning to their units in Category A, Major Duthie and Captain Macleod[6,7] demanded that each soldier should do a physical assault course, a 3-mile cross-country run, and a 15-mile route march. Of the 120, 103 or 85.8% were classified as A1. The average time for all 120 from admission to the hospital to return to the unit was 63 days (W. R. Bristow, 1944*). Many rugby players have played first class (major league) rugby in 6 weeks without harm, and two have taken their places in international teams 6 weeks after meniscectomy.

Older people return to normal activities, housework, golf, and tennis. They lose their pain and no longer suffer recurrent attacks of aching and swelling after activity.

This is the group in which recovery of full extension of the knee (which includes exter-

* Personal communication.

nal rotation of the tibia) is of greatest importance. Until full extension is easy and natural and the rotation signs have disappeared, the knee is not always comfortable, and restoration of adequate muscle power and tone is difficult.

POSTOPERATIVE COMPLICATIONS

Synovial Effusion

The reaction to operation is a mild effusion in most knees. Usually it has resolved by the tenth day and does not recur if all exercise and activity is carried out progressively within the compass of the strengthening muscles. Occasionally, the reaction is excessive, and tense effusion results which may require aspiration. If so, injection of 1% procaine in saline simplifies the aspiration and promotes absorption. When the effusion is due to fatigue or strain, rest, followed by graduated exercise, is advocated. Forcing exercise and physiotherapy often aggravates the condition.

Hemarthrosis and Pain

Early in the Middle East campaign in the last war, many meniscectomies were performed by young and inexperienced surgeons. The postoperative hemarthrosis rate in some military hospitals varied between 60% and 80%. Three factors, not always coincident, were no doubt responsible:

1. The quality of the surgery. As anywhere else, inexperience or rough operating techniques lead not only to postoperative hemorrhage, bruising, and swelling but to increased pain and delayed healing as well.

2. The prevalent teaching that the whole meniscus must be removed. This leads to damage to the vascular synovium and to the uncontrolled and untutored use of special meniscectomy knives to remove the posterior horn. It is essential that each stroke of the knife should be within the vision of the surgeon. On the lateral side, also, the vulnerability of the geniculate artery was demonstrated. A gentle atraumatic technique, leaving a rim of meniscus and using a hemostatic suture for

the synovium, prevents hemarthrosis and leads to a relatively painless and rapid convalescence.

3. The cult of early movement. There is no need to flex the knee for the first 5 days, by which time the vessels are sealed. In this connection it was remarkable that even in some of these hospitals that used postoperative splinting by plaster-of-paris slab or cylinder for 2 weeks, the operation acquired the reputation of causing severe pain and rough convalescence—an accurate reflection of the surgeon's technique.

Hemarthrosis and pain are considered under one heading, for hemorrhage is associated with, and is probably the most common factor in, postoperative distress.

Smillie[12] contends, with justification, that hemarthrosis occurring as a complication of operation has more serious consequences than that resulting from simple trauma. It is more liable to be followed by protracted convalescence due to adhesions, synovial thickening and persistent effusion. He ascribes this to the presence of a large area of raw synovial membrane from which the meniscus has been dissected.

This, the author contends, is the very factor that can be avoided by leaving a narrow rim of meniscus. Each incision should be made into the substance of the cartilage. In this way the operation is practically bloodless, and hemarthrosis becomes an exceedingly rare complication of meniscectomy.

Division of the Infrapatellar Branch of the Saphenous Nerve

The incision described and recommended invariably divides the infrapatellar branch of the saphenous nerve. Therefore, the operation is followed by a patch of anesthesia over and lateral to the lower end of the patellar tendon and the tibial tubercle. Sometimes this is permanent, but often in a few months partial or complete sensation is recovered. After explanation, the patient realizes that a patch of anesthesia is no disability. In no instance has a painful neuroma complicated the scar from this incision. The only painful scars result from a more vertical incision (Fig. 12-6) which divides a branch of the nerve as it crosses the lower edge of the femur. The scar with the nerve end adheres to the bone. Irritation by repeated tension on the adhesions results in a painful neuroma. Stretching the scar reveals the neuroma, for the small segment that contains the nerve ending blanches. The finding may be confirmed by the hypersensitive reaction to tapping with a blunt point. The scar should be surgically freed from the bone, and the neuroma and the nerve isolated and divided well away from the scar.

Healing of the Wound

Great care should be exercised in assessing the condition of the skin before operation. If abraded or infected, operation should be delayed until all signs of inflammation have disappeared. With this proviso, healing is seldom delayed.

The late Professor T. P. McMurray once told me that Sir Robert Jones believed that synovial fluid delayed wound healing and that he took great care to wipe all traces of synovial fluid from the skin edges before suturing.

With modern theater and surgical techniques, joint sepsis following meniscectomy is almost unknown. Routine postoperative chemotherapy or antibiotics are unnecessary and in this series have been prescribed only in a few instances when wound discomfort and a niggling temperature have suggested stitch infection. When the dressings are removed for the first time on the tenth day, the skin wound occasionally is found to be moist or inflamed around a suture.

Residual Tags

The patient with a residual posterior fragment gives the history of recurrent internal derangement of the knee in spite of previous operation. The symptoms may be similar or changed in character, but the patient remains disabled, either by recurring stabs of pain, always in the same place, or by the knee giving way. The incidents may or may not be followed by effusions. Examination reveals finger-point tenderness over the fragment plus an easily elicited diagnostic click and, frequently, pain on complete flexion or on squatting. Occasionally, stabs of pain in the region of the collateral ligaments are due to pedicled or frondlike tags. The pain and tenderness are always over the tag, and, with the characteristic momentary nature of the incidents, are diagnostic.

Mistaken diagnosis before the first operation, a missed cartilaginous loose body, and a recurrent subluxation of the patella must all be considered in the differential diagnosis, but the detection of a residual fragment is usually simple.

Experienced surgeons using the preoperative criteria described in Chapter 7 coupled with careful inspection and assessment during the operation seldom miss an unstable posterior fragment or tag. The treatment is always excision of the fragment.

REFERENCES

1. **Annandale T:** An operation for displaced semilunar cartilage. Br Med J 1:779, 1885
2. **Bruser DM:** A direct approach to the lateral compartment of the knee joint. J Bone Joint Surg 42B:348, 1960
3. **Bunnell S:** Surgery of the Hand. Philadelphia, JB Lippincott, 1956
4. **Dandy DJ,** Br Med J 1:1099, 1978
5. **Dandy DJ, Jackson RW:** J Bone Joint Surg 578:346, 1975
6. **Duthie JJR, Macleod JG:** Rehabilitation after meniscectomy. Lancet 244:197, 1943
7. **Duthie JJR, Macleod JG:** Meniscectomy in soldiers. Lancet 246:182, 1944
8. **Fairbank TJ, Jamieson ES:** A complication of lateral meniscectomy. J Bone Joint Surg 33B:567, 1951
9. **Jones Sir Robert:** Notes on derangements of the knee. Ann Surg 50:969, 1909
10. **Jones Sir Robert:** Notes on Military Orthopaedic Surgery. London, Cassell, 1918
11. **Mayer L:** The physiological method of tendon transplantation. III. Experimental and clinical experiences. Surg. Gynecol Obstet 182:472, 1916
12. **Smillie IS:** Injuries of the Knee Joint. Baltimore, Williams & Wilkins, 1962

CHAPTER 13
OSTEOARTHRITIS

Louis Solomon
Arthur J. Helfet

Osteoarthritis (OA) is defined as primary when it occurs without any known cause, and as secondary when it can be traced to a demonstrable abnormality in the anatomy and mechanics of the joint. More and more evidence is accumulating to suggest that most OA in the middle-aged and elderly is secondary in nature, although to the mechanical abnormalities must be added certain metabolic disorders such as gout and chondrocalcinosis.

Several well-defined clinical patterns have long been recognized in patients with OA of the knee. There is the overweight woman with bilateral genu valgum and patellofemoral OA; more common is the patient with progressive varus deformity who presents with pain and tenderness localized to the anteromedial joint line and radiographic signs of OA confined, at least in the early stages, to the medial compartment of the knee. A significant number of patients give a history of meniscal tears or ligamentous injury with joint instability, resulting in OA some years later; in others, usually elderly women, the OA appears to be second-

ary to degeneration and detachment of the medial meniscus, which results in a traumatic erosion of the juxtaposed femoral condylar surface and the opposing facet of the patella. In all of these, however, there does appear to be a common factor: absolute or relative overload of a focal area of articular cartilage. Initially, cartilage destruction is confined to either the medial compartment, the lateral compartment, or the patellofemoral surfaces, and only when instability ensues does the rest of the joint become involved.

PATHOGENESIS

Notwithstanding the introductory remarks, OA of the knee should not be thought of as a disease resulting from a purely mechanical disorder of the joint in all cases. As with OA elsewhere, it is not a single, circumscribed disease entity but rather a manifestation of joint failure due to a number of factors in various combinations. There is increasing evi-

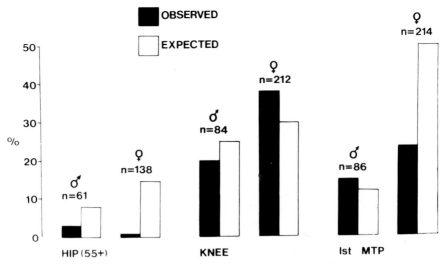

FIG. 13-1. Prevalence of osteoarthritis in South African blacks (35+) compared with the expected prevalence based on previous surveys in Caucasians.

dence of an inflammatory component in OA of the knee, and undoubtedly many patients have polyarticular involvement of some degree.[5] Nevertheless, even in these cases the joint is almost always affected asymmetrically, and the surfaces most severely eroded are those subjected to the greatest load.

Anthropometric studies carried out on patients with OA predominantly of the hip or knee show that the former tend strongly toward mesomorphy, whereas the latter (especially woman with OA of the knee) tend towards endomorphy and are often markedly overweight. This observation is complemented by epidemiologic findings in South African blacks and whites.[13] Osteoarthritis is generally much less common in blacks than in whites (Fig. 13-1), yet for OA of the knee the highest frequency occurs in urban African women, the next highest in urban white women, the next in white men, and the lowest in African men; this distribution is closely paralleled by the Ponderal Index in the four groups.[13]

The apparently conflicting claims of "inflammatory" versus "mechanical" factors in the pathogenesis of OA of the knee can be reconciled by the concept of *absolute or relative*

overload of articular cartilage. This involves the proposition that there are basically three types of OA, in the knee as elsewhere:

Type I. Absolute overload of normal articular cartilage, for example, due to varus or valgus instability, patellofemoral subluxation, or localized meniscal impingement on articular cartilage.

Type II. Relative overload of abnormal cartilage that fails even under physiologic loads; for example, OA secondary to gout or chondrocalcinosis, or in joints previously damaged by inflammatory arthritis. Recent work on the ultrastructure of osteoarthritic cartilage has shown the presence of hydroxyapatite in the midzone of articular cartilage,[16] emphasizing again that even histologically "normal" cartilage may be functionally disturbed.

Type III. Overload due to abnormalities of the subchondral bone; for example, subarticular sclerosis after fracture healing or acromegaly, both of which expose the overlying cartilage to peak overload due to loss of resilience in the subchondral bone.

THE BIOMECHANICS OF COMPARTMENTAL OVERLOAD

Maquet has presented a convincing analysis of the mechanical disturbance in OA of the knee.[10] In the normal unilaterally loaded knee (Fig. 13-2) the force resulting from the residual body mass (P) passes medial to the joint and is balanced by an equal force (L) on the lateral side produced by muscle contraction. The resultant force (R) normally passes through the center of the knee in the coronal plane. Theoretically, any of the following can cause medial displacement of force R and consequent medial compartment overload:

Increase of force P due to increased body mass

Varus deformity of the knee will displace force P further from the center of the knee and so increase the lever arm on the medial side of the joint; again, the resultant force R will shift medially.

Decrease of force L due to weakness or abnormal action of the lateral muscles, gluteus maximus, tensor fascia lata, and the iliotibial band. Because these muscles also control the hip, any disorder that produces a Trendelenburg dip at the hip will also weaken lateral stability of the knee.

Similarly, lateral displacement of force R may be caused by a valgus deformity of the knee, or by relative overaction of force L. It is a common observation that displacement osteotomy at the hip may be followed by valgus stresses on the knee and lateral compartment OA. The explanation is probably that the medial displacement of the femur diminishes the lever arm between the center of the joint and force P, resulting in relative overaction of force L.

These positions are further aggravated when force R is displaced so far medially or laterally that the deforming forces cannot actually be compensated by the contralateral force, because then the ligaments are stressed beyond their tolerance and eventually give way, resulting in increasing instability of the joint.

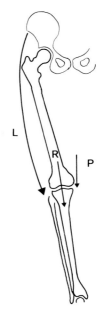

FIG. 13-2. Diagrammatic representation of forces acting on the knee in the coronal plane. (After Maquet, 1968)

Forces acting in the sagittal plane also have a determinant effect on knee function (Fig. 13-3). During normal gait the resultants of forces at both the ankle and the hip pass behind the knee and tend to flex the joint. This is counterbalanced by contraction of the quadriceps mechanism, which affects both the femorotibial and the patello femoral joints. The resultant of the flexor and extensor forces (R1) passes through the axis of flexion of the knee joint and exerts a compressive force on the femorotibial joint. Any increase in R1 will cause excessive loading of the articular surfaces; this would happen, for example, if full passive extension of the joint were impossible and stability had to be maintained by the quadriceps during weight-bearing on a partially flexed knee. It follows, therefore, that a medial or lateral compartmental overload is further aggravated by development of a flexion deformity.

The extensor effect on the patellofemoral joint is produced by the complementary forces of the quadriceps muscle (M) and the patellar tendon (P); the resultant of these two

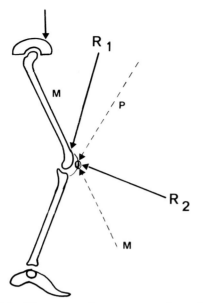

FIG. 13-3. Diagrammatic representation of forces acting on the knee in the sagittal plane. (After Maquet, 1968)

forces (R2) produces compression of the patellofemoral joint (Fig. 13-3). Here again, any increase in the moments of forces involving M or P (as would occur when walking on a partially flexed knee) will cause an increase in R2 and a tendency to overload the patellar and femoral condylar surfaces.

Though oversimplified, this explanation gives some idea of the ways in which abnormal mechanics at the knee or hip or ankle might contribute to the development of femorotibial and patellofemoral OA.

THE RELATIONSHIP OF MENISCAL INJURY TO OA OF THE KNEE

A traumatic tear of the medial or lateral meniscus may result in the entrapment of a firm, mobile wedge of fibrocartilage between the articular surfaces of the joint. It is surprising how quickly this may lead to cartilage fibrillation and progressive OA of that part of the femoral condyle in contact with the torn meniscus.

Unfortunately, meniscectomy offers no guar-

antee that OA will not ensue anyway, especially in the somewhat older patient. In a follow-up of patients over 40 years who had undergone meniscectomy, Jones and associates found that 75% of those with "traumatic" tears had postoperative knee pain, and signs of OA were significantly more severe on the side operated on than in the contralateral knee.[7] It is our belief that this result is partly due to the gradual development of rotatory instability after meniscectomy, especially in active sportsmen who continue to place heavy physical demands on the joint. This is less likely to occur if the peripheral part of the meniscus is retained, and for this reason partial meniscectomy, and even meniscal repair when possible, is advocated instead of the thorough dissections practiced in previous years.

Others have shown experimentally that the menisci play an important part in load distribution across the joint, and local stresses on articular cartilage are significantly increased after total meniscectomy.[8]

More controversial is the relationship of degenerative meniscal lesions to osteoarthritis. With aging the meniscus becomes less pliable, and minor (perhaps unnoticed) injuries may cause either horizontal cleavage lesions or partial detachment from the anterior tibial spine.

The young meniscus is white, elastic, and firm but pliable. It is avascular, except where it is attached to the capsule of the joint. Microscopically, it consists of highly cellular fibrocartilage. As it ages the meniscus becomes harder, loses its pearly color, and turns yellowish and translucent, especially at its thin free border. Microscopically, there is a gradual loss of cellularity, and the tissue becomes more fibrous and inelastic. Such a degenerated meniscus is less capable of adapting to abnormal stresses, and relatively minor rotational injury may pull it from its attachment to the tibia.

It is tempting to suggest that the fibrotic, partially detached meniscus can act as an impactor on the opposite articular surface, thus causing the typical cartilaginous destruction frequently seen at arthrotomy in these patients (Fig. 13-4). On the other hand, it could be argued equally cogently that meniscal degeneration is the *result* of long-standing OA.[9] Noble and Hamblem, who studied these changes in 100 necropsy examinations, found that the patterns of degenerative meniscal lesions and OA were quite distinct and came to the conclusion that the two disorders are coincidental rather than causally related.[12]

OSTEOARTHRITIS AND LONG-DISTANCE RUNNING

With the increasing popularity of jogging and more serious long-distance running, many athletes are concerned about the possibility that these activities might predispose them to OA of the knees. Undoubtedly, knee pain due to one cause or another often occurs in these people, and they surely suffer a higher incidence of meniscal lesions and other soft-tissue injuries than the population at large. In this sense, therefore, they are somewhat predisposed to the later development of OA of the knee. It is also likely that, once early OA is present, persistent long-distance running on hard surfaces will hasten the cartilage destruction, and this is especially likely to occur in elderly enthusiasts.

On the other hand, it is equally true that no good evidence has yet appeared that long-distance running *per se* initiates OA in anatomically sound knees.

OSTEOARTHRITIS OF THE KNEE AS AN INFLAMMATORY DISORDER

Osteoarthritis is still widely regarded as a "degenerative" disease, and the paucity of signs of inflammation has in recent years prompted the introduction of the term "osteoarthrosis." That OA is quite different from inflammatory joint diseases such as rheumatoid arthritis remains undisputed. However, to hold that there is *no* inflammatory component is to ignore the features of pain, stiffness, swelling, and effusion that commonly accompany the disorder.

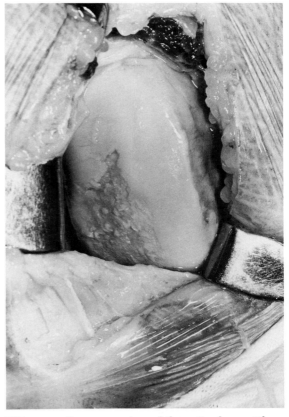

FIG. 13-4. Severe erosion of the articular cartilage on the medial femoral condyle in a patient with detachment of the medial meniscus.

Huskisson and co-workers have recently presented a well-documented account of the evidence suggesting inflammation and polyarticular involvement, sometimes associated with some metabolic abnormality causing hydroxyapatite crystal deposition, OA.[5] Of 74 patients with OA of the knee, 85% had bilateral involvement, 73% had effusions, and 26% had increased warmth of one or the other knee. Synovial fluid aspirated from the knee in 34 patients also showed inflammatory changes with increased cell counts.

All of these features could, of course, be the result of OA rather than its cause. For the moment their true significance remains unresolved. However, even if it is accepted that metabolic and inflammatory disorders are involved in the *initiation* of OA, it still seems true that mechanical factors determine the *progression* of the disease in the majority of cases.

PATHOLOGY

The natural progress of human OA has been well described in recent years,[3,4,14,15] and the accompanying molecular changes have been minutely observed in a reliable animal model.[11]

The earliest detectable abnormality, prior to any macroscopic change, is an increase in water content of the articular cartilage; this is followed by disaggregation of the macromolecular chondromucoprotein and loss of glycosaminoglycans from the cartilage matrix. At this stage the articular surface is softer than normal on direct pressure, and there may be some splitting of the superficial layers of cartilage. Gradually, these clefts become more marked until there is obvious fraying, or fibrillation, of the normally smooth and glistening articular cartilage. The early changes correspond to the clinical disorder of chondromalacia, and, although they are not actually reversible, neither do they necessarily progress to complete articular destruction. In other words, it is useful to picture OA as occurring in two merging phases, (1) the initiation of cartilage fibrillation and (2) the progression to clinically symptomatic OA. It is significant that, although areas of early fibrillation may be found in minimally loaded parts of the joint, progressive cartilage loss advances most rapidly in the more heavily loaded surfaces.

Even at a comparatively early stage of progressive OA there are reactive changes in the subchondral bone. Active osteogenesis and trabecular thickening may produce an absolute increase in bone mass, which is apparent on radiography as subchondral sclerosis in the overloaded segment of the joint. At the edge of the articular cartilage endochondral ossification leads to osteophyte formation, which appears in the radiograph to be most marked at the medial or lateral joint margins and adjacent to the tibial spines. All these changes can be looked upon, in some sense, as *repair* phenomena, attempts on the part of the bone to support the increasingly punishing load transferred to the metaphysis and to stabilize the crumbling joint.

Later, subchondral cysts appear, and these are also manifestations of joint overload. Ultimately, when the bone is completely denuded of cartilage, trabecular fragmentation may occur (Fig. 13-5), resulting in major distortion of the joint architecture. Clinical experience suggests that this late stage of bone fragmentation may actually be hastened by oversolicitous prescribing of powerful anti-inflammatory agents or repeated intra-articular injection of corticosteroids.

With bone destruction the joint becomes unstable due to collapse of the affected compartment rather than to any stretching of the ligaments on the opposite side; however, once the deformity reaches the point where the resultant of loading forces passes medial or lateral to the center of rotation of the affected femoral condyle, the opposite side of the joint will "open up," and those ligaments will then be permanently damaged (Fig. 13-6).

The changes in cartilage and bone are accompanied by a low-grade synovitis and intra-articular effusion. In the late stages meniscal degeneration and capsular fibrosis are almost inevitable; together with osteophytic hypertrophy they lead to loss of full extension and impairment of the normal helicoid movements of the femorotibial surfaces, thus contributing further to the vicious cycle of abnormal joint loading and progressive articular destruction.

CLINICAL AND RADIOLOGIC FEATURES

The commonest symptom in OA of the knee is pain. This is usually felt over the anteromedial aspect of the joint, but sometimes it is parapatellar, sometimes vaguely "inside the joint," and occasionally confined to the popli-

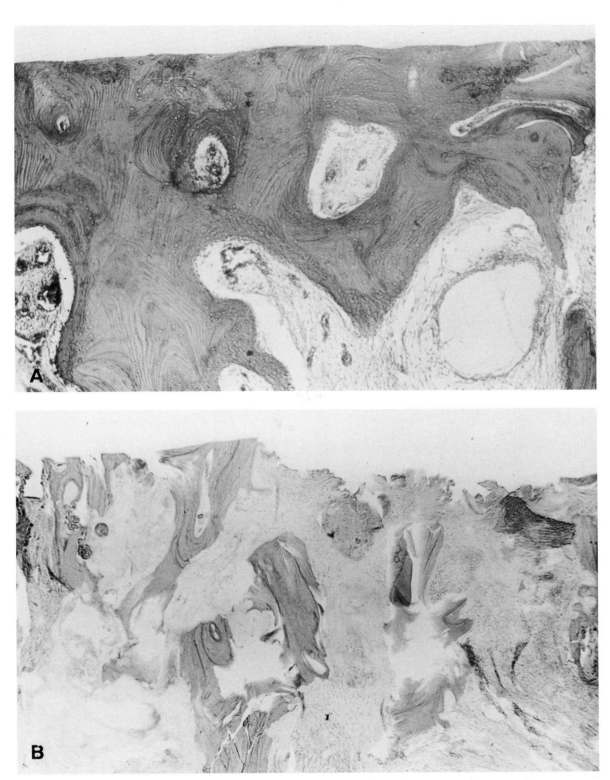

FIG. 13-5. Photomicrographs showing advanced stages of osteoarthritis. In *A* there is complete loss of articular cartilage and sclerosis of the subchondral bone. In *B* there is fragmentation of the subchondral trabeculae.

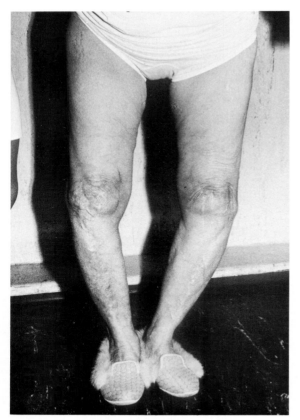

FIG. 13-6. Patient with bilateral osteoarthritis of the knees. In addition to the varus and slight flexion deformities, there is also some fixed internal rotation of the tibia and prominence of the medial femoral condyle, particularly noticeable on the right side.

teal fossa. Often it follows a regular diurnal rhythm, worse at the end of the day and immediately after rising from bed. It may also be aggravated by going up or down stairs or by some sudden unaccustomed movement. In the beginning it is usually relieved by rest or by limiting activity, but in time relief comes more slowly and is less complete. The ultimate phase is bone pain in bed at night, and the patient has difficulty finding any position of comfort.

Stiffness, too, is common and is felt typically in the early morning and after periods of inactivity. It may be accompanied by swell-ing, which often varies from day to day and may cause a feeling of "tightness" in the joint.

Clinical findings depend on the stage of the disease. There may be an obvious deformity, usually varus and slight internal rotation of the tibia (Fig. 13-6). As the condition progresses, full extension becomes more and more difficult, and in the late stage there is almost invariably some fixed flexion deformity.

Tenderness along the anteromedial joint line, a slight increase in local warmth, intra-articular effusion, and some limitation of the range of movement complete the picture. This may remain unchanged for many years, and, if the hypertrophic osteophyte formation is marked, the knee will continue to be stable. Ligamentous instability is a bad prognostic sign and heralds rapid progression of articular destruction.

Radiologic changes are often missed because the knee is radiographed with the patient lying down. The radiographic investigation should always include weight-bearing views (Fig. 13-7), which will show the early signs of narrowing of the articular cartilage and subchondral sclerosis in the zone of overload. The other classic features are cyst formation and osteophytes at the joint margins and on the tibial spines. In the late stages bone loss and joint instability may be marked (Fig. 13-8).

Whatever the mode of onset, the later stages of OA often involve the patellofemoral joint as well, and this may be the greatest source of pain (Fig. 13-9). It is important to bear this in mind when planning treatment; many patients have been subjected to total joint replacement when conservative treatment of patellofemoral pain might have given a similar degree of relief.

Occasionally, a single large subarticular cyst may raise the suspicion of a primary bone lesion (Fig. 13-10). The associated features of OA should make the true diagnosis clear.

Additional features such as chondrocalcinosis, calcification of the menisci, loose bodies, and preceding abnormalities like subchondral fractures may be present as well.

FIG. 13-7. Radiograph of the knees, with the patient standing. In the right knee there is diminution of the articular "space" on the medial side; in the left knee the articular cartilage of the medial compartment is completely absent and there is marked subchondral sclerosis in the zone of maximum loading.

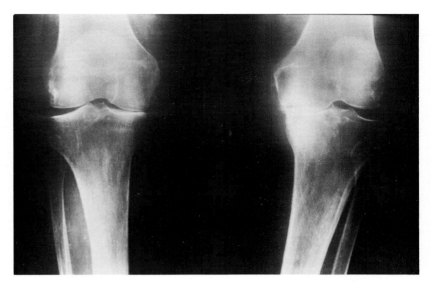

TREATMENT

Once cartilage fibrillation is established, the progress of the disorder is determined largely by mechanical factors, and it is on these factors that one must concentrate if the destructive changes are to be arrested or slowed down.

The principles of treatment in the early stages, preferably before instability ensues, are fairly straightforward—(1) treat the pain and inflammation, (2) stabilize the joint, and (3) reduce the load. This approach is most likely to be effective when the radiographic changes are confined to one compartment (usually the medial compartment), the articular "space" is not completely lost, and extension with concomitant rotation of the knee joint and consequent relief of tension of the patella in the trochlear groove, even if not complete, is still possible, and the knee is still

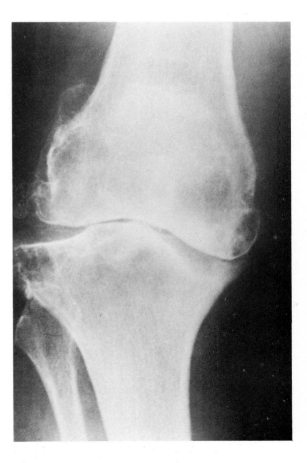

FIG. 13-8. Anteroposterior radiograph showing rotatory subluxation of the joint, varus deformity, and opening up of the lateral compartment in advanced osteoarthritis of the knee. Note that there is also some calcification of the articular cartilage in the lateral part of the joint.

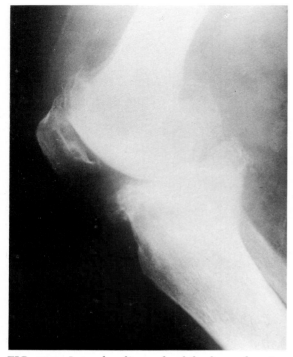

FIG. 13-9. Lateral radiograph of the knee showing advanced osteoarthritis of both femorotibial and patellofemoral compartments.

stable on clinical examination. Indeed, it is at this stage that "prophylactic surgery" in the form of realignment procedures might be justified to transfer load away from the severely affected part of the joint before total articular destruction leads to progressive instability.

PAIN AND INFLAMMATION

Pain, swelling, and intra-articular effusion are part of the low-grade inflammatory process that usually accompanies OA. Appropriate analgesic and anti-inflammatory therapy can offer control of these symptoms for many years. Such treatment may even necessitate the occasional (once or twice a year) injection of intra-articular substances such as corticosteroids, nitrogen mustard, or radiocolloids. However, one should beware of overmedication for pain while articular destruction grinds on relentlessly, and even with effective symptomatic treatment the progress of joint stability and architectural integrity should be carefully observed at regular intervals, so that other measures may be introduced in good time.

PREVENTION OF TRAUMATIC ARTHRITIS

It is questionable whether conservative treatment is really worthwhile. Once the arthritic process is in progress, is it possible to stay further erosion without surgery? One can sometimes teach patients to reduce displacement of the meniscus themselves; if this is possible, by limiting activity and by prevention of all strain, conservative treatment, when circumstances demand it, may be practicable. The patient must exercise assiduously to maintain muscle strength and bulk, for the stronger muscles can allow greater activity and withstand more strain before discomfort and effusion result.

For the knee with limited movement, when operation is contraindicated, the wearing of a caliper fitted with a knee-spring is helpful.

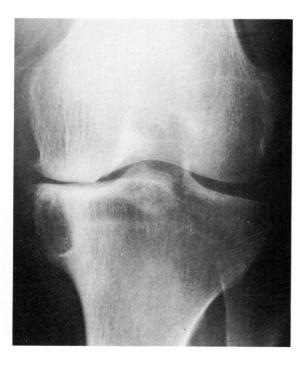

FIG. 13-10. Radiograph showing a large osteoarthritic cyst of the medial tibial condyle, and loss of the adjacent articular cartilage.

This is a light caliper fitted into the heel of the shoe, with an extension spring at the level of the knee joint. The spring is loaded by flexion of the knee. When the leg is raised and weight is taken on the other foot, the spring is released and reinforces the quadriceps in extending the knee. In this manner it helps the patient to maintain full extension of the knee—the important movement—and also limits untoward flexion and rotation strains.

When a good range of movement is possible but with a measure of instability, the knee brace described in Chapter 5 is helpful.

THE USE OF INTRA-ARTICULAR INJECTIONS

At the end of the last war, Waugh advised intra-articular injections of a solution of lactic acid with a pH of 5.8.[17] His thesis was that because synovial fluid in osteoarthritic knees is slightly alkaline, it would be neutralized by the acid solution. The technique used is the injection, once a week, of 10 ml of a saline solution of lactic acid with 0.5% procaine into and around the joint, followed by gentle passive movements and exercise. These injections are comforting, and the effect may last for a week or more.

The injection of the latest preparations of corticosteroids into swollen and painful joints is generally regarded as a valuable measure in the treatment of rheumatoid arthritis. Hollander and his colleagues[12] and Chandler, Wright, and Hartfall,[4,5] of the University of Leeds, carried out a controlled trial of hydrocortisone tert-butyl-acetate on 24 patients whose main incapacity arose from involvement of the knees.[5] They found that significant relief of pain and tenderness and improvement in movement and walking time appeared for periods lasting from 4 to 8 weeks. However, every success carries with it potential dangers, for deterioration was observed by roentgenography in another trial in 13 of 25 knee joints despite clinical improvement in the majority of cases. Chandler and Wright[4] therefore were of the opinion that cortisone interferes with the normal protective processes natural to inflammatory disease. Functional improvement and the relief of pain, being the most important features, encourage a degree of activity and weight-bearing that is frankly traumatic. They commented on the production of a virtual Charcot's arthropathy in an osteoarthritic hip treated over an 18-month period by monthly injections of hydrocortisone. The patient had obtained almost complete relief of pain when treatment was discontinued.

It has been my practice over a number of years to inject only acutely painful swollen osteoarthritic knees with a mixture of 10 ml of 1% procaine in saline and 1.0 ml to 1.5 ml of prednisolone (25 mg to 37.5 mg). This local injection of hydrocortisone into osteoarthritic joints is of value when there is an acute exacerbation of the chronic condition, that is, when the knee is swollen and painful. When the joint is not swollen or inflamed, the clinical condition is not significantly changed. In other words, intra-articular injections are of value for pain but not in the treatment of the underlying arthritic lesion.

Injections carry the not inconsiderable danger of increased and significant destruction of articular cartilage, because as noted above, the pain-free joint permits undue activity without the protection of a painful inflammatory reaction.

We are now observing the long-term results of injections of hydrocortisone in the knees of adults. After a variable period of comfort, symptoms recur, and the roentgenograms show erosion of articular cartilage and the separation of loose bodies. Joseph Milgram reports several instances of more acute lesions (see Chap. 28). A sudden twist of a flexed weight-bearing knee has resulted in a tangential fracture of the medial femoral condyle with separation of a disk of articular cartilage. This lesion from limited trauma would be almost impossible in any knee with normal articular cartilage.

In 1965 Jocelyn Hill* crystallized the opinion of many that

The use of hydrocortisone for the relief of joint pain should be stopped. Symptoms are masked, producing a local steroid honeymoon in a manner similar

* Hill J: Personal communication, 1965

to that produced more often in the rheumatoids. Destruction proceeds not because of any local malignant activity on the steroid's part but simply because the weight-bearing joint, like a Charcot's, is pounded to destruction. Since many of these elderly bones are also osteoporotic, the addition of steroids to the diet can sometimes produce a central hip protrusion, for example, in a bed-ridden patient. This suggests that unguarded muscle pull is sufficient to cause this damage. Experience in the treatment of rheumatoid arthritis suggests that much joint pain and stiffness (viz, elbows, wrists, feet, and knees) can be relieved by simple surgical measures, and the more generalized symptoms relieved by less dangerous drugs.

Corticosteroids probably exert their effect by countering the deleterious enzyme reactions that are a feature of OA, and this provides the initial benefit. But normal enzyme reactions may be affected as well, leading to long-term deterioration of articular cartilage.[4]

Other protease inhibitors have been tested in the treatment of OA of the knee, often with immediate relief of pain and improvement of movement. But in a week, or at most two, symptoms have usually recurred. After further injections, improvement tended to be less and of shorter duration, simulating the course after corticosteroids and probably for the same reason, which has led us to discontinue this as therapy.

Endre A. Balazs reports in Chapter 4 on the considerations behind the use of a pure, high-molecular-weight hyaluronic acid, the principle constituent of synovial fluid, in joint diseases. In OA the concentration of hyaluronic acid is very often lower than in normal joints, and both the viscosity and elasticity of the synovial fluid is decreased. Clinical trials of replacement of synovial fluid by intra-articular injection of a pure, pyrogen-free, and sterile large-polymer hyaluronic acid is giving most promising results. In principle, it is an ideal form of therapy—the replacement of a natural constituent by a natural product. It is not a drug, and in no instance have we had any immediate or long-term undesirable effects.

The clinical trial of Healon, as this high-polymer hyaluronic acid preparation has been

called, produced the following preliminary results in our hands. Sixty-two injections were given to 45 patients in 22 hips and 40 knees, all with varying severity of arthritis. Most were selected with fair range of movement without instability. No follow-up was possible on two hips and four knees. There was immediate improvement with painless movement in all but one knee and two hips. The improvement in 14 hips and 33 knees after each injection lasted from 1 week to 12 months. The average duration of improvement after injection was 6 weeks for hips and 10 weeks for knees.

RAISED HEEL

The osteoarthritic knee finds comfort in slight flexion. Once fixed flexion has developed, attempts to force extension are painful. The patient tends to walk with the knee flexed a few degrees short of this painful extreme. Raising the heel of the shoe on the side of the injured knee eases the effort of walking, which becomes less fatiguing. However, it must be realized that raising the heel is an admission of resignation. It is always preferable to attempt the recovery of full extension by manipulation or meniscectomy.

STABILIZATION

Ligamentous instability may precede the onset of OA and should be corrected as far as possible by physiotherapy, external bracing, or, in more severe cases, reconstructive surgery. If it occurs later as part of the osteoarthritic process, the same principles apply.

Patients can be taught to exercise regularly by themselves to maintain muscle strength. In more advanced cases in which physiotherapy is ineffectual and surgery is contraindicated, the use of a knee brace is often helpful (see Chap. 5, Fig. 5-4).

Incomplete extension of the joint causes a particular type of instability that was discussed earlier. Walking on a partially flexed knee calls for excessive quadriceps action, resulting in increased compression of both the femorotibial and the patellofemoral surfaces. If full extension is prevented by a displaced meniscus, this may be corrected by gentle manipulation in flexion and rotation. This simple maneuver may give relief of pain and improved mobility for long periods. Patients may even be taught to do this themselves. While sitting on a raised surface, the knee is pulled up into full flexion. The leg is then rotated medially and laterally on the thigh until a full range is obtained, often with an audible click. Finally the leg is kicked out as if at an invisible ball so that the knee is jerked into full extension. If the manipulation is successful, pain is immediately relieved. Manipulation for adhesions between fat pad or menisci and tibia, which may follow a traumatic incident, are discussed in Chapters 26 and 27.

In patients with clear-cut features of meniscal degeneration and detachment, in whom simple conservative measures no longer bring relief, meniscectomy and removal of blocking osteophytes may restore a full range of extension and rotation.

REDUCTION OF LOAD

Several common-sense measures suggest themselves as a means of reducing articular load. Weight loss (when necessary), the use of a walking stick, maintenance of full extension by exercises or physiotherapy, prevention of muscle wasting, avoidance of unnecessary stresses (such as jogging or climbing stairs), and even intermittent periods of complete rest, are all part of the stock-in-trade of the concerned therapist. Again, though, the trap to be avoided is the obsessive perseverance with such "conservative" measures in the face of progressive articular destruction when a judiciously timed operation can effectively prevent this.

The surgical approach to load reduction involves osteotomy and realignment of either the tibia or the femur *before* joint instability is present. Our policy has been to perform high tibial osteotomy for medial compartment overload with varus deformity and low femoral osteotomy for lateral compartment over-

load with valgus deformity. Maquet (1976) has presented sound mechanical reason for choosing these particular sites for osteotomy,[10] and the theoretical considerations are borne out in practice by the results in 94 patients recently assessed after 6 to 10 years following surgery. Pain relief and radiographic "arrest" of the disease were achieved in 70%; factors that appeared to improve the likelihood of success were (1) early disease, (2) joint stability, (3) angular deformity of less than 20°, and (4) the age of the patient—younger patients (those under 50 years) do much better than the elderly.

The "double osteotomy" of Benjamin in which both femur and tibia are divided close to the joint, has gained some popularity in recent years.[2] There is no sound evidence, however, that it is any more effective than a carefully planned realignment procedure on one side of the joint.[6]

Once joint destruction has progressed to both compartments and instability is marked, the only effective treatment is either arthrodesis or total joint replacement.

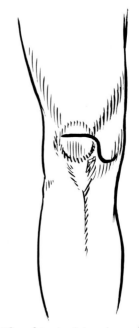

FIG. 13-11. The skin incision is prolonged transversely across the patella.

THE PATELLA

Intraarticular examination of the patella is required if any of the following conditions are present:

Postpatellar pain on walking up and down stairs or slopes

Tenderness of the medial border of the patella

Radiographic evidence of osteophytic or erosive changes on skyline views of the patella

An extended skin incision is necessary, and treatment is dictated by the stage and extent of the degenerative changes in the articular cartilage of the patella. If the changes are moder-

ate, the release of tension with recovery of full extension after meniscectomy is sufficient to relieve pain. As soon as the patella can achieve its normal and balanced position in the trochlear groove, climbing and descending stairs are comfortable.

DÉBRIDEMENT OF THE PATELLA

Patellar débridement is a helpful procedure when the osteophytes are young and not too massive and desiccated, and when patches of articular cartilage are frayed and fissured. If the edges of the eroded areas are ragged, they should be trimmed carefully until a smooth, almost transparent surface is obtained.

The effectiveness of the débridement may be gauged by a simple test. If the knee is flexed and extended before débridement, the impingement of the patellar osteophytes on the femoral edge is obvious. After adequate removal, movement of the patella is free and without friction or tension.

When the typical medial compartment OA is accompanied by patellofemoral disease, the patella may be "decompressed" at the time of high tibial osteotomy by either displacing the entire distal tibial fragment and patellar tendon anteriorly, or by combining the tibial osteotomy with a formal anterior displacement osteotomy of the tibial tubercle as described by Maquet.[10] (See Chap. 14.) This effectively reduces loading of both the femorotibial and the patellofemoral joint.

PATELLECTOMY

Removal of the patella is rarely required but is indicated if the articular cartilage of the patella or the trochlea is widely and grossly affected. The skin incision is prolonged transversely (Fig. 13-11), and the bone is removed subperiosteally. The synovial layer usually approximates without tension and may be closed with fine plain catgut. The repair of the capsule and the fascial and periosteal coverings of the patella must be meticulous. As in all knee surgery, the keynote is the restoration of function of the patellar mechanism and the

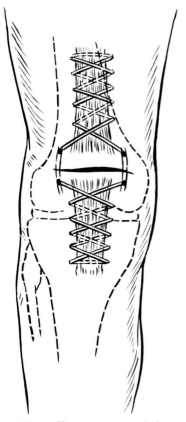

FIG. 13-12. Bunnell-type suture of chromic catgut or linen thread is used to pull the quadriceps and the patellar tendons together.

medial capsule so that complete, active extension and rotation are recovered. Therefore, the knee is extended completely with full lateral rotation of the tibia before the capsule is sutured with No. 1 chromic catgut or linen thread. If necessary, to achieve proper tension in the medial capsule the edges are overlapped, and to tighten the whole mechanism, a Bunnell-type suture of the same material is used to pull the quadriceps and patellar tendons together (Fig. 13-12). Postoperatively, the patient should stay in bed for 2 weeks with a compression bandage and a plaster-of-Paris splint that includes the foot with the leg in external rotation. After removal of the skin sutures, a back splint is applied for 6 weeks; for the first 4 weeks the patient walks on crutches without bearing weight on the leg. During the last 2 weeks the back splint is removed for periodic active flexion exercises. Thigh drill is commenced 2 weeks after operation. Comfort is restored by this operation, and satisfactory movement is usually recovered in a few weeks. Occasionally, gentle manipulation under Pentothal is necessary to recover or accelerate recovery of movement. The manipulation should not be undertaken until the adhesions are ''dry.'' If done too soon, the vascular adhesions bleed, and the joint reacts with swelling and pain. Generally speaking, adhesions are dry when deep tenderness is localized, and reaction to deep heat and active use results in minimal pain and swelling. Good judgment in this regard is the criterion of success. Manipulation at the wrong time delays recovery, but at the right time it may result in dramatic relief.

Because these older patients are happy to be without pain and do not seek violent activity, the short-term results of patellectomy are good and the long-term prognosis is usually better than in younger patients.

THE FUTURE

Recently attention has turned to the possibility of resurfacing osteoarthritic joints with osteocartilaginous allografts. This has already been done in several centers in experimental animals and, somewhat more hesitantly, in human knees with large osteocartilaginous defects. Technically, the knee joint is ideally suited to this procedure. An appropriately chosen allograft can restore both the shape and the height of the femoral or tibial articular surface; the grafted cartilage remains viable, and, once the bone has been fully incorporated, it functions as a true biologic articular replacement.

REFERENCES

1. **Ali SY, Wisby A:** Ultrastructural aspects of normal and osteoarthritic cartilage. Ann Rheum Dis Suppl 2 34: 21–23, 1975
2. **Benjamin A:** Double osteotomy for knee pain in rheumatoid arthritis and osteoarthritis. J Bone Joint Surg 51B:694, 1969
3. **Byers PD, Pringle J, Oztop F et al:** Observations on osteoarthrosis of the hip. Semin Arthritis Rheum 6:277, 1977
4. **Chandler GN, Wright V, and Hartfall SJ:** Deleterious effect of intra-articular hydrocortisone. Lancet, 2:661, 1958
5. **Freeman MAR, Meachim G:** Adult articular cartilage —aging and degeneration. In Freeman MAR (ed): Adult Articular Cartilage, 2nd ed. Pitman, London, 1979
6. **Hill, Jocelyn:** Personal Communication, 1965
7. **Hollander JL, Brown EM, Jessar RA, and Brown CY:** Hydrocortisone
8. **Huskisson EC, Dieppe PA, Tucker AK et al:** Another look at osteoarthritis. Ann Rheum Dis 38:423, 1979
9. **Iveson JMI, Longton EB, Wright V:** Comparative study of tibial (single) and tibiofemoral (double) osteotomy for osteoarthrosis and rheumatoid arthritis. Ann Rheum Dis 36:319, 1977
10. **Jones RE, Smith EC, Reisch JS:** Effects of medial meniscectomy in patients older than forty years. J Bone Joint Surg 60A:783, 1978
11. **Krause WR, Pope MH, Johnson RJ et al:** Mechanical changes in the knee after meniscectomy. J Bone Joint Surg 58A:599, 1976
12. **Lidge RT:** Medial meniscectomy in the osteoarthritic knee. Clin Orthop 68:63, 1970
13. **Maquet PGJ:** Biomechanics of the Knee. Berlin, Springer-Verlag, 1976
14. **Muir H:** Molecular approach to the understanding of osteoarthrosis: Heberden Oration, 1976. Ann Rheum Dis 36:199, 1977
15. **Noble J, Hamblen DL:** The pathology of the degenerative meniscus lesion. J Bone Joint Surg 57B:180, 1975

16. **Solomon L, Beighton P, Lawrence JS:** Rheumatic disorders in the South African Negro. Part II. Osteoarthrosis. S Afr Med J 49:1737, 1975

17. **Sweet MBE, Thonar EJ-MA, Immelman AR et al:** Biochemical changes in progressive osteoarthrosis. Ann Rheum Dis 36:387, 1977

18. **Venn M, Maroudas A:** Chemical composition and swelling of normal and osteoarthrotic femoral head cartilage. I. Chemical composition. Ann Rheum Dis 36:121, 1977

19. **Waugh, WG:** Monoarticular osteoarthritis of the hip. Brit Med J 1:873, 1945

CHAPTER 14

OSTEOTOMY FOR OSTEOARTHRITIS AND RHEUMATOID ARTHRITIS OF THE KNEE

R. J. Furlong

In osteoarthritis and rheumatoid arthritis of the knee, osteotomy of the tibia or the femur has no effect on the arthritic joint other than a mechanical one. It follows, therefore, that these kinds of arthritis of the knee have at least a mechanical component. It is by altering the mechanical forces acting on the knee that the surgeon hopes to ameliorate the symptoms. The assumption is that osteoarthritis is the consequence of too great a stress on the joint. This increased stress provokes functional adaptation in the subchondral, which evolves through its apposition stage and, entering the stage of resorption, displays all the changes embraced in the term osteoarthritis. Osteotomy is performed to reduce this unit-loading by realigning the forces and increasing the load-transmitting area. In rheumatoid arthritis increased mechanical pressure plays no part in the etiology of the condition, though the deformity that develops worsens the clinical state. This can be ameliorated by

osteotomy. Osteoarthritis of the knee, from whatever cause, generally is divided into two regional types (1) primary or generalized and (2) secondary, resulting from altered stress on the joint.

PRIMARY OSTEOARTHRITIS

Primary osteoarthritis is the consequence of an inherent insufficiency of the articular cartilage to withstand physiologic stress. All three compartments of the knee are affected, and no deformity is characteristic except fixed flexion. The x-ray film shows subchondral sclerosis in both the tibial plateau and the patella. Later, as the condition evolves it loses its etiologic identity and becomes nonspecific osteoarthritis. Because the condition develops in a previously normal knee and no deformity is yet present, the only biomechanical remedy would be to reduce the total overall loading in

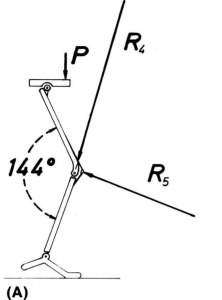 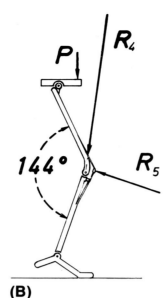

FIG. 14-1. Modification of the forces produced by anterior displacement of the patella tendon. **(A)** Normal knee. **(B)** After displacement of the patellar tendon. R_4 and R_5 are vectorial. (After Maquet)

(A)   **(B)**

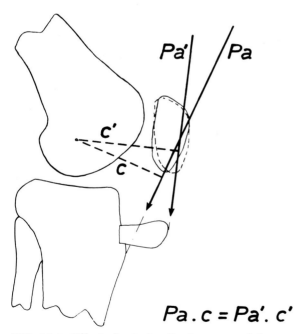

$$Pa \cdot c = Pa' \cdot c'$$

FIG. 14-2. Effect of anterior displacement of the patella tendon, or force Pa. Pa is the force normally transmitted by the patella tendon. Pa[1] is the force transmitted by the patella tendon when displaced forward. C is the lever arm of Pa; C[1] is the lever arm of Pa.[1] (After Maquet)

the joint. No increase in the weight-transmitting area is possible because it is not anatomically reduced. The patella is an exception, however, as will be described later. This aim is achieved by anterior displacement of the patellar tendon.

ANTERIOR DISPLACEMENT OF THE TIBIAL TUBERCLE

This is not the place to describe in detail the biomechanical stresses acting on the knee. Figure 14-1A shows R_4 and R_5, which are the resultants of the forces acting on the knee. R_4 is the resultant of body weight P and of the hamstring muscles (which prevent the pelvis from tipping forward), and the gastrocnemius group (which prevent the foot from dorsiflexing). Both these muscle groups tend to flex the knee so that the quadriceps muscle and its counterpart, the patellar tendon, produce equilibrium by powerful contraction that prevents the knee from flexing; hence, the magnitude of R_4, which in the diagram is vectorial.

Because of the angle of the knee, the patella (Fig. 14-1B) is pressed against the lower end of the femur, represented by the vector R_5. It is

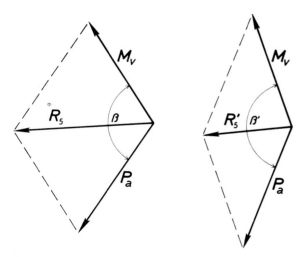

FIG. 14-3. Opening of the angle formed by the pull of the quadriceps M_v and the patella tendon Pa decreases the magnitude of resultant force R_5. (After Maquet)

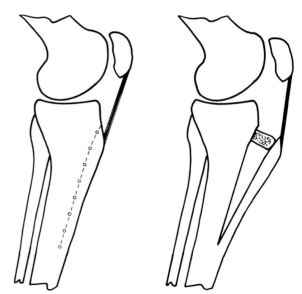

FIG. 14-4. Anterior displacement of the patella tendon by splitting the tibial crest and wedging it forward. (After Maquet)

the object of anterior displacement of the patellar tendon to reduce both R_4 and R_5.

By altering the line of action of the patellar tendon Pa to Pa¹, the lever arm C¹ is lengthened by about 10% (Fig. 14-2). Therefore, the quadriceps muscle can do the same work for 10% less effort, and this reduces the force across the femorotibial joint proportionally.

Reduction of the patellofemoral pressure is even more striking in Fig. 14-3. A forward displacement of this tibial tubercle by 2 cm reduces the patellofemoral pressure by as much as 50% (this is useful in the treatment of the patella in chondromalacia). The altered direction of Pa brings the upper facet of the patella into contact with the femur earlier in the arc of flexion. Because the upper facet is larger than the middle, the weight-transmission area is usually enlarged.

Indications for Surgery

If tricompartmental osteoarthritis, developing in a previously normal joint, is the consequence of inability of the articular cartilage to withstand physiologic stress, a pressure-reducing operation should be performed as soon as the diagnosis is evident. This is the essential indication for surgery.

Physiotherapy may be advisable initially as a matter of convenience for treating the patient before the knee joint is treated surgically.

The Operation

An anteromedial incision is made 1 cm posterior to the crest of the tibia extending from the tibial tubercle (often recessive) downward for about 10 cm. The periosteum is divided, and many holes are drilled transversely with Kirschner wire a little more than 0.5 cm behind the crest for the entire length of the incision. The holes are drilled through the opposite cortex (Fig. 14-4); they are connected by a fine osteotome, and the whole sliver of bone is pried forward, retaining the origin of the anterior tibial muscles. The elevated position—up to 2 cm according to the availability of skin—is maintained by wedging in a piece of bone taken from the iliac crest. Drainage and careful suture of the skin are important. If osteoarthritis of the patellofemoral joint is ac-

A   **B**

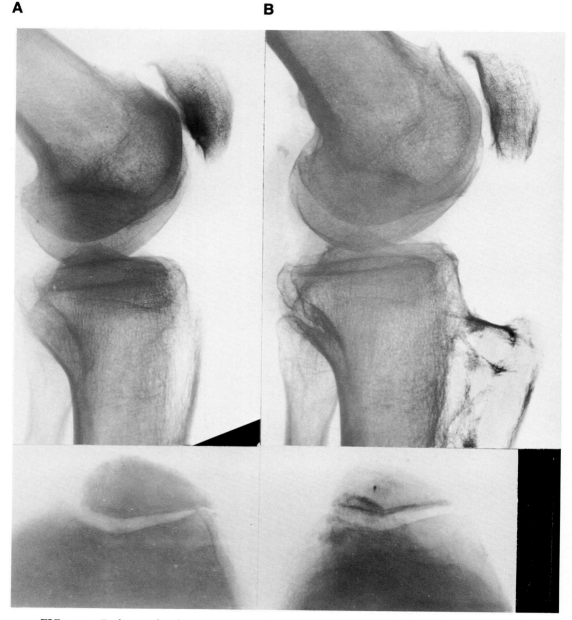

FIG. 14-5. Radiographs show the patient **(A)** before an anterior and medial displacement of the tibial tubercle, and **(B)** 3 years following the operation. (After Maquet)

centuated in the lateral facet of the femoral groove, the upper end of the sliver is displaced slightly medially to equalize the pressure in the groove.

In the experience of surgeons who have used this operation, the results are good and are maintained (Fig. 14-5). In practice, it should replace physiotherapy and Indocid.

Results

Maquet lists 60 operations of this type carried out since 1963, of which 57 are available for analysis. The operations were carried out for patellofemoral osteoarthritis, chondromalacia patellae, and tricompartmental osteoarthritis without deformity. Of the 57 patients receiving follow-up care, results are described as excellent in 48, good in 8, and poor in 1.

SECONDARY OSTEOARTHRITIS

Secondary osteoarthritis, as distinct from the primary form, results from "something." This event either reduces the load-transmitting area or increases the total loading, or both. During unilateral stance the resultant R of the compressive forces (body weight and muscular forces producing equilibrium) passes through the center of gravity of the joint in the frontal plane (Fig. 14-6). Anything that moves the point of intersection of force R with the joint line is therefore the precursor of osteoarthritis. To obtain a balanced distribution of compressive stresses over the weight-bearing surfaces, the load R must be recentered, and osteotomy accomplishes this.

INDICATIONS FOR SURGERY

Osteoarthritis of the knee with a varus deformity is as subject to surgical correction as any osteoarthritic joint showing evident reduction of the load-transmitting area.

OSTEOARTHRITIS OF THE KNEE WITH VARUS DEFORMITY

If in the anteroposterior x-ray film, a dense triangle of bone is present subchondrally beneath the medial tibial plateau, and if in the film taken with the patient standing, there is sclerosis in the medial femoral condyle, it is clear that the resultant R has shifted medially, reducing the load-transmitting area. If no varus deformity is present at this time, it is

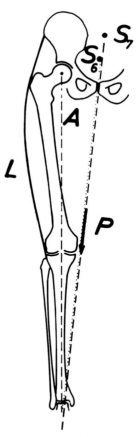

FIG. 14-6. Standing on one foot. S_6 is the center of gravity of the body. S_7 is the center of gravity of that part of the body supported by the knee. P is the line of body weight. L is the muscular stay balancing P. The resultant R will pass through the center of the knee. (After Maquet)

equally clear that one will develop. The load has to be recentered by an upper tibial osteotomy, and the degree of valgus to be obtained must be decided during preoperative biomechanical planning.

Preoperative Planning

A full-length frontal x-ray film, extending from the femoral head to the talus, is taken with the patient standing. A line is drawn from the center of the femoral head to the tibial tubercle. Another line is drawn from the

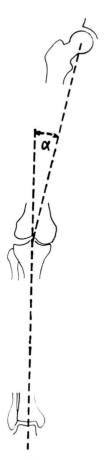

FIG. 14-7. Tracing of lines to show angle in a case of osteoarthritis with varus deformity. (After Maquet)

middle of the talus to intersect the first at the tubercle. This second line is prolonged upward for 5 cm to 6 cm. The angle between these lines is measured (Fig. 14-7). This is the basic angle used for correction, but to correct this angle alone would merely put the knee back to the state in which it was when the osteoarthritis developed originally. Often it is impossible to know whether the varus deformity demonstrated by angle α is primary or secondary, that is, whether it is the cause of the arthritis or the result of it. Therefore, the varus angle must be overcorrected, and it is wise to add between 3° and 5° of overcorrection to angle α; the smaller figure is used for the younger and stronger patient.

At this point fixed flexion deformity must be mentioned. In this deformity a smaller area of both femoral condyles are bearing weight on an equally reduced area of the tibial plateaux. No correction of a varus deformity of the knee can be effective in the presence of a fixed flexion deformity. This can be corrected at the same operation by a posterior capsulotomy carried out through lateral and medial incisions, but not by extending the osteotomy.

When the degree of correction has been determined (angle α + 3° to 5°), the local geometry of the knee level is drawn on tracing paper for reference during surgery.

Maquet Barrel-Vault Osteotomy

It is important that the operation be carried out without a tourniquet. Through an appropriate incision 1 cm of the fibula is resected from its middle third. The fibular vein and peroneal nerve must be avoided, and the wound is sutured over drainage. An incision 5 cm long is made centered over the tibial tuberosity. The patellar ligament is lifted and freed down to the most proximal point of its insertion into the tibial tubercle. The sickle guide is inserted as shown in Figure 14-8. Using a Kirschner wire, as many holes as possible are power-drilled through both tibial cortices, extending completely across the bone in a semicircular outline. The sickle is removed. Using the pin guide protractor set at angle α + 3° to 5°, a 5-mm Steinmann pin is inserted transversely across the tibia; its position will be indicated by the protractor (Fig. 14-9). The higher Steinmann pin is inserted above the marked osteotomy line at the angle dictated by the protractor and as close to the knee joint line as possible. Image-intensifier or radiographic control is necessary to determine the level of the upper pin and to verify the angle to be corrected.

Using a narrow osteotome, the multiple drill holes are connected. The osteotomy is now completed through both cortices, and the deformity is easily corrected manually. At this point the lower fragment of the tibia is pulled forward at the osteotomy line. This ensures

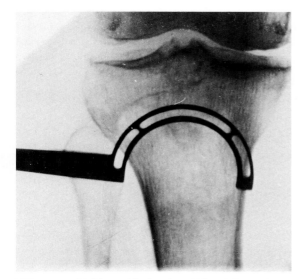

FIG. 14-8. Sickle guide in site. (After Maquet)

that the knee enjoys in addition all the advantages of a tibial tubercle anterior displacement, in that patellofemoral pressure is further reduced by up to 50%, and femorotibial pressure by 10%.

The Steinmann pins are clamped together using two A-O type compression devices. Because the protractor was set at angle $\alpha + 3°$ to 5°, when the Steinmann pins are made parallel and compressed, the original varus deformity is overcorrected by the predetermined amount. The wound is then sutured over drainage. Knee movement is encouraged at once. The patient is ambulatory, with partial weight-bearing for a few days. The Steinmann pins (they must be 5 mm in diameter with a 4 mm bend) are removed at 8 weeks, and crutches are abandoned as soon as possible.

The value of osteotomy to correct a varus deformity in patients with osteoarthritis of the knee is now generally accepted. The Maquet barrel-vault operation is the outward expression of the high biomechanical thinking and planning that has taken place previously. It is not just lining up the leg. It has been known for many years that careful preliminary planning, for instance, in the Pauwels intertrochanteric osteotomies, ensures a lasting result in the great majority of cases (Fig. 14-10).

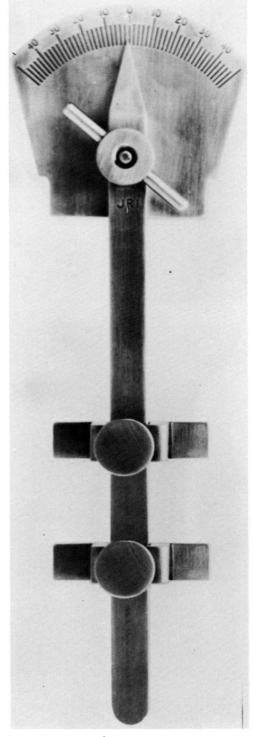

FIG. 14-9. Pin guide protractor.

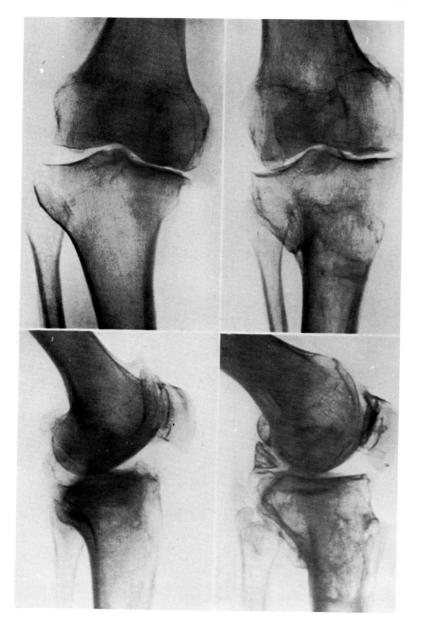

FIG. 14-10. X-ray films before and 5 years after correction of a varus deformity by barrel-vault osteotomy. (After Maquet)

Results

According to Maquet's published results, in 86 barrel-vault procedures, excellent results were obtained in 68, and good results were achieved in 9. These were cases in which overcorrection of the varus deformity was obtained and maintained. In addition, there were two cases with fair results, three with poor results, and one patient died. In three instances in which the original correction was lost, all had poor results—surely an endorsement of the operation.

OSTEOARTHRITIS WITH VALGUS DEFORMITY

In a valgus deformity accompanying osteoarthritis the line of action of load R lies laterally to the center of gravity of the weight-bearing surfaces. The origin of the valgus deformity that leads to osteoarthritis may be congenital, or it may be the result of some disequilibrium at the hip, for example, a hip ankylosed in adduction. Furthermore, if the disorder of equilibrium at the hip requires an augmented abductor muscular effort, the tensor fascia lata, being a bi-articular muscle, has the effect of increasing the power of the lateral muscular stay L. The result, in conformity with the parallelogram of forces, is a lateral shift of resultant R to the external plateau of the tibia. A localized increase of pressure takes place (Fig. 14-11), and a cup-shaped subchondral area of dense bone forms under the lateral plateau. Pauwel's theories are fulfilled, and osteoarthritis develops.

Once the osteoarthritic process occurs in the lateral compartment of the knee and valgus deformity is present, the resultant R must be recentered. It is now generally accepted that correction of a valgus deformity at the knee is best achieved by a low femoral osteotomy through the condyles. The imprecise wedge osteotomies without geometry are not advised for the same reason that caused the barrel-vault osteotomy to replace them in tibial corrections—because they are imprecise.

Preoperative Planning of Osteotomy Through the Lower End of the Femur

A full-length, standing x-ray film is taken, the two axes are drawn, and the degree of valgus deformity is accurately measured. At this point careful planning is necessary. If the deformity (and most are) is due to hyperactivity of the lateral muscular stay L, the valgus angle must be overcorrected by between 2° and 3°, because the same force will continue to operate after correction. If the osteoarthritis is the result of local causes—as, for instance, previous removal of the external meniscus—theoretically, a simple correction of the angle is all that is required. Unnecessary overcorrection should be avoided since it is unscientific and because if a varus deformity is produced, the length of the lever arm of body weight P is in-

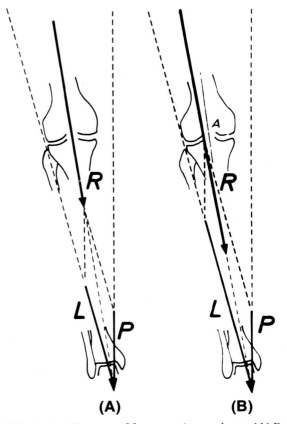

FIG. 14-11. Diagram of forces acting on knee. **(A)** P is body weight. L is lateral stay (i.e., tensor fasciae latae). R is resultant (vectorial). **(B)** If L is increased to maintain equilibrium at hip (to avoid a Trendelenburg gait), R is inevitably shifted laterally so that it no longer passes through the center of the knee. (After Maquet)

creased at the knee. This obviously should be avoided because it can lead to osteoarthritis of the medial compartment.

When the degree of overcorrection has been decided, that is, angle α + 1° to 3°, the preoperative drawing is made. The x-ray film of the knee is traced on paper, and the position and direction of the osteotomy line through the metaphysis is indicated. The position of the two central Steinmann pins is also indicated—they lie divergent from each other by the angle of overcorrection required, open medially.

Technique Lower Femoral Osteotomy

A 5-cm incision is made longitudinally over the medial femoral condyle between the vastus internus muscle and the hamstring group to give access to the femur at the step between the condyle and the metaphysis— that is, the adductor tubercle. Using the protractor, two 5-mm Steinmann pins are drilled across the condyle parallel to each other and to the articular surface of the femur. The pin-inserting protractor is set at the correct angle of overcorrection ($\alpha + 1°$ to $3°$). The two upper Steinmann pins are now drilled across the diaphysis in accordance with the device. The osteotomy (Fig. 14-12) is now carried out, and the line is made parallel to the lower Steinmann pins. It is completed up to but not through the lateral cortex. The lower edge of the proximal fragment is nibbled off, because this makes it easier for the bone to sink into the cancellous bone of the condyle. The four Steinmann pins are now made parallel and are clamped under compression with an A-O clamp on each side. The whole assembly is checked by radiographs. The wound is sutured over drainage. The patient is mobilized within a few days, and walking using two crutches with partial weight-bearing is encouraged from the first. The advantages of not using external fixation either in this or in the barrel-vault osteotomy are manifest. The pins are removed 8 weeks later when radiography confirms that union is sound.

Good results are predictable and occur if resultant R is recentered so that it passes through or a little beyond the center of gravity of the tibial plateaus, thereby ensuring the use of the maximum weight-transmitting area— that is, the normal anatomic area (Fig. 14-13).

Results

Excellent and good results can be obtained with a valgus deformity by performing a high tibial osteotomy. This osteotomy is not recommended when a correction of greater than 15° is required. However, in 21 knees excellent or good results were obtained in 13 cases, fair results in 1 case, and poor results in 4 cases. Three patients had died at the time of follow-up. On the other hand, results in those patients with a valgus deformity who were treated by a low femoral osteotomy (these included patients with a greater or lesser deformity), were only marginally better. In a series of 20 low femoral osteotomies 14 had excellent or good results. The difficulties of the surgery and the greater chances of complications inherent in correcting a valgus deformity with previous techniques are reflected in the results.

PATELLOFEMORAL OSTEOARTHRITIS

Not all aspects of patellofemoral osteoarthritis are clear. Adolescent chondromalacia patellae can be a troublesome entity. When the patella is centrally placed in the femoral groove, the condition is evidently the consequence of cartilaginous inadequacy for the loading stress (often, but not always, athletic) placed upon it. Usually the condition is self-limiting, although it may merge imperceptibly into patellofemoral mechanical arthritis. Strictly, an entity of this nature with a centrally placed patella should be classified as primary osteoarthritis because it is clear that chondromalacia and patellofemoral osteoarthritis must have a similar etiology.

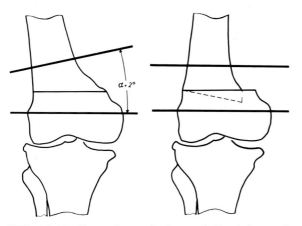

FIG. 14-12. Operative technique of distal femoral osteotomy. Only the two central pins are shown. (After Maquet)

FIG. 14-13. 58-year-old patient before and 5 years after over-correction of a valgus deformity. (After Maquet)

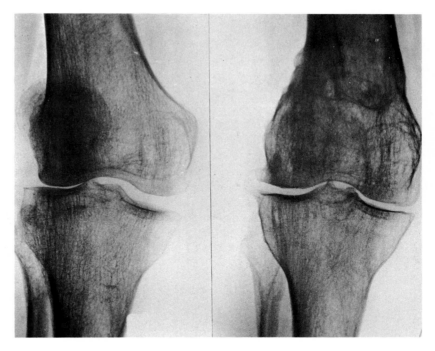

FIG. 14-14. (A) Flexed knee. **(B)** Extended knee. **(C)** Extension following osteotomy.

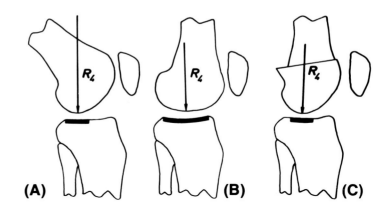

(A)   (B)   (C)

More often in patellofemoral osteoarthritis the patella lies laterally in the femoral groove; because the load-transmitting area is reduced, it is a secondary osteoarthritis. It is a persistent subluxation and therefore a minor stage of recurrent dislocation of the patella.

Indications for Surgery

Surgery is indicated when a tangential patellar x-ray film shows subchondral density be-neath the lateral facets of the patella and diminution of the lateral joint interspace, thus demonstrating mechanical arthritis that is the result of reduced load-transmission area.

The Operation

Merely to recenter the patella in the femoral groove is insufficient. The tibial tubercle should be elevated to reduce the load on the femorotibial joint and also on the patellofemoral joint generally. However, the tibial tubercle should also be displaced medially to equalize the load.

THE PLACE OF OSTEOTOMY IN THE TREATMENT OF DEFORMITIES RESULTING FROM RHEUMATOID ARTHRITIS

Only when rheumatoid disease is no longer active does osteotomy have any part to play. If a useful range of movement remains and full functional enjoyment is hampered by a correctible deformity, osteotomy should be considered. Within this framework the preoperative planning and the operation itself are similar to those for osteoarthritis.

If there is a fixed flexion deformity following rheumatoid arthritis that hampers activity, it is better corrected. This correction should, however, be carried out by posterior capsulotomy rather than by a lower femoral osteotomy. As the knee flexes from the fully extended position, the weight-transmitting area is rapidly reduced. After a lower femoral osteotomy, the knee remains flexed as previously, although the leg is straight; that is, the weight-transmitting area remains reduced. This state encourages the development of osteoarthritis in a previously rheumatoid joint (Fig. 14-14). Posterior capsulotomy should be carried out in such instances, thereby increasing the load-transmitting area.

CHAPTER 15
THE CLINICAL BIOMECHANICS OF THE HELICOID KNEE PROSTHESIS

Arthur J. Helfet

The evolution and nature of the helical system of joints of the leg are discussed in Chapter 5. Based on the premise that the helical movement of the knee is inherently stable while under the active control of the muscles of the thigh, a helicoid brace has been developed. By doing no more than keeping the tibia in its normal track on the femur during flexion and extension of the knee, it has proved successful in permitting participation in sports after ligamentous injury and in allowing many patients with osteoarthritis of the knee to recover comfortable function.

A prosthetic implant must maintain the same helical motion if it is to be stable. If designed to conform to the demands of the muscles of the thigh, it will simulate the function of the normal knee in stability and in range of movement. The main problem with most implantable knee prostheses is that they do not conform to the movement of the normal knee; instead, the knee has to follow the unnatural

shape of the prosthesis with unnecessary mechanical stress on the knee and implanted prosthesis.

The development of knee endoprosthesis design is admirably described by Peter Walker in the next chapter. He discusses the problems that each type has endeavoured to solve, including materials, movement, stability, wear, loosening, and so on.

If the knee of a person with a *hinged or straight-path unhinged prosthesis twists or turns or bends and straightens without rotation,* the movement is resisted by the mechanical design, thus creating a stress either at the interface of bone and bone cement, or that is transmitted to the implant as metal or plastic fatigue. The abnormal movement, moreover, usually results in pain. These malfactors could be obviated if the replacement unit achieved anatomic or near-anatomic movement—that is, synchronous rotation with flexion and extension.

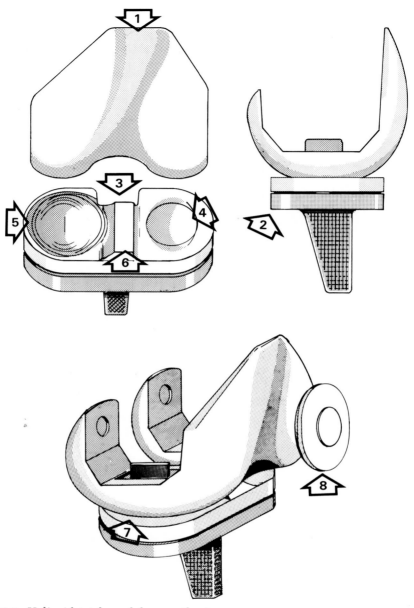

FIG. 15-1. Helicoid total condylar prosthesis.

(1) The trochlear surface of the femoral component is tracked to allow synchronous movement of the patella.

(2) A metal tray for the tibial component spreads compressive load bearing.

(3) A gap for the posterior cruciate ligament.

(4 and 5) The lateral **(4)** and medial **(5)** facets differ to allow the medial to rotate on the lateral.

(6) A central eminence contributes to medial-lateral stability.

(7) The tibial component is slightly wider than the femoral to permit transfer of semitendinosis or a strip of the iliotibial band when necessary.

(8) A plastic button to surface the patella.

212

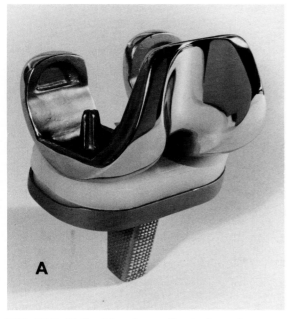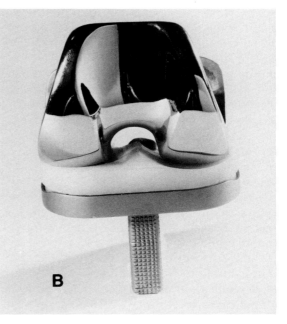

FIG. 15-2. Helicoid endoprosthesis, two views.

The new helicoid design (Figs. 15-1 and 15-2) is unhinged and allows rotation and also flexion, extension, and lateral movement, plus lateral tilt, but only as dictated by the voluntary muscles in control of its movements. The design of the prosthesis does no more than facilitate this movement, which occurs without abnormal tensions.

The lead to the new prosthesis was the realization that the femur and tibia in concert in any phase of voluntary movement must follow a definite track, that is, the muscles acting on the knee joint will insist on helical excursion of the knee joint, and as long as the tibia is firmly on this track, the knee joint is stable and without tension in any position of flexion or extension. The muscles acting on the joint constitute the main control, with the capsular ligaments as subsidiary check straps.

Any factor that upsets this balance, either extrinsic, as in applied force from outside, or intrinsic, as in a displaced meniscus or an implant that does not permit this normal pattern of movement, will produce derangement which will cause either instability or blocked movement. The *blocked movement* arises

from a conflict between the direction of muscle action and the displaced or deformed or misjudged inherent design structure of the implant. This is a frequent reason for failure of knee prostheses, for the recurrent impact at approximately 90° leads to loosening of the prosthesis and instability of the joint.

A second reason for the failure that is common to all prostheses is incorrect insertion.

Most previous prostheses do not lend themselves to the natural excursion of the joint and therefore suffer unnecessary mechanical stresses as described above.

The new helicoid version of the knee prosthesis incorporates all the features found advantageous. It is a total condylar device designed for stability and maximum movement of near normal character. Because movement is helicoid the tibial component need not be raised in front to prevent anterior subluxation. Instead, a central eminence prevents excessive rotation.

Provision is made for retaining the posterior cruciate ligament should it be present. Semitendinosus or iliotibial band transfer, as appropriate, is recommended for lateral instability, the tibial component being slightly wider then the femoral to allow for this.

The trochlear surface of the femoral component is tracked obliquely to encourage synchrony of patellar and tibial movement during helical excursion. This aspect of the design should add stability to the joint and prevent the development of retropatellar pain.

A metal tray for the tibial component spreads compressive load-bearing over a wider area of the trabecular surface of the upper tibia.

It is expected that the helicoid design will ensure an improved range of flexion with less tension. The posterior slope of the tibial component adds 5° or more.

The ideal unit, therefore, while unprogrammed, should simulate in as many aspects as possible the natural joint. These may be summarized as follows:

1. The centers of rotation of the knee should not change materially. The prosthesis should replace all movement of the knee joint but not necessarily the anatomic patterns of changing centers of rotation.
2. The main muscle groups and ligaments should be retained in their original positions and intact.
3. Minimum bone should be removed.
4. During insertion it should be possible to correct abnormalities, such as valgus and varus.
5. A metal tray for the plastic tibial component spreads compressive load-bearing over a wider area of the cut upper tibia, thus protecting the trabecular bone surface.
6. The design should facilitate the normal synchrony of movement.
7. As in the original limb, the movement of the prosthesis should be in sinuous adaptation with the joints above and below. Otherwise, friction, limitation of range and movement, and eventual loosening of the prosthesis will ensue. In all, the knee joint should have a flexion–extension range of between 130° and 135° synchronised with 15° to 20° of rotation; but I repeat that these movements must be synchronous and must occur only on muscle demand and not because of the structure of the implant.

8. As long as the collateral ligaments are intact, loss of the cruciate ligaments would not necessarily result in instability. Disruption of the lateral ligaments as well, however, would lead to the same marked instability that occurs after injury in the normal knee. But although stable collaterals are necessary, the patient's ligaments are not indispensable. They can be replaced quite simply and dynamically by using the tendon of the semitendinosus hooked into the femoral condyle on the inner side of the biceps or a strip of iliotibial band on the lateral side. (See Chap. 15.)

The function of the cruciates is not clear. I believe they act as guide ropes and not as check straps. (See Chap. 1.) It is known that with stable lateral ligaments we can do without at least the anterior cruciate. The importance of the posterior cruciate has not been proved one way or the other, and therefore, if the design of the implant, aided by the capsular ligaments, is sufficient to maintain a stable excursion of the joint, retaining the cruciates is not essential. In this prosthesis design a gap in the surface of the tibia may be used for knees in which the posterior cruciate has survived.

9. It should allow retention or replacement of the patella. The patella is necessary to ensure the additional stability of the knee joint. This is achieved when the patella, moving in the trochlear groove on the femoral component, maintains its excursion synchronously with the rotation of the tibia on the femur. Normally, as the knee straightens, the patella moves from the lateral edge of the medial condyle of the femur in helical fashion upward and outward into the tensionless comfort of the trochlear groove. A hinge-joint implant would not permit this kind of movement. The patella would move straight up and down, leading to irritation of the surfaces and eventual erosion of the articular carti-

lage of the patella and femoral condyle. Most implants of the hinge type develop the complication of retropatellar pain. The trochlear groove of the new implant allows for normal synchronous excursion of the patella, and retropatellar pain should not develop.

Whether or not the patellar surface or the trochlear groove is found to be eroded or irregular, the insertion of a plastic button for the surface of the patella (Fig. 15-1) should be considered whenever a tricompartmental replacement is used. It is unlikely that the shapes of the articular surface of the patella and a replacement trochlear groove or vice versa will fit exactly. Erosion of the normal surface is likely and eventually retropatellar pain.

The factor producing the greatest stress on the joint is unnatural movement. A prosthesis that conforms to anatomic function need not be as strong physically as a hinge or straight-path prosthesis. When sinuous synchronous movement is achieved, potential lateral instability is of secondary importance because it would produce, at most, increased wear on the prosthesis. But nonsynchronous movement and consequent recurrent impact and friction produces failure due to fracturing or metal fatigue or cement-bone failures that are infinitely worse. It is calculated that with this new prosthesis, loads are distributed more evenly to the muscle and ligament groups that constrain the knee from deviating from the normal pattern; therefore, transmitted loads to the prosthesis are less.

The common methods of injury produce, instead of fracture or metal fatigue or cement-bone failure, a muscle or ligament injury as in the normal knee, or in more severe injury, the prosthesis will be part of a dislocation of the whole joint.

THE PROSTHESIS

This implant replaces the three compartments of the knee. The radii of the medial and lateral facets on the tibial component differ so that the medial may rotate on the lateral. A central eminence contributes to medial-lateral and rotational stability. The trochlear surface of the femoral component has a groove running from below upward and laterally for the normal excursion of the patella, whose surface is embellished by a plastic button. The jigs are designed to cut a posterior slope on the upper surface of the tibia to increase the range of flexion. Separate models are required for the right and left knees.

The "triple deformity" that may be present in the rheumatoid knee presents an added problem. As noted previously, internal derangement leads to fixed medial rotation and flexion of the tibia on the femur. The medial femoral condyle protrudes over the edge of the tibia. Spasm of the iliotibial band acting on the flexed rheumatoid knee acts as a posterior retractor of the lateral tibia, so that both condyles of the femur protrude anteriorly. Movement of the tibia on the femur now takes place by angulation without glide.

To mobilize the knee to facilitate insertion of the prosthesis, it is necessary to divide the iliotibial band and to excise the adherent meniscus, or both menisci, and any adhesions that obstruct rotation. It is then possible to restore alignment by pushing the upper end of the tibia forward and derotating and extending the joint.

CHAPTER 16
THE BIOMECHANICS OF KNEE PROSTHESES*

Peter S. Walker

There are numerous designs of artificial knee joints available to the orthopaedic surgeon. Many of these designs are so similar that a number of specific types or classes can be identified. These types are aimed at dealing with particular pathologies, or they reflect different philosophies about what functions the prosthesis should perform. In addition to devices for primary cases, there is a growing demand for special or custom-made designs to revise failures of a previous implant.

The principles behind any design must be tested by the criteria of analysis and clinical performance. The latter, however, also depends upon the instrumentation and the technical skill of the surgeon. The alignment and spacing of the components will have an effect on the force distribution, stability, and motion. When cement is used for fixation, the durability of the cement-bone and cement-implant interfaces will depend on the proper-

ties of the cement and on the technique. The biologic reaction to the implant and the regenerative abilities of atrophied tissues are still largely unpredictable. Accurate follow-up methods are thus needed to test the validity of the devices.

Hence, a complete approach to artificial knee joints should include all aspects of the design, surgical technique, and follow-up. This chapter will concentrate mainly on the design aspects.

EVOLUTION OF KNEE PROSTHESES

Before discussing the biomechanical aspects of today's prostheses, it will be useful to study their evolution[18] (Fig. 16-1). Among the first designs were metallic surfaces for the femur or for the upper tibia, such as those designed by Virgin and Carroll (1941) and by Townley. The center-board insert of Smith-Peterson and Aufranc (1940), was an attempt to extend the principle of mold arthroplasty to the knee. All

* Howmedica, Inc., is thanked for permission to publish this chapter. The illustrations are by Mr. Bill Thackeray.

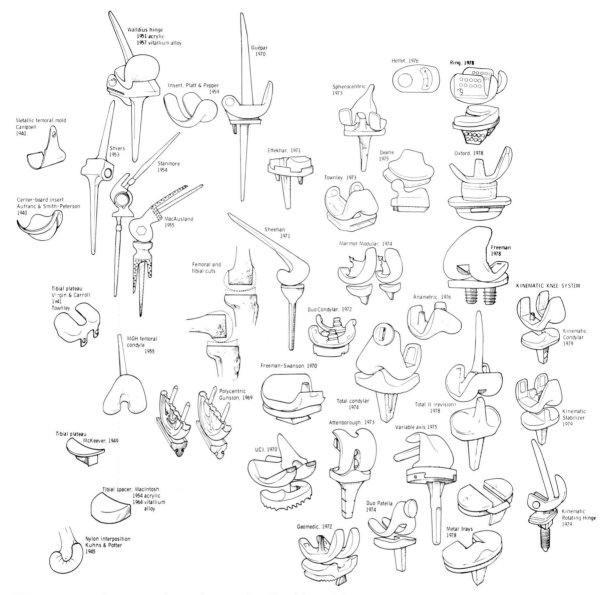

FIG. 16-1. Key designs in the evolution of artificial knee joints.

these devices were limited in application and gave variable results. Kuhns and Potter (1945) tried interposition using a nylon stockinette around the lower end of the femur, but this failed owing to tearing and shredding. Unicondylar tibial plateaus of different heights were designed by McKeever in 1949 for the correction of varus or valgus deformity. The MacIntosh plateaus, introduced later, were widely used up to the early 1970s. They were more successful in rheumatoid arthritis than in osteoarthritis, for which osteotomy was the treatment of choice.

In the early 1950s, various hinges were introduced. The Walldius (1951) was made in acrylic, a material in vogue at the time, and was not changed to Vitallium alloy until about 1957. The stainless steel hinge of Shiers, without a patellar flange, was introduced in 1953. These hinges and others like them were intended for severe cases but required large bone resection and gave unpredictable results. There were many cases of excessive settling, and infection was a problem with sometimes serious consequences. A classic custom hinge of this period was used on a tumor patient at Stanmore. It was actually bolted to the bones and has withstood over two decades of usage.

Two other hemiarthroplasties were used in the mid to late 1950s—the MGH femoral condyle and the Platt-Peppler knee insert. The former was closely anatomical and had an intramedullary stem. When inserted accurately successful long-term results were often obtained. The Platt-Peppler device was more geometrical in shape for ease of manufacture but fared poorly because it blocked motion.

Thus until the late 1950s, the available treatments for arthritis were osteotomy, particularly for varus osteoarthritis; MacIntosh tibial plateaus, particularly for valgus rheumatoid arthritis; and the Walldius or Shiers hinge for severe cases. It was inevitable that, following Charnley's striking results with the metal-polyethylene-acrylic cement combination in the hip, a knee would be developed using the same system. This was accomplished in 1969 by Gunston who worked with Charnley at Wrightington. The concepts involved were to replace only the femorotibial load-bearing surfaces, to embed the components in slots for fixation, and to allow laxity for polycentric motion. This design was called the Gunston, or the Polycentric.

Within the next 2 to 3 years, several variations were designed, each with different principles. Eftekhar enclosed the polycentric components in metallic trays with intramedullary stems for enhanced fixation. The Geometric was much more conforming, gave uni-axial motion, and was intended to cope with mild to severe cases. The Freeman-Swanson used components of a large surface area to maximize fixation, cylindrical bearing surfaces for

simplicity, and low stresses on the plastic, and introduced the idea of cruciate ligament sacrifice. Also, the use of square bone cuts and the application of tension to obtain collateral ligament balance were important advances. The cuts were made in sequence with special spacers to create a gap in both extension and flexion equal to the thickness of the prosthesis. The approach in the design of the Duocondylar was to approximate normal anatomy and function; it used a bicondylar femoral component and separate flat (except for the tibial spines) plastic tibial plateaus. The UCI was somewhat similar but used a one-piece plastic component with a circular track to allow freedom of rotation. An entirely modular design enjoyed widespread use based on the ease of surgery and the satisfactory early results.

This group of devices, the "first generation," had a number of problems. Loosening occurred after a few years, particularly in the constrained designs such as the Geometric, or in those with low surface area and high flexibility such as the modular tibials. Patellofemoral pain occurred frequently, either from the beginning or after a time lapse. Recurrence of deformity could occur, sometimes associated with inadequate instrumentation and technique. The average range of motion in the more constrained designs was about 90°, and in the unconstrained it was about 105°.

Townley's design was probably the first to deal with the patellofemoral problem by adding a patellar flange. The Duopatella was evolved from the Duocondylar, still preserving the cruciates and using a plastic patellar button. The Total Condylar replaced all surfaces including that of the patella. The cruciates were sacrificed, and the bone cuts and technique were derived from the Freeman-Swanson concept. The plastic tibial component was one piece with a stout central peg for enhanced fixation. The femorotibial surfaces were partially conforming to give stability with laxity. The Duopatella, as well as several other prostheses introduced recently, added a similar central-peg tibial component but with a cutout for posterior cruciate retention.

This group of prostheses, the "second generation," were great improvements upon the earlier models, reducing the frequency of problems or retarding their occurrence. Although there are a number of other interesting ideas undergoing trials today, the majority of prostheses in current use are of this second generation. They consist of a femoral component with a patellar flange, a plastic patellar button, a one-piece tibial component with a central peg, partially conforming bearing surfaces, and a cutout for posterior cruciate retention or no retention at all. Two problems today are whether to retain the posterior cruciate and whether a metal tray is an improvement in fixation over the all-plastic component. These issues will be discussed later in this chapter.

The problem of anterior subluxation was recognized as a drawback with the posterior cruciate sacrificing types such as the Total Condylar. This problem has recently been countered in two ways—by increasing the height of the anterior tibial component and by adding intercondylar stops or guiding surfaces, such as in the Kinematic Stabilizer. The overall problem of achieving sufficient stability while allowing laxity and a full range of motion was addressed in Helfet's helicoid design.

There were a number of advances in the linked designs for treating severe cases. The Guépar (1970) was intended to be used with cement and was more acceptable in shape and size than the Walldius. The Attenborough and the Spherocentric were intercondylar lax hinges, which allowed some rotatory freedom and avoided long intramedullary stems. Accurate alignment was necessary to avoid loosening. The Sheehan hinge allowed laxity but needed collateral ligaments for varus-valgus support. The Stabilo-Condylar was later modified to produce the Total II, an unlinked intercondylar "hinge." Custom long-stem versions of some of these have been made to deal with the growing need to revise previous failures.

I have recently designed the Kinematic Knee System, a group of devices intended to deal with various knee problems. The System comprises a condylar replacement with provision for the retention of either the posterior, or both anterior and posterior cruciate ligaments; a stabilized, noncruciate design for patients in whom the cruciates cannot be preserved; and a rotating hinge for severe and revision cases.

The Oxford knee is a design departure that attempts to obtain low stress on the plastic tibial surfaces by close conformity with the femoral condyles but without compromising freedom of motion and compatibility with the cruciate ligaments. The plastic pieces are wedge-shaped discs that are free to slide back and forth on metal surfaces on the top of the tibia. Current clinical experiments with noncemented designs include the Kodama-Yamamoto, the Freeman, and the Ring.

Undoubtedly, the evolutionary process in knee prostheses will continue for many years to come.

CONCEPT OF THE NORMAL KNEE—FUNCTIONAL ELEMENTS

The normal knee is required to bend to one and a half right angles and to carry external forces and moments either statically or dynamically. An ideal knee prosthesis would allow the knee to do the same, taking of course the age and general condition of the patient into account. The approach to prosthesis design expounded in this chapter is to specify the functional requirements (e.g., load-bearing, motion) of the knee, to identify the functional elements that perform those functions, to determine which elements are damaged, and then to design the prosthesis to replace those elements. This does not imply that the elements are replaced anatomically; for example, varus-valgus stability, normally borne by the collateral structures, can be replaced by a hinge with intramedullary stems.

NORMAL KNEE FUNCTION

Motion may be linear or rotational. The linear motions are anterior-posterior, medial-lateral, and distraction-compression; rotational motions are flexion-extension, internal-external, and varus-valgus.

In the normal knee joint, the anteroposterior laxity (or drawer) is about 4 mm to 8 mm, the lower value being with the knee in extension. The laxity is reduced under load-bearing to approximately half these values, depending on the loads acting and the constraints against other motions such as transverse rotation while the anteroposterior test is being carried out.[5] The medial-lateral motion is only a few millimeters and is also reduced on load-bearing.

The varus-valgus motion varies in a similar way with angle of flexion and with external loads. In walking, the angular range has been measured at about 5°,[13] which is similar to that measured passively (around 7°).[5]

In the unloaded flexed knee, there is considerable rotational laxity of the femur about the long axis of the tibia, amounting to 20° to 30°. However, as the knee is brought up from flexion to full extension even under light loads, there is a continuous internal rotation of the femur, particularly in the last few degrees of extension.[2,18] Such a motion pattern has been found to occur in walking and in other activities, the range in walking being about 10°.[13] This synchrony of transverse rotation with flexion is apparently due to the relative geometry of the femoral and tibial surfaces and is particularly apparent at the terminal external rotation of the tibia, the so-called screw-home motion. The cruciate ligaments are not primary guides to this motion; Blacharski and associates found no significant change in motion after they were cut. The muscles are likely to play a part in guiding this motion and to be in harmony with the joint surfaces. In extending the knee, the quadriceps have a force component that externally rotates the tibia; in flexion the semitendinosus, semimembranosus, and popliteus internally rotate the tibia. The muscle actions are clearly complex, however, and their description requires considerations of electromyography and muscle mechanics that are beyond the scope of this chapter.

The principal motion of the knee is, of course, flexion-extension. The normal range

of flexion in men is 0° to 143° and varies little with age.[3] In level walking, the knee flexes to 60° in the swing phase, while in sitting and rising and in ascending and descending stairs, flexion is 80° to 90°. The range beyond 90° is used for rising from a low sitting position, kneeling, crouching, and so on.

To summarize, the principal motion is flexion-extension, while the other linear and rotational motions depend on the following factors:

The angle of flexion

The compressive load across the joint down the tibial axis

The applied shear forces and rotational moments

This is explained in the laxity curves shown in Figure 16-2. Assume that with the knee at a particular angle of flexion, a push and pull drawer force is applied to the tibia. The knee is lax in the midregion of its motion but tightens at each extreme. If a compressive force is initially applied down the tibial axis, the laxity is reduced.

The forces and moments acting on the knee in different activities can be expressed in relation to axes set in the tibia (Fig. 16-3).

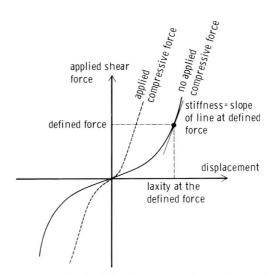

FIG. 16-2. Typical laxity curves for a knee, depicted for anteroposterior drawer.

F_x = anterior or posterior force
F_y = medial or lateral force
F_z = compressive or distractive force
M_x = varus or valgus moment
M_y = internal or external rotational torque
M_z = flexion or extension moment

All of M_z will be carried by muscle forces, except at the extremes of motion when pas-sive soft structures are operative. All of the other forces and moments will be carried by muscles and by passive soft tissues. The original studies of Morrison[7,8] provided values for some of these forces in different activities. The peak compressive forces at heel strike and toe-off averaged three times body weight for level walking, with the average center of pressure disposed 10 mm to 15 mm to the medial side, with a medial to lateral force ratio of up to about 2:1. This is consistent with the larger area and the stronger bone of the medial side. Further determinations for various activities, where antagonistic muscle activity was accounted for, were carried out by Seireg and Arvikar.[11] Force values for rising from a chair were determined by Seedhom and Terayama.[10]

Approximate maximum values of the forces and moments determined by these investigators for different activities are shown in Figure 16-4. The forces are shown acting on the tibia; for example, the anterior force of 0.2 times body weight (Morrison) would be resisted by the anterior cruciate ligament. The anterior and posterior shearing forces were described by Morrison as "ligament forces."

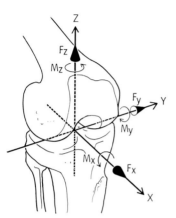

FIG. 16-3. Axes fixed with respect to the tibia, and the different components of force and moment.

FORCES AND MOMENTS ACTING ON THE TIBIA

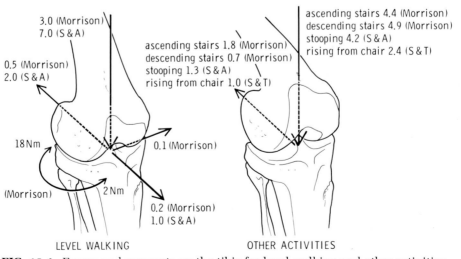

FIG. 16-4. Forces and moments on the tibia for level walking and other activities. ("S & A" refers to Seireg and Arvikar; "S & T" refers to Seedhom and Terayama [see references].)

Several observations can be made from this data. The predominant force component is compressive, reaching several times body weight in everyday activities, and has a changing medial-to-lateral distribution. The shearing force pulling the tibia backward is significant because it is up to twice body weight, due partly to the action of the hamstrings. This implies the importance of the posterior cruciate ligament. The shear force in the other direction appears to be less in magnitude and frequency. The medial-lateral shear forces are relatively small. The varus-valgus moments will normally be carried by appropriate distribution of the forces on the medial and lateral condyles and by the collateral ligaments and muscles when the point of overbalance is reached. Torques about the tibial axis are significant, particularly those that rotate the tibia externally. Such torques will be carried by a combination of structures, including the geometry of the condylar surfaces, the cruciate ligaments (particularly in internal rotation of the tibia), the medial collateral ligament, the posterior oblique ligaments, and the patella-tendon combination.

Thus, the concept of *functional elements* is introduced, whereby different structural elements act to resist the various forces and moments. In the arthritic knee, some of the functional elements are damaged. The purpose of the prosthesis, then, is to replace only those elements that are damaged. The five major elements are listed as follows:

1. Compressive forces down the axis of the tibia—resisted by the condylar surfaces and menisci
2. Anteroposterior shearing forces on the tibia—resisted by the cruciate ligaments and surface geometry
3. Varus-valgus moments—resisted by the collateral ligaments
4. Rotational moments—resisted by several structures
5. Medial-lateral forces—resisted by the tibial spines

The first three of these elements are illustrated in Figure 16-5.

BIOMECHANICAL ASPECTS

The following discussion is concerned mainly but not exclusively with the standard condylar replacement type of knee prosthesis. The first three functional elements will now be discussed.

FIG. 16-5. Three functional elements of the knee. A prosthesis should replace the deficient elements.

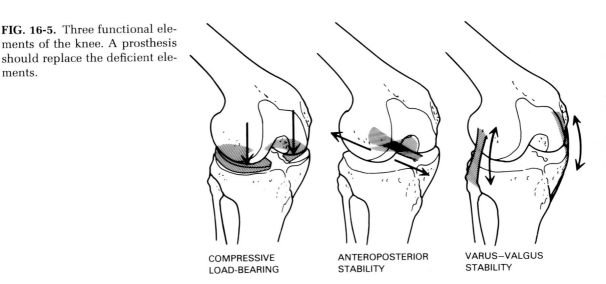

COMPRESSIVE
LOAD-BEARING

ANTEROPOSTERIOR
STABILITY

VARUS–VALGUS
STABILITY

COMPRESSIVE LOAD-BEARING ELEMENTS

In a prosthesis, the aim should be to transmit the compressive forces to the bone over the areas used in the normal knee, avoiding excessively high or low contact stress. In partially conforming devices, where the contact is localized, the load can be spread to the bone over a wide area by using the more rigid materials such as metal.

The use of plastic on the femoral side requires thick pieces unless they are slotted into the bone as in the Polycentric prosthesis. However, assuming metal runners, they should cover all of the femoral condyles to maximize use of the trabecular bone. Rocking of the component in the sagittal plane is reduced by a patellar flange and by pegs entering the condyles or the lower medullary canal. Undesirable shear and tensile stresses can be avoided by attention to the fit on the bone and cement technique (Fig. 16-6). Joining of the medial and lateral sides prevents rocking of the individual runners but causes tilting in extreme varus or valgus loading. However, particularly with the presence of a patellar flange, a one-piece femoral component is, on the whole, an advantage for surgical simplicity and alignment. The same reasons justify making square cuts on the bone, even if the cut surfaces are not perpendicular to the trabeculae.

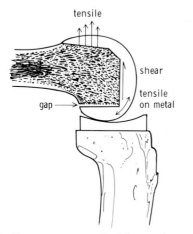

FIG. 16-6. Stresses on a typical femoral component which are increased by lack of support posteriorly.

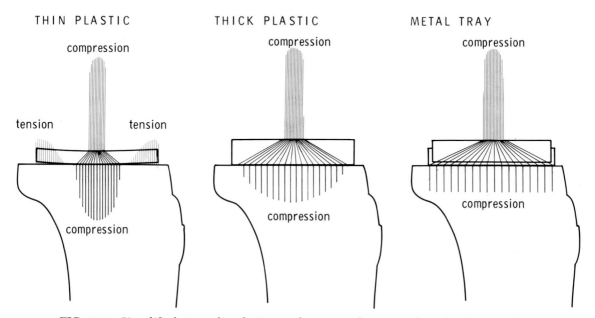

FIG. 16-7. Simplified stress distribution at the cement-bone interfaces for three configurations of tibial component. A "point contact" situation on the upper surface is assumed.

FIG. 16-8. The effect of a cemented central-peg type of tibial component on the strains on the proximal outer surface of the bone. The ratios are relative to the intact knee.

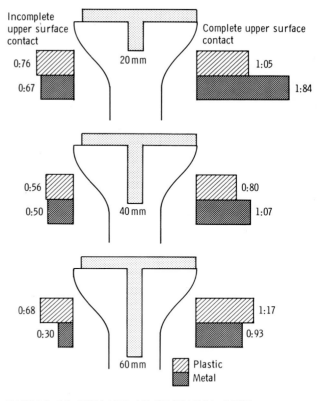

RATIOS OF STRAINS IN PROXIMAL BONE
COMPONENT INSERTED: NORMAL KNEE
DIRECT COMPRESSION
AVERAGE OF 4 BONES, LEVEL 1

Partial conformity of the metal-plastic surfaces results in localized contact areas. The contact stresses on the surface should be dissipated to avoid stress concentrations on the underlying bone. Figure 16-7 shows three cases. With thin plastic, the stresses are poorly distributed, causing high compressive stresses under the load and tensile stresses at the sides. Thickening the plastic relieves this situation to some degree. However, the addition of a metal tray can spread the load almost evenly over the entire area. The actual distribution will depend upon the stiffness pattern of the trabecular bone.

Experiments were carried out[9] to determine in more detail the effects of tibial components on load transfer. Strain gauges were attached around the tibia 10 mm below the upper sur-

face. The strains were measured for compressive loads on the intact knee and then again after tibial components were cemented in place. The components required 5 mm of bone to be cut. The central peg type of component was used. The variables were the length of the central peg, all-plastic or a metal tray, and complete versus incomplete upper surface contact. The ratios of strains after component insertion, to the strains of the intact knee, were calculated. The results for one knee specimen are shown in Figure 16-8.

Incomplete upper surface contact bypassed the peripheral bone, leaving much lower strains than normal. This could lead to long-term atrophy, which would weaken the soft tissue attachments. Complete upper surface contact restored normal or even higher strain

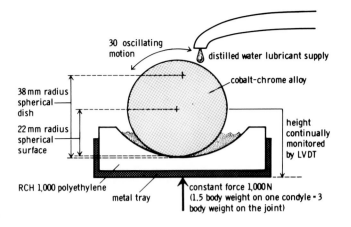

FIG. 16-9. The experimental arrangement for measuring wear and deformation in a "partially conforming" bearing.

with a metal tray. The central peg did not seem to bypass the load, except for the 60-mm-long metal peg. In this case, the cortex was being reached. The plastic would be too soft axially to give such load bypassing. The long metal pegs would be chosen if cortical load transfer was required in cases of serious proximal bone deficiency.

Deformation and Wear

Wear is affected by many factors including contact stress. The less conforming the femorotibial surfaces, the smaller the area of contact and the higher the contact stresses on the plastic. There are several basic types of wear. Adhesive wear is material removed at small adhesive points between the sliding surfaces. Abrasive wear results from a hard material cutting microasperities in a softer. If hard loose particles intervene, this produces three body abrasive wear. Finally, if the stresses are high and there is oscillating load or motion, fatigue wear can occur, releasing large fragments or sheets. All these types of wear have been observed in removed knee prostheses.[18] However, fatigue wear is of particular significance in knees.

Wear tests have been carried out specifically to study the high-stress conditions. A geometry was chosen to represent a typical conforming knee in flexion (Fig. 16-9). The variable chosen was the thickness of the plastic

(RCH-1000). The significance was that when plastic is backed by metal, the thinner the plastic, the higher the contact stress because the femoral condyle "feels" the metal tray. The depth of penetration (wear plus deformation) was found to increase with the number of cycles as expected, but the rate was greater as the plastic became thinner.

The thicknesses of plastic were 2 mm, 3 mm, 4.5 mm, and 6 mm. The slopes of the penetration-time curves were reasonably constant, so that average penetration rates could be taken. Using the data from Seedhom and associates,[10] who estimated about 3000 walking cycles per day, or about 1 million cycles per year for an arthritic patient, the rates were calculated as shown in Table 16-1.

The penetration rates may be underestimated because in the real joint the load is pulsating, the motion multidirectional, and the effect of loose debris probably greater. However, it was clear that the thinner the plastic, the higher the rate and, by implication, the higher the stress, the higher the rate. About 4 mm should be regarded as the lowest desirable plastic thickness, using the present-day high-molecular-weight polyethylene.

ANTEROPOSTERIOR FORCE ELEMENTS

It is clear from Figure 16-4 that in normal functions, considerable anteroposterior forces

TABLE 16-1. FATIGUE WEAR IN PLASTIC KNEE PROSTHESES

Plastic Thickness	Penetration per Million Cycles (μ)	Years per mm Penetration
2 mm	50	20
3 mm	40	25
4.5 mm	27	37
6 mm	14	71

are carried. The options in a prosthetic replacement are as follows:

None of the forces are carried by the prosthesis.

All of the forces are carried by the prosthesis.

A proportion of the forces are carried by the prosthesis.

The first solution implies that the tibial plateaus are close to flat in the anteroposterior direction, and that the cruciate ligaments carry almost all of the forces. Even in this situation, there will be friction at the metal-plastic surface, but for a coefficient of friction of 0.05 and a compressive force of 3.0 body weight, the frictional force is only about 110 newtons.* This solution minimizes the shearing force on the components that will enhance fixation, as long as the anteroposterior laxity is not so excessive that the contact points move close to the front or the back.

To avoid instability, the bone cuts, the component thicknesses, the design, and the size of the prosthesis all become critical, and accuracies within a few millimeters are called for. There are other disadvantages of the flat plateau system. The contact stress on the plastic is high, increasing the penetration rate. In the normal knee the condylar surfaces carry a significant part of the anteroposterior forces, particularly when compressive loads are acting, and thus total reliance on the cruciate ligaments would stress them excessively.

The second solution, in which all of the anteroposterior forces are carried by the prosthe-

sis, implies that there is complete conformity between the femoral and tibial components in the sagittal plane or that some form of hinged prosthesis is used. An example of the former is the early Geomedic knee. One of the consequences of this arrangement is that there is a fixed center of rotation at the center of curvature of the surfaces. In the normal knee the center of rotation changes with the angle of flexion because of the geometry of the surfaces and the constraints of the cruciate ligaments. Hence, there is an incompatibility in that, as flexion increases, the femoral condyles, which normally move posteriorly due to the pull of the posterior cruciate, are prevented from doing so. The result is restriction of range of motion and posterior tilting moments on the tibial component. The only solution is to place the components in such a way that the cruciate ligaments are loose. In any case, conforming geometry is incompatible with cruciate retention and ensures that all of the anteroposterior forces (as well as torques) are transmitted between the components, maximizing the stresses at the implant-bone interface. Furthermore, transverse rotation, necessary for normal function, is prevented.

In many cases, however, the cruciate ligaments are absent or cannot be preserved. If collateral stability can be obtained, it is possible to provide anteroposterior stability in a condylar replacement. Two methods have been used.

1. The first method relys on partial conformity of the femoral and tibial surfaces, as in the Freeman-Swanson and Total Condylar. The stabilizing mechanism has been explained previously.[18] Briefly, when there is a compressive load acting, applying, say, an ante-

---

* 1 kilogram-force = 9.8 newtons = 2.2 pounds-force.

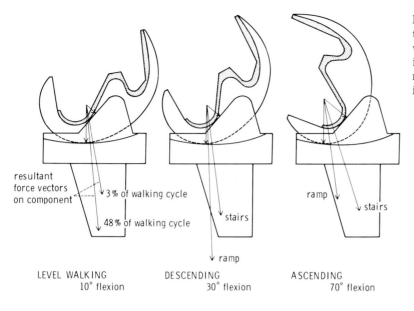

FIG. 16-10. The forces acting on the Kinematic Stabilizer Knee, which has a-p stability and guiding surfaces in the intercondylar notch. Note the femoral roll-back in flexion.

resultant force vectors on component

3% of walking cycle

48% of walking cycle

stairs

ramp

ramp

stairs

LEVEL WALKING
10° flexion

DESCENDING
30° flexion

ASCENDING
70° flexion

rior force, this leads to anterior movement of the femur on the tibia to an equilibrium point.

At this point, the femorotibial force is no longer vertical but is angled backward in such a way that the backward component balances the anterior force. Even with no compressive force, the uphill motion as the femur slides forward tenses the collateral structures, producing a femorotibial compressive force. The stabilizing mechanism is then the same as before. Nevertheless, anterior femoral subluxation of the femur is sometimes a problem.[4]

2. The second method involves adding a guiding or stabilizing mechanism in the intercondylar area. Two examples of this are shown in Figure 16-1, the Total II and the Kinematic Stabilizer. Another example, which preceded both, is the Deane Knee. The principle of the Stabilizer is illustrated in Figure 16-10. The major load-bearing is still on the condylar surfaces as normal, but the anteroposterior forces are carried by the guiding surfaces. In extension, the condylar surfaces closely conform, and both anterior and posterior stability are provided. As the knee is flexed beyond about 30°, posterior femoral stability is lost, but anterior stability is provided throughout the remaining motion. Another important feature is that the femorotibial contact point rolls backward with flexion as in the

normal knee. This is intended to avoid posterior soft tissue restraint and allow a full range of motion.

The net force vector on the tibial component can be shown to lie within the outline of the central peg (Fig. 16-10), so that only in extreme or traumatic events should there be a high rocking moment. At the time of writing, the clinical experience with such devices is limited.

Many condylar replacements today use partially conforming surfaces to carry a proportion of the anteroposterior forces. Either both cruciate ligaments are preserved or, more commonly, only the posterior. Few clinical deficiencies have been evident thus far due to sacrifice of the anterior cruciate. Because compatibility with the posterior cruciate implies that the femorotibial contact point rolls backward with flexion, this must be allowed by a shallow posterior plastic surface (Fig. 16-11). A raised surface can cause excessive tightness and restriction of the range of motion.

VARUS-VALGUS ELEMENTS

It was stated earlier that in the frontal plane the resultant line of force moves from side to side during activity, mainly on the medial side. The disposition will be affected by the

FIG. 16-11. Femorotibial contacts in a condylar replacement knee which preserves the posterior cruciate ligament.

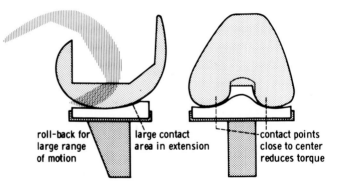

roll-back for large range of motion

large contact area in extension

contact points close to center reduces torque

FIG. 16-12. The test rig for measuring component-to-bone tilting deflections when various loads and moments are applied to the tibial component.

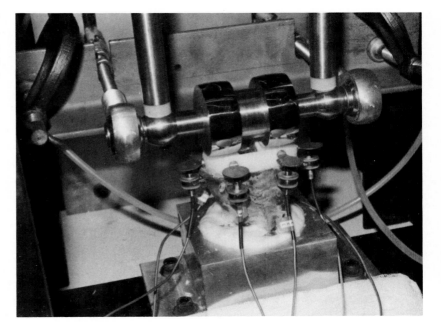

individual gait and by the alignment of the prosthetic components.

With respect to the tibial component, such a force causes an uneven distribution of the stresses at the implant—bone interface. If the resultant force is excessively to one side, there can be high compressive stresses beneath the force and tensile stresses on the opposite side. With plastic components not supported by a metal tray, bending or buckling can occur additionally.

Such effects were investigated for different designs of tibial component by experimenta-

tion,[17] and by finite element analysis.[1,14] In the experiments the components were cemented to the bone, and compressive load combined with varus-valgus moments, anteroposterior forces, and rotational moments were applied (Fig. 16-12). Anteroposterior forces and rotation lead to uneven stress distribution in a way similar to varus-valgus loading. The tilting, either distraction or compression, between the component and the bone was measured at points around the periphery. It was clear that certain features of components reduced the degree of tilting:

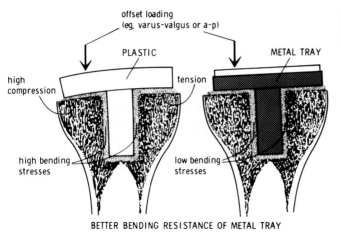

FIG. 16-13. Bending and stress characteristics of all-plastic and metal tray components in response to an off-center load.

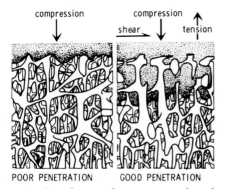

FIG. 16-14. Interfaces of cement and trabecular bone, with low and high intertrabecular penetration.

Large surface area

A central post, or two separate posts

A rigid connection between the medial and lateral sides (a disadvantage in extreme varus-valgus)

Further studies were carried out to determine in more detail the characteristics of the central-peg type of component, namely, the strain gauge experiments referred to earlier in this chapter. As well as strain-gauging the tibia, the central peg itself was gauged at three levels. Various combinations of forces and moments were applied as in the tilting experiments described above.

The effects of varus-valgus, and of the other types of loading that redistributed the stress,

were striking when the all-plastic and the metal tray units were compared. If the plastic peg is well cemented in trabecular bone, it does not provide a great deal of bending resistance to an offset force on the condyles. However, the strain or amount of bending can be marked. In contrast, a metal peg provides considerable bending resistance, but the strain will be low.

This is illustrated in Figure 16-13. The low bending resistance of the all-plastic component leads to high compressive stresses beneath the load and high bending strains in the peg, particularly near the top. The latter will be reflected in relatively high stresses in the surrounding acrylic cement and at the cement—bone interfaces. The metal tray reduced both the compressive stresses and the bending stresses around the peg. The strain-gauge measurements indicated nearly ten times the reduction in bending around the peg compared with the plastic.

Long-term clinical results will be needed to assess the effects of some of the variables discussed fully, although the laboratory data narrow down the valid types of design and can explain some of the clinical observations.

FUTURE ADVANCES

Today, most knee prostheses used are condylar replacements, on the grounds that, when accompanied by suitable surgical technique, most knees can be restored to satisfactory stability and function, and pain relief will ensue. The longevity of the prostheses has not yet been established because of the limited follow-up time, particularly of the newer designs. However, the reasons for failure include:

Infection. The incidence is usually less than 1% primary cases.

Instability. This problem occurs mainly when the cruciate is sacrificed, although excessive bone removal can cause it even when the cruciates are present. Poor varus-valgus alignment can also be responsible.

Patellofemoral problems. Pain has been virtually nonexistent with patellar flanges and plastic buttons. However, superior pole bone fracture remains a problem due to excessive bone removal with the buttons.

Loosening, particularly on the tibial side. This problem has affected all designs to a greater or lesser degree. Contributing factors (other than design) may be poor cement technique, poor alignment, or excessive activity level.

Wear and deformation. Gross deformation or change of shape of plastic should be reduced with metal trays, but wear with the present RCH-1000 promises to be a long-term problem, greater than that in the hip.

Hopefully, future advances will address the above problems. Instrumentation and technique need to provide greater accuracy and reproducibility. When cement is used, it should penetrate the cleansed spaces of trabecular bone (Fig. 16-14) to provide shear and tensile, as well as compressive, resistance. Fixation without using cement, either by bone ingrowth surfaces or by other interfaces, may reduce loosening, but it cannot be expected to do so entirely. Wear may be reduced by the "floating bearing" type of designs, but they may introduce other problems. In any case, a material with more resistance to stress and deformation than high-molecular-weight polyethylene would be a great advantage. Continued cooperative efforts between the surgeon, biologist, and engineer will be needed to deal with the multifaceted problems involved.

REFERENCES

1. **Askew MJ, Lewis, JL, Keer LM:** The effect of post geometry material and location on interface stress levels in tibial components of total knee prostheses. Proc Orthop Res Soc, San Francisco, February, 1979
2. **Blacharski PA, Somerset JH, Murray DG:** A three-dimensional study of the kinematics of the human knee. J Biomechanics 8:375, 1975
3. **Boone DC, Azen SP:** Normal range of motion of joints in male subjects. J Bone Joint Surg 61A:756, 1979
4. **Insall JN, Scott WN, Ranawat CS:** The total condylar knee prosthesis. J Bone Joint Surg 61A:173, 1979
5. **Markolf KL, Graff-Radford A, Amstutz HC:** In-vivo measurements of knee stability. Proc Orthop Res Soc, Dallas, February, 1978
6. **McLeod PC, Kettelkamp DB, Srinivasan V et al:** Measurements of repetitive activities of the knee. J Biomech 8:369, 1975
7. **Morrison JB:** Function of the knee joint in various activities. Med Biol Eng 4:573, 1969
8. **Morrison JB:** The mechanics of the knee joint in relation to normal walking. J Biomech 3:51, 1970
9. **Reilly D, Walker PS, Ben-Dov M et al:** Effects of tibial components on load transfer in the upper tibia. Proc Orthop Res Soc, Atlanta, February 1980
10. **Seedhom BB, Terayama K:** Knee forces during the activity of getting out of a chair with and without the aid of arms. Biomed Eng 278–282, 1976
11. **Seireg A, Arvikar RJ:** A mathematical model for evaluation of forces in lower extremities of the musculo–skeletal system. J Biomechanics 6:313, 1973
12. **Seireg A, Arvikar RJ:** Muscular load-sharing during walking. J Biomech 8:89, 1975
13. **Townsend MA, Izak M, Jackson RW:** Total motion knee goniometry. J Biomech 10:183, 1977
14. **Vichnin HH, Hayes WC, Lotke PA:** Parametric finite element studies of tibial component fixation in the total condylar knee prosthesis. Proc Orthop Res Soc, San Francisco, February, 1979
15. **Walker PS:** Wear and fixation of condylar replacement knee prostheses. In Evarts M (ed): Current Status of Total Knee Replacement, Chap 25. Chicago, C.V. Mosby, 1977
16. **Walker PS:** Human Joints and Their Artificial Replacements. Springfield, Charles C Thomas, 1977
17. **Walker PS, Greene, D, Ben-Dov M et al:** Fixation of tibial components of knee prostheses. Proc Orthop Res Soc, San Francisco, February, 1979
18. **Walker PS Hsieh H-H:** The conformity of condylar replacement knee prostheses. J Bone Joint Surg 59B:222, 1977

CHAPTER 17
TOTAL KNEE ARTHROPLASTY— INDICATIONS AND TECHNIQUES

David G. Mendes

Although surface replacement of the knee has been carried out only during the past 10 years, it has proved to be a very satisfactory procedure.[1] During that time many new designs have been developed to overcome problems that caused failures originally.

Replacement arthroplasty should be limited to the physiologically older age group with severe involvement of the knee joint when other methods of treatment are unlikely to help. For younger patients and for the less affected knee, a conservative procedure is a better choice.

The need for surface replacement arthroplasty should be measured against the potential benefit expected from other surgical procedures such as one of a variety of osteotomies, arthrotomy and drilling arthroplasty, replacement by allograft, replacement by prosthetic hinge, or arthrodesis.

INDICATIONS

TRICOMPARTMENTAL INVOLVEMENT OF THE KNEE JOINT

Pathologic conditions involving the three compartments, namely, the medial, lateral, and patellofemoral compartments, are indications for surface replacement. Such conditions include rheumatoid arthritis, psoriatic arthritis, dermatomyositis and other collagen diseases, gouty arthritis, chondrocalcinosis, degenerative osteoarthritis, and traumatic arthritis. When the primary disease, such as rheumatoid arthritis, has been arrested, it may be complicated by secondary degenerative changes affecting the three compartments. This too is an indication for surface replacement.

BIOCOMPARTMENTAL INVOLVEMENT OF THE KNEE JOINT

Severe structural changes in two compartments may necessitate replacement of the knee even if the third compartment is not involved. The extent of the structural changes is expressed in the resulting angular deformity, either valgus or varus, fixed or unstable.

A fixed deformity cannot be corrected by stress. A deformity of more than 10° to 15° that can be fully corrected or overcorrected by stress is an unstable deformity.

Valgus deformity responds less favorably to high tibial osteotomy, and the supracondylar osteotomy carries a higher incidence of morbidity; therefore a patient with a significant lateral and patellofemoral involvement might be a suitable subject for replacement arthroplasty.

Varus deformity, when in excess of 15°, is frequently accompanied by rotatory deformity, lateral subluxation of the tibia, and abnormal weight-bearing on the intercondylar eminence. The patellofemoral joint is also frequently involved. This bicompartmental involvement does not respond well to high tibial osteotomy, and replacement arthroplasty should be the surgical procedure of choice.

The rotatory deformity that accompanies the angular deformity is in external rotation as a rule and is also corrected by replacement arthroplasty.

Instability accompanying an angular deformity is determined by stress correction or overcorrection of the deformity. It reinforces the indications for replacement arthroplasty. With instability of unusual magnitude, such as 25° or more, especially if accompanied by recurvatum, a hinge replacement arthroplasty should be considered, although surface replacement with a thicker component may suffice.

FAILURE OF PREVIOUS PROCEDURE

A previous procedure such as osteotomy, drilling arthroplasty, or hemireplacement that has failed may be salvaged by replacement arthroplasty.

RELATIVE INDICATIONS

Osteonecrosis. In the elderly patient with unicompartmental involvement such as osteonecrosis of the medial condyle of the femur, replacement arthroplasty can be an alternative procedure to an allograft or high tibial osteotomy.

Stiff knee. A limited arc of motion of less than 60° or 70° may improve after replacement arthroplasty, particularly if it is associated with a flexion contracture.

Flexion contracture. Significant flexion contracture (over 30°) can be corrected effectively at the time of replacement arthroplasty.

CONTRAINDICATIONS

Infection. A recent or old infection of the knee may flare up after replacement arthroplasty owing to the large amount of foreign material involved.

Neuropathy. A neuropathic joint, such as Charcot's joint, or a meningomyelocele, may cause loosening and disintegration of the prosthesis due to injudicious use of the joint.

Paralysis. A paralytic limb, such as occurs in poliomyelitis, may loosen the prosthesis if submitted to excessive and unprotected demands from the prosthetic knee.

Instability. Significant recurvatum instability may cause loosening of the prosthesis.

Age. A physiologically young and otherwise healthy patient is a contraindication to the procedure.

The surgical procedure is planned pre-operatively on roentgenograms. The anteroposterior view is taken with the patient standing to reproduce the full deformity, and then with the patient lying down, applying a stress to correct the deformity and to demonstrate the instability of the knee. Routine lateral, skyline, and tunnel views are also taken. The bony cuts are drawn on the anteroposterior, lateral, and skyline views to mark the inclination of the cuts to the long axis of the bones and the estimated level of each cut (Fig. 17-1*A*, *B*, *C*).

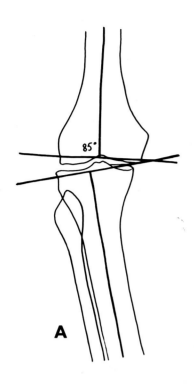

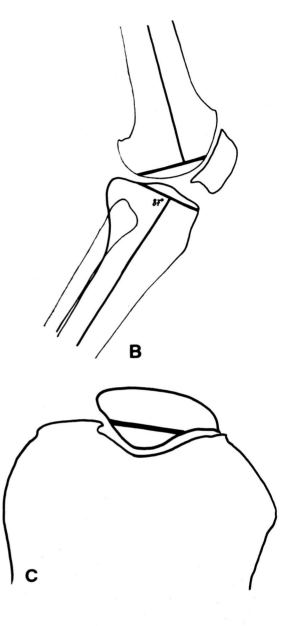

FIG. 17-1. (A) Diagram of the typical measurements made on an anteroposterior radiograph of the knee. This was a patient with varus instability about to undergo arthroplasty. **(B)** Measurements made on the lateral radiograph. **(C)** Diagram of a skyline view showing the mark made for removal of the posterior patellar surface.

The patient lies supine. A sterile tourniquet, if available, is placed on the thigh; the leg is prepared and draped routinely. When a sterile tourniquet is used, the leg is draped free, exposing the tourniquet and the hip joint to ease the realignment of the knee during the operation.

A medial parapatellar hockey stick incision is preferred, carried proximally through the fibers of the vastus medialis. The medial half

of the insertion of the patellar tendon is sharply elevated from the tibial tuberosity. The pad of fat is preserved to protect the inferior patellar blood supply.

The "femoral jig" is used to mark the anterior and posterior cuts of the femur. There is no need to drill the femoral canal (Fig. 17-2A, B, C). The jig marks the anterior cut (first cut) flush with the anterior cortex of the femur and parallel to the plane of the posterior aspect of

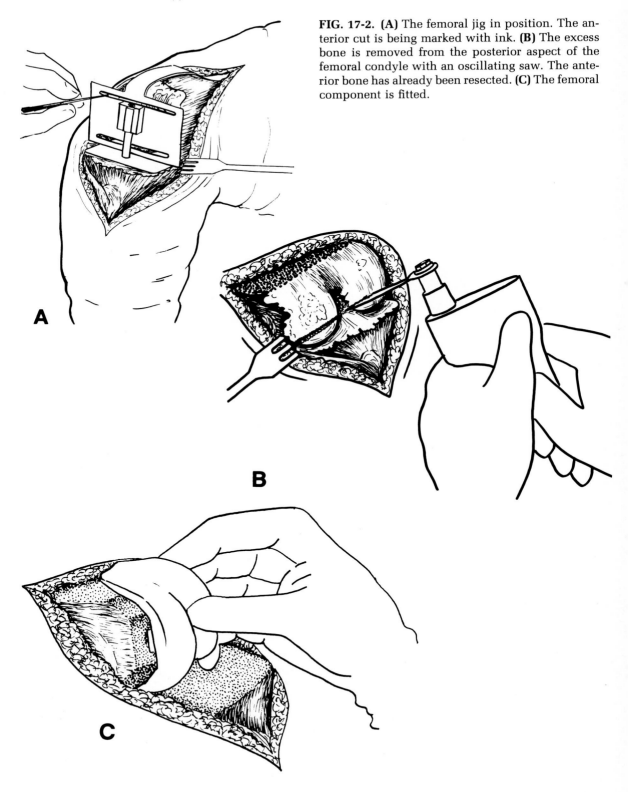

FIG. 17-2. (A) The femoral jig in position. The anterior cut is being marked with ink. **(B)** The excess bone is removed from the posterior aspect of the femoral condyle with an oscillating saw. The anterior bone has already been resected. **(C)** The femoral component is fitted.

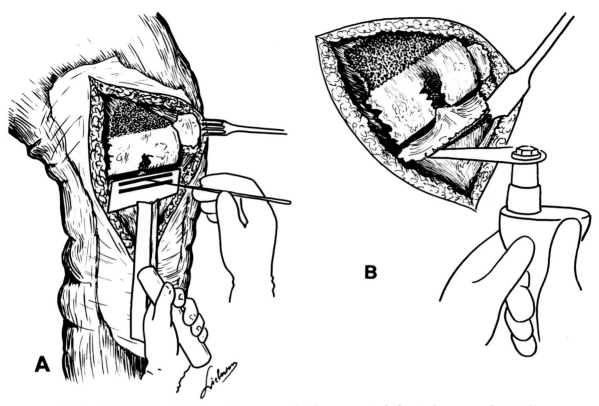

FIG. 17-3. (A) The third cut. The pen marks the amount of tibia to be resected. **(B)** The appropriate amount of bone is removed from the tibia with an oscillating saw.

the femoral condyles; thus it properly orients the prosthesis in the frontal plane. If the anterior cut is misplaced it may either cut into the femoral cortex and eventually result in a fracture, or it may interfere with closure of the retinaculum at the end of the procedure.

The jig also marks the posterior cut (second cut) of the femur to fit the width of the femoral prosthesis. If a small prosthesis is used, this cut is modified according to the width of the femoral component. In a patient with an external rotation deformity, the leg should be internally rotated to realign the tibial tuberosity, with the tibial jig used to mark the cut of the proximal tibia (third cut). The cut should be made perpendicular to the axis of the tibia in the frontal plane and at 2° to 3° of posterior inclination in the sagittal plane. It should resect a minimal amount of bone from the tibial pla-

teau (Fig. 17-3A , B). The anterior cruciate ligament is sacrificed; the posterior cruciate may be retained. Then the cut for the stem of the tibial component is made close to and in the inclination of the posterior wall to accept the stem with an exact fit. This cut is also oriented to correct the leg malrotation and to keep the tibial tuberosity a few degrees out of rotation in relation to the prosthetic intercondylar ridge.

The cut of the distal femur (fourth cut) is marked using the alignment jig (third jig). This is placed intimately over and along the distal femur and the femoral cut is marked 7° in valgus in relation to the long axis of the femur (Fig. 17-4A). The level of the cut is then determined by the spacer, which represents the thickness of the prosthetic knee; this is placed over the tibial cut with the leg pulled

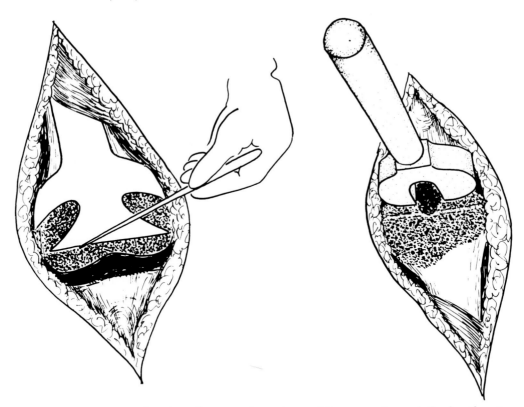

FIG. 17-4. Diagrams showing alignment jig and use of the spacer to mark the fourth cut, that is, for removal of the distal end of the femur. The leg is extended and traction applied. (See text for description.)

distally (Fig. 17-4*B*). The level of 7° valgus mark is adjusted according to the spacer. An alternative to that simple method is the use of a long wire extending from the hip joint to the ankle. This is best done with a sterile tourniquet and under TV control.

The cut of the patella (fifth cut) is made with the patella turned over. The cut is made parallel to the nonarticulating surface of the patella, maintaining a thickness of bone of 10 mm to 15 mm. The circumference of the prosthetic patella is marked, and the bony excess is cut with a saw. The anchoring hole is shifted slightly medially from the center to allow the effect of a lateral release. The depth of the hole is gently undermined with a tiny curette (Fig. 17-5*A*, *B*).

It is emphasized that the jigs and the spacer are used to allow resection of a minimal amount of bone, and the prosthesis should fit to give a stable joint in full extension and in 90° of flexion. The alignment of the knee of 7° of valgus is produced by the laterally tilted cut in the distal femur and the perpendicular cut in the proximal tibia. In replacement of the valgus knee, an alignment of 2° of valgus rather than 7° is the aim.

The prosthetic components should be cemented on bone that is as dry as possible. The tibial component is seated peripherally on the posterior cortex of the tibia and is firmly fixed on the tibial cortices through the stem and two anchoring 12-mm holes. The tibial and patellar components are cemented in one stage. Attention is given to the accurate placement first of the tibial components and then of the patellar, and a constant pressure should be applied until the cement hardens.

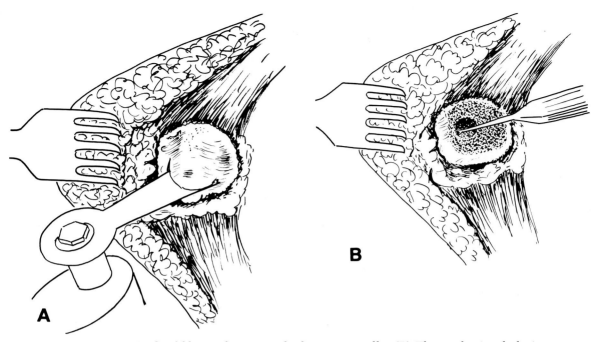

FIG. 17-5. (A) The fifth cut for removal of excess patella. **(B)** The anchoring hole is placed medial to the center of the patella and is undermined with a curette.

The femoral component is cemented in the second stage. Polymethylmethacrylate is placed on the anterior and distal surfaces of the femur and within the posterior part of the prosthetic condyles. The prosthesis is firmly placed and the excess cement removed from the intercondylar notch and around the prosthesis. The knee is extended, and the cement is left to harden with the knee in full extension.

In a knee with a fixed angular deformity, the tibial cut often removes bone mainly from one part of the plateau (Fig. 17-6*A*, *B*, *C*). For example, in a fixed varus deformity only the lateral part of the tibial plateau is cut. The eburnated bone on the medial part of the plateau is roughened by multiple drill holes, using a 4.5-mm drill. The holes are interconnected with a fine rongeur. Eburnation of the patellar surface is handled in a similar way to allow a better grip for the cement. A fixed angular deformity of the knee can be fully corrected by careful subperiosteal release of the stabilizing structures. In the varus knee, the medial liga-ment and the pes anserine are partly or fully released as necessary from their tibial insertion (Fig. 17-7*A*, *B*, *C*). In the valgus knee, the lateral ligament is detached from its femoral origin, and the iliotibial band is detached anteriorly from its tibial insertion; alternatively, it can be lengthened by a Z-plasty. Excessive or unnecessary release and overcorrection should be avoided, and the more posterior stabilizers should be preserved to avoid recurvatum.

There are two conditions in which the overall alignment of the knee should be modified to aim for 0° to 2° of valgus: the first is the preoperative valgus knee, in which it is presumed that the lateral musculotendinous structures are stronger than those on the medial side; the second occurs when the ipsilateral hip is medialized, such as after McMurray's osteotomy. The knee alignment of 0° to 2° is determined by the distal cut of the femur.

External rotation deformity of the tibia is commonly seen in advanced degenerative os-

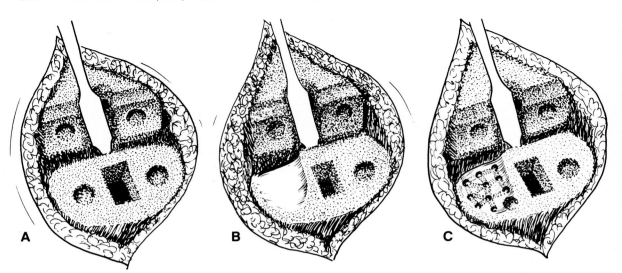

FIG. 17-6. (A) Diagram showing prepared femoral and tibial surfaces with cancellous bone and the holes and notches that have been cut. A spike has been inserted behind the tibial plateau to push it forward. **(B)** In a fixed varus deformity, eburnated bone remains on the medial plateau after the cuts have been made. **(C)** Drill holes are made in the eburnated bone and connected to provide a roughened area for attachment of the cement.

teoarthritis of the knee and is also corrected by subperiosteal stripping of the stabilizers until the tibial tuberosity faces just lateral to the center.

Instability of the knee is usually countered by resecting as little bone as possible and taking up the ligamentous slack by fitting a prosthesis of the right thickness. A point is made of using a tibial component nearly 10 mm thick. If it were thicker the shearing stress on the cement–bone junction would be increased; a thinner component might become deformed because of cold flow.

Mild flexion deformity is easily corrected by cutting the distal femur slightly more proximally than usual, using the spacer in the routine way. When flexion deformity is more than 20°, posterior capsulotomy should be done transversely prior to cutting the distal femur; this will prevent unnecessary resection of larger amounts of bone. The femur and the tibia may be held apart with a lamina spreader, and the capsule is cut over a Kelly clamp with a knife.

Lateral retinacular release is routinely done when correcting a valgus deformity; otherwise, recurrent dislocation of the patella may occur soon after surgery or as a late complication. Lateral release is performed when subluxation of the patella tends to occur laterally at time of closure. It may also be done if closure of the retinaculum is too tight. Technically, the release should avoid the lateral geniculate vessels if possible. Occasionally, in a very deformed knee, realignment of the quadriceps mechanism should be carried out proximally and distally.

Occasionally, excess bone from the tibial plateau may protrude under the tibial component in spite of the correction of rotation deformity. This excess bone is removed gently with a rongeur.

Closure of the wound includes meticulous repair of the fascia of the vastus medialis. Hemovac drainage is instituted. The limb is protected in a cylinder cast for 5 days. Straight leg raising is routinely done, assisted by a sling. Full weight-bearing is allowed on the second postoperative day and knee motion on the sixth day, emphasizing full extension. If

FIG. 17-7. **(A)** Detachment of the pes anserinus. **(B)** Release of the medial ligament. **(C)** Lengthening of the iliotibial band by Z-plasty.

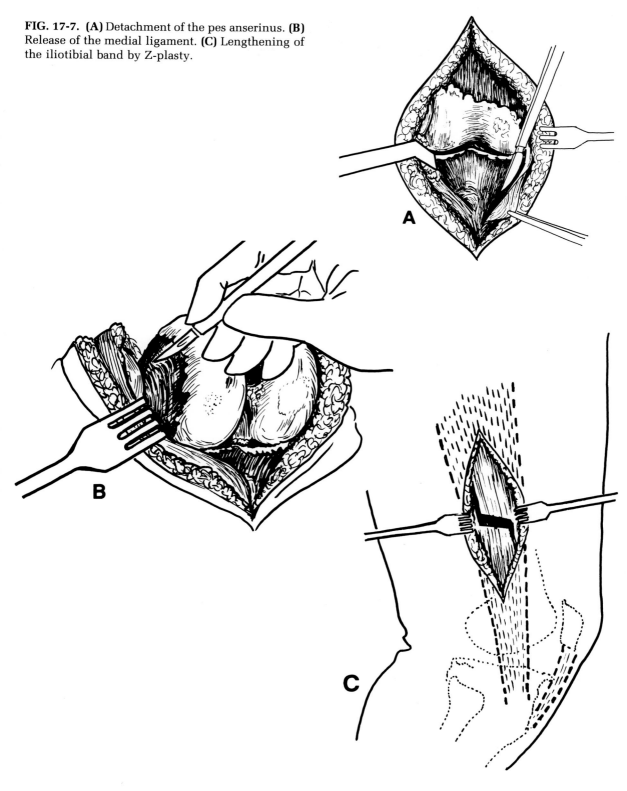

range of movement does not exceed 60° to 70° by the third week, manipulation is indicated. All patients receive prophylactic antibiotics and anticoagulation (low-dose Coumadin).

REFERENCE

1. **Gunston FH:** Polycentric knee arthroplasty. J Bone Joint Surg 53B:272, 1971

CHAPTER 18
COMPLICATIONS OF
TOTAL KNEE ARTHROPLASTY

Edward T. Habermann

HISTORICAL BACKGROUND

In 1860 Verneuil introduced the concept of an arthroplasty to improve knee function by interposing tissues between resected bone ends to prevent fusion.[143] Ferguson, in 1861, reported on the achievement of successful early movement between the newly created surfaces.[38] These were the first documented reports of an ever-increasing number of knee arthroplasties that used different designs and techniques in an attempt to maintain motion and provide good joint function.

In early 1950, Walldius described the hinge arthroplasty;[147,148] he was followed by Young[159] and Shiers,[132] and later by the GUEPAR[28,101] group. The early results of Walldius and Young were successful in about 50% of cases, which would be considered unacceptable in the present era of total joint arthroplasty. The major problems of infection and loosening led to further investigation into design and the use of different materials for the prosthetic knee joint replacement.

After total hip arthroplasty had become a standard procedure with relatively predictable results, new concepts of total knee replacement could be developed. In 1968, Gunston pioneered the use of high-density polyethylene and stainless stell to resurface the tibiofemoral joint,[50] using methylmethacrylate for fixation, a substance that had already proved effective in total hip replacement. In 1970, Freeman and Swanson developed a prosthesis that was nonrestrained and that sacrificed the cruciate ligaments.[41] This type of prosthesis allowed better knee motion and better surgical exposure and alignment. Since that time, many modifications of the nonconstrained type of prosthesis have been made. Early results of the present designs of total knee arthroplasty have been reported by various authors as successful in 80% to 90% of cases. It is vital, however, that long-term follow-up investigation be available in the evaluation of total knee arthroplasty, so that definitive changes in design and technique can be made to overcome the multiple problems encountered. Problems include loosening, alignment difficulties, wear, future salvage procedures, and many others.

One major problem is the lack of uniformity in the grading system used in comparing results from series to series. Many factors play a critical role in the success of any arthroplasty, including the initial diagnosis, the type of deformity, the degree of bone destruction, and what the patient expects from his arthroplasty. A standard method of assessing the long- and short-term results of total knee arthroplasty would be most valuable in comparing the different types and in determining the factors that might decide the choice of one type over another. Many questions are still without answers, and large numbers of total knee replacements of varying designs are being clinically tested in an attempt to provide a uniformly desirable total knee arthroplasty. Not all surgeons are able to achieve the 80% to 90% success rate reported by some authors, and long-term follow-up by the initial evaluators has shown that complications increase significantly with the passage of time.[8]

TYPES OF PROSTHESIS

At present there are many types of total knee replacements. They may be characterized as completely restrained, semirestrained, and nonrestrained; although the terminology may be confusing. Conceptually, the character of the prosthesis depends on whether the stability of the reconstructed knee is due to the prosthesis, the ligamentous structures, or a combination of both.[151] A completely constrained prosthesis has no need of ligamentous structures, whereas the total nonconstrained prosthesis depends on ligamentous support. In addition, the shaping, primarily of the tibial combonent,[147] offers varying degrees of stability ranging from the totally flat tibial surface, which offers little stability, to the very deeply "dished" tibial component, which provides moderately significant stability. When the cruciate ligaments are retained, they afford the stability required, and the

prosthesis used has a relatively flat tibial surface. Those prostheses employed where the cruciate ligaments are usually sacrificed, such as the total condylar, variable axis, or ICLH type in common use today, depend upon the prosthetic components to provide some degree of stability. Prostheses such as the Spherocentric,[84,100,140] Stabilocondylar, or Attenborough[4] are condylar-bearing with an intercondylar stabilizing mechanism and are used most frequently when ligamentous laxity or significant bony destruction is present. They provide more stability and yet allow motion in a rotational plane, which makes them significantly different from the hinged prostheses. These moderately restrained total knee replacements have been advocated for use in the more severely destroyed knee or in revision surgery when a less restrained prosthesis may have failed. The more constrained the prosthesis, the more bone resection is required. These semi-restrained prostheses have largely obviated the need for the hinge prosthesis, thereby allowing some rotational components and avoiding some of the complications of the hinged prosthesis.[22,23,45,65,73,74,75,88,95,99,109,110]

LOOSENING

Loosening is a major problem in total knee arthroplasty (Table 18–1). A number of factors may contribute, including (1) failure to correct the deformity, (2) infection, (3) failure in technique of alignment and cement, (4) improper selection of prosthesis to provide stability, (5) synovial reaction to products of wear and excess cement, (6) fracture, (7) abnormal loading, (8) poor patient selection, and (9) tibial component sinkage.[23,38,72,74,75,76,145]

Loosening must be defined carefully so that meaningful data on frequency and severity can be collected from reports on different types of total knee arthroplasties. As defined by Kaufer,[83] loosening is categorized into four types:

Simple loosening, which appears as a par-

TABLE 18-1. INCIDENCE OF LOOSENING

Author	Type of Prosthesis	%
Sledge	Duocondylar	1.2
Murray	Variable axis	0
Habermann	Geometric	8
Finerman	Anametric	0
Insall	Total condylar	1
	Total condylar II	4
Skolnick	Polycentric	2.4
Coventry	Geometric mark II	5
Cracchiolo	Geometric	8
Cracchiolo	Polycentric	4
Kaufer	Spherocentric	8
Freeman	ICLH	12.5
Attenborough	Attenborough	1
Insall	Unicondylar	10
Insall	Duocondylar	5
Riley	Geometric	2
Lacey	UCI	10
Gschwind	GSB	0.6
Gunston	Gunston	2
Skolnick	Geometric	10
Evanski	UCI	5.8
Ducheyne	UCI	7.0
Jones	Unicondylar	5.8
Insall	Guepar	12
Phillips	Walldius	3.6
Freeman	Walldius	5
Arden	Shiers	7
Deburge	Guepar	15

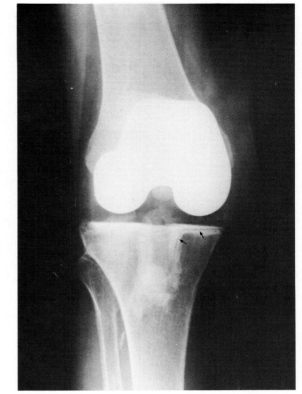

FIG. 18-1. Early radiolucency at medial tibial plateau and along upper portion of tibial stem in total condylar knee replacement 6 months after operation. This radiolucency was nonprogressive and the patient was asymptomatic. Also note radiopaque methylmethacrylate in posterior recess of knee.

tial or complete radiolucent zone between implant and bone. It is painless, and clinical functioning is satisfactory (Fig. 18-1); physical loosening on stress views or arthrography may be absent or present.

Symptomatic loosening, characterized by a radiolucent zone, discomfort aggravated by activity and relieved by rest, and the absence of other causes of symptoms such as infection or fracture.

Progressive loosening, characterized by a documented increasing length or width of the radiolucent zone in a patient with good clinical function; it may be painful or not (Fig. 18-2A–D).

Functional loosening, which reveals a radiolucent zone and progressive displacement of the implant, leading to malalignment of the limb and instability or other malfunction, with or without pain (Figs. 18-2D, 18-3A–G).

Loosening of the hinge prostheses has long been recognized, and radiographic evidence of such loosening has approached 100%.[149,159] In the early Walldius series, in which no cement was used, only those patients who showed clinical evidence of loosening had symptoms.[80,81,153,154] Loosening of the cemented prosthesis caused more symptoms than loosening of noncemented implants. This has been our own experience with the Walldius prosthesis, and it is borne out by the reports of Bain[5] and Freeman.[46]

Arden reported 7% loosening with the Shier prosthesis.[3] Deburge and associates found that 13% showed aseptic loosening after 2 years with the GUEPAR, and 15% after 5 years.[29] Forty-three percent of these patients had

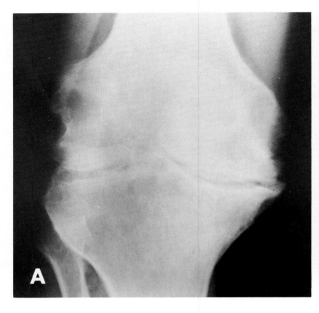

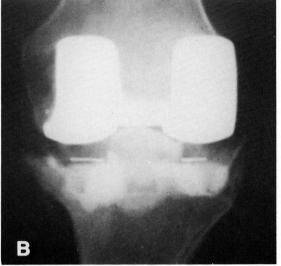

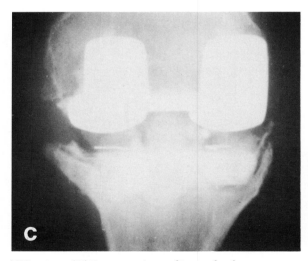

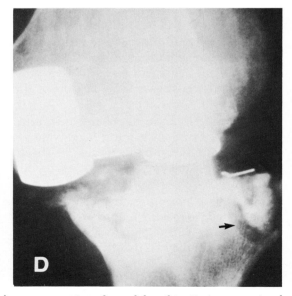

FIG. 18-2. (A) Preoperative radiograph of a 64-year-old obese woman with osteoarthritis of the knee. **(B)** One year postoperatively, there is no radiolucency at the bone cement interface of the tibia. Patient is asymptomatic and functioning well. **(C)** At 2 years, there is progressive radiolucency at the bone cement interface of the tibia. Patient remained asymptomatic. **(D)** At 4 years there was functional loosening with eventual subluxation as depicted on this anteroposterior radiograph. Note marked increase in the radiolucency at the bone cement interface compared with previous radiographs.

symptoms caused by their loose prosthesis and required revision surgery.

The GUEPAR hinge prosthesis showed a radiolucent line around the femoral component in 45% of patients described by Insall and colleagues,[73] but loosening was documented in only one tibial, two femoral, and three axial components. Witvoet, in an early review of 210 cases, reported aseptic loosening of the GUEPAR prosthesis in 2% of cases.[156]

Articulated knees show more femoral loosening than tibial, in marked contrast to nonarticulated knees. In a series of 292 knees with GUEPAR prostheses, however, 2% showed loosening, all involving the tibial component. The GUEPAR II knee is being utilized without cement, making any required revision surgery easier to perform.

Loosening of the nonrestrained prosthesis approaches 10%.[70,71] This has been our experience of tibial loosening with the geometric prosthesis after 5 years, and between 2 and 5 years the incidence increased significantly. Femoral loosening in the nonrestrained prosthesis is infrequently encountered.

Patients with osteoarthritis have a higher incidence of loosening[6,28,70,71,73,85] than those with rheumatoid arthritis; a result probably related to the different activity levels of these two groups. Riley and Hungerford reported only one case of loosening in 54 geometric total knee replacements in rheumatoid arthritic patients.[123] Osteoporosis does not seem to play a significant role. Its incidence in the literature has been variously reported, depending upon each author's definition of loosening.[6,30,34,44,51,54,70,71,73,85]

Insall and his colleagues, in their review of 461 total condylar prostheses, reported a 2% loosening rate, and their results did not seem to deteriorate with time.[77] The femoral component of the total condylar knee is derived from the duocondylar prosthesis, and the tibial component is similar to that of the geometric prosthesis, providing for close conformity in extension to provide stability. This conformity is lost when the knee goes into flexion, allowing for sliding and rotary movements. Intercondylar stability to prevent transloca-

tion is provided by a tibial eminence between the grooved articular depressions. This articular pattern allows for excision of the cruciate ligaments.

The total condylar II model provides anteroposterior stability by a tapered tibial post. The total condylar II prosthesis, when used for revision, provides both anteroposterior and medial-lateral stability and is more constrained than the total condylar II.

In our hands, the total condylar knee prosthesis can be used in most knees if careful attention is paid to balancing the ligamentous structures and to the demanding technique of insertion.

Loosening of the patellar component has not been a problem.[128] Both Insall and associates and Sledge and Ewald have reported large series without loosening.[77,136]

The consequences of loosening are significant. Though all loose prostheses are not necessarily symptomatic, a certain number produce pain and deformity requiring revision surgery, which has inherent technical difficulties, increased risk of sepsis, and the risk of repeated loosening.

LOOSENING FACTORS AND MODES OF FAILURE

Failure of fixation of total knee implants may occur in a number of ways.

Resorption of bone is seen frequently around the stems of constrained prostheses and is probably the result of high loads placed on the bone–cement interface, leading to micromotion, resorption, and gross loosening.

Collapse or fracture of supporting bone may result from poor distribution of forces. Overload is often due to malalignment (Fig. 18-4A–C), excessive removal of subchondral bone, or atrophy of cancellous bone.

Malalignment has been a major problem in our hands, especially in the early geometric series. Failure to correct for varus malalignment led to a higher incidence of failures than for valgus malalignment. Correction in the anteroposterior plane is also important. Mala-

(text continued on p. 251)

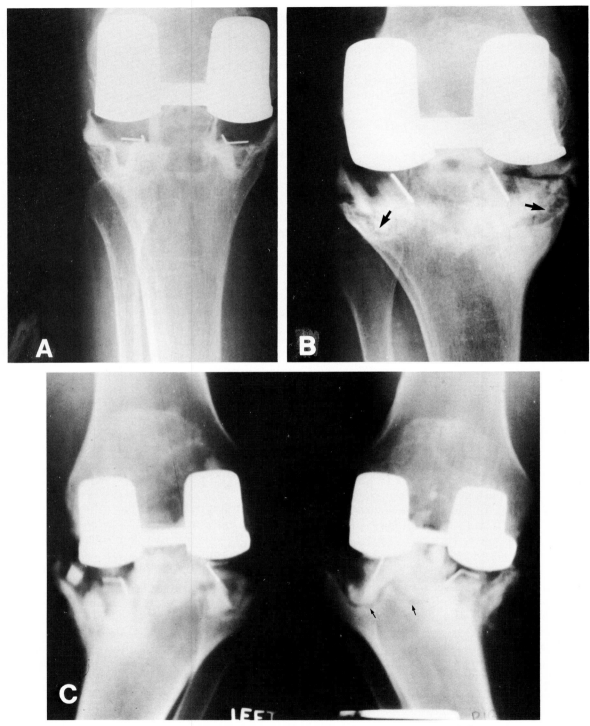

FIG. 18-3. (A) Anteroposterior radiograph of a geometric total knee. **(B)** Progressive loosening and cracking of methylmethacrylate at 2 years. **(C)** Bilateral symptomatic functional loosening with failure. Note severe varus deformity and tibial loosening at 3½ years.

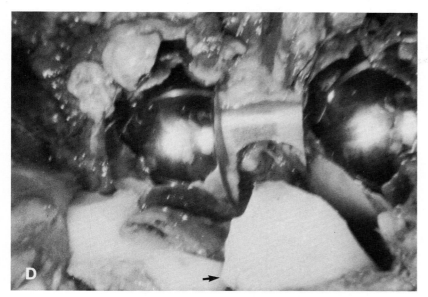

FIG. 18-3. (D) Loosening and fracture of one tibial component at transverse bar (*arrow*) connecting the condylar surfaces in this geometric total knee replacement.

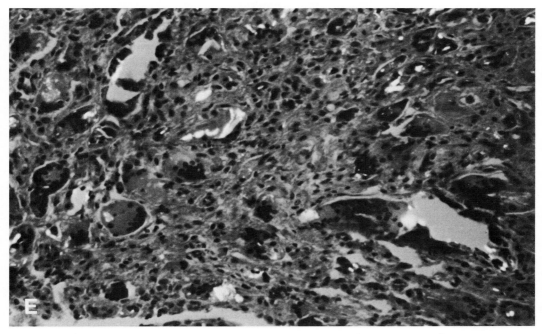

FIG. 18-3. (E) Gross appearance of the tibial component. There is severe polymethacryate impregnation on the condylar surfaces of the tibial component.

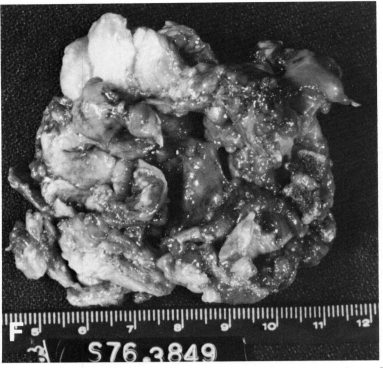

FIG. 18-3. (F) Gross appearance of a polypoid reactive synovium at time of revision surgery.

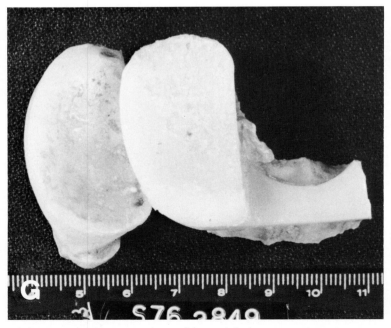

FIG. 18-3. (G) Microscopic appearance of synovial tissue reaction as seen under polarized light microscopy. Birefringent particulate debris of high density polyethylene and methylmethacrylate is visible with giant cell reaction. The large clear clefts represent areas of leached-out methylmethacrylate surrounded by giant cells.

lignment brings excessive local force concentrations to bear on the articular surface. Lotke and associates have shown a statistically significant positive correlation between a good clinical result and a well-aligned prosthesis.[94]

There is no ideal alignment for all knees and all types of prostheses, but 0° to 7° of valgus alignment, with the tibial component at near right angles to the long axis of the tibia, seems most appropriate. Asymmetrical loading of the knee joint creates a tendency for the tibial plateau to tilt, resulting in a compressive state on one side of the prosthesis and a tensile state on the opposite side. Stress in tension may contribute significantly to loosening because both methylmethacrylate and bone perform poorly under tensile stress compared with compressive stress.

Bone, cement, metal, and polyethylene all have a different Poisson's ratio, which is the number derived by dividing the change in length by the change in width that occurs in a material when it is loaded.[40] When loaded, each composite material alters differently, thereby creating shear stress at every different material interface. These stresses are significantly large because the physiologic loads, as described by Morrison,[108] are three to four times body weight, and the Poisson's ratio between the components used in total knee arthroplasty are all markedly dissimilar.[31]

Kaufer and associates have shown that as one goes deeper into the cancellous bone of both the tibia and the femur, the compressive breaking strength is significantly less.[83,84] The strongest bone is closest to the articular surface; the bone on the femoral side being stronger than that on the tibial, and bone on the medial side of the tibia being stronger than that on the lateral side. This correlates with the clinical preponderance of loosening on the tibial side compared with the femoral. In removing the tibial bone careful attention must be paid to staying as close to the joint surfaces as possible (Fig. 18-5).

Separation of cement from bone due to weak bone cement interface and fracture of the cement play a major role in loosening. Miller and associates have shown that as a re-sult of thermal contraction methylmethacrylate shrinks after polymerization.[104] This results in a less than perfect fit between the cement and the bone, and micromotion may occur.[103] Reckling and his colleagues demonstrated that the temperatures created at the bone–cement interface were lower than the 56°C at which protein is thought to be irreversibly damaged.[79,120,122] He suggested that if necrosis was present at the bone–cement interface it was due to factors other than thermal trauma, such as mechanical injury to bone or its blood supply, or the cytotoxic or lipolytic effects of nonpolymerized polymer.[13,115,137,152,155] The presence of blood and moisture at the interface, as well as the large surface area and poor heat conductivity of methylmethacrylate, may prevent the interface from experiencing the high rise in temperature that occurs at the center of the polymerizing cement mass.

Infection must be eliminated as a cause of loosening. Identification of the causative organism by bacteriological culture is important. Radiographic studies may be helpful. There is often increased resorption of bone about the site of infection and less sclerosis than is seen with loosening from other causes. Bone scans, especially with gallium, might give additional information. A frozen section made at the time of revision surgery will show acute inflammatory cells if sepsis is present, in contrast to other histological features as described by Mirra and colleagues.[106]

RADIOLUCENT ZONE

The radiolucent line between cement and bone is commonly seen and justifies concern (Table 18–2). It may be the earliest sign of loosening. In our series of geometric prostheses, it was seen in 80% of cases, varying from an incomplete radiolucent line measuring less than 1 mm to a progressive zone of more than 5 mm. This radiolucent zone has had a reported incidence of from 2% to 100%. Simple, nonprogressive radiolucent lines do not necessarily denote looseness or failure of fixation and in most cases are not associated with symptoms.[1,12,15,42,48,59,79,102,120,121,125,137,144,152]

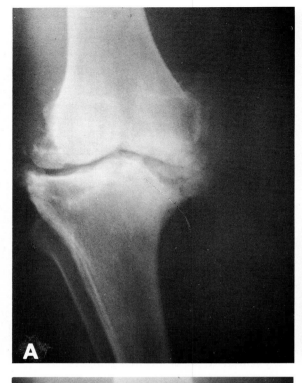

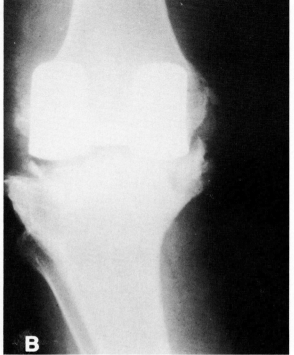

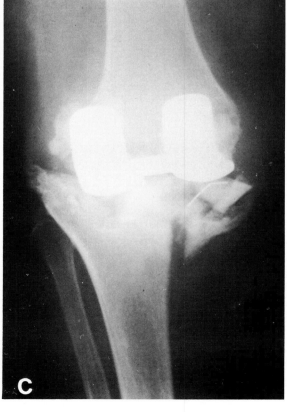

FIG. 18-4. (A) Anteroposterior radiograph of a 72-year-old woman with severe varus deformity and osteoarthritis. Note deficiency of medial tibial plateau. **(B)** Geometric prosthesis was inserted, but overall alignment was not corrected and varus remained. Patient was asymptomatic with good function for 2 years. **(C)** After 2 years and 5 months, she developed progressive pain and subsequent failure with fracture of the medial tibial plateau secondary to malalignment and stress overload, as depicted on this anteroposterior radiograph.

When, however, the line becomes progressively larger, wider, and longer and when symptoms ensue, loosening must be suspected. The radiolucent line is not unique to total knee replacements. It is frequently observed in other joint replacements, especially the hip, where it is most often asymptomatic. It may be present about the acetabulum in more than 50% of cases.

The radiolucent line, when present on the immediate postoperative radiograph, is highly suggestive of poor preparation and packing of cement into the prepared tibial bed. The bone–cement interface, therefore, is mechanically incompetent from the moment of implantation. Cement introducers, water-pik cleansing of the trabecular bone, application of the cement in a more liquid state, cement pressure injection, porous coated implants, and other techniques are being studied to achieve a better cement–bone interface.

It is postulated that poor fixation leads to micromotion which, in turn, leads to bone resorption and the development of a fibrous membrane.

Miller and associates have shown, experimentally and clinically, that when a low-viscosity cement is used under pressure injection and careful attention is paid to preparing the cancellous beds, loosening and the development of a radiolucent line are rarely observed.[105]

TABLE 18-3. HINGED PROSTHESES: INCIDENCE OF SEPSIS

Author	Type of Prosthesis	%
Insall	Guepar	6
Phillips	Walldius	4.8
Habermann	Walldius	6
Freeman	Walldius	5
Jones	Walldius	6.5
Bain	Walldius	10
Arden	Shiers	14
Jackson	Shiers/Walldius	3
Deburge	Guepar	6.6
Lettin	Stanmore hinge	3
Watson	Shiers	2.5
Hui	Guepar/Walldius/Hebert	7

TABLE 18-2. INCIDENCE OF RADIOLUCENCY

Author	Type of Prosthesis	%	
Insall	Unicondylar	70	
	Duocondylar	50	
	Guepar	45	femoral component
	Geometric	80	
Lacey	UCI	90	
Finerman	Anametric	22	osteoarthritis
Sledge	Duocondylar	28	
	Duopatellar	45	
Coventry	Geometric mark II	70	
Sheehan	Sheehan	2	
Kaufer	Spherocentric	37	femoral
		40	tibial
Reckling	Geometric	71	
Laskin	Marmor	86	
Ranawat	Duocondylar	76	tibial
		25	femoral
Ilstrup	Polycentric	41	osteoarthritis
		31	rheumatoid arthritis
	Geometric	100	osteoarthritis
		70	rheumatoid arthritis
Habermann	Geometric	80	
Inglis	Duopatellar	45	

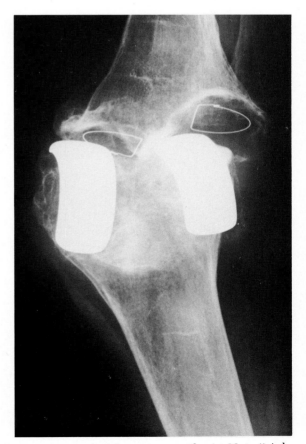

FIG. 18-5. Failed four-part prosthesis. Note "sinking" of lateral tibial plateau and subsequent valgus deformity.

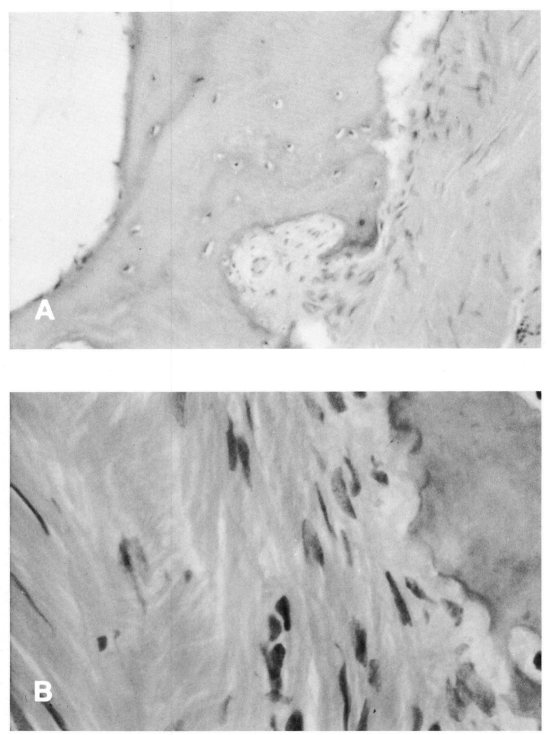

FIG. 18-6. (A) Fibrous tissue membrane at interface between methylmethacrylate and bone. Note fibrous tissue invading bony trabeculae. **(B)** Higher magnification of fibrous tissue membrane at bone cement interface. Note the absence of any inflammatory process and normal osteocytes in the lacunae of the trabecular bone.

The radiolucent line at the interface between the bone and cement corresponds to a fibrous tissue membrane. In some of our specimens it was several millimeters thick (Fig. 18-6*A*, *B*), mature or immature, with certain areas showing fibrocartilage. There is no inflammatory process at this fibrous tissue interface. Osteoclasts are rarely seen, although some foreign body giant cells may be present. Necrotic bone trabeculae are uncommon. In autopsy specimens of total knee replacements in which there was no radiolucent line on the x-ray film, sections taken from the bone—cement interface revealed no fibrous tissue or fibrocartilaginous membrane. The trabecular bone was alive, and there was no inflammatory process. Mechanically, this fibrous tissue membrane clearly represents an area of weakness between the cement and bone and is a potential site of loosening. Micromovement must occur at these interfaces when a fibrous tissue layer is interposed.

It is clear that the pathogenesis of loosening is multifactoral and remains the single most important long-term problem associated with total knee arthroplasty.

Proper patient selection, choice of prosthesis, alignment criteria, and meticulous attention to the preparation of the bony bed are critical in keeping this problem to a minimum (Fig. 18-7*A*—*G*).

TABLE 18–4. NONHINGED PROSTHESES: INCIDENCE OF SEPSIS

Author	Type of Prosthesis	%
Finerman	Anametric	1
Sledge	Duocondylar	0
Habermann	Geometric	2
Murray	Variable axis	4
Yamamoto	Kodama	0.6
Skolnick	Polycentric	2.8
Laskin	Modular	4
Pelty	Geometric/Polycentric	2
Skolnick	Geometric	1.8
Cracchiolo	Geometric	4
Moreland	ICLH	5
Sheehan	Sheehan	0.3
Kaufer	Spherocentric	2.2
Attenborough	Attenborough	1.6
Lacey	UCI	3
Riley	Geometric	0
Gschwind	GSB	2
Gunston	Gunston	5
Insall	Total condylar	1.3

INFECTION

Infection is of great concern to the orthopaedic surgeon performing implant surgery. The ravaging consequences of infection mar the expected results for both patient and surgeon (Fig. 18-8*A*—*D*).

Reports of sepsis in total knee arthroplasty vary widely, but it seems clear that a significantly higher incidence of sepsis occurs with the hinged type of prostheses compared with the less restrained types (Tables 18–3, 18–4). Theoretically, the rate of infection is influenced by the size of the implant, the foreign material used, the presence of a hematoma, the lack of viable tissue in areas adjacent to the implant, the avascular bone around the implant, the length of the surgical procedure, the operating room environment, and the experience of the surgeon.[25,92,111,117] There is also the possibility that wear on high-density polyethylene and methylmethacrylate produces reactive changes that are more conducive to infection. Dead space and hematoma formation act as sources of sepsis and frequently remain unrecognized until it has developed. Often little living tissue is directly in contact with large orthopaedic implants to combat infection. Avascularity around the bone adjacent to surgical implants and acrylic cement may exist for a considerable period of time and may be a precursor of early and even of late infections. Other significant factors in the high-risk, elderly patient who undergoes implant surgery include the patient's host-defense mechanisms, generalized nutritional status, obesity, steroid therapy, and systemic illnesses such as diabetes, chronic pulmonary and genitourinary disease, and rheumatoid arthritis.[111] All these factors have been implicated in the increased incidence of sepsis. All patients undergoing total knee replacement should be treated for any clearly defined infection, such as that of the genitourinary tract (which may not be symptomatic) prior to operation.

PROPHYLACTIC ANTIBIOTICS

In the past there has been great controversy regarding the use of prophylactic antibiotics.

(*text continued on p. 258*)

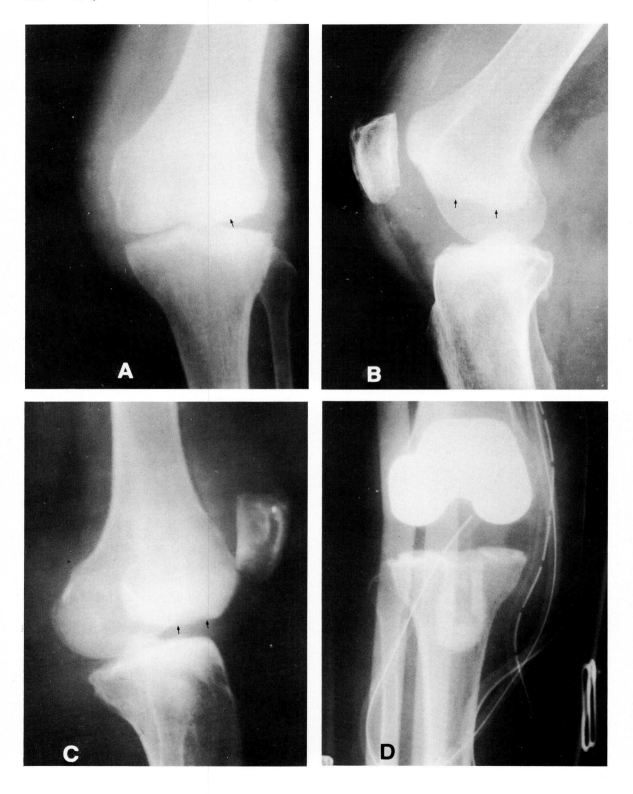

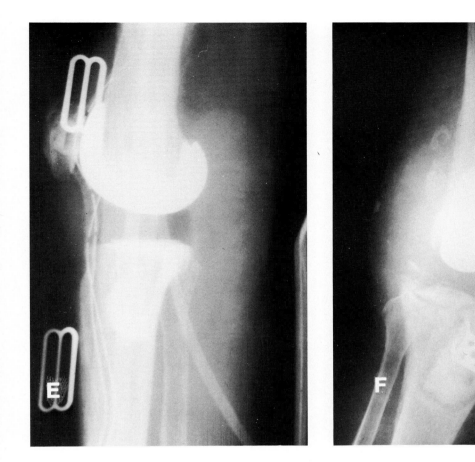

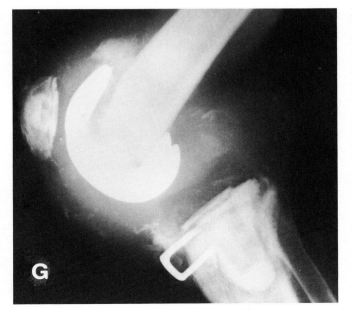

FIG. 18-7. **(A–C)** Anteroposterior, lateral, and oblique preoperative radiographs of a 60-year-old woman with loss of lateral femoral condyle in the absence of other significant arthritic changes. The radiographs are suggestive of a neuropathic joint. However, this was not suspected, and a total condylar knee replacement was performed. **(D, E)** Anteroposterior and lateral radiographs showing the postoperative appearance of the total condylar knee replacement. **(F, G)** Anteroposterior and lateral radiographs 9 months postoperatively revealing marked radiolucency at the bone cement interface of the tibial component, marked instability, soft tissue swelling with synovial hypertrophy, and heterotopic bone embedded in the synovium (seen histologically). This was subsequently found to be a neuropathic joint with infection. The staple was previously introduced when the patient sustained a patellar tendon rupture.

258

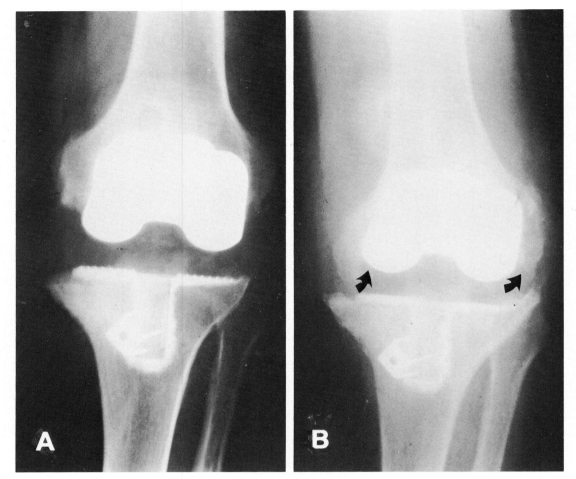

FIG. 18-8. (A) Initial anteroposterior radiograph showing total condylar knee replacement. **(B)** Late infection. Note resorption of bone about femoral component (*arrows*) and generalized soft tissue swelling. Also note high-riding patellar button compared with original placement.

The regimen for this therapy varies. Our present protocol includes 1 g of cephalosporin given intravenously just prior to the surgical incision, and 1 g given intraoperatively. This is continued intravenously for 48 hr, 1 g every 6 hr, and then discontinued unless longer use is indicated. Bacitracin, neomycin, or polymixin solution is used for irrigation intraoperatively. Opening cultures are taken routinely. Postoperatively, the drains are removed after 24 hr to 48 hr, depending on the amount of outflow. The tourniquet normally used is released prior to closure to obtain the best possible hemostasis. The compression bandage is left in place for approximately 5 days.

It is recognized that most commonly used antibiotics produce antibacterial concentrations within inflamed joints.[113] It has been shown that antibiotics are capable of penetrating wound fluid and hematomas even into the depths of the hip.[112] However, less data are available about the antibiotic penetration into deep taut hematomas around wound sites. This is obviously an area of great concern, because hematomas provide an ideal setting for bacterial growth. Some variation in serum and bone concentrations occurs with different antibiotics owing to the lower protein level in the intercellular fluid of bone. A bactericidal level is reached in bone only 30 min after in-

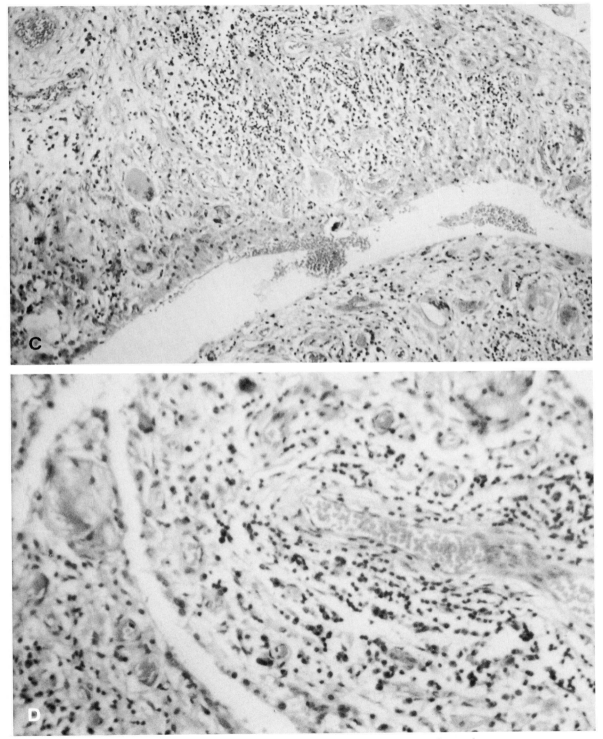

FIG. 18-8. **(C)** Microscopic appearance of infected synovium with polymorphonuclear infiltration in infected total knee replacement. **(D)** High power view of (C).

travenous administration of antibiotics. It does not, therefore, seem necessary to give antibiotics several days prior to surgery to penetrate normal bone. Whether local antibiotics play a significant role in the prevention of subsequent infection is not clear, but they may be of value.[66,126] One of the beneficial effects of local irrigation is débridement. When irrigating an elderly patient with an antibiotic such as polymixin, bacitracin, or neomycin, caution is needed because local absorption of the antibiotic may be dangerous. Antibiotic-impregnated cement has been more widely used in Europe than in the United States. The antibiotic is released from the cement over a long period of time and is apparently affected by the concentration gradient—that is, material lodged within the interstices of the cement is exposed to body fluids and, if not bound, passes into the surrounding fluids and tissues. When used in this manner, antibiotics should be in powder form and not in aqueous solution because the latter decreases the strength of the composite. Studies by Levin and Marks and associates have shown local effectiveness of various antibiotics used in the cement without significant alteration in the cement properties.[91,98]

Antibiotic-Impregnated Cement

Hill and his co-workers feel that intravenous and topical antibiotics play a more important role in achieving a bactericidal concentration in the exposed tissues during surgery and that antibiotic-impregnated cement does not fulfil this role.[66] Elson and associates reported that the concentrations of gentamicin and furadin in antibiotic-impregnated cement were sufficient to penetrate dead cortical tissue.[32] Buchholz and Engelbrecht have shown that antibiotic cement reduced the incidence of infection in patients with total hip replacement.[10] Significant data in total knee arthroplasty using antibiotic-impregnated cement have not yet appeared.

RISK FACTORS

Fitzgerald and his colleagues found 30% positive intraoperative cultures in total hip re-

placement.[39] The number rose to 38% when there had been prior surgery. Our experience with total hip replacement also revealed a significant percentage of positive cultures, higher when surgery had already been performed. Peterson and associates, in reviewing 1597 consecutive total hip arthroplasties, concluded that there was a significant risk factor in those patients who had a positive intraoperative culture and had undergone previous surgery.[116] In 2-yr to 5-yr follow-ups, this group of patients had a higher incidence of infection. We have not found a similar occurrence of positive intraoperative cultures in our patients after total knee replacement.

The incidence of deep sepsis reported in total knee replacements of all types ranges from less than 1% to 14%. If superficial infections, delayed wound healing, and wound drainage are included, this rate increases significantly.

Scott and co-workers reported wound drainage in 21% of patients after total condylar knee replacement,[127] and Cracchiolo noted 12% wound drainage after geometric arthroplasty.[24] Skolnick and his associates reported delayed wound healing in 16% after polycentric knee arthroplasty;[138] Lettin and colleagues described delayed healing in 28% with the Stanmore Hinge;[90] and Moreland and co-workers noted a delay in wound healing in 22% with the ICLH prosthesis.[107] The newer designs of metal-to-plastic total knee replacements apparently have a lower incidence of infection than the older hinged-type of prosthesis.[68] Our overall infection rate in over 200 cases of nonhinged arthroplasties is approximately 2%.

Since we have begun utilizing a straight, longitudinal skin incision over the midpatella instead of a median parapatellar incision, we have been able to decrease local wound complications of superficial skin slough and delayed healing. Care must be taken when planning an incision if the patient has had prior knee surgery. Use the prior incision if possible to avoid devitalizing an area of skin between two incisions. We have had two skin sloughs in patients who had prior median parapatellar incisions and straight longitudinal incisions on their second surgical procedure, creating an area of skin between the two incisions that sloughed and required skin grafting.

If a lateral release is anticipated, we place the straight, longitudinal incision slightly lateral to the midline of the patella. Undermining of the skin should be avoided, especially in patients with rheumatoid arthritis, and the skin flaps should be kept as thick as possible to obtain adequate coverage of the prosthetic components.

LATE INFECTIONS

Late infections in total knee arthroplasty have not been as common as they are in total hip arthroplasty but do occur in sufficient numbers to present problems. If the infection is diagnosed early, an attempt should be made to salvage the knee by thorough débridement and an effective irrigation system, together with appropriate antibiotic therapy. If this fails, reoperation is necessary for the removal of the components, including the methylmethacrylate, and for a thorough débridement of all tissues. We have not revised these infected prosthetic failures with immediate replacement arthroplasty but have instituted any reconstructive surgery on the basis of the clinical and laboratory findings. Often an immediate arthrodesis is attempted, especially when there is marked involvement of bone and gram-negative organisms are cultured. We find that patients infected with gram-negative organisms have a worse prognosis. This has also been the experience of others in salvage of infected total hip replacements.[67,93] Compression arthrodesis can be used as a salvage procedure in failed total knee replacement; however, it is not often easily achieved.

We have had two failures out of five attempts at arthrodesis, both following removal of a hinged prosthesis. Failure is due to the amount of bone destruction after the prosthesis and cement have been removed. Often one is left with a cortical shell on the tibial and femoral sides. The more constrained the original prosthesis, the more difficult the arthrodesis or any other salvage procedure. Hagemann and associates reported failure of fusion in 5 out of 14 patients.[56] Deburge, in reviewing 292 GUEPAR prostheses, reported 12 attempted arthrodeses resulting in three solid fusions, seven nonunions, and two deaths.[28] The successful arthrodesis rate following failed total knee arthroplasty is markedly lower than when the knee is fused by other conditions.

We have encountered late hematogenous infections in three cases. Two patients with rheumatoid arthritis became acutely ill 28 months and 50 months, respectively, after total knee replacement. Both patients were elderly and presented with toxicity and septicemia. Aspiration of the knee joint, which was asymptomatic at the time of admission, revealed no abnormal findings suggesting infection, but the knee subsequently became infected. One patient who was diabetic had an infected carbuncle, which was the source of subsequent seeding into the knee. The other two patients had urinary tract septicemia with subsequent seeding into the knee arthroplasty. In two of these patients the joint was salvaged by antibiotic therapy, débridement, and aspiration, and the third patient had a successful arthrodesis.

D'Ambrosia and associates[27] reported three fatal cases following spread of hematogenous infection.[11,26] Hall reported a late infection of a total knee replacement secondary to a urinary tract infection.[57] It is clear that the prosthetic joint is at risk during an episode of bacteremia. The rheumatoid patient on steroids may be especially susceptible. We insist that all patients after total joint replacement take prophylactic antibiotics when undergoing any surgical procedure such as dental extractions or genitourinary surgery or manipulation, much like the patient with rheumatic heart disease. Careful attention to eradication of all septic foci is important, and long-term antibiotic therapy may be necessary.

THROMBOPHLEBITIS AND PULMONARY EMBOLISM

Thromboembolism is a common complication of lower extremity surgery.[19,36,60,61,97,114,142] The elderly patient who undergoes extensive surgery of the lower extremity and subsequent immobilization is at high risk for thromboembolic disease. The incidence of thrombophlebitis following knee operations was reported by Cohen and co-workers to be 57%.[19] Nine percent of this group developed pulmonary emboli. McKenna and associates reported thromboembolic disease in 53% of patients undergoing total knee replacement, of whom 10% had pulmonary emboli.[97] The diagnosis was made by ^{125}I fibrinogen scanning and venography. Nylander reported 87% of patients with tibial fractures had venographic abnormalities.[114] Lynch's findings showed that thrombophlebitis occurred in 40% of patients after total knee replacement and pulmonary emboli in 12%.[96]

The unreliability of clinical diagnosis of deep venous thrombosis has been emphasized repeatedly.[55,62,87] Physical examination of the extremities fails to detect 50% to 90% of thrombi in the deep venous system; conversely, Hull and co-workers have shown that when physical signs of thrombosis are present, the diagnosis is incorrect in as many as 50% of cases.[69] The clinical diagnosis of pulmonary emboli is equally treacherous. The initiating mechanisms of thromboembolism are obscure, the clinical recognition is elusive, the recurrence rate is high, and the mortality is unpredictable.

A firm diagnosis of deep vein thrombosis must be established by an objective test. Modern diagnostic methods differentiate between potentially dangerous thigh thrombi and less dangerous calf thrombi. The latter are less prone to cause clinically significant pulmonary emboli unless they extend into the popliteal area or the thigh. Orthopaedic patients are more prone to develop thigh and pelvic thrombi, which may be life-threatening, than are general surgical patients, and many patients undergoing total knee replacement are in the high-risk category—elderly, obese, and having cardiovascular or venous disease.

Improved methods of detection employing fibrinogen uptake show that most thrombi form shortly after surgery (within 48 hr) and may be present intraoperatively. The recorded incidence of pulmonary emboli varies according to the method of detection. Autopsy studies of patients with tibial fractures revealed pulmonary emboli in 60%.[129] Cases of fatal pulmonary emboli in orthopaedic patients have ranged from 0 to 38%.[124]

Techniques available for the diagnosis of deep venous thrombosis include venography, which gives the highest accuracy rate in the diagnosis of deep venous thrombosis, greater than 95%. Iodine-125 fibrinogen uptake and its incorporation into the fibrin of a developing blood clot allow the recognition of early thrombi by external scanning of the lower limbs.[82] This procedure is essentially noninvasive and has an accuracy rate approaching 90%. It is less accurate, however, in the proximal thigh; a significant shortcoming for the orthopaedic surgeon.[63]

Cuff impedence phlebography, pneumatic plethysmography, and Doppler ultrasound methods can detect obstruction of venous outflow. These tests are somewhat less reliable in the diagnosis of deep venous thrombosis but are noninvasive and therefore appealing. They have an accuracy rate of approximately 70% to 80%. The diagnosis of pulmonary emboli can be established definitively by selective pulmonary angiography, pulmonary perfusion, and ventilation scanning. Arterial blood gas determination is useful as a screening test for pulmonary embolism, because PO_2 is rare in the presence of this condition. Preoperative blood gas studies are frequently helpful as a baseline in patients with pulmonary disease. The diagnosis of pulmonary emboli should be established by objective tests to avoid long-term anticoagulation that might be given inappropriately.

Prophylactic measures in the form of anticoagulation treatment should be taken after total knee arthroplasty. These include antithrombotic drugs such as warfarin and other oral anticoagulants. The merit of these agents is well recognized. Heparin is highly effective in the prevention of thrombosis and pulmonary emboli; whether it is equally serviceable in the form of "mini heparin" in the high-risk orthopaedic patient is questionable.[35,47,58,63] Dextran, however, appears to answer the purpose. The use of aspirin is attractive because it is relatively easy to administer and has few complications as a rule. Various reports indicate its usefulness in low and high doses, but the latter need further investigation.

Hemorrhagic complications remain the major side-effect of prophylactic antithrombotic agents. When such agents are used, one must carefully monitor the dosage and critically evaluate whether their administration is indicated in certain patients. Physical measures such as early ambulation, elastic stockings, and elevation of the legs should be carried out routinely, but they will not eliminate venous thromboembolism. Calf pneumatic compression and electrical stimulation of the calf muscles have also been evaluated.[20]

Prevention is the hallmark of the treatment of thromboembolic disease. Unless definitive studies such as venography or fibrinogen scanning tests are performed, there will be inadequate data for judging the incidence of thromboembolic disease following total knee arthroplasty.

PERONEAL PALSY

Peroneal nerve injury following total knee arthroplasty was more frequent when hinged prostheses were used.[2,5,49,52,78] Sheehan reported five transient peroneal palsies in 135 cases,[131] and Insall and associates noted four —a rate of less than 1% in their total condylar knee series.[77] Moreland and his colleagues had one case in 84 ICLH knees.[107]

The condition is more likely to occur in patients with significant flexion and valgus deformities,[138] when it follows traction on and stretching of the nerve. Postoperative dressings, splints, or traction apparatus must be applied carefully because they may be causative factors, as may pressure on the nerve while lying in certain positions of external rotation. An effort should be made to control external rotation and to check the patient carefully for nerve dysfunction in the recovery room. We have encountered peroneal nerve palsy primarily with the hinged prostheses; all cases have been transient and the patients subsequently recovered fully. Caution must be used with the tightly applied knee immobilizer

with Velcro straps about the head of the fibula.

If peroneal function has not returned by the time the patient is ready for discharge, a simple ankle–foot orthosis should be applied to prevent deformity.

PENETRATION OF THE SHAFT BY THE PROSTHESIS

Penetration of the shaft has been more of a problem when large intramedullary stems are used, and these are more frequently seen with the Walldius and Shiers hinged prosthesis. We reported a case of a Walldius prosthesis penetrating the femoral shaft that was not recognized until an x-ray film had been taken (Fig. 18-9).[52] Intraoperative radiographs are helpful if there is any significant preoperative deformity or when there is difficulty in inserting the stem. A spherocentric implant penetrated the posterior aspect of the tibia in one of our patients but did not influence the final result. Loosening of the cement mass can lead to erosion of the intramedullary canal with subsequent penetration, and loosening of the prosthesis itself can create a similar situation. Freeman, Phillips, and Wilson have all reported femoral penetrations.[46,118,154]

PATELLAR PROBLEMS
PATELLOFEMORAL PAIN

It has been our recent policy to resurface the patella in all total knee replacements. The clinical results showed that patellofemoral pain decreased and we have not encountered significant problems with this procedure. Patellofemoral pain has been reported in virtually all series in which the patella was not replaced. Sledge and Ewald, using the duocondylar prosthesis, reported a 3.5% incidence of patellofemoral pain,[136] which was the reason for half the revisions in that series. Marmor and Ranawat and associates also reported a significant number of patellofemoral problems with similar prosthetic designs.[99,119] In 300 patellar resurfacings, however, Sledge and Ewald report that none has loosened.[136] Insall and his colleagues had three patellar loosenings and one fracture, accounting for a complication rate of less than 1%.[77] Reoperation of the total condylar knees for other reasons revealed no evidence of wear on the polyethylene patellar replacement. In 39 cases in which the patella was not replaced, three required subsequent revision because of patellar pain. Freeman and his colleagues, using the ICLH prosthesis, reported front-of-the-knee pain suggestive of patellofemoral pain in 42% of cases.[43]

Patellectomy should be avoided, because the problems after this procedure, which is associated with tibiofemoral replacement, have been significant.

PATELLAR SUBLUXATION AND DISLOCATION

Subluxation of the patella is a problem when inadequate attention is given to patellar stability and position at the time of surgery and is especially apt to occur with the GUEPAR prosthesis because routine lateral release was usually performed in conjunction with its insertion to allow the patella to assume an appropriate position. Transplantation of the tibial tubercle had to be performed on a 72-year-old woman who had a chronically dislocated patella after a lateral release had failed.

Reefing of the medial retinacula is performed in certain cases. The GUEPAR hinge has been modified for better adaptation to the shape of the patella. The use of a patellar implant with the GUEPAR prosthesis has relieved the problem of pain.[29,101] Moreland and associates reported 5% patellar subluxation with the ICLH prosthesis.[107] A significant degree of valgus deformity or flexion contracture as well as external rotation deformity is frequently associated with tight lateral contractures, and these must be surgically released.

Erosion of the patella against the femoral component can cause symptoms and requires revision surgery. Lacey reported lateral patellar erosion in 25% of cases with the UCI prosthesis.[86] On rare occasions a patellectomy is necessary because there is insufficient bone stock for a replacement.

QUADRICEPS AND PATELLAR TENDON RUPTURE

Our one case of quadriceps tendon rupture occurred 3 years after inserting a Walldius prosthesis and was related to wear of the tendon against the femoral metallic component. On exploration, the entire quadriceps mechanism was greenish gray in color and necrotic.

Arden had five cases of quadriceps tendon rupture and nine (4.7%) with significant extensor lag.[2,3]

Patellar tendon rupture occurred in two cases of total condylar knee replacement—

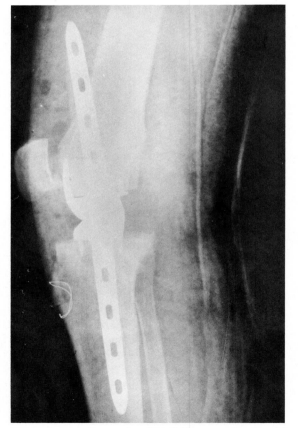

FIG. 18-9. Radiograph of Walldius prosthesis with femoral stem protruding through anterior cortex of femur. This problem was recognized postoperatively and subsequently revised.

one required stapling after a fall, and another followed strenuous exercise in a stiff knee that resulted in a 35° extensor lag. Avulsion of the patellar tendon has been reported by others.[43,101,154,158]

PATELLAR FRACTURE

Moreland and co-workers reported five patellar fractures with 84 ICLH prostheses.[107] Insall and his associates had one patellar fracture in over 400 total condylar prostheses.[77] We have not encountered this complication.

WEAR AND TISSUE REACTION

A certain degree of wear occurs in all metal-to-polyethylene total knee articulations, primarily in the high-density polyethylene. Major factors responsible for this type of wear are the amount of stress per unit area of contact and the range and rate of excursion of the articulating surfaces. Wide contact areas are advantageous in reducing the stress per unit area, but a broad area of contact increases the chance of entrapment of wear particles. Determining the ideal size for the contact area is difficult because there are advantages and disadvantages for the varying sizes of the components. Stress concentrations seem to have a greater effect and may be more detrimental

than particulate matter entrapment on the "runner" surface of the tibia. Both, however, probably play a significant role in failure.

Shearing effects occur when the load is asymmetrically concentrated on one side of the tibial surface and not in a vertical direction to the prosthesis. In our review of geometric prostheses,[53] malalignment of the component parts, primarily in varus, was a significant factor in failure and wear. In three of four failed polycentric prostheses studied by Shoji and associates the cause was malalignment.[135] We have observed extensive wear on our geometric prostheses that were removed because of symptomatic loosening. Marked erosion and loss of polyethylene were evident on the edges of the tibial component (Fig. 18-10).

Wear can be defined as removal of material from a bearing surface, which can be damaged without removal of material when a polymer surface suffers local deformation or flows owing to high stresses in a nonconforming situation. This may reduce the effectiveness of the bearing but is not wear in the true sense of the term.

Mechanical wear includes the following: (1) Adhesive wear occurs when local contacts on opposing gliding surfaces form a junction that fractures, and particle matter is either released or transferred from one surface to another. Manifestations of adhesive wear are

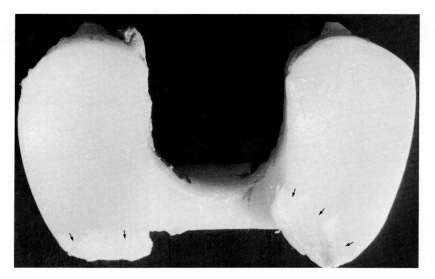

FIG. 18-10. Tibial surface of geometric prosthesis showing gross deformation and wear at anterior aspect of condylar surfaces (*arrows*). Also note methylmethacrylate impregnation.

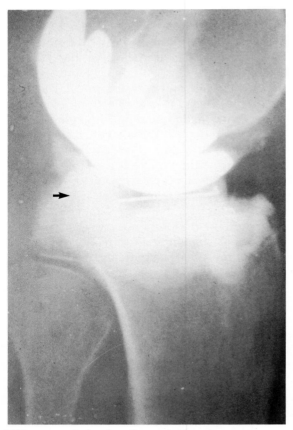

FIG. 18-11. Lateral radiograph showing excess cement posteriorly in geometric total knee replacement.

seen on the polyethylene surface as "scoring" or "scuffing." (2) Two-body abrasive wear occurs when changes on the metal surface cut or burrow into the softer polyethylene material. (3) Three-body abrasive wear indicates a third body in the form of interposed particles between the two gliding surfaces that act on one or both of the surfaces, depending on their hardness. These particles may originate from the original surfaces, or they may be remnants of methylmethacrylate on the tibial polyethylene surface.

Meticulous removal of all excess methylmethacrylate around the component parts is imperative to decrease the potential for remnants of methylmethacrylate to adhere to the tibial runners, thereby producing increased wear and friction between the bearing sur-

faces. Often excess cement gets into the posterior recesses of the knee joint and cannot be visualized without a radiograph (Fig. 18-11). Excess cement confers no benefit but is detrimental because it is a potential cause of future failure of the knee arthroplasty (Fig. 18-12*A*, *B*). Particles (cementophytes) break away and fall into the joint, impregnating the tibial polyethylene. In reviewing our failed geometric knees, we found marked evidence of methylmethacrylate impregnation, with extensive wear and deformation of the tibial components and pitting and gouging up to several millimeters in width and 1 mm to 2 mm in depth (Fig. 18-13). Scoring in all the tibial surfaces was seen. The extent of the area of wear showed that the contact was localized in some cases, while in others there was marked shearing and loss of substance. To avoid leaving excess cement posteriorly, we routinely cement the tibial component first, so that adequate access to the posterior recesses of the joint can allow removal of all excess cement. If there are any doubts, an x-ray film will visualize the cement. Freeman and associates showed that cement was present behind the knee in 60% of cases.[45]

Scanning electron microscopy of the tibial surfaces revealed rippling, cracking, scuffing, and three-body abrasive wear (Fig. 18-14*A*– *C*). When methylmethacrylate becomes embedded on the polyethylene surface it has a very abrasive effect, and sheets of polyethylene are drawn up from the surface. The use of carbon-impregnated, high-density polyethylene is being evaluated to see if this will enhance the wear properties of the polyethylene.

SOFT TISSUE REACTION

There were extensive changes in the soft tissues surrounding the failed implants we retrieved. One failed geometric prosthesis removed for aseptic loosening revealed macroscopically a polypoid mass of synovium resembling pigmented villonodular synovitis (Fig. 18-3*F*). Microscopic examination under polarized light (Fig. 18-15*A*, *B*) revealed large amounts of debris of polyethylene and methylmethacrylate, marked histiocyte and giant

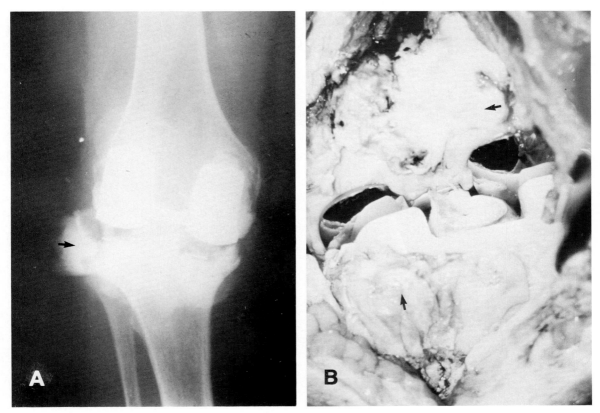

FIG. 18-12. (A) Radiograph of geometric total knee arthroplasty. There is malalignment and excessive amount of methylmethacrylate, especially around the tibial component. **(B)** At time of revision surgery, excessive amounts of methylmethacrylate are visible outside the confines of the prosthetic components.

FIG. 18-13. Tibial surface of geometric prosthesis showing gross pitting and methylmethacrylate impregnation as well as deformation of condylar surfaces.

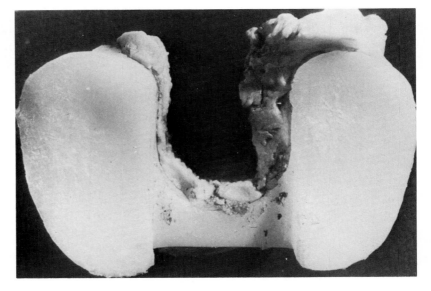

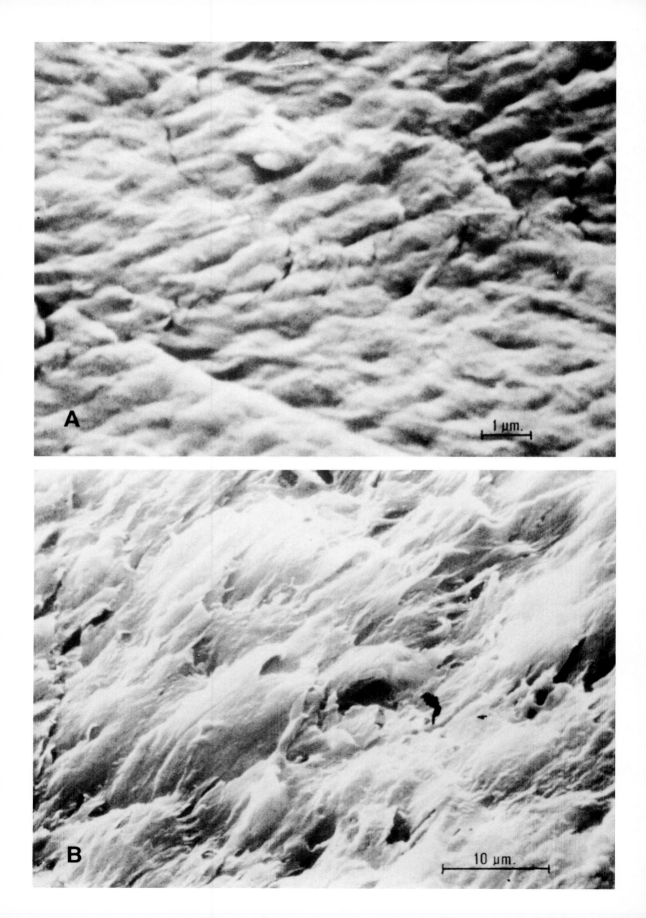

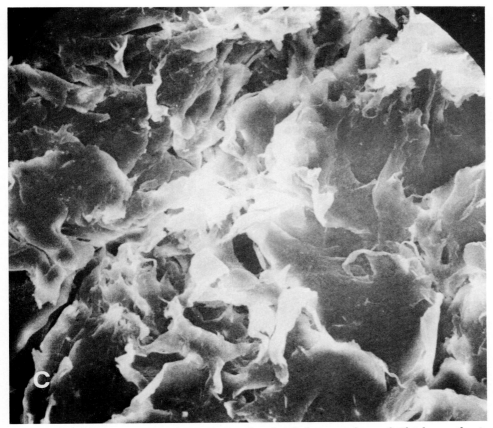

FIG. 18-14. (A–C) Electron microscopy of polyethylene surface of tibial prosthesis showing evidence of (A) rippling, (B) scuffing, and (C) disorganization.

cell reactions, and large clefts (where methylmethacrylate particles were leached out in the preparative process) surrounded by flattened giant cells (Fig. 18-16).

The same microscopic picture was seen in all our aseptic failed geometric knees. An extensive foreign body giant cell reaction but no acute inflammatory response was present around the debris of polyethylene and methylmethacrylate. The polyethylene particles, which were easily visualized under polarized light, varied in size and shape but were usually smaller than the methylmethacrylate particles. The methylmethacrylate was abundant, and when the prostheses were grossly loose, sheets of histiocytes were frequently seen. A fibrous tissue membrane was found in most cases at the bone–cement interface. It was noninflammatory, and the surrounding

trabecular bone was alive. It varied in thickness up to several millimeters.

Wroblewski reported that wear of high-density polyethylene, resulting from contact by bone and cartilage, shed large volumes of polyethylene into the knee joint.[157] The synovium had a polypoid appearance. Polyethylene does not react well to articulation with cortical bone or with degenerative cartilage. Shedding of the polyethylene and a giant cell synovitis were described when a patellar polyethylene resurfacing was allowed to articulate with degenerated cartilage.[37]

METAL SENSITIVITY

In three cases of hinged prostheses (two Walldius and one GUEPAR), the tissue surround-

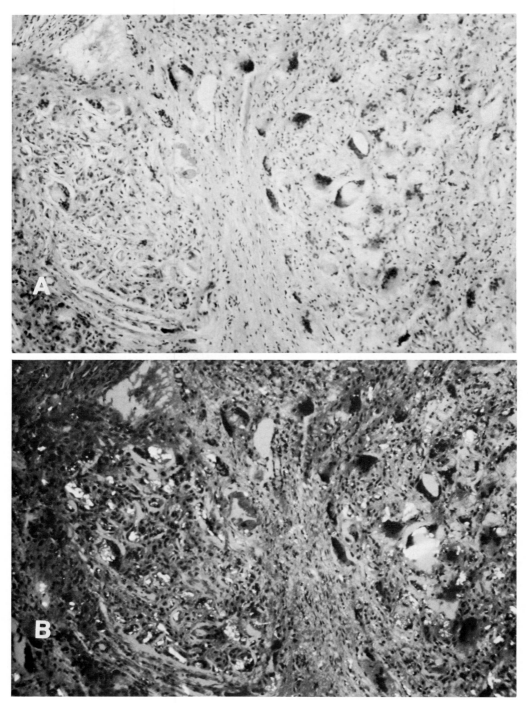

FIG. 18-15. **(A)** Microscopic view of synovium with hematoxylin and eosin stain under regular light shows marked giant cell reaction. **(B)** Same specimen under polarized light reveals birefringent particulate debris of high-density polyethylene and methylmethacrylate.

ing the loose implant was black or blackish gray, and in one case the intramedullary canals were black, as was every area of bone and soft tissue in contact with the metal components (Fig. 18-17A –C). Both tissues and capsule were blackish in color and showed signs of necrosis. Joint fluid revealed evidence of metallic debris measuring 1 μm to 5 μm, and under electron microscopy the metallic particles were being phagocytized. These cases apparently represent a severe sensitivity to metal. All the prostheses were loose, but there was little evidence of inflammation. Whether the loosening was secondary to metal sensitivity has not been conclusively shown.

Metal sensitivity as a cause of sterile loosening has been reported by Evans and associates.[33] The studies of Brown and his colleagues did not support this conclusion.[7]

Sensitive lymphokine assays for migration inhibition factor and bastogenic factor were done but were positive in only 1 out of 20 assays. Their histological specimens revealed findings similar to ours. Patch tests to chromium, nickel, cobalt, and methylmethacrylate monomer were negative in Brown and associates' series. These materials are all capable of causing skin sensitivity.

MASSIVE OSTEOLYSIS

Massive osteolysis has been reported by Harris and co-workers as localized bone resorption following total hip replacement.[64] We have encountered it on a number of occasions around both the femoral and acetabular components. It is less frequently seen follow-

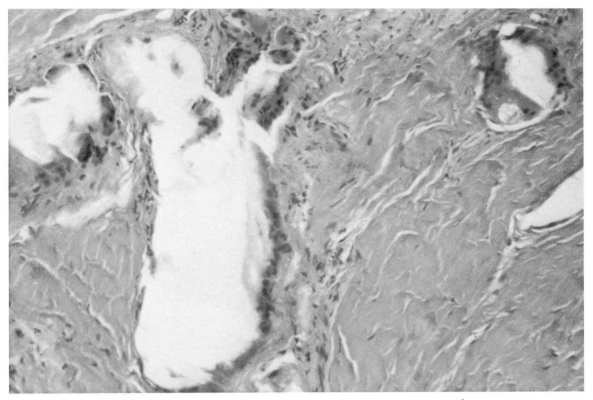

FIG. 18-16. High power microscopic appearance of synovial tissue reaction in a loosened geometric tibial component showing a large cleft (representing methylmethacrylate that had been dissolved in preparation) surrounded by flattened giant cells.

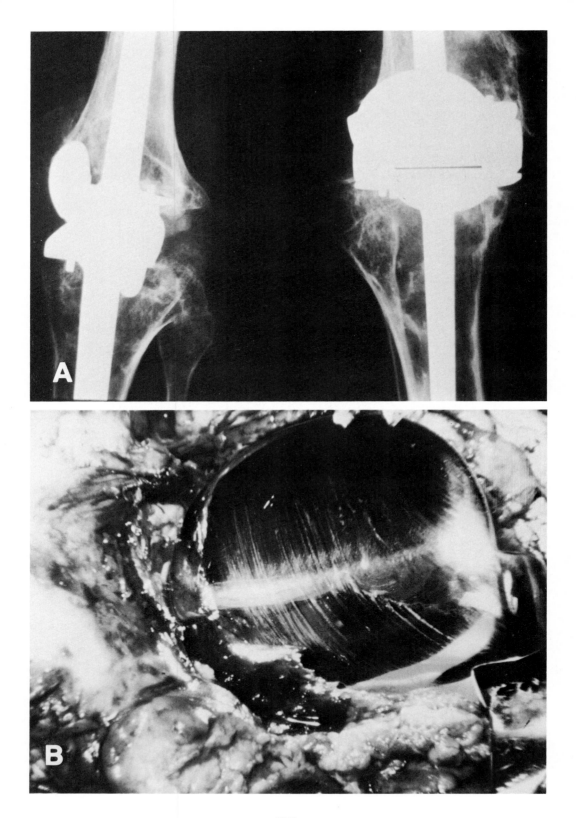

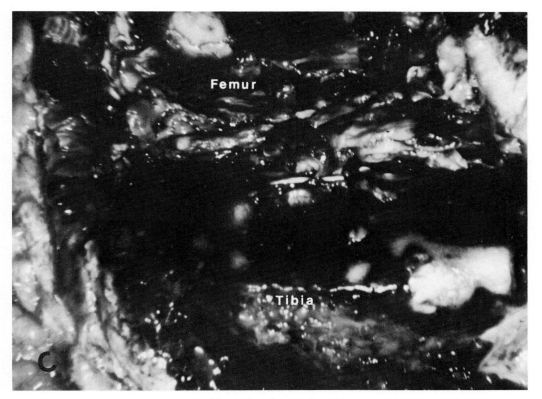

FIG. 18-17. (A) Anteroposterior and lateral radiographs of knee in a 56-year-old man who had a painful Walldius prosthesis. Note generalized radiolucency around the femur and tibia. (B) Severe metal reaction at time of exploration. (C) Blackened areas at all sites of contact of the metallic prosthesis with bone and soft tissues were seen at surgery after the prosthesis was removed from the tibia and femur.

ing total knee arthroplasty. The exact cause is not known, but Scales and Harris and associates believe that the differential motion between the cement and bone, coupled with some effect of the fragmented cement, plays a role in stimulating resorption.[64,125] Methylmethacrylate sensitivity was considered unlikely by Charnley and associates.[14,16,18] Infection must always be considered and excluded.

We encountered a 52-year-old man with generalized rheumatoid arthritis who had a Walldius prosthesis 8 years old; the prosthesis functioned well for some time and then started causing pain. Radiographs demonstrated massive osteolytic loosening and failure (Fig. 18-18A–E). It is possible that when the bone–cement interface fails and the cement and prosthesis become excessively loose within

the medullary canal, a "sandpaper"-like effect is created, abrading the bone in its path by excessive motion. Microscopically, there is no evidence of acute infection. Massive amounts of loose methylmethacrylate are found in the soft tissues, capsule, and synovium.

FRACTURES

Fractures of the prostheses have been observed by many authors.[81,89,132,133,134] They have occurred primarily with the hinged prostheses. The Herbert prosthesis suffered a number of fatigue fractures at the stem–prosthesis junction,[110] but this has not been a significant problem in the nonconstrained designs. We

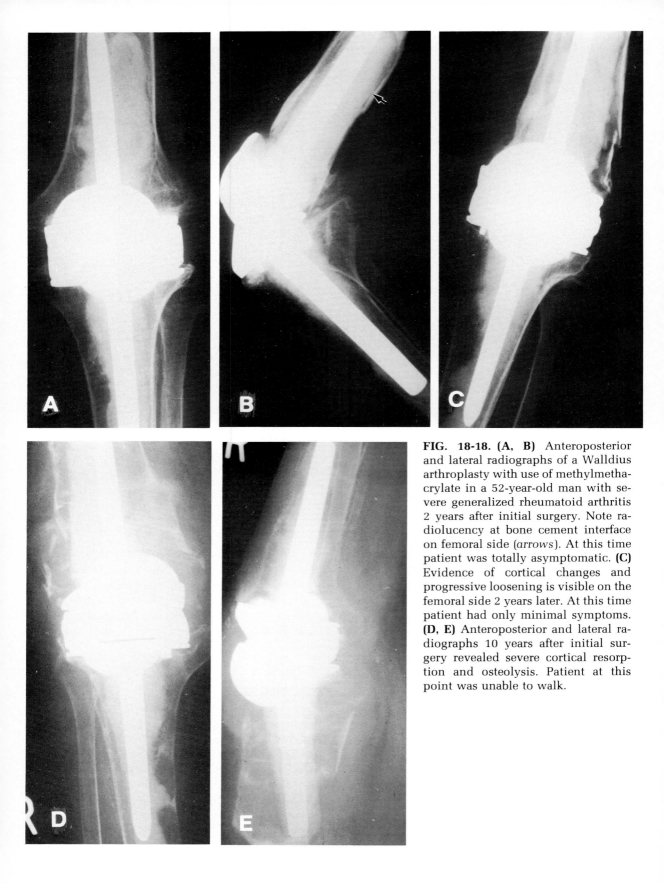

FIG. 18-18. (A, B) Anteroposterior and lateral radiographs of a Walldius arthroplasty with use of methylmethacrylate in a 52-year-old man with severe generalized rheumatoid arthritis 2 years after initial surgery. Note radiolucency at bone cement interface on femoral side (*arrows*). At this time patient was totally asymptomatic. **(C)** Evidence of cortical changes and progressive loosening is visible on the femoral side 2 years later. At this time patient had only minimal symptoms. **(D, E)** Anteroposterior and lateral radiographs 10 years after initial surgery revealed severe cortical resorption and osteolysis. Patient at this point was unable to walk.

have encountered two fatigue fractures of the tibial component in geometric prostheses that were loose.

FRACTURES OF THE FEMUR AND TIBIA

Shaft fractures were frequently associated with intramedullary hinged prostheses[3,46,78,118,154] and can usually be treated with traction. However, we have utilized internal fixation with a plate when necessary. If the prosthesis is loose, revision surgery is often necessary.

Supracondylar fractures have been treated by traction, casting or bracing, or internal fixation. It is critical to revise knees in which the prosthesis has become loose.

We have seen several stress fractures of the tibial shaft without loosening or displacement of the prosthesis; these have healed with splinting or casting.

Fractures that are secondary to overload of the tibial component are obvious and often result in sudden onset of pain. However, the exact cause of pain related to such activities as getting up from a sitting position or beginning ambulation may be difficult to analyze. These symptoms may well be caused by fractures that are not obvious on routine radiographs, and tomograms may be helpful. Simple immobilization or rest for a period of time with external support may allow these small fractures or microfractures to heal, and further loosening may not occur. Collapse or compression fracture of the supporting bone may result from weakening due to the poor quality of the subchondral bone, a condition especially characteristic of the rheumatoid patient.

Rand and Coventry, reviewing stress fractures seen at the Mayo Clinic, found 18 fractures after total knee arthroplasty—9 of the tibial plateau following geometric arthroplasty and 9 following polycentric arthroplasty.[120] Three had stress fractures of the tibia, and 15 had fractures of the medial tibial plateau. Varus malalignment was seen in a significant number of these fractures. Lotke and Ecker reported five fractures of the medial tibial plateau with the geometric knee.[94] These experiences as well as ours indicate that stress overload occurs on the medial side of the tibia when varus malalignment is pres-

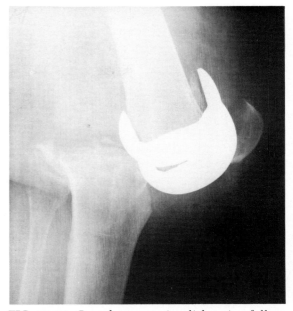

FIG. 18-19. Complete posterior dislocation following knee arthroplasty.

ent. It must be emphasized that meticulous attention to alignment and ligamentous balance would reduce the incidence of these stress fractures.

INSTABILITY

True dislocation following total knee arthroplasty is rare but does occasionally occur (Figs. 18-19, 18-20A–C).[8,9,21] Skolnick and associates reported dislocations (1.4%) in the polycentric knee and concluded that severe preoperative instability is a contraindication for this type of prosthesis.[138] We have encountered one such case following trauma. However, subluxation is not uncommon.[8,9,21] Insall and associates reported a 1.3% subluxation rate in the total condylar knee (Fig. 18-21A, B).[77]

Depending on the degree of instability, conservative management may suffice. Minimal laxity may be controlled by proper strengthening of the quadriceps and hamstrings. An orthosis or revision surgery for the more unstable knee may be necessary.

Proper selection of the prosthesis in the unstable knee should provide stability without

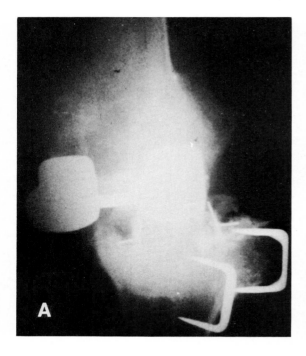

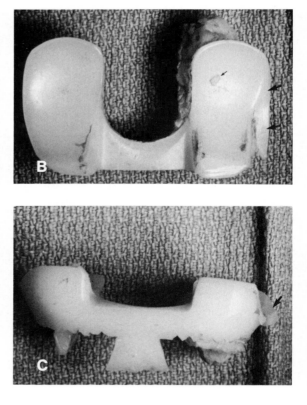

FIG. 18-20. (A) Radiograph revealing lateral dislocation following geometric total knee replacement. **(B, C)** Two views of this failed geometric tibial component. Note methylmethacrylate impregnation on condylar surfaces (*small arrow*) and marked flaring and distortion of condylar surface (*large arrow*) secondary to dislocation.

the need to use a hinged design. The stabilo-condylar, spherocentric, and Attenborough prostheses are suitable for this type of knee, as is the helicoid design.

Care taken at the time of surgery to balance the ligamentous structures and to use a tibial component of the proper height may well reduce the incidence of instability (Fig. 18-22).

There is controversy about whether the posterior cruciate ligament should be saved or sacrificed. The main advantage in saving the ligament is not stability but to achieve a greater range of motion.[77] The posterior cruciate ligament causes the femoral condyles to roll backward upon the tibia, thereby increasing flexion.

INFREQUENT COMPLICATIONS

Myositis ossificans occurred in the distal femur in two cases, one following manipulation of a total condylar knee arthroplasty (Figs. 18-23, 18-24). After further manipulation, the patient was able to maintain full extension and 90° of flexion.

Synovial herniation presented in one patient with a Walldius prosthesis 7 months after the procedure. Attempted repair resulted in a synovial fistula that closed spontaneously without incident.[52]

Bolt extrusion, seen with the hinged prosthesis, has not been a recent problem.[2]

FIG. 18-21. (A) Total condylar knee replacement shows no subluxation when anterior stress is applied. **(B)** When posterior stress is applied, there is posterior subluxation of the tibia.

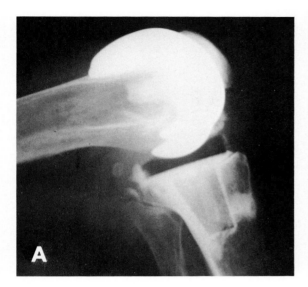

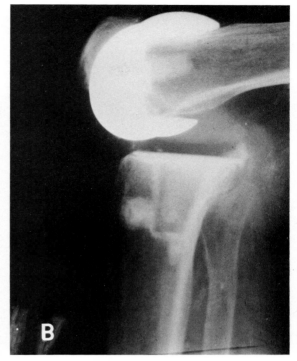

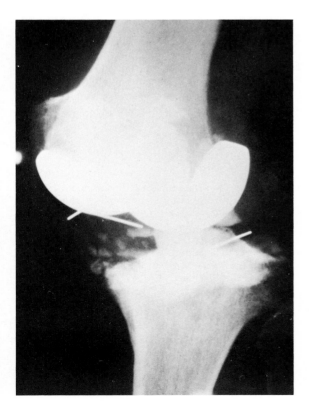

FIG. 18-22. Rotary instability of the knee following arthroplasty. Note loss of congruence of the wire markers on the tibial component. The tibial component was also fractured.

CONCLUSION

Great strides in the design, technique, and understanding of total knee arthroplasty have been made during the last 10 years, but much remains to be done. The results and complications of total knee replacement need to be continually assessed. The knee is a more complex joint than the hip and requires precision in its replacement. In the words of one author, "Remarkable advances have been made and there is now reason for cautious optimism."[150]

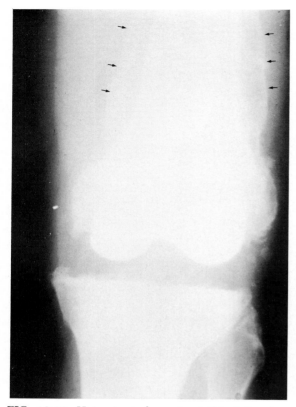

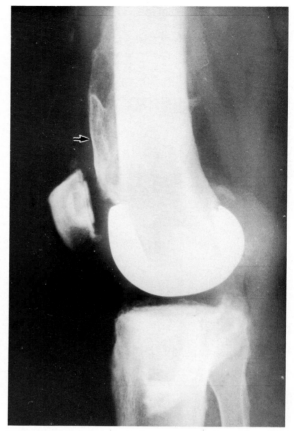

FIG. 18-23. Heterotopic bone is visible following manipulation of a total condylar knee arthroplasty in a very obese man with osteoarthritis. After manipulation he had extensive bleeding into the knee. Two years after surgery, he had 90° of flexion and full extension without symptoms.

FIG. 18-24. Heterotopic bone seen on lateral radiograph in a 65-year-old woman who had an uneventful total knee arthroplasty. She was asymptomatic and had 90° of flexion and complete extension.

REFERENCES

1. **Andersson GBJ, Freeman MAR, Swanson SAV:** Loosening of the cemented acetabular cup in total hip replacement. J Bone Joint Surg 54A:590, 1972
2. **Arden GP:** Total knee replacement. Clin Orthop 94:92, 1973
3. **Arden GP:** Complications of total knee replacement and their treatment. In: The Knee Joint. International Congress Series, 324:221. Amsterdam, Excerpta Medica, 1974
4. **Attenborough CG:** The Attenborough total knee replacement. J Bone Joint Surg 60B:320, 1978
5. **Bain AM:** Replacement of the knee joint with the Walldius prosthesis using cement fixation. Clin Orthop 94:65, 1973
6. **Bargren JH, Freeman MAR, Swanson SAV et al:** ICLH (Freeman, Swanson) arthroplasty in treatment of arthritic knee. Clin Orthop 120:65, 1976
7. **Brown GC, Lockshin MD, Salvati EA et al:** Sensitivity to metal as a possible cause of sterile loosening after cobalt–chromium total hip arthroplasty. J Bone Joint Surg 59A:164, 1977
8. **Bryan R, Peterson LFA:** Polycentric total knee arthroplasty: A prognostic assessment. Clin Orthop 145:23, 1979
9. **Bryan RS, Peterson LFA, Combs JJ:** Polycentric knee arthroplasty. A preliminary report of postoperative complications in 450 knees. Clin Orthop 94:148, 1973
10. **Buchholz HW, Engelbrecht H:** Uber ide Depotwirkung einiger Antibiotica bei Vermischung mit dem Kunstharz Palacos. Chirurg 41:511, 1970

11. **Burton DS, Schurman DJ:** Hematogenous infection in bilateral total hip arthroplasty. J Bone Joint Surg, 57A:1004, 1975

12. **Charnley J:** Anchorage of the femoral head prosthesis to the shaft of the femur. J Bone Joint Surg 42B:28, 1960

13. **Charnley J:** The bonding of prostheses to bone by cement. J Bone Joint Surg 46B:518, 1964

14. **Charnley J:** Sensitivity to acrylic resins. In Acrylic Cement in Orthopaedic Surgery, pp 79–85. Baltimore, Williams & Wilkins, 1970

15. **Charnley J:** Acrylic Cement in Orthopaedic Surgery, pp 24–26. Baltimore, Williams & Wilkins, 1970

16. **Charnley J:** The histology of loosening between acrylic cement and bone. In Proceedings of the British Orthopaedic Research Society. J Bone Joint Surg, 57B:245, 1975

17. **Charnley J, Follacci FM, Hammond BT:** The long-term reaction of bone to self-curing acrylic cement. J Bone Joint Surg 50B:822, 1968

18. **Charnley J, Follacci FM, Hammond BT:** The long-term reaction of bone to self-curing acrylic cement. J Bone Joint Surg 55A:49, 1973

19. **Cohen SH, Ehrlick GE, Kauffman MS et al:** Thrombophlebitis following knee surgery. J Bone Joint Surg 55A:106, 1973

20. **Collins REC:** Physical methods of prophylaxis against deep vein thrombosis. In Fràntantoini J and Wessler S (eds): Prophylactic Therapy of Deep Vein Thrombosis and Pulmonary Embolism, pp. 158–172. Washington, D.C., U.S. Department of Health, Education and Welfare, Publication No. (NIH) 76-866, 1975

21. **Coventry MD, Upshaw JE, Riley LH et al:** Geometrical total knee arthroplasty II. Patient data and complications. Clin Orthop 94:117, 1973

22. **Coventry MB:** Two-part total knee arthroplasty: Evolution and present status. Clin Orthop 145:29, 1979

23. **Cracchiolo A III:** Statistics of total knee replacement. Clin Orthop 120:2, 1976

24. **Cracchiolo A III, Benson M, Finerman GAM et al:** A prospective comparative clinical analysis of the first-generation knee replacements: Polycentric vs. geometric knee arthroplasty. Clin Orthop 145:37, 1979

25. **Cruse JPE, Foord R:** A five-year prospective study of 23,649 surgical wounds. Arch Surg 107:206, 1973

26. **Cruess RL, Bickel WS vonKessler KLC:** Infections in total hips secondary to a primary source elsewhere. Clin Orthop 106:99, 1975

27. **D'Ambrosia RD, Shofi H Heater R:** Secondarily infected total joint replacements by hematogenous spread. J Bone Joint Surg 58A:450, 1976

28. **DeBurge A, GUEPAR:** Guepar hinge prosthesis. Complications and results with two years' follow-up. Clin Orthop 120:47, 1976

29. **Deburge A, Aubriot JH, Genet JP et al:** Current status of a hinge prosthesis (GUEPAR). Clin Orthop 145:91, 1979

30. **Ducheyne P, Kagan A II, Lacey JA:** Failure of total knee arthroplasty due to loosening and deformation of the tibial component. J Bone Joint Surg 60A:384, 1978

31. **Dumbleton JH, Black J:** An introduction to orthopaedic materials. Springfield, Charles C Thomas, 1975

32. **Elson RA, Jephcott AE, McGechie DB et al:** Antibiotic-loaded acrylic cement. J Bone Joint Surg 59B:200, 1977

33. **Evans EM, Freeman MAR, Miller AJ et al:** Metal sensitivity as a cause of bone necrosis and loosening of the prosthesis in total joint replacement. J Bone Joint Surg 56B:626, 1974

34. **Evanski PM, Waugh TR, Crofina CF et al:** UCI knee replacement. Clin Orthop 120:33, 1976

35. **Evarts CM, Alfidi RJ:** Thromboembolism after total hip reconstruction. Failure of low doses of heparin in prevention. JAMA 225:515, 1973

36. **Evarts CM, Feil EJ:** Prevention of thromboembolic disease after elective surgery of the hip. J Bone Joint Surg 53A:1271, 1971

37. **Ewald FD, Sledge CF, Corson JM et al:** Giant cell synovitis associated with failed polyethylene patellar replacements. Clin Orthop 115:213, 1976

38. **Fergusson W:** Excision of the knee-joint. Recovery with a false joint and a useful limb. Med Times 1:601, 1861

39. **Fitzgerald RH Jr, Peterson LFA, Washington JA II et al:** Bacterial colonization of wounds and sepsis in total hip arthroplasty. J Bone Joint Surg 55A:1242, 1973

40. **Frankel VH, Burstein AH:** Orthopaedic Biomechanics. Philadelphia, Lea & Febiger, 1970

41. **Freeman MAR, Swanson SAV:** Total prosthetic replacement of the knee. J Bone Joint Surg 54B:170, 1972

42. **Freeman MAR, Swanson SAV, Todd RC:** Total replacement of the knee using the Freeman-Swanson knee prosthesis. Clin Orthop 94:153, 1973

43. **Freeman MAR, Sculco T, Todd RC:** Replacement of the severely damaged arthritic knee by the ICLH (Freeman–Swanson) arthroplasty. J Bone Joint Surg 59B:64, 1977

44. **Freeman MAR, Todd RC, Cundy AD:** The presentation of the results of knee surgery. Clin Orthop 128:222, 1977

45. **Freeman MAR, Todd RC, Bamert P et al:** ICLH Arthroplasty of the knee: 1968–1977. J Bone Joint Surg 60B:339, 1978

46. **Freeman PA:** Walldius arthroplasty: A review of 80 cases. Clin Orthop 94:85, 1973

47. **Gallus AS, Hirsh J, Tuttle RJ et al:** Small subcutaneous doses of heparin in prevention of venous thrombosis. N Engl J Med 288:545, 1973

48. **Gibson R:** Radiological evaluation of replacement arthroplasty of the hip. In Proceedings of the Combined Meeting of Australian and New Zealand Orthopaedic Associations. J Bone Joint Surg 55B:433, 1973

49. **Gschwend N:** GSB knee joint: A further possibility, principle, results. Clin Orthop 132:170, 1978

50. **Gunston FH:** Polycentric knee arthroplasty—prosthetic stimulation at normal knee movement. J Bone Joint Surg 53B:272, 1971

51. **Gunston FH, MacKenzie RI:** Complications of polycentric knee replacement. Clin Orthop 120:33, 1976

52. **Habermann ET, Deutsch SD, Rovere GD:** Knee arthroplasty with the use of the Walldius total knee prosthesis. Clin Orthop 94:72, 1973

53. **Habermann ET, Hirsh DM:** Wear, tear and tissue reaction in failed geometric knee arthroplasty. Ortho Transactions 1:162, 1977

54. **Habermann ET, Hirsh DM:** Geometric total knee arthroplasty—evaluation and analysis of failures. Ortho Transactions 2:194, 1978

55. **Haeger K:** Problems of acute deep venous thrombosis. I. The interpretation of signs and symptoms. Angiology 20:219, 1969

56. **Hagemann WF, Woods WG, Tullos HS:** Arthrodesis in failed total knee replacement. J Bone Joint Surg 60A:790, 1978

57. **Hall AJ:** Late infection about a total knee prosthesis. J Bone Joint Surg 56B:144, 1974

58. **Hampson WGJ, Harris FC, Lucas HK et al:** Failure of low-dose heparin to prevent deep-vein thrombosis after hip-replacement arthroplasty. Lancet 2:795, 1974

59. **Harris WH:** Traumatic arthritis of the hip after dislocation and acetabular fractures: Treatment by mold arthroplasty. An end-result study using a new method of result evaluation. J Bone Joint Surg 51A:737, 1969

60. **Harris WH, Salzman EW, DeSanctis RW:** The prevention of thromboembolic disease by prophylactic anticoagulation. Controlled study in elective hip surgery. J Bone Joint Surg 49A:81, 1967

61. **Harris WH, Salzman EW, DeSanctis RW et al:** Prevention of venous thromboembolism following total hip replacement. JAMA 220:1319, 1972

62. **Harris WH, Salzman EW, Athanasoulis et al:** Comparison of warfarin, low-molecular-weight dextran, aspirin, and subcutaneous heparin in prevention of venous thromboembolism following total hip replacement. J Bone Joint Surg 56A:1552, 1974

63. **Harris WH, Salzman EW, Athanasoulis, C et al:** Comparison of ^{125}I fibrinogen count scanning with phlebography for detection of venous thrombi after elective hip surgery. N Engl J Med 292:665, 1975

64. **Harris WH, Schiller AL, Scholler JM et al:** Extensive localized bone resorption in the femur following total hip replacement. J Bone Joint Surg 58A:612, 1976

65. **Herbert JJ, Herbert A:** A new total knee prosthesis. Clin Orthop 94:202, 1973

66. **Hill J, Klenerman L, Trustey S et al:** Diffusion of antibiotics from acrylic bone-cement in vitro. J Bone Joint Surg 59B:197, 1977

67. **Hughes PW, Salvati EA, Wilson PP Jr et al:** Treatment of subacute sepsis of the hip by antibiotics and joint replacement criteria for diagnosis with evaluation of twenty-six cases. Clin Orthop 141:143, 1979

68. **Hui FC, Fitzgerald RH:** Hinged total knee arthroplasty. Ortho Transactions 2:195, 1978

69. **Hull R, VanAken WG, Hirsh J et al:** Impedance plethysmography using the occlusive cuff technique in the diagnosis of venous thrombosis. Circulation 53:696, 1976

70. **Ilstrup DM, Coventry MB, Skolnick MD:** A statistical evaluation of geometric total knee arthroplasties. Clin Orthop 120:27, 1976

71. **Ilstrup DM, Combs, JJ Jr, Bryan RS et al:** A statistical evaluation of polycentric total knee arthroplasties. Clin Orthop 120:18, 1976

72. **Insall J, Aglietti P:** A five to seven year follow-up of unicondylar arthroplasty. Presented at the International Society of the Knee, Lyon, France, 1979

73. **Insall J, Ranawat CS, Aghetti P et al:** A comparison of four models of total knee replacement prostheses. J Bone Joint Surg 58A:754, 1976

74. **Insall J, Ranawat CS, Scott WN et al:** Total condylar knee replacement. Preliminary report. Clin Orthop 120:149, 1976

75. **Insall J, Scott WN, Ranawat CS:** The total condylar knee prosthesis. A recent report of two hundred and twenty cases. J Bone Joint Surg 61A:173, 1979

76. **Insall J, Tria AJ:** The total condylar knee prosthesis type II. Presented at AAOS meeting, San Francisco, 1979

77. **Insall J, Tria AJ, Scott NW:** The total condylar knee prosthesis. The first 5 years. Clin Orthop 145:68, 1979

78. **Jackson JP, Elson RA:** Evaluation of the Walldius and other prostheses for knee arthroplasty. Clin Orthop 94:104, 1973

79. **Jefferiss CD, Lee AJC, Ling RSM:** Thermal aspects of self-curing polymethylmethacrylate. J Bone Joint Surg 57B:511, 1975

80. **Jones GB:** Walldius arthroplasty of the knee. J Bone Joint Surg 52B:390, 1970

81. **Jones GB:** The Walldius hinge. Clin Orthop 94:50, 1973

82. **Kakkar V:** The diagnosis of deep vein thrombosis using the ^{125}I fibrinogen test. Arch Surg 104:152, 1972

83. **Kaufer H, Matthews LS, Sonstegard DA:** Symposium on Reconstructive Surgery of the Knee, pp 308–336. St. Louis, CV Mosby, 1978

84. **Kaufer H, Matthews LS:** Spherocentric knee arthroplasty. Clin Orthop 145:110, 1979

85. **Kaushal SP, Galante JO, McKenna MD et al:** Complications following total knee replacement. Clin Orthop 121:181, 1976

86. **Lacey JA:** A statistical review of 100 consecutive UCI low friction knee arthroplasties with analysis of results. Clin Orthop 132:163, 1978

87. **Lambie JM, Mahaffy RG, Barber DC et al:** Diagnostic accuracy in venous thrombosis. Br Med J 2:142, 1970

88. **Laskin RS:** Modular total-knee replacement arthroplasty. J Bone Joint Surg 58A:766, 1976

89. **Letournel E, Lagrange J:** Total knee replacement with the "LL" type prosthesis. Clin Orthop 94:249, 1973

90. **Lettin AWF, Deliss LJ, Blackburne JS et al:** The Stanmore hinged knee arthroplasty. J Bone Joint Surg 60B:327, 1978

91. **Levin PD:** The effectiveness of various antibiotics in methylmethacrylate. J Bone Joint Surg 57B:234, 1975

92. **Lidgren L, Lindberg L:** Post-operative wound infections in clean orthopaedic surgery. Review of a 5-year material. Acta Orthop Scand 45:161, 1974

93. **Lindberg L:** Exchange of infected total hip arthroplasties with gentamicen cement: A multicentre investigation in Scandinavia. In the Hip Society Proceedings of the fifth open scientific meeting of the Hip Society. St. Louis, CV Mosby, 1977

94. **Lotke PA, Ecker ML:** Influence of positioning of prosthesis in total knee replacement. J Bone Joint Surg 59A:77, 1977

95. **Lotke PA, Ecker ML, McCloskey J et al:** Early experience with total knee arthroplasty. JAMA 236:2403, 1976

96. **Lynch JA:** Total knee replacement arthroplasty. In The Knee Joint. International Congress Series, No. 324:271. Amsterdam, Excerpta Medica, 1974

97. **McKenna R, Bachmann F, Kaushal SP et al:** Thromboembolic disease in patient undergoing total knee replacement. J Bone Joint Surg 58A:928, 1976

98. **Marks KW, Nelson CL, Lautenschlayer EP:** Antibiotic impregnated bone cement. J Bone Joint Surg 58A:358, 1976

99. **Marmor L:** The modular (Marmor) knee. Clin Orthop 120:86, 1976

100. **Matthews LS, Sonstegard PA, Kaufer H:** The spherocentric knee. Clin Orthop 94:234, 1973

101. **Mazas FB, GUEPAR:** Guepar total knee prosthesis. Clin Orthop 94:211, 1973

102. **Mendes G:** Roentgenographic evaluation in total hip replacement. A study of 100 McBee-Farrar prostetic replacements. Clin Orthop 95:104, 1973

103. **Miller J, Burke DL, Stachniewicz J et al:** The fixation of major load-bearing metal prostheses to bone. An experimental study comparing smooth to porous surfaces in a weight bearing mode. Trans Orthop Res Soc, p 54, 1976

104. **Miller J, Burke DL, Stachniewicz JW et al:** A study of the interface between cortical bone under conditions of load-bearing. Trans Orthop Res Soc p 191, 1976

105. **Miller J et al:** Improved fixation of knee arthroplasty components to prevent loosening. 47th Annual Meeting, American Academy of Orthopaedic Surgeons, Atlanta, 1980

106. **Mirra JM, Amstatz HC, Matos M et al:** The pathology at the joint tissues in prosthetic failure and its clinical relevance. Clin Orthop 117:221, 1976

107. **Moreland JR, Thomas RJ, Freeman MAR:** ICLH replacement of the knee, 1977–1978. Clin Orthop 145:47, 1979

108. **Morrison JB:** The mechanics of the knee joint in relation to normal walking. J Biomech 3:51, 1970

109. **Murray DG, Webster DA:** Variable axis total knee replacement—clinical experience with a two year follow-up. Orthop Trans 2:193, 1978

110. **Murray DG, Wilde AH, Werner F et al:** Herbert total knee prosthesis combined laboratory and clinical assessment. J Bone Joint Surg 59A:1026, 1977

111. **National Research Council, Postoperative Wound Infections:** The influence of ultraviolet radiation of the operating room and of various other factors. Ann Surg (Suppl) 160:1, 1964

112. **Nelson CL, Bergfeld JA, Schwartz J et al:** Antibiotics in human hematoma and wound fluid. Clin Orthop 108:138, 1975

113. **Nelson JD:** Antibiotic concentrations in septic joint effusions. N Engl J Med 284:349, 1971

114. **Nylander G:** Phlebographic diagnosis of acute deep leg thrombosis. Acta Chir Scand (Suppl) 387:30, 1968

115. **Ohnsorge J:** Some aspects of polymerizing bone cement. In Proceedings of the British Orthopaedic Assoc, J Bone Joint Surg 53B:758, 1971

116. **Peterson L, Fitzgerald R, Coventry M et al:** The relationship of operative wound culture to deep wound sepsis following total hip arthroplasty. Orthop Trans 2:210, 1978

117. **Petty W, Bryan RS, Coventry MB et al:** Infection after total knee arthroplasty. Orthop Clin North Am 6:1005, 1975

118. **Phillips RS:** Shiers alloplasty of the knee. Clin Orthop 94:122, 1973

119. **Ranawat CS, Insall J, Shine J:** Duo-condylar knee arthroplasty. Clin Orthop 120:76, 1976

120. **Reckling FW:** The measurement of the bone–cement interface temperature during total joint replacement procedures. In Transactions of the Twenty-second Annual Meeting of the Orthopaedic Research Society, 1:59, 1976

121. **Reckling FW, Asher MA, Dillon WL:** A longitudinal study at the radiolucent line at the bone–cement interface following total joint-replacement procedures. J Bone Joint Surg 59A:355, 1977

122. **Reckling FW, Dillon WL:** The bone cement interface temperature during total joint replacement. J Bone Joint Surg 59A:80, 1977

123. **Riley LH, Hungerford DS:** Geometric total knee replacement for treatment of the rheumatoid knee. J Bone Joint Surg 60A:523, 1978

124. **Salzman EW, Harris WH:** Prevention of venous thromboembolism in orthopaedic patients. J Bone Joint Surg 58A:903, 1976

125. **Scales JT:** Acrylic bone cement—Bone or plug? J Bone Joint Surg 50B:698, 1968

126. **Scheer DD, Dodd TA, Buckingham WW Jr:** Prophylactic use of typical antibiotic irrigation in unin-

fected surgical wounds, a microbiological evaluation. J Bone Joint Surg 54A:634, 1972

127. **Scott N, Insall J, Ranawat C:** Total condylar prosthesis. Ortho Trans 1:102, 1977

128. **Scott WN, Rosbruch JD, Otis JC et al:** Clinical and biomechanical evaluation of patellar replacement in total knee arthroplasty. Orthop Trans 2:203, 1978

129. **Sevitt S, Gallagher N:** Venous thrombosis and pulmonary embolism. A clinico-pathological study in injured and burned patients. Br J Surg 48:475, 1961

130. **Sheehan JM:** Arthroplasty of the knee. J Bone Joint Surg 60B:333, 1978

131. **Sheehan JM:** Arthroplasty of the knee. Clin Orthop 145:101, 1979

132. **Shiers LGP:** Arthroplasty of the knee, preliminary report on a new method. J Bone Joint Surg 36B:553, 1954

133. **Shiers LGP:** Arthroplasty of the knee, interim report. J Bone Joint Surg 42B:31, 1960

134. **Shiers LGP:** Hinge arthroplasty of the knee. J Bone Joint Surg 47B:506, 1965

135. **Shoji H, D'Ambrosia RD, Lipscomb PR:** Failed polycentric total knee prostheses. J Bone Joint Surg 58A:773, 1976

136. **Sledge CB, Ewald FC:** Total knee arthroplasty experience at the Robert Breck Brigham Hospital. Clin Orthop 145:78, 1979

137. **Sloop TJJH:** The influence of acrylic cement: An experimental study. Acta Orthop Scand 42:465, 1971

138. **Skolnick MD, Bryan RS, Peterson LFA et al:** Polycentric total knee arthroplasty. J Bone Joint Surg 58A:743, 1976

139. **Skolnick MD, Coventry MB, Ilstrup DM:** Geometric total knee arthroplasty. A two-year follow-up study. J Bone Joint Surg 58A:749, 1976

140. **Sonstegard DA, Kaufer H, Matthews LS:** The spherocentric knee. J Bone Joint Surg 59A:602, 1977

141. **Swanson SAV, Freeman MAR:** A new prosthesis for the total replacement of the knee. Acta Orthopaedica Belgica (Suppl 1) 38:55, 1972

142. **Tubiana R, Duparc J:** Prevention of thromboembolic complications in orthopaedic and accident surgery. J Bone Joint Surg 43B7, 1961

143. **Vernevil A:** De la creation d'une fausse articulation par section ou resection partielle de l'os maxillaire inferieur comme moyen de remedier a l'ankylose vraie ou fausse de la machoire inferieure. Arch Gen Med 15:174, 1860

144. **Walker PS, Bienenstock M:** Fixation properties of acrylic cement. Rev Hosp Spec Surg 1:27, 1971

145. **Walker PS, Ranawat CS, Insall J:** Fixation of the tibial components of condylar replacement knee prostheses. J Biomech 9:269, 1975

146. **Walter PS, Hsieh HH:** Conformity in condylar knee prostheses. J Bone Joint Surg 59B:222, 1977

147. **Walldius B:** Arthroplasty of the knee joint using an acrylic prosthesis. Acta Orthop Scand 23:121, 1953

148. **Walldius B:** Arthroplasty of the knee using an endoprosthesis. Acta Orthop Scand 24:1, 1957

149. **Watson JR, Wood H, Hill RCJ:** The Shiers arthroplasty of the knee. J Bone Joint Surg 58B:300, 1976

150. **Waugh W:** Knee replacement 1978. J Bone Joint Surg 60B:301, 1978

151. **Werner F, Foster D, Murray DG:** The influence of design on the transmission of torque across knee prostheses. J Bone Joint Surg 60A:342, 1978

152. **Willert HG, Ludwig J, Semlitsch M:** Reaction of bone to methacrylate after hip arthroplasty. A long-term gross, light microscopic, and scanning electron microscopic study. J Bone Joint Surg 56A:1368, 1974

153. **Wilson FC:** Total replacement of the knee in rheumatoid arthritis. A prospective study of the result of treatment with the Walldius prosthesis. J Bone Joint Surg 54A:1429, 1972

154. **Wilson FC:** Total replacement of the knee in rheumatoid arthritis. Part II of a prospective study. Clin Orthop 94:58, 1973

155. **Wiltse LL, Hall RH, Stenehjem JC:** Experimental studies regarding the possible use of self-curing acrylic in orthopaedic surgery. J Bone Joint Surg 39A:961, 1957

156. **Witvoet J, GUEPAR Group:** GUEPAR total knee prosthesis. In The Knee Joint, International Congress, Series No. 324:305. Amsterdam, Excerpta Medica, 1974

157. **Wroblewski BM:** Wear of high density polyethylene on bone and cartilage. J Bone Joint Surg 61B:498, 1979

158. **Yamamoto S:** Total knee replacement with the Kodama–Yamamoto knee prosthesis. Clin Orthop 145:60, 1979

159. **Young HH:** Use of a hinged vitallium prosthesis for arthroplasty of the knee, a preliminary report. J Bone Joint Surg 45A:1627, 1963

CHAPTER 19
THE RHEUMATOID KNEE

Louis Solomon

Until fairly recently the surgical treatment of the rheumatoid knee consisted essentially in radical synovectomy in the early stages and arthroplasty in the late, derelict joint. Better understanding of the pathologic progress of the disease and *earlier participation of the surgeon in the total management of the patient* have led to a more rational approach.

THE NATURAL PROGRESS
OF THE DISEASE

The progress of rheumatoid arthritis in the knee may be visualized in three stages (Fig. 19-1 and Plates 19-1, 19-2, 19-3). The disease may be arrested, or may even subside spontaneously, at any of these stages. In most cases, however, once the joint is involved, lack of effective treatment will result in a relentless progression to articular destruction.

Stage 1 consists of a subacute synovitis, with proliferation of the lining synoviocytes and inflammatory cell infiltration of the subsynovial layers. There is thickening of the capsular structures and a cell-rich effusion

into the joint. The knee is painful, swollen, and tender, but mobility is retained and the joint is stable (Fig. 19-2). At this stage the pathology is potentially reversible, provided the synovitis is brought under control.

During the stage of synovitis, and particularly in the more active individual with powerful muscles, intra-articular pressures may rise sufficiently to produce a rupture of the posterior capsule with extrusion of the joint contents into the calf, usually by communication with one of the anatomical bursae associated with the joint (Fig. 19-3A, B). This presents as a painful episode resembling thrombophlebitis and is frequently misdiagnosed as such by the unwary practitioner.

Stage 2 shows a progression of the inflammatory process, with the formation of granulation tissue in the vascular folds of the synovial reflection. This vascular reaction produces the periarticular erosions that are the hallmark of the disease in its later stages (Fig. 19-4). In addition, there is surface destruction of the articular cartilage, probably due to the effects of proteolytic enzymes in the effusion. Thickening and fibrosis of the subsynovial tis-

283

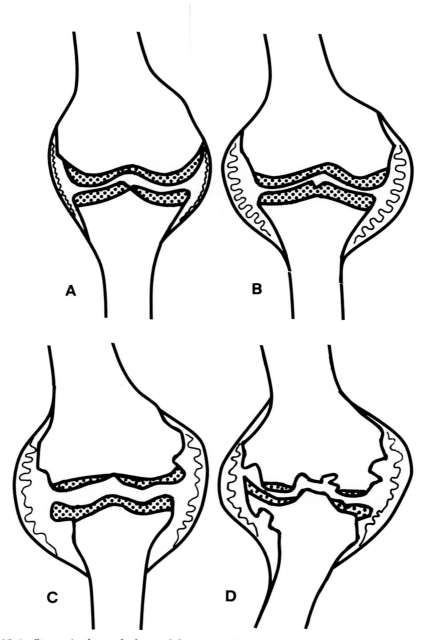

FIG. 19-1. Stages in the pathology of rheumatoid arthritis: **(A)** The normal joint. **(B)** Early sub-acute synovitis. **(C)** Chronic synovitis and cartilage erosion. **(D)** Late articular and peri-articular destruction with joint instability.

FIG. 19-2. Synovitis and intra-articular effusion in a patient with early rheumatoid arthritis.

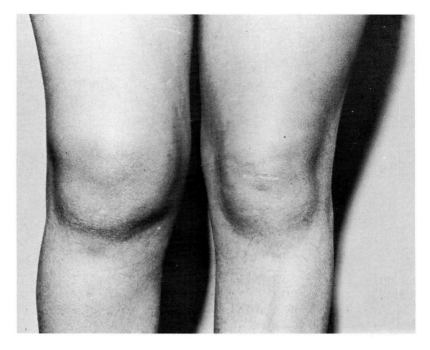

sues lead to increasing stiffness of the joint, which is manifested first as an inability to extend the knee completely. Added to the destructive effects of the synovitis there are now the mechanical forces of the muscles concerned with stabilization during weight-bearing; the powerful lateral stabilizers, the tensor fascia lata and the iliotibial band, now act partially as flexors and external rotators, with the result that the tibia starts to drift into posterior luxation, valgus, and external rotation (Fig. 19-5).

Stage 3 is characterized by increasing destruction of the articular surfaces, the intra-articular ligaments, and the menisci. The major feature now is instability of the joint, with laxity in both anteroposterior and mediolateral planes. This is a painful joint, and typically the patient holds it immobile during the swing phase of walking. If deformity is marked, there may be lateral subluxation or even complete dislocation of the patella, thus further interfering with stability during weight-bearing.

DERANGEMENT OF THE KNEE JOINT AND "TRIPLE DISPLACEMENT"

The progress of derangement of the knee joint in rheumatoid arthritis follows fairly consistent patterns. As a bicondylar helicoid joint, the lateral articular surface of the tibia pivots on the roundish lateral condyle of the femur while the medial articular surface follows the longer winding course on the medial femoral condyle. In rheumatoid arthritis adhesions in the joint and adherence of the menisci or fat pad hamper rotation as well as flexion–extension, which are evident in the extended knee by the medial position of the tibial tubercle and *protrusion of the medial femoral condyle* —that is, the first deformity of the rheumatoid knee is fixed flexion and medial rotation of the tibia on the femur. This stage cannot be distinguished from the osteoarthritic knee in which the same deformity and limitation occurs.

The addition of posterior displacement of

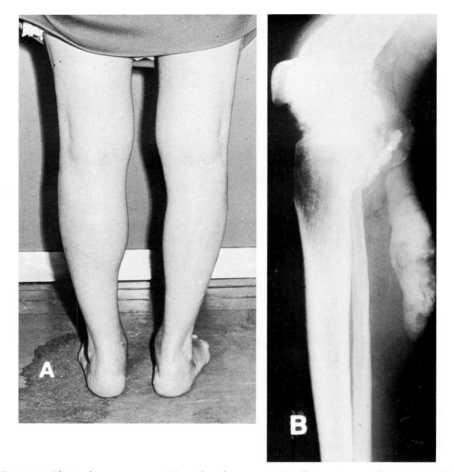

FIG. 19-3. Clinical appearance **(A)** and arthrogram **(B)** of a patient with rupture of the knee joint and extrusion of synovial contents into the calf.

the tibia on the femur with lateral rotation of the leg completes the so-called triple displacement of the rheumatoid knee. This interesting development is induced by overaction of the iliotibial band on the flexed knee.

Normally, the iliotibial band and biceps femoris are the stabilizers of the leg on the thigh. The tibia must rotate on the femur in flexion and extension. To do this while bearing weight would produce lateral instability if it were not for the stabilizing control of the biceps acting directly on the fibula and tibiofibular joint, and for the iliotibial band on the outer border of the tibial tuberosity, the point of pivot of the rotating tibia.

Once fixed flexion–internal rotation deformity of the knee is established, however, the iliotibial band acts as a posterior retractor of the tibia. The flexed tibia is pulled backward, leaving *both the lateral and the medial femoral condyles protruding* beyond the anterior margin of the tibia (see Fig. 19-7). This distinguishes the rheumatoid from the osteoarthritic knee, in which only the medial femoral condyle protrudes.

At the same time, since the center of the tibia is behind that of the femur, the pull of the laterally fixed iliotibial band will externally rotate the retracted tibia. The primarily internally rotated tibia is now rotated laterally

FIG. 19-4. Radiograph showing peri-articular erosion characteristic of rheumatoid arthritis.

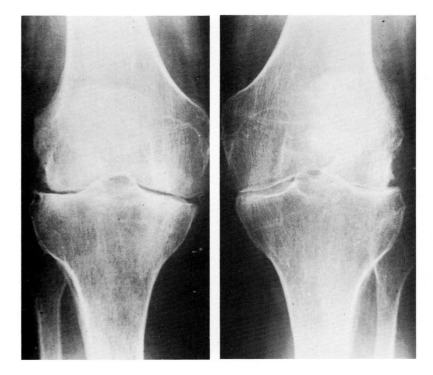

but at a different point of pivot. A similar deformity and for the same reason occurs after poliomyelitis owing to unbalanced muscle action. Yount devised the simple operation of division and release of this muscle to correct the deformity.

PAIN IN RHEUMATOID ARTHRITIS

The acute phase of rheumatoid arthritis is always painful. Pain is associated with the red inflammatory process and indicated by hot swelling and muscle spasm. Patients complain of a constant ache aggravated by activity with acute pain on movement. Pain is relieved by rest and support and by excision of all inflamed synovium.

As the acute phase subsides, the pain and disability depends on the extent of derangement of the joint. If the rotator mechanism is tethered with limitation of the extremes of extension and flexion, the manner and type of

pain is exactly the same as in comparable derangement in the osteoarthritic knee. And similarly, pain is relieved by rest and support, or by excision of the remaining inflamed synovium plus surgical correction of the derangement. Once the normal pattern of movement is recovered, pain disappears dramatically even though the ulcers and eroded areas of articular cartilage remain, a fact that supports the assumption that articular cartilage is relatively insensitive. Pain in the deranged joint derives from abnormal tensions in the soft tissues and not from abnormal pressures on articular cartilage.

The insensitivity of the articular cartilage is also apparent in the finally fibrosed inactive joint. Now the knee joint is stiff but not painful. Because the articular surfaces are insensitive, movement recovered by division of adhesions and release of the rotator mechanism and infrapatellar pad of fat is painless. Thirty degrees to 60° of movement may be so recovered; this makes a great difference to the pa-

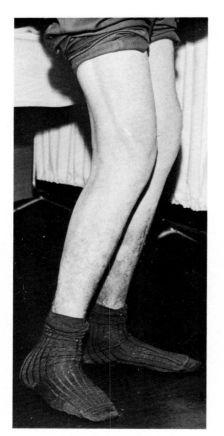

FIG. 19-5. Typical deformity of the knee in late rheumatoid arthritis.

tient, especially in bilateral cases. The patient is able to get in and out of motor cars and to drive.

MANAGEMENT

During stage 1 treatment is directed entirely at control of the synovitis. Systemic therapy with nonsteroidal anti-inflammatory drugs seldom reduces the synovial thickening and effusion in the knee. Local measures consisting of rest and splintage and synoviorthesis are usually necessary.

In milder cases, and especially in patients without joint deformity, splintage may consist of a simple plaster cylinder that is worn for a few weeks. For the really painful joint, how-

ever, the patient should be admitted to the hospital for a period of bed rest and plaster immobilization. The knee joint itself is left exposed to allow daily examination, to facilitate physiotherapy, and to permit aspiration or intra-articular injection if necessary.

Total rest alone will reduce the inflammatory reaction in the majority of cases, but if this fails to bring improvement within a week it is advisable to go on to synoviorthesis— that is, the intra-articular injection of agents that will effectively counteract the synovitis. Three types of preparation are commonly employed: (1) an effective, quick-acting anti-inflammatory agent, usually a corticosteroid or a combination of a corticosteroid and nitrogen mustard; (2) a more potent preparation such as osmic acid, which actually causes destruction of the surface layers of the synovium; (3) radiocolloid preparations such as ^{90}Y, which, though slow acting, produce an anti-inflammatory effect over a longer period of time than is usually achieved with corticosteroids.

Our own preference is for a combination of corticosteroid and nitrogen mustard in patients with florid synovitis, reserving ^{90}Y for those with really long-standing chronic synovitis predominantly of a single joint. The nitrogen mustard (mustine hydrochloride BP) is dissolved in normal saline to make a 0.02% solution (1 mg in 5 ml of saline); this is then mixed with corticosteroid and novocaine in the following proportions: 1 ml of the mustine solution plus 2 ml of Depo-Medrol plus 2 ml of 1% novocaine. If there is marked effusion this is first aspirated, and then 3 ml to 5 ml of the mustine mixture are injected into the joint. When ^{90}Y is used it is injected in a dose of 5 mc in 5 ml of saline.

Controlled trials, in which synoviorthesis was compared with surgical synovectomy, have shown that intra-articular radiocolloid injection is at least as effective as surgical synovectomy and has the advantage of avoiding the complications of surgery.[1] Synovectomy of the knee is now rarely carried out in multidisciplinary rheumatology units, where a range of alternative treatment programs are available.

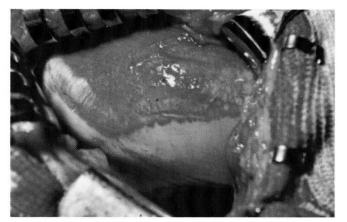

PLATE 19-1. The synovium of acute rheumatoid arthritis is uniformly red and swollen.

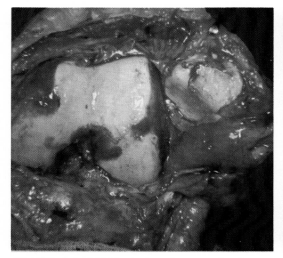

PLATE 19-2. **(A)** Operative photograph of pannus invading the articular cartilage.

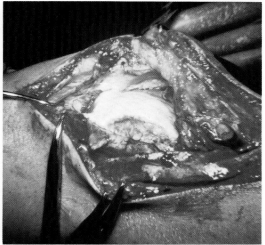

(B) Healing by fibrosis has commenced. Patches of articular cartilage are dull and yellow.

PLATE 19-3. The articular cartilage of the patella has been destroyed. The menisci are degenerated, ragged and partially absorbed. The medial meniscus has been transfixed by an osteophyte.

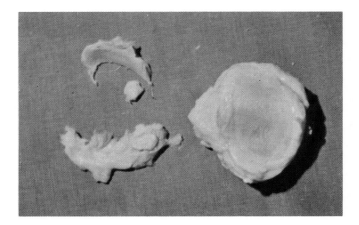

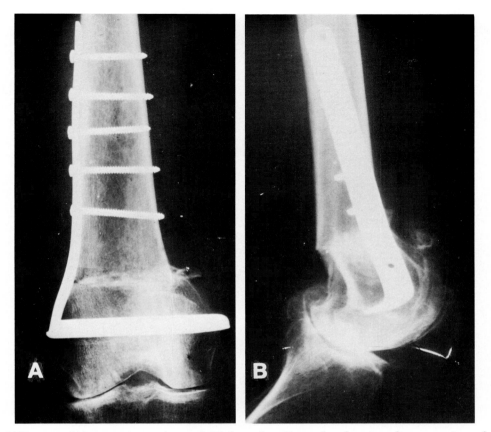

FIG. 19-6. (A) Anteroposterior and **(B)** lateral radiographs showing the correction of both valgus and flexion deformities by supracondylar osteotomy and internal fixation.

Rupture of the knee joint was formerly treated by surgical excision of the synovial sac and repair of the defect in the posterior capsule.[2] However, in recent years we have treated these patients also by simple immobilization and synoviorthesis, and surgical intervention is seldom if ever required.

In stage 2 it will still be necessary to control the synovitis, but in addition the impending deformity of the knee will require treatment. Here again the most effective measure is immobilization in a plaster-of-Paris cast, with increasing correction of the flexion and rotatory deformity. Once correction is achieved, physiotherapy is important to help restore physiologic muscle control of the knee. Early or mild valgus deformity may be corrected by division of the iliotibial band (Yount's operation), *provided the knee joint is not yet unstable.* More severe valgus deformity in the essentially stable knee calls for surgical correction, and the procedure of choice is a supracondylar osteotomy with internal fixation, *which must correct both the valgus and the slight flexion deformity.* The results of this procedure in the stable knee, even after articular erosion has begun, are extremely good (Figs. 19-6*A*, *B*, 19-7*A*, *B*, 19-8*A*, *B*, *C*).

In patients with advanced articular destruction and instability of the knee (stage 3), conservative surgery is unlikely to succeed. It is in these patients that the recent advances in total joint replacement have been most appreciated.

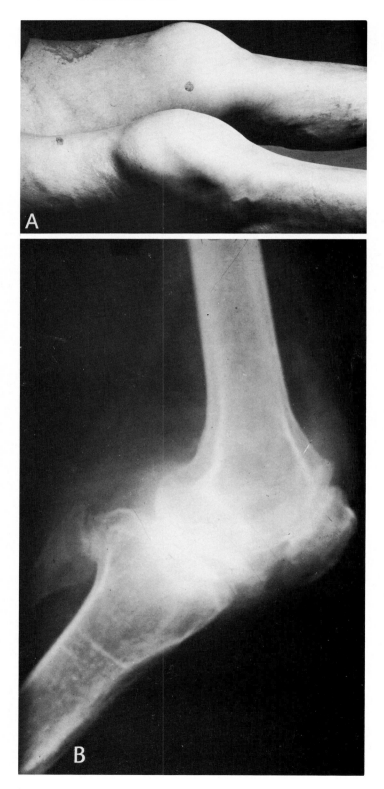

FIG. 19-7. (A) The swollen knees of rheumatoid arthritis with both the medial and femoral condyles protruding beyond the anterior margin of the tibia. **(B)** Lateral roentgenogram of triple displacement of the rheumatoid knee.

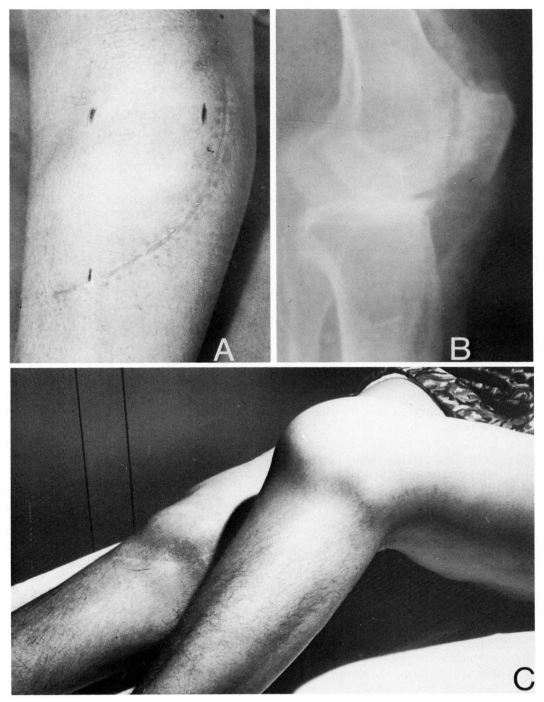

FIG. 19-8. (A) After release of the iliotibial band and the rotator mechanism of the right knee (including the fat pad and obstructing intra-articular adhesions) the menisci shown in Plate 19-3 were excised. The maneuver of reduction was performed. The knee is now extended. Protrusion of the femoral condyles has been minimized. **(B)** In the anterior view, the alignment of the right knee is satisfactory. Normal external rotation of the tibia on the femur is possible. **(C)** The lateral view of the right knee in Figure 19-7**B** after operation compared with the unreduced triple displacement in the left knee.

PLANNING OF TREATMENT

One is seldom allowed to forget that rheumatoid arthritis is a systemic disorder with polyarticular involvement. If the general disease activity is inadequately controlled, the results of surgery on any one joint will be less impressive, and functionally less useful, than when the systemic disease is quiescent. Therefore, although it is theoretically quite feasible to operate even in the presence of marked disease activity, it is preferable to achieve optimal general management before undertaking surgery on the knee. Moreover, the state of the other joints must always be taken into account. If both hip and knee require surgery, it is better to tackle the hip first; a painful, deformed hip, if left untreated while the knee is reconstructed, may well force the patient into compensatory deformity at the knee during the postoperative phase. Thus, a patient with fixed flexion at the hip will want to walk with the knee in flexion as well, making post-operative rehabilitation very difficult. On the other hand, if both knee and foot require reconstructive surgery, the knee should be attended to first, so that foot surgery can be planned with the limb in its optimal anatomical position. Indeed, the correction of deformity at the knee sometimes improves foot posture to the extent that further surgery is unnecessary.

REABLEMENT OF THE KNEE AFTER SURGERY

An interesting and most important phase in the management of the rheumatoid knee is the restoration of power and function after surgery. A Jones compression dressing is applied with the knee fully reduced and is supported by a light plaster of Paris cast with the foot in external rotation. Isometric thigh drill with the patient consciously attempting to hold the leg in forced active extension is started next day and practiced regularly.

After the stitches have been removed, foam rubber traction is applied, and the patient begins active flexion exercises using Guthrie-Smith slings or Russell traction. Aided by the apparatus, each flexion movement is followed by active full extension. Between the exercise periods the back splint is reapplied.

The main problem is recovery of full extension. Frequently intrinsic weakness, fibrosis, and stretched extensors leave an extension lag however hard the patient practices. Passive extension is full and comfortable, but active extension may lag by as much as 20°. The patient has usually recovered sufficient control to walk with crutches and a back splint in 3 weeks or less. However, walking without support should not be permitted before full, strong, active extension is recovered. Otherwise extension lag, signalled by a feeling of insecurity or of actual "givingway" followed by pain and swelling after effort, is not prevented. These effects are relieved by rest or support but recur with stress.

Soon after the operation the patient is usually comfortable, and if the recovery of muscle power and excursion copes with carefully graduated activity, the patient is content and requests surgery for the other knee. However, if extension lag and inadequate power persist, and they may do so because of intrinsic changes in the muscle, recurrent strain obstructs recovery postoperatively.

Finally, a word of caution is necessary: in planning multiple reconstructive procedures always set realistic goals. The patient who has not walked for 2 years is unlikely to be restored to a state of walking unaided outside his home, and heroic efforts on the part of an overoptimistic surgeon may not be worth the risks involved in gaining a comparatively small improvement in function. The patient should always be given a severely realistic estimate of the probable results of multiple joint surgery and should participate actively in the decision to embark on what may be the first step on a long and difficult road.

REFERENCES

1. **Gumpel JM, Roles NC:** A controlled trial of intraarticular radiocolloids versus surgical synovectomy in persistent synovitis. Lancet 1:488–489, 1975
2. **Solomon L, Berman L:** Synovial rupture of the knee joint. J Bone Joint Surg 54B:460–467, 1972

CHAPTER 20
HEMOPHILIC ARTHRITIS
OF THE KNEE

John E. Handelsman

Advances in the understanding and management of hemophilia and related inherited bleeding disorders have altered the emphasis placed on the disease. The major focus is now on the associated orthopaedic deformities, commonly the result of repeated hemarthroses and intra-muscular bleeding. More effective replacement of the deficient factors has enabled the orthopaedic surgeon and therapist to apply standard methods of treatment so that the deformities that occur may be appropriately treated.

The knee is affected in approximately half of all cases of hemarthrosis in hemophilia. Recurrent knee hemorrhage may commence before walking is established, and a boggy, chronically swollen knee joint may present at an early age (Fig. 20-1). The prevention of the significant joint disintegration that may follow demands an energetic prophylactic and therapeutic regimen.

BASIC CONSIDERATIONS

A clear understanding of the etiology of the disease is recent. As late as 1932, clinicians were treating repeated hemorrhages in hemophilic patients by injecting maternal blood taken during the menstrual cycle in the belief that ovarian extract provided protection.[5] In 1937 Pohle and Taylor established that hemophilia was due to a lack of an "antihemophilic factor in the blood clotting mechanism."[25] Deficiency of Factor IX, called also Christmas disease or hemophilia B, behaves in a similar manner and will not be discussed as a separate entity.

Both conditions are sex-linked recessive disorders, occurring in men but carried by clinically normal women. Approximately 30% of men with hemophilia have no family history of the disease. In some instances the defective gene is present but not apparent be-

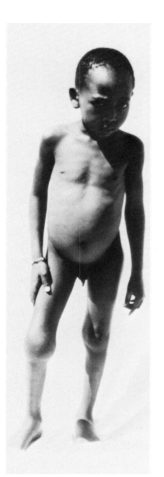

FIG. 20-1. Subacute hemophilic arthropathy in a young boy. The right knee is chronically swollen, and there is a fixed flexion contracture.

cause families in previous generations have produced few sons. A high mutation rate, however, is probable. In the United States, the incidence of hemophilia A and B combined is estimated to be 1 per 10,000 male births. The mutation rate in hemophilia A is 25% per year, which is one of the highest among genetic diseases.[22] Von Willebrand's disease, in which there is both a Factor VIII deficiency and a functional platelet abnormality, affects both sexes and may produce similar joint and muscle hemorrhages.

Reliable methods of assaying the deficient factor are now available, and it is established that the level is related to the clinical severity of the disease. When the circulating plasma level is under 1%, the patient is severely affected, and spontaneous hemarthroses and hemorrhages are common. Moderately affected patients have a level of between 1% and 5%, and in this category spontaneous bleeding is less frequent but may be severe after minor injuries. Mildly affected individuals have a deficient factor level of between 5% and 30% and may lead normal lives, bleeding only after severe accidents or surgery. However, no absolute correlation of factor level and the frequency of hemarthroses exists. With comparable factor level concentrations, one patient may sustain crippling deformities following multiple episodes of joint bleeding while another may retain well-preserved joints. Furthermore, more patients experience a seasonal or phasic susceptibility to hemarthroses.[20]

The significance of hemophilia is not reflected in the incidence of the disease. Although the victims of the condition are numerically few, its chronicity imposes a disproportionate strain on both patients and medical resources.

HEMOPHILIC ARTHROPATHY

PATHOLOGY

A hemorrhage that becomes intra-articular occurs initially in the synovium with subsequent rupture into the joint space. Hemophilic blood within the joint remains partly fluid; the cell count is somewhat elevated and the sugar content slightly reduced. The red cells slowly break up, hemoglobin disintegrates, and hemosiderin is released. The iron-containing pigment is phagocytosed by the superficial cells indefinitely while the rest aggregates in macrophages found in the deep portions of the synovial membrane.[10] Repeated hemorrhages progressively increase the synovial hemosiderosis, and ultimately the iron content may be as much as 70% of the ashed weight of the synovial tissue.[29]

Iron deposition irritates the synovium,

which proliferates markedly and becomes convoluted, thus increasing the surface area. This fact, coupled with a marked increase in vascularity, makes the synovium more prone than ever to repeated hemorrhage. A vicious cycle is thus established.[2] The joint lining ultimately resembles that seen in rheumatoid arthritis except that it is stained a deep chocolate-brown color by iron pigmentation. Some of the joint swelling in chronic cases is probably the result of effusions produced by the irritable synovium. It is certain, however, that once more than one hemorrhage has occurred, the joint becomes predisposed to further bleeding (Fig. 20-2). Furthermore, the affected knee joint is less well protected because of disuse atrophy of the associated muscles and thus becomes more liable to suffer injury from minor trauma. Ultimately, the florid synovium becomes fibrosed and contracted. Hemarthroses and effusions diminish, but progressive stiffness occurs, regardless of the condition of the articular cartilage.

The most significant feature of chronic hemophilic arthritis is disproportionate destruction of the articular cartilage. Changes occur early in the disease process, and when the dis-

ease is progressive, articular cartilage may ultimately be completely lost over wide areas. Subchondral bone may become cystic and sclerotic and may eventually collapse.

The postmortem changes in hemophilic arthropathy have been well described.[15,34] Much less is known about the early disease process. For this reason, material was obtained at surgical synovectomy from seven patients and examined closely.[13,26] The macroscopic appearance at surgery was similar in all knee joints examined. Synovial fluid was dark and more viscous in consistency than usual. The synovium was a deep chocolate-brown color and was markedly thickened. Convolutions on the irregular inner surface penetrated into the joint crevices (Fig. 20-3). The articular cartilage, however, was usually unchanged in color except for patchy areas of discoloration associated with pannus formation. On the periphery, cartilage appeared normal except for some loss of sheen, but in other areas there was visible fibrillation and palpable softening. Over most weight-bearing areas and in the intercondylar region, cartilage was diseased and frequently shelved sharply away to expose bone that was covered

FIG. 20-2. The vicious cycle of hemophilic arthritis.

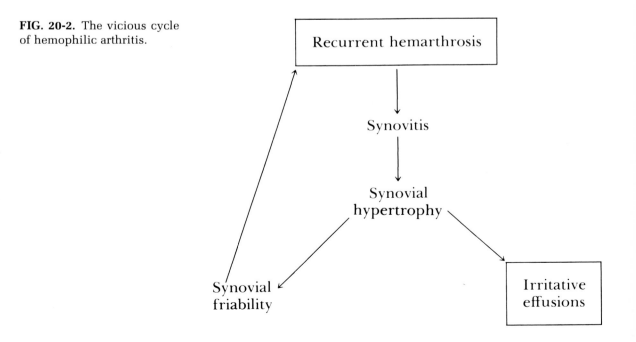

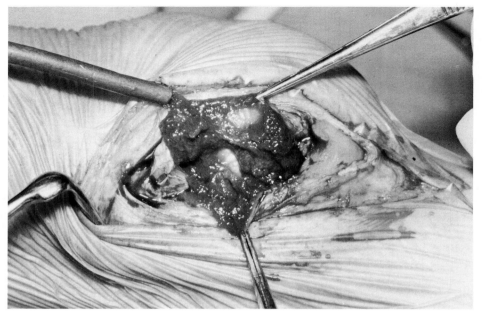

FIG. 20-3. Florid synovitis in a hemophilic knee at surgical synovectomy. The synovium is convoluted and dark in color.

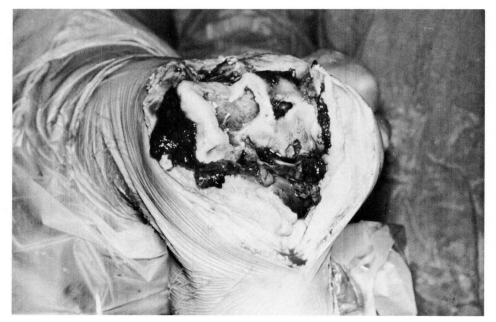

FIG. 20-4. The distal femur of a 12-year-old hemophilic boy at surgery. There is a central punched-out area of articular cartilage loss, typical of chronic hemophilic arthritis.

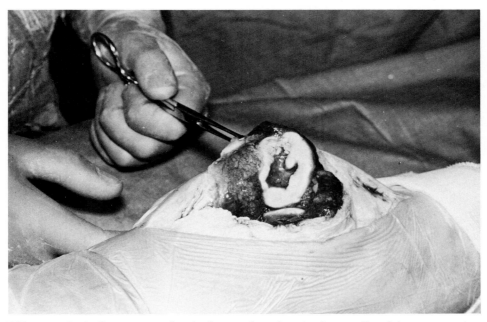

FIG. 20-5. A similar pattern of articular cartilage loss in the patella of the same patient shown in Figure 20-4. The heavily pigmented fibrous covering in the floor of the crater contrasts sharply with the almost unstained surrounding articular cartilage. The synovium is frondlike and deeply pigmented.

by no more than a thin layer of pigmented fibrous tissue (Fig. 20-4). Contact areas of the femur, tibia, and patella were usually affected (Fig. 20-5). In some joints a thin pannus formed over softened articular cartilage. In no instance was this continuous with the surrounding synovium.

The microscopic appearance of the synovium showed that the villus-like proliferation affected both lining and subsynovial cells (Fig. 20-6). Hemosiderin deposits could be seen as granules of golden brown pigment that stained for iron. These occurred predominantly in the more superficial cells of thickened synovium but were also evident in the deeper synovial layers and in underlying macrophages. There was a patchy infiltration of inflammatory cells in the subsynovial tissues where capillary proliferation and congestion were prominent. In some specimens, a diffuse infiltration of plasma cells was seen toward the surface, associated with aggregates of lymphocytic cells in the deeper subsynovial areas (Fig. 20-7).[26] Fresh hemorrhage into the synovial membrane sometimes occurred (Fig. 20-6).

The histologic appearance of articular cartilage varied according to the site and extent of the disease process. When the macroscopic appearance of the articular cartilage was nearly normal, the changes consisted of horizontal splitting of articular cartilage and crowding of chondrocyte nuclei toward the surface (Fig. 20-8). These nuclei were oval or spindle-shaped and were positioned with their long axes parallel to the surface, thus presenting an appearance of fibrous metaplasia. Pannus was seen as a fibrous vascularized overgrowth that was contiguous with these areas of articular cartilage change. Hemosiderin was present in the cells of the pannus but could not be demonstrated in the adjoining articular cartilage matrix or superficial chondrocytes (Fig. 20-9).

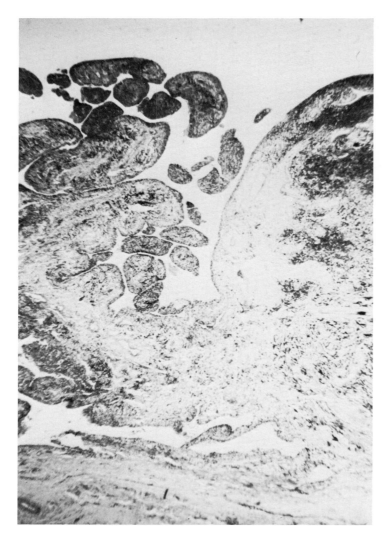

FIG. 20-6. Microphotograph of synovium from a patient with hemophilic arthritis. The villous proliferation is shown. The dark areas on the right are recent hemorrhages.

In the deeper layers of damaged cartilage, chondrocytes came together to form groups of 8 to 12 cells (Fig. 20-10). In contrast to the superficial chondrocytes, the presence of iron pigment in these deep cell aggregations could be demonstrated by Perls' iron stain. Except in the immediate area of the chondrocyte aggregations, the articular cartilage matrix was deficient in glycosaminoglycans, as shown by poor staining with alcian blue (Fig. 20-9).

In more severely affected areas, the cartilage was deeply fissured at right angles to the surface (Fig. 20-11). The deep chondrocyte clusters were larger, containing up to 40 cells. These were frequently necrotic and contained large quantities of stainable iron (Figs. 20-12, 20-13).

The chondrocyte response in hemophilic arthropathy appears to be twofold. Superficially, cells proliferate, become horizontally oriented, and resemble fibroblasts. In some areas, these cells appear to be intimately involved in the production of a superficial fibrous pannus overgrowth of the articular cartilage. Deep cartilage cells aggregate, proliferate initially, and ultimately die. The

FIG. 20-7. Hemophilic synovium. The distribution of hemosiderin deposits in proliferated synovial cells and the subsynovial area is shown by Perls' iron stain. There is markedly increased vascularity as well as lymphocytic and plasma cell infiltrations.

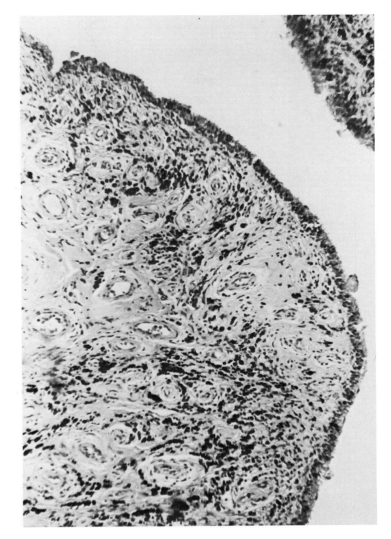

latter process is associated with the presence of considerable iron pigment.

The cause of disproportionate articular cartilage breakdown and hemophilic arthritis has been the subject of considerable speculation. Lysosomal enzymes are known to injure cartilaginous matrix, and these may play a part in hemophilia. This view is supported by Hilgartner,[14] who considers that articular cartilage destruction in this condition is due in part to the release of lysosomal hydrolases, which are found in high concentration in the synovial membrane, macrophages, and polymorphonuclear leukocytes. The levels of cathepsin D, acid phosphotase, and collagenases are all abnormally high in chronic hemophilic joints. In particular, cathepsin D damages the extracellular matrix of the chondrocyte. Because these hydrolytic enzymes are present only in small quantities in normal individuals with acute traumatic hemarthroses, it is thought that they are produced primarily by the hypertrophic synovium in hemophilia.

Niemann believes that pressure phenomena in joints are important.[23] This view correlates with the finding that maximal damage to ar-

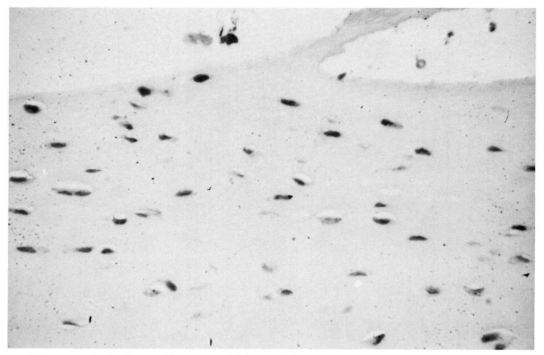

FIG. 20-8. Articular cartilage in mild hemophilic arthropathy. The surface chondrocytes are crowded and spindle-shaped and lie horizontally. A superficial layer of cartilage has split horizontally.

ticular cartilage occurs in weight-bearing areas. An interaction of mechanical and enzymatic mechanisms has been postulated by Kisker and associates[19] and supported by Sokoloff.[30]

The evidence that iron penetrates the articular cartilage and appears within the chondrocyte is almost certainly significant. Brighton and his co-workers suggested that iron might damage mitrochondrial or other oxidative mechanisms,[7] and our study produced evidence of chondrocyte death with increasing hemosiderin content. Furthermore, Sokoloff suggests that the addition of ferrous iron, a polyvalent cation, directly weakens the articular cartilage matrix.[30]

It is thus probable that a number of factors account for the severe articular cartilage damage seen in hemophilic arthritis. These factors include excessive lysosomal enzymes from the abnormal synovium, mechanical factors, and the direct effect of iron penetration into the components of articular cartilage.

CLINICAL ASPECTS

Spontaneous and post-traumatic hemorrhages occur predominantly in the knee joints.[33] The elbow, presumably because of its anatomy and exposure to minor trauma, is also frequently affected. Other weight-bearing joints are less commonly involved, the ankle being more susceptible than the well-protected hip joint. Hemarthrosis of the shoulder joint is relatively uncommon, and the spine and hand are rarely involved without significant trauma.

Hemophilic arthropathy of the knee can be divided into three clinical categories—acute, subacute, and chronic.

Acute. A sudden hemorrhage into an otherwise normal knee joint constitutes acute he-

FIG. 20-9. The articular cartilage in advancing hemophilic arthritis. A cellular pannus overgrowth, contiguous with cartilage, is seen on the upper right. Vertical fissuring has occurred, and the ground substance is glycosaminoglycan-depleted, as shown by irregular staining with Alcian blue.

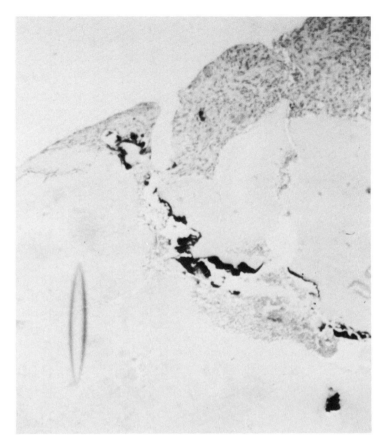

mophilic arthropathy. After an initial period of some stiffness and pain, the joint becomes rapidly swollen. Pain may be severe, and motion, particularly extension, is restricted. The joint is usually tense, warm, and very tender.

Subacute. Multiple hemorrhages into a joint sooner or later produce subacute hemophilic arthropathy. At this stage the joint is always swollen to some extent even when there has been no recent hemorrhage. It presents a boggy feel, partly the result of synovial hypertrophy and partly because of persisting fluid in the joint. This fluid may be an actual hemarthrosis but is frequently an irritative effusion produced by the diseased synovium. Relative overgrowth of the epiphyses that follows constant local hyperemia produces some true enlargement, which is accentuated by wasting of the quadriceps and other periarticular muscles.

Chronic. A joint that has been constantly swollen and thickened for 6 months or more falls into the category of chronic hemophilic arthropathy, but this classification covers a wide spectrum of disease. The joint space is lost as articular cartilage fragments, and in some instances it may be totally destroyed. The thickened inflamed synovium slowly fibroses as adulthood is reached, and ultimately the combination of synovial contraction and articular cartilage destruction may result in a stiff, severely disorganized knee joint. At this stage hemarthrosis is uncommon, but when it does occur, a small amount of bleeding may make this contracted joint very tense, painful, and immobile.

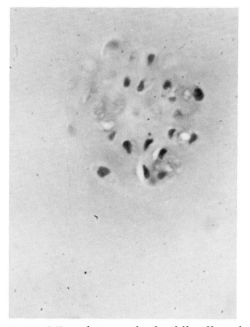

FIG. 20-10. Microphotograph of mildly affected articular cartilage in hemophilic arthropathy. A small aggregation of chondrocytes has formed in the deeper layers of the matrix.

Radiographic Appearances

A useful classification has been suggested by Arnold and Hilgartner.[4]

Stage I. No skeletal abnormalities are apparent on the x-ray film, although there may be soft tissue swelling due to hemarthrosis or periarticular bleeding. This appearance coincides with an otherwise normal joint that has sustained an acute hemorrhage.

Stage II. The feature at this stage is some epiphyseal overgrowth at the lower femur and upper tibia compared with a normal opposite knee (Figs. 20-14, 20-15). There may be mild osteoporosis on the affected side, and the thickened synovium may be outlined by a relative radiodensity of the contained hemosiderin (Fig. 20-14). This is the radiographic appearance of subacute hemophilic arthropathy with thickened synovium, chronic effusion, and muscle wasting. Chronic hyperemia

is probably responsible for the epiphyseal overgrowth.[6]

Stage III. Specific subchondral bone changes in the form of cyst formation and sclerosis occur, although there is usually no significant narrowing of the cartilage joint space (Fig. 20-16). At this stage, both the patella and the overgrown condyles may take on a squared appearance.

Large condylar cysts, usually situated marginally, are occasionally seen. These probably result from subperiosteal bleeding and, like any large bone cyst, may grow to form a hemophilic pseudotumor (Fig. 20-17).

These radiographic appearances are seen when a knee joint has been chronically swollen and thickened for several years (Fig. 20-18).

Stage IV. The features of advancing osteoarthritis are now present radiologically. Articular cartilage destruction is evidenced by a narrow joint space, subchondral bone sclerosis is more marked, and there may be some lateral shift of the tibia under the femur (Fig. 20-19). Typically, the intercondylar notch appears deepened and widened. This may be due to destructive erosion in the area, but the appearance may in some instances be apparent because a flexion contracture of the knee throws the notch into greater relief in the x-ray projection.*

This radiographic appearance coincides with a stiff and painful knee joint in which fibrosis is commencing in the previously thickened synovium.

Stage V. This is the end stage of progressive hemophilic arthritis, and joint disorganization is the radiographic characteristic. There is almost complete loss of the joint space, eburnation and sclerosis of exposed subchondral bone, and osteophyte formation. Except for the deepened intercondylar notch, the appearance is similar to that of severe degenerative arthritis (Fig. 20-20).

This appearance coincides with a stiff contracted joint in which the synovium is very fibrous. If the fibrous ankylosis is firm, pain

* Murray RO: Personal communication, 1972.

FIG. 20-11. Microphotograph of severely affected articular cartilage in hemophilic arthropathy. There are vertical fissures in the superficial layer, the matrix stains irregularly, and several clusters of chondrocytes have formed in the deeper layers.

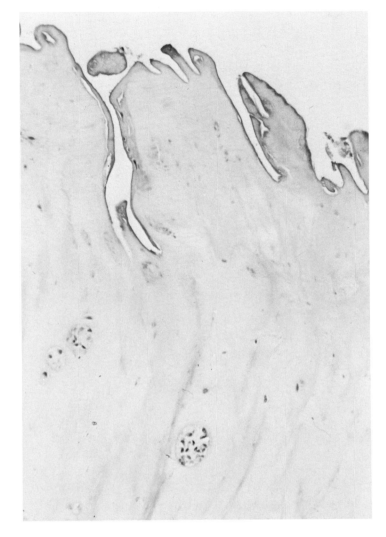

may not be a feature, but movement if present is painful. Contractures are usual, but hemarthroses may be infrequent or virtually absent.

Diagnosis

The sudden onset of a painful swelling in the knee joint of a 3- or 4-year-old boy might be the first indication of hemophilia and must be distinguished from septic arthritis or monarticular rheumatoid disease. The lack of sys-

temic illness and a previous history of bleeding from other sites establish the diagnosis.

Recurrent bleeding into a knee joint in which chronic hemophilic arthropathy already exists is usually obvious. An acute hemarthrosis should be distinguished from an irritative effusion. In the latter case joint tension is not a feature, and therefore pain may be mild or absent.

A fresh hemarthrosis is a severely disorganized knee joint in an adult is usually acutely painful because of tension within a contracted

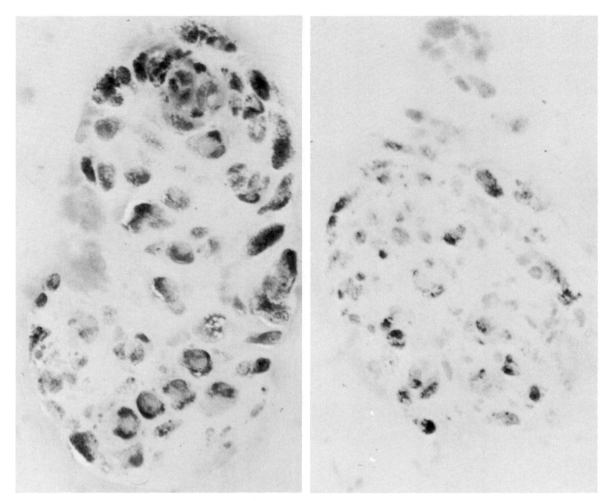

FIGS. 20-12 and 20-13. Microphotographs of severely affected articular cartilage in hemophilic arthropathy. The chondrocyte clusters have multiplied and many cells are necrotic. The iron content is demonstrated with Perls' stain (Fig. 20-13).

capsule. Movement previously present is invariably lost.

TREATMENT

Principles

The essential features of the management of hemophilia are two-fold: prevention of further hemorrhage by replacement of the deficient factor, and local treatment of the affected joint. Management requires a multidisciplinary approach—in particular, close cooperation between the hematologist and the ortho-

paedic surgeon. The hemophilic patient and his parents soon learn to recognize the hemarthroses that require active management. It is probable that in many minor episodes of bleeding, recovery occurs after 2 or 3 days of rest without specific therapy. It is now appreciated, however, that immediate replacement with deficient factor may control the hemarthrosis very early, thus lessening the amount of blood in the joint for the already overtaxed synovium to clear. In the past, every acute bleeding episode required hospitalization, but with effective home therapy programs,

FIG. 20-14. Subacute hemophilic arthropathy. There is mild epiphyseal overgrowth of the affected right knee. The synovium is outlined by a deposition of hemosiderin.

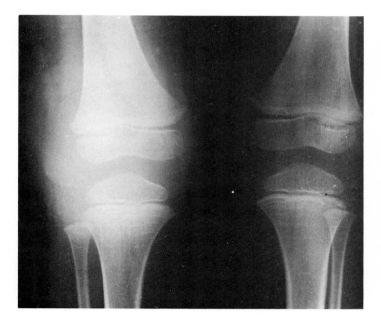

FIG. 20-15. Subacute hemophilic arthropathy. The lower femoral and upper tibial epiphyses of the hemophilic left knee are larger than those of the normal knee because of chronic hyperemia.

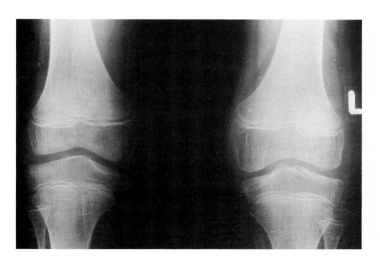

early treatment in the home may be both safe and effective. A combination of early replacement therapy and proper treatment of the affected joint provides the best insurance against ultimate joint destruction.

Replacement of Deficient Clotting Factor

Administration of Factor VIII or IX is best undertaken under the direction of a competent hematologist working in cooperation with other members of the multidisciplinary team. Details of the substances available and methods of use will not be discussed here, but some comments on the principles of replacement therapy are appropriate.

Historically, an intravenous infusion of fresh plasma was used to replace the deficient clotting factor. Because Factor VIII in particular degrades rapidly at ordinary refrigerator temperatures, the technique of rapidly freezing fresh plasma to $-30°$ was developed. The

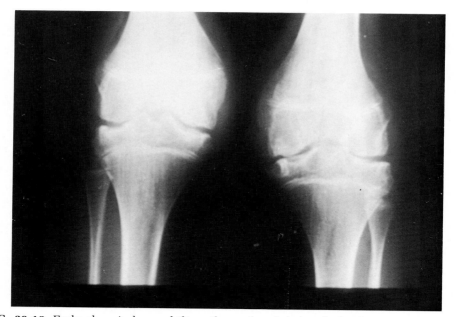

FIG. 20-16. Early chronic hemophilic arthropathy. Subchondral sclerosis, cyst formation, and early loss of articular cartilage space can be seen in this roentgenograph. The epiphyses are squared, and lateral subluxation of the tibia is commencing on the more affected left knee (*right*).

concentration of missing factors remains satisfactory if fresh frozen plasma is administered soon after reconstitution. Its usefulness is limited, however, by the quantity that must be administered to achieve an adequate level of the missing factor. Should this need to be between 10% and 20% of the normal circulating volume, it is necessary to administer 10 ml to 15 ml per kilogram of body weight of fresh frozen plasma during a period of 45 to 60 minutes.[28] Since the half-life of Factor VIII is only 12 hr, a plasma level of 20% of normal will drop to 5% within 24 hr. Thus a high plasma level, such as may be needed during surgery, cannot be obtained using fresh frozen plasma without over-loading the circulation and possibly producing renal embarrassment because of an excess of circulating protein. Furthermore, anemia may follow significant dilution of the red cells.

Methods of concentrating the antihemophilic globulins are now available. The easiest and least expensive way of concentrating Factor VIII commercially is by cryoprecipitation.

When fresh frozen plasma is reconstituted from $-30°$ to $+4°C$, an undissolved portion remains behind. This "cryoprecipitate" is rich in Factor VIII and fibrinogen. It is possible to give sufficient doses of this concentrate during surgery to maintain the required level of Factor VIII without causing circulatory overload. However, there is considerable variation in the concentration of products of different blood transfusion services, and blood-level assays are thus necessary to estimate the dosage. Nevertheless, cryoprecipitates are very useful in home therapy and in the treatment of spontaneous hemarthroses and muscle bleeding.

More recently, techniques that will precipitate the antihemophilic globulin (AHG) are available. These concentrates were in short supply until recently and are still very expensive. At one time animal precipitates of bovine or porcine origin were tried. These have the advantage of being about 15 times as potent as human AHG, but animal globulins are highly antigenic, often causing thrombocyto-

FIG. 20-17. A large marginal cyst is present in the tibial condyle. This probably began as a subperiosteal hematoma and may progress to form a hemophilic "pseudotumor." For this reason, and because the knee was painful and fixed in flexion, arthrodesis was subsequently performed. Note squaring of the patella in this lateral x-ray projection.

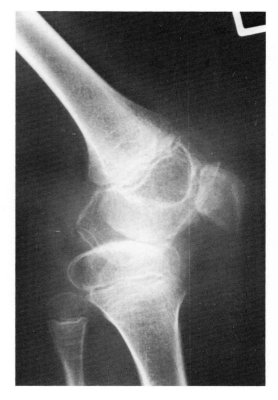

FIG. 20-18. Chronic hemophilic arthropathy. The joint is large because of intra-articular fluid, a thickened synovium, and epiphyseal overgrowth. The appearance is accentuated by wasting of the quadriceps muscles.

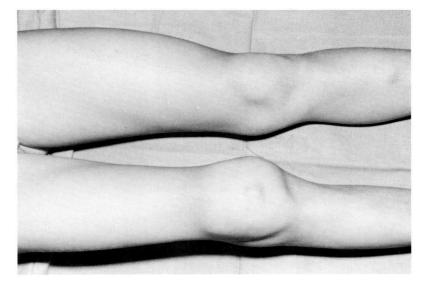

penia and the rapid development of resistance. Their administration should be reserved for life-saving procedures.

The currently available antihemophilic glob-ulin concentrates are of two types. The first contains Factor VIII and fibrinogen and is effective in the treatment of hemophilia A and Von Willebrand's disease. The second con-

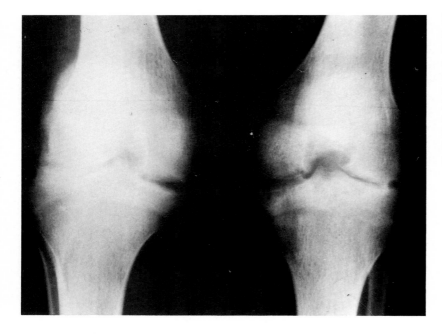

FIG. 20-19. Advancing hemophilic arthropathy. There is loss of joint space bilaterally, and subchondral cyst formation and sclerosis have occurred in the left knee (*right*). The intercondylar notches present a deepened and widened appearance typical of the knee joint in hemophilia.

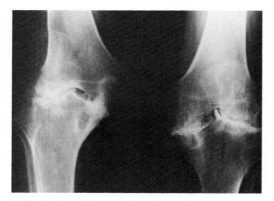

FIG. 20-20. Advanced arthropathy in an adult hemophiliac with gross disorganization of both knees. Articular cartilage is completely absent, exposed bone is eburnated and sclerotic, and some osteophyte formation suggests degenerative arthritis. The deepened intercondylar notch on the left and a degree of subluxation of the tibia on the right establish the cause as hemophilia.

tains Factor IX and also Factors II, V, and X and is used in the treatment of hemophilia B.

These concentrates are complex to manufacture and cannot be produced in ordinary blood banks. Furthermore, their use has been associated with a high incidence of hepatitis,

and disseminated intravascular coagulation has also been reported. In spite of these disadvantages and the added cost when compared to cryoprecipitate, the antihemophilic globulin concentrates have been widely accepted by both physicians and patients because of dose standardization and ease of administration.

An International Unit of Factor VIII or Factor IX is defined as the amount of activity found in 1 ml of fresh normal pooled plasma and is equal to 100% factor activity. The dose required is based on the patient's weight and assumed plasma volume. One unit of Factor VIII per kilogram of body weight will raise the patient's plasma level by 2%. The same quantity of Factor IX will raise the patient's plasma level by only 1.5% because a greater amount of this factor goes into the extravascular space.

The plasma level required depends upon the severity of the bleeding episode and its location—that is, whether it is intra-articular or intramuscular or in a danger area such as the central nervous system, retroperitoneal area, or nasopharynx. The biologic half-life of the infused factor must be taken into account. It may thus be necessary to achieve an initial plasma level of 40% to 50% if a 20% level is to be maintained for 24 hr.[1]

There is considerable variation in the plasma levels of antihemophilic globulin recommended by different clinics. Arnold and Hilgartner use an initial level of 30% to 40% for hemarthrosis and joint aspiration.[4] The level is raised to 40% or 50% for muscle bleeding, and further elevated to a level between 80% and 100% for a serious soft tissue hemorrhage such as bleeding into the central nervous system. At surgery they aim to achieve 100% plasma levels and to maintain a level of more than 60% for the first 4 postoperative days and 40% for the following 4 days. Following major surgery, the level is maintained at 20% for 4 to 6 weeks to provide a cover for postoperative physiotherapy. This concept is at variance with the practice of Pietrogrande and co-workers, who maintain a level as low as 30% during an operative procedure and 5% subsequently until the ninth postoperative day.[24] It has been our experience that in most instances the clinical response is a good guide for continuing therapy. We have kept the level at over 50% during surgery followed by a maintenance level of about 20% for 10 days.[13]

The use of any blood derivative is not without risk. The danger of hepatitis, particularly hepatitis B, is always present. Furthermore, many patients develop a low-titer inhibitor, particularly after the long-term high-dosage therapy required to cover surgical procedures. Before elective surgery, a patient should be thoroughly investigated for the presence of inhibitor substances, and the antihemophilic globulin efficacy in each patient should be individually tested.

Analgesics and Anti-inflammatory Agents

Pain relievers in the treatment of hemophilic arthropathy must be used with caution. Aspirin, antihistaminics, and certain other drugs inhibit platelet aggregation and prolong the bleeding time in patients with hemophilia.[17] Furthermore, aspirin may irritate the gastric mucosa and even produce ulceration and hemorrhage. Medications containing an aspirin compound should thus be avoided.

Corticosteroids have been used following acute hemarthroses, the dose being limited to 1 mg or 2 mg per kilogram of body weight for 5 days.[18] Side-effects have not been reported following these short courses of steroid therapy. Other common anti-inflammatory agents such as phenylbutazone, indomethacin, and ibuprofen may inhibit platelet function and produce liver disease in hemophilic patients.[1] Furthermore, any of these substances may cause gastric irritation with the danger of peptic ulcer formation and gastrointestinal bleeding. They must therefore be used with the greatest care.

ORTHOPAEDIC MANAGEMENT OF ACUTE HEMARTHROSIS
Assessment

In order to establish a baseline, an exact assessment of the degree of hemarthrosis should be made. The knee joint lends itself to precise monitoring.

The circumference of the joint is measured at the point of maximal swelling, using an ordinary tape measure, and the findings are recorded on a chart. The opposite knee is used as a control, care being taken to make the measurement with both knees equally flexed.

Using a goniometer, the range of movement of the affected knee is measured, charted, and compared with that of the opposite knee. The standard international method of joint range measurement is followed whereby full extension of the knee is equivalent to 0°. Fixed flexion contracture is thus accurately reflected by a record of the reading. For example, a range of 35° to 100° represents a fixed flexion contracture of 35° and an actual range of movement of 65°.

Joint Immobilization

Once an intravenous infusion of the deficient factor is established, the joint should be treated by rest. Any form of long leg splint, including a well-padded plaster-of-Paris back-slab, might suffice, but our experience is that the knee tends to flex out of flat splints unless bandaging is made uncomfortably firm. On that account the Robert Jones pressure bandage is preferred. This consists of a generous layer of wool applied from the groin to the ankle, followed by an Ace or crepe bandage. A second layer of wool and bandage is then applied. This method provides reasonable immobilization, comfort, and a degree of even compression. It is easily removed by the nursing staff and the physiotherapists for daily inspection and assessment of the knee joint. Furthermore, daily reapplication ensures that compression and immobilization remain satisfactory. When necessary, the degree of immobilization may be increased by incorporating four thin wooden slats situated on the anterior, posterior, medial, and lateral aspects, deep to the last turn of bandage.

Physiotherapy

It is important to commence muscle rehabilitation as soon as possible. Once the knee is held extended, hemarthrosis is not a contraindication to static quadriceps exercises. Irritation of the knee joint synovium produces reflex quadriceps inhibition with loss of protective tone and early diminution of muscle bulk (Fig. 20-18); thus an immediate energetic regimen is essential to prevent wasting, provide joint protection, and speed rehabilitation.

The Role of Knee Joint Aspiration

Ideally, blood should be completely removed from the joint. In current practice many hemarthroses are now treated at home. In the hospital environment, aspiration is rarely fully successful because large doses of deficient factor will have been given prior to the time of proposed joint aspiration, ensuring that some of the hemarthrosis will be clotted.

In most instances, the combination of immobilization, deficient factor replacement, and graded exercises produces rapid absorption of the hemarthrosis and speedy recovery.

For this reason, knee joint aspiration is only occasionally indicated, a view that accords with the work of Crock and Boni.[9] Aspiration, however, should be considered when the hemarthrosis remains very tense in spite of adequate conservative management or when the size of the knee joint, although not tense, remains static for 10 days or more. When measurements indicate that the knee joint is actually increasing in size in spite of formal treatment, aspiration must be performed.

Joint aspiration is regarded as a formal surgical procedure and must be undertaken in an operating room under full aseptic conditions. Replacement factor should be administered during and not immediately prior to the aspiration procedure to minimize intravascular clotting.[11,20]

An irritative effusion should be differentiated from an acute hemarthrosis in the chronically affected knee joint. When present, some fluid will remain in the joint for a protracted period, but pain will be absent and the range of motion unimpaired. Thickening of the synovium will be palpable. Aspiration of these joints is not helpful.

Rehabilitation

When daily joint measurements establish that the hemarthrosis is resolving, knee movement is encouraged under physiotherapeutic supervision. Isotonic exercises of both quadriceps and hamstring muscles against light resistence are now commenced. When good muscle control has returned, weight-bearing is permitted but only with the affected joint supported. A Robert Jones bandage or light plaster-of-Paris splint is suitable, and crutches are used in the first instance.

The patient who has had recurrent bleeding needs a more protracted form of support. A lightweight orthosis, which maintains the knee straight during walking but permits flexion for sitting, should be used until the knee is completely quiescent. This support is particularly important during the potentially traumatic school hours or working day.

TREATMENT OF FIXED FLEXION
CONTRACTURE OF THE KNEE

Significant knee flexion contractures are common in subacute and chronic hemophilic arthropathy. Apart from the cosmetic deformity, the relative shortening that results may secondarily affect both ankle and hip joints, producing equinus and hip flexion contracture respectively. A short leg limp then develops (Fig. 20-21).

When joint damage and capsular contraction makes stiffness inevitable, treatment should be directed at keeping the knee as straight as possible—that is, in a position of function. Once fixed flexion becomes established, relative shortening of the collateral ligaments of the knee occurs.[8] Straightening of the knee, whether by traction or by casting techniques, may then be accompanied by posterior subluxation of the tibia on the femur (Fig. 20-22).

Several methods have been devised for the treatment of fixed flexion contracture. Simple skin traction with the limb held on a padded splint can be used successfully to straighten the joint but will not prevent backsetting of the knee. To overcome this problem, Stein and Dickson devised a modification of balanced Thomas traction using a Pearson knee flexion attachment to support the tibia.[31] A reverse sling is passed over the patella and under each limb of the Thomas splint. Each end of the sling is then directed anteriorly and attached to a cord so that traction can be applied upward at a right angle to the distal femoral shaft. Increasing this traction thus pushes the distal femur posteriorly while the upper end of the tibia is held in place by slings under the Pearson knee piece. This technique can not only prevent but correct backward subluxation as the knee joint is slowly straightened.

Traction techniques, however, require hospitalization, and therefore casting methods that allow the patient to be treated at home are usually preferred. A turnbuckle cast composed of leg and thigh sections connected by

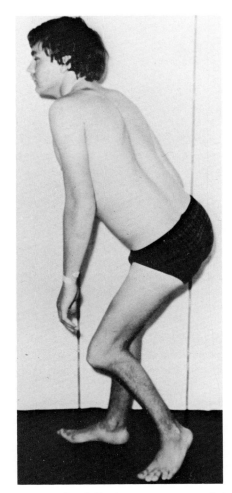

FIG. 20-21. A fixed flexion contracture of the left knee has produced a short leg limp. The hip on that side is held flexed and the foot is in equinus. Contractions in these otherwise normal joints will ultimately develop.

an eccentric hinge with a locking mechanism can be effective, and some designs do control posterior tibial subluxation. Wedging of plaster casts or the use of a turnbuckle with simple hinge mechanisms are not recommended because both of these methods aggravate backsetting of the tibia. In our experience, a method used by Conner in correcting knee flexion contractures in poliomyelitis, in which a similar problem of tightness of the collateral

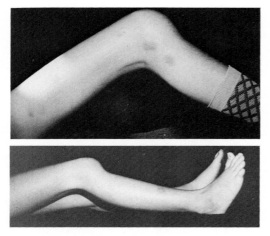

FIG. 20-22. A severe fixed flexion contracture of the knee in hemophilia was corrected by a combination of traction on a Thomas splint and a hinged turnbuckle plaster cast (A). Marked back-setting of the tibia resulted (B).

ligaments exists, is effective.[8] At each weekly cast replacement the knee is gently straightened and the tightness of the collateral ligaments overcome by a deliberate anterior pull under the upper tibial shaft as extension of the leg is achieved.

When these methods fail, a Quengel cast may be used.[16] This consists of a short hip spica to which is attached an outrigger over the front of the flexed tibia. A separate short tibial cast is applied, which is then connected to the outrigger at each end by a Spanish windlass (Fig. 20-23). Tightening each windlass enables traction to be applied to both the proximal and distal ends of the tibia simultaneously. Care must be taken to prevent the occurrence of a valgus deformity as the knee straightens.

If these techniques are carried out gently, deficiency factor replacement is only rarely required. It should be emphasized that as correction is achieved, active mobilization and quadriceps exercises must be encouraged. Furthermore, it is important to maintain the correction that is achieved, and the use of a lightweight splint at night and a walking orthosis during the day is necessary. As the quadriceps muscles strengthen, day supports

may be abandoned, but a night splint should be used until the knee is completely mobile and extension is virtually complete and easily maintained by the powerful quadriceps muscles.

TREATMENT OF SUBACUTE ARTHROPATHY

Once a pattern of repeated hemarthrosis has become established, the physical changes of palpable synovial thickening and epiphyseal overgrowth are certain to be present. Control of further hemarthroses at this stage is mandatory if the long-term integrity of articular cartilage is to be preserved.

Nonsurgical Management

Six to 8 weeks of intensive therapy is warranted in these patients in an endeavor to break the cycle of repeated hemarthroses. Duthie recommends initial hospitalization.* During the first 10 to 14 days, deficient factor is replaced daily, the affected knee is rested with a Robert Jones pressure bandage for much of the time, and intensive physiotherapy is administered in the form of static muscle exercises and controlled movement out of the bandage. During the following period, deficient factor replacement should be given three times a week in a dose sufficient to raise the patient's plasma level to between 20% and 30% of normal. Immediately after each transfusion and on the following morning, when the antihemophilic globulin level is still high, active quadriceps muscle and range of motion exercises should be undertaken. Swimming should also be encouraged, and the patient should be prepared to graduate to bicycle riding, hiking, and other noncontact sports.

Surgical Synovectomy

Pietrogrande and co-workers first reported the results of a significant series of surgical synovectomies.[24] They were encouraged because the incidence of hemarthroses was greatly di-

* Duthie RB: Personal communication

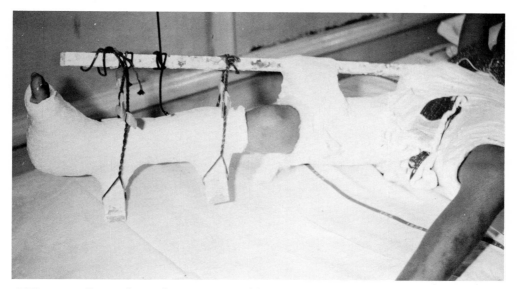

FIG. 20-23. Quengel cast for correction of fixed flexion contracture of the knee in hemophilia. The femur is stabilized by a short hip spica, and the tibia with a below-the-knee, plaster-of-Paris cast. Spanish windlasses connect suitable outriggers attached to both casts so that steady traction can be applied to both proximal and distal ends of the tibia simultaneously.

minished and the procedure did not reduce the range of motion of the joint. Since then, the operation has been carried out in small numbers at many centers. Its role, however, is still controversial. One of the reasons for this is the lack of stringent indications for the procedure. Storti and associates performed a large number of synovectomies after only three or four joint hemorrhages.[32] Most workers agree that the principal clinical indication for the operation is the morbidity associated with recurrent hemorrhages and effusions that cannot be controlled by nonoperative methods, and will undertake surgery only when chronicity is established. Using these criteria, the operation is usually successful in that subsequent hemarthroses are infrequent. The synovium that regrows is very fibrous and relatively avascular.[21] Our current knowledge suggests that synovectomy should also be considered as a prophylactic procedure to preserve the longevity of the articular cartilage.

Synovectomy of the knee may be satisfacto-

rily performed through a lateral parapatellar incision that avoids the infrapatellar branch of the saphenous nerve. With the patella dislocated and the knee flexed, almost all of the synovium can be resected (Fig. 20-24). A small rongeur is useful for removing synovium from the posterior recesses and the intercondylar notch. The procedure must be carried out under the protection of proper deficient factor replacement as outlined earlier. Manipulation of the knee is usually required two weeks postoperatively to help restore motion.

Surgical synovectomy was conducted on eight knees in patients ranging in age from 8 to 12 years (one boy was 6 years old). In the seven older patients, craterlike defects were found in the articular cartilage (Figs. 20-4, 20-5). The 6-year-old patient had advanced chondromalacia of all articulating surfaces (Fig. 20-25). Postoperatively, in spite of joint manipulation, all patients had an extremely limited range of motion for the first 6 to 12 months. Ultimately, seven of the eight knees

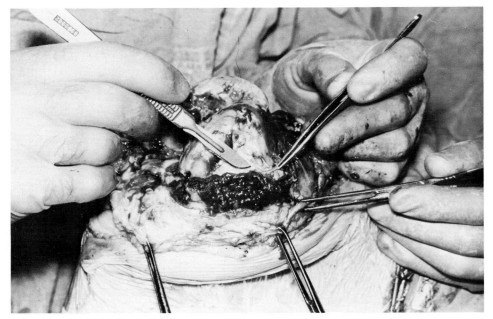

FIG. 20-24. Surgical synovectomy of the knee. Dislocation of the patella and flexion of the knee provide access to almost all of the synovium.

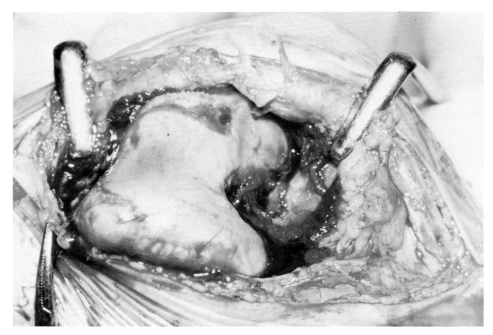

FIG. 20-25. Femoral condyles in a 6-year-old boy at surgical synovectomy. The articular cartilage was softened, presenting the feel and appearance of severe chondromalacia. There are two strips of pannus formation on the weight-bearing surfaces of the femoral condyles.

regained 90° or more of flexion. In spite of the protracted postoperative course, every patient was pleased with the results because subsequent hemarthroses were almost nonexistent. Freedom from the need for treatment is important, and from this point of view the operations must be regarded as successful. The long-term prognosis for seven of the eight joints, however, was thought to be poor because of the severe loss of articular cartilage. One patient in this group died at the age of 15 of a cerebral hemorrhage following a head injury. We were thus able to examine the synovectomized knee at postmortem three years after the operation. The previous craters from the articular cartilage had filled with fibrocartilage and there were many fibrous bands between the articular surfaces of the tibia, femur, and patella. The synovium was very thin, fibrous, and contracted. In spite of this appearance, the patient had enjoyed a pain-free range of flexion to 90° during life.

Surgical synovectomy is a major undertaking that taxes the resources of the hemophilic center. Although it should not be undertaken lightly, it certainly has a place when the morbidity of the chronically affected knee joint is severe. When performed early enough, it may well prevent the disproportionate amount of articular cartilage breakdown that is a feature of the disease.

TREATMENT OF THE SEVERELY DISORGANIZED KNEE

As joint destruction progresses, both pain and stiffness usually increase. Fortunately, a short, firm, fibrous ankylosis is often the eventual outcome. The capsule is usually fibrosed, and hemarthroses are rare. If the knee is nearly straight and functionally satisfactory for walking, no treatment may be required. On the other hand, the knee joint with a painful range of motion presents a serious therapeutic problem because of the danger inherent in the use of simple analgesics such as salicylates and the common anti-inflammatory agents. In some instances, the use of a block leather or plastic knee gaiter during the day may keep the patient comfortable at work and may permit pain-free weight-bearing. Removal of the orthosis can enable the patient to use the available range of motion for sitting during his leisure hours (Fig. 20-26). When an orthosis does not control pain or when a fixed flex-

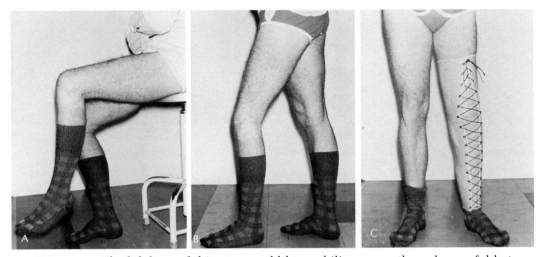

FIG. 20-26. The left knee of this 26-year-old hemophiliac moves through a useful but very painful range **(A,B)**. A close-fitting knee orthosis, worn only to work, allows pain-free weight-bearing **(C)**. At home, he is able to sit with the knee comfortably flexed.

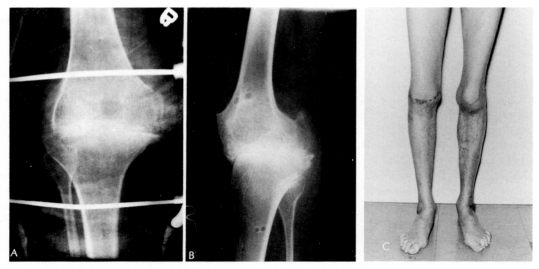

FIG. 20-27. Minimal excision of bone and the use of Charnley compression clamps **(A)** have produced a sound arthrodesis of the right knee in a good functional position **(B,C)**.

ion or other deformity exists, surgery is usually indicated.

Corrective osteotomies have a limited role in the surgical management of knee deformities, provided the patient has a good range of painless knee motion. A supracondylar osteotomy should not be used to correct a fixed flexion deformity because further contractions frequently occur postoperatively. In general, the severely disorganized knee is better corrected at the knee joint itself. In the hemophiliac, arthrodesis is the most reliable and satisfactory procedure.

A standard Charnley technique using compression clamps has resulted in rapid fusion without complications in four instances. Any deformity may be easily corrected (Fig. 20-27). Excision of the patella is not necessary. A painless stable knee, particularly when other joints are significantly involved, is much appreciated by the hemophilic patient. At the present time, total knee replacement procedures in the hemophiliac are viewed with caution because complications are severely aggravated by the bleeding diathysis. Nevertheless, a significant number of total knee arthroplasties have been undertaken in some centers. Kostuik in Toronto has performed 13

total knee replacements and 4 MacIntosh arthroplasties.* He believes that total replacement is contraindicated in simple joint arthritis in a young man but that it has a place in the treatment of severe joint destruction in an older patient, particularly when there is ipsilateral knee joint involvement. Ideally, preoperative knee joint motion should be 40° or greater. When multiple joint involvement prevents the patient from imposing much stress on the arthroplasty, Kostuik would undertake the operation in younger patients.

The procedures were performed in a clean-environment operating room. When possible, a tourniquet was applied but deflated before skin closure, and hemostasis was achieved. Hemovac wound suction and compression dressings were used, and pain was controlled by instilling long-acting anesthetic agents through a fine epidural catheter left in the knee joint for up to 10 days after surgery. The Gunston polycentric and total condylar duopatellar prostheses were used except for one early Marmor prosthesis. This subsequently loosened and the joint was arthrodesed. In a short-term follow-up examination Kostuik

---

* Kostuik JP: Personal communication

noted four cases with excellent results (motion was increased and there was no pain), a further four were categorized as good (motion was preserved and pain was relieved), and three cases had fair results (postoperative motion was decreased but pain was relieved). Knee manipulation was undertaken 10 days postoperatively in all patients. No significant operative complications developed.

MUSCLE HEMATOMAS

Knee joint deformity is not infrequently of extra-articular origin. Damaged fibers in nearby musculature are replaced by fibrous tissue that slowly contracts and produces permanent shortening of the overall muscle length. The quadriceps and the calf, particularly the triceps surae, are frequently damaged by deep-seated hemorrhages (Fig. 20-28). A hematoma under tension within a fascial compartment may occlude the arterial flow and produce a true muscle infarction of the Volkmann type with subsequent muscle necrosis and contracture. This overt form of compression is uncommon but has occurred on two occasions in the forearm flexor musculature in which infarction and nerve damage produced the typical peripheral deformity.

In our experience a less well recognized but nevertheless severe form of muscle necrosis occurs more commonly in hemophilia, particularly in the calf muscle. This follows a slow, insidious hemorrhage deep to the fascia of a group of muscles or within an individual muscle compartment. Arterial occlusion does not occur, the peripheral pulse is not occluded, and the doctor is wooed into a sense of false security. Tension gradually builds up within the closed compartment, and capillary blood flow becomes obstructed. The ischemic muscle fibers swell and further strangle their own blood supply. The result is a patchy necrosis of muscle fibers followed by round cell infiltration and ultimately an irregular fibrous tissue replacement (Fig. 20-29). If left untreated, this fibrous tissue steadily contracts over a period of months and may result in se-

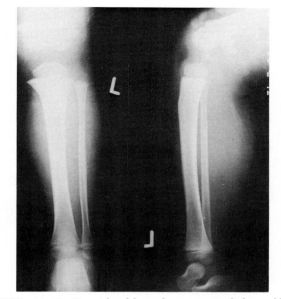

FIG. 20-28. Considerable enlargement of the calf shadow is evident on this radiograph of a 7-year-old boy's left leg. This was caused by a large, almost painless hematoma within muscle deep to the fascia.

rious shortening of the affected muscles. When the gastrocnemius muscles are involved, a flexion contracture of the knee as well as an equinus deformity of the foot will follow (Fig. 20-30). Contractions of the quadriceps may produce fixed extension or even hyperextension of the knee. These contractures become rigid and are resistant to nonoperative correction.

The clinical importance of this insidious form of relatively painless hemorrhage cannot be overemphasized. Bleeding into the calf, quadriceps, and other large muscle groups must be watched even more closely than the more obvious hemarthroses. Pain is a feature during the early phase of deep muscle hemorrhages and should never be ignored. Later, as nerve fibers become ischemic, tension within a muscle fascia may increase with little discomfort. These episodes of muscle bleeding warrant hospital admission, immediate immobilization of the limb in a position of function, and the infusion of large doses of he-

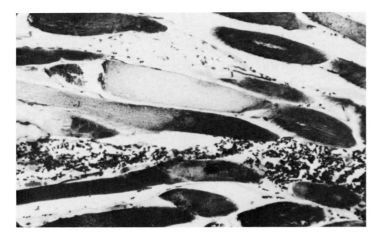

FIG. 20-29. Patchy areas of muscle fiber death and marked round cell infiltration are illustrated in this biopsy specimen of gastrocnemius muscle obtained during decompression of subfascial hemorrhage into the calf.

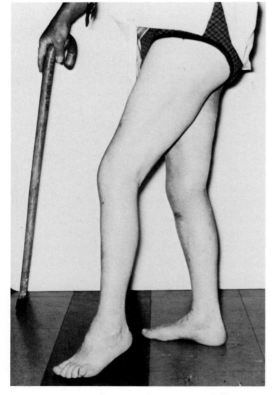

FIG. 20-30. Patchy muscle necrosis following subfascial muscle hemorrhages has left this patient's left calf thin and contracted. Shortening of the gastrocnemii caused a fixed equinus deformity of the ankle and a flexion contracture of the knee even though both joints are essentially normal.

mophilic concentrate. The affected muscle should be closely observed and circumferential measurements made over the point of maximal swelling every hour. Unless there is rapid reduction in size and subsidence of pain within 8 hours, full surgical decompression is indicated forthwith. This must be undertaken as a formal surgical procedure with full deficient factor cover. The hematoma should be completely evacuated and tense ischemic muscles fully decompressed. When skin closure is achieved, the use of sealed suction drainage is favored. Prolonged postoperative splinting in a position of function is imperative. A splint for both knee and ankle at night and a suitable orthosis during the day should be used for months after the ischemic episode. As in the treatment of hemarthrosis, physiotherapy plays an important role (Fig. 20-31).

GENERAL MANAGEMENT OF THE HEMOPHILIAC

The regimen outlined for the management of the hemophilic knee requires a multidisciplinary team approach involving the hematologist, pediatrician, orthopaedic surgeon, and physiotherapist. Access to a sophisticated blood transfusion service and the availability of cryoprecipitate and antihemophilic globulin concentrates are essential.

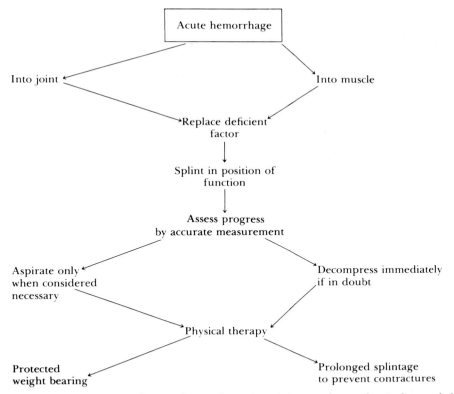

FIG. 20-31. Management of acute hemorrhage into joints and muscles in hemophilia.

The general environment of the hemophilic patient must not be neglected. The disease lasts a lifetime; sufferers can expect to lose a great deal of time from school work, and the possibility of progressive and permanent crippling is ever present. The social and economic implications must be taken into account, and emphasis should be placed on a full education and subsequent job placement for the afflicted patient. The medical team must thus seek collaboration with social workers and teachers so that treatment will disrupt schooling as little as possible.

The patient should carry a card that states that he is a hemophiliac and provides essential data such as his address, telephone number, blood group, and deficient factor levels. The name, address, and telephone number of his family practitioner should also be recorded. Any allergies, particularly to drugs,

and the presence or absence of inhibitors should be noted on the card.

Education of the parents and in due course the patient is important to achieve their cooperation. They must understand the implications of the disease and be able to recognize the signs and symptoms that call for active treatment either at home or in the hospital.

Proper schooling arrangements are essential. Although a few severely crippled boys do better at schools for the physically handicapped, the average hemophiliac patient should attend a regular school where arrangements have been made to avoid areas of potential trauma. The knee joint is particularly susceptible to damage in sports, and suitable advice for participation in sports is necessary. Although body contact sports should be avoided, it is essential to maintain muscle tone, and swimming, cycling, riding, and hiking can be encouraged. Some gymnastic activities may be safely performed. A powerful quadriceps femoral muscle is the best protection against knee hemarthroses.

THE FUTURE

The long-term prognosis of the knee joint depends upon maintaining the integrity of the articular cartilage. The chronically swollen knee with a thickened friable and hyperactive synovium is at risk, and attention must be given to reducing synovial hypertrophy and activity.

The role of surgical synovectomy has been discussed. This major surgical procedure is expensive and taxing for both patient and medical staff. For this reason alternative methods of inactivating the synovium are being investigated.

Several workers have injected osmic acid into hemophilic joints.[3,27] This substance reduces synovial hypertrophy by destroying its superficial layers, but the procedure has met with only partial success in hemophilic arthropathy. At the present time its use in patients is not permitted in the United States.

Ahlberg first reported the use of radioactive gold in an effort to achieve a "medical synovectomy".[2] More recently, Erken and co-workers used intra-articular doses of ^{90}Y in patients with continuing hemophilic arthropathy.[12] The ages ranged from 9 to 32 years; half were under 16 years. In an effort to limit the spread of the radioactive substances beyond the injected joint, the procedure was always performed on Friday afternoon and the patient was instructed to rest the joint until Monday morning. At present 27 joints have been injected. Fifteen have been followed for up to 2 years, and the early results are most encouraging. In all, the bleeding frequency has been much reduced, particularly in five joints in which synovial thickening was palpably less. The response in seven joints was considered to be good, and only three have remained swollen even though acute hemarthroses have diminished. Yttrium-90 is a beta-emitter with a very limited penetration. Because of this and its short half-life of 63 hr, its intra-articular use is considered safe even in young children.

Nonsurgical destruction of the diseased synovium will probably be the most important future form of therapy for the chronically afflicted knee joint.

The ultimate aim of management should be prophylaxis. Home infusion programs that enable the patient to receive antihemophilic globulins as soon as possible may prove to be a major advance in the treatment of the condition. The severely afflicted patient whose deficient factor level is under 1% may benefit from the prophylactic administration of antihemophilic globulin concentrates once or twice a week. Vigorous quadriceps-building exercises should be performed at the time of the intravenous infusion. Besides the cost considerations, it is yet to be established whether the risk of inhibitor development outweighs the value of prophylactic therapy.

SUMMARY

Early recognition and an energetic interdisciplinary approach to the hemophilic patient can to a large extent prevent knee joint destruction and deformity. When significant damage has already occurred, deficient factor replacement has enabled the surgeon to proceed confidently with the procedures necessary to rehabilitate his patient.

REFERENCES

1. **Abildgaard CF:** Current concepts in the management of hemophilia. Semin Hematol 12:223, 1975
2. **Ahlberg A:** Radioactive gold in treatment of chronic synovial effusion in haemophilia. In Ala F, Denson KWE (eds): Haemophilia. Amsterdam, Excerpta Medica, 1973
3. **Allain JP:** Synoviorthesis as treatment of chronic haemophilic arthropathy. Talk presented at the Eighth Congress of the World Federation of Haemophilia, Tehran, Iran, 1970

4. **Arnold WD, Hilgartner MW:** Hemophilic arthropathy: Current concepts of pathogenesis and management. J Bone Joint Surg 59A:287, 1977

5. **Bernstein MA:** The treatment of joint lesions in haemophilia by means of whole blood from menstruating women. J Bone Joint Surg 14:659, 1932

6. **Boldero JL, Kemp HS:** The early bone and joint changes in haemophilia and similar blood dyscrasias. Br J Radiol 39:172, 1966

7. **Brighton CT, Bigley EC Jr, Smolensky BI:** Iron induced arthritis in immature rabbits. Arthritis Rheum 13:849, 1970

8. **Conner AN:** Treatment of flexion contracture of the knee in poliomyelitis. J Bone Joint Surg 52B:138, 1970

9. **Crock HV, Boni V:** The management of orthopaedic problems in the haemophiliac. A review of 21 cases. Br J Surg 48:8, 1960

10. **Curtiss PH Jr:** Changes produced in synovial membrane and synovial fluid by disease. J Bone Joint Surg 46A:873, 1964

11. **Duthie RB, Matthews JM, Rizza CR et al:** The Management of Musculoskeletal Problems in the Haemophilias, p. 45. Oxford, Blackwell Scientific Publications, 1972

12. **Erken EHW, Schepers A, Sweet MBE et al:** The use of radioactive colloids (yttrium 90) in the treatment of haemophilic arthropathy. Paper presented at the 24th Congress of the South African Orthopaedic Association, Bloemfontein, South Africa, September, 1978

13. **Handelsman JE, Lurie A:** Pathological changes in the juvenile haemophilic knee. S Afr J Surg 13:243, 1975

14. **Hilgartner MW:** Pathogenesis of joint changes in hemophilia. In McCollagh NC III (ed): Comprehensive Management of Musculoskeletal Disorders in Hemophilia. Washington, D.C., National Academy of Sciences, 1973

15. **Jaffe HL:** Metabolic Degenerative and Inflammatory Diseases of Bones and Joints, p 721. Philadelphia, Lea & Febiger, 1972

16. **Jordan HH:** Hemophilic Arthropathies. Springfield, Ill. Charles C Thomas, 1958

17. **Kasper CK, Rapaport SI:** Bleeding times and platlet aggregation after analgesics in hemophilia. Ann Intern Med 77:189, 1972

18. **Kisker CT, Burke C:** Double-blind studies on the use of steroids in the treatment of acute hemarthrosis in patients with hemophilia. N Engl J Med 282:639, 1970

19. **Kisker CT, Perlman AW, Benton C:** Arthritis in hemophilia. Semin Arthritis Rheum 1:221, 1972

20. **Lurie A, Bailey BP:** The management of acute haemophilic haemarthroses and muscle haematoma. S Afr Med J 46:656, 1972

21. **Mitchell NS, Cruess RL:** The effect of synovectomy on articular cartilage. J Bone Joint Surg 49A:1099, 1967

22. **National Heart and Lung Institute:** National Heart, Blood Vessel, Lung and Blood Program, Vol 4, Part 4. Report of the Blood resources Panel. DHEW Pub. No. (NIH) 73-515-73-524. Bethesda, Department of Health, Education, and Welfare, 1973

23. **Neimann KMW:** Pathogenesis of hemophilic arthropathy. In McCollagh NC III (ed): Comprehensive Management of Musculoskeletal Disorders in Hemophilia. Washington, D.C., National Academy of Sciences, 1973

24. **Pietrogrande V, Dioguardi N, Mannucci PM:** Short-term evaluation of synovectomy in haemophilia. Br Med J 2:378, 1972

25. **Pohle FJ, Taylor FHL:** The coagulation defect in hemophilia. The effect in hemophilia of intramuscular administration of a globulin substance derived from normal plasma. J Clin Invest 16:741, 1937

26. **Rippey JJ, Hill RRH, Lurie A et al:** Articular cartilage degradation and the pathology of haemophilic arthropathy. S Afr Med J 54:345, 1978

27. **Risse JC, Menkes CH, Allain JP et al:** Synoviorthesis in the treatment of chronic haemophilic arthropathy: A preliminary report. In Ala F, Denson KWE (ed): Haemophilia. Amsterdam, Excerpta Medica, 1973

28. **Rizza CR:** The management of haemophilia. Practitioner 204:763, 1970

29. **Rodman GP:** Experimental hemarthrosis: The removal of chromium-51 and iron-59 labelled erythrocytes injected into the knee joint of rabbit and man. Arthritis Rheum 3:195, 1962

30. **Sokoloff L:** Biochemical and physiologic aspects of degenerative joint diseases with special reference to hemophilic arthropathy. Ann NY Acad Sci 240:285, 1975

31. **Stein H, Dickson RA:** Brief notes. Reversed dynamic slings for knee-flexion contractures in the hemophiliac. J Bone Joint Surg 57A:282, 1975

32. **Storti E, Traldi A, Tosatti E et al:** Synovectomy in hemophilia: a new therapeutic approach and efficient technique in hemostasis. Gaz San 29:11, 1970

33. **Stuart J, Davies SH, Cummings RA et al:** Haemorrhagic episodes in haemophilia: A 5-year prospective study. Br Med J 2:1624, 1960

34. **van Creveld S, Hoedemaeker PJ, Kingma MJ et al:** Degeneration of joints in haemophiliacs under treatment by modern methods. J Bone Joint Surg 53B:296, 1971

CHAPTER 21
PATHOLOGIC ANATOMY OF KNEE JOINT LIGAMENT INJURIES

E. L. Trickey

The way to understand the complex movement of the normal and abnormal knee joint is by examining freshly amputated specimens. Such an examination enables the observer to investigate closely the pattern of normal movements and the complex abnormal ones which are produced by ligament division, singly and in combination. Such investigations should be undertaken by anyone who is seriously interested in the subject. Without them the detailed results that are described often appear too complex to understand.

The pathologic understanding and treatment of knee ligament injuries have been hampered by dogmatic statements from clinicians that have no pathologic proof. If one particular abnormal movement can be produced constantly by the division of a particular ligament, it stands to reason that this fact must be of clinical importance. It is recognized that in practice there are various grades of severity of knee ligament damage and that it is impossible to sustain the complete tearing of one ligament without some damage to

another structure. Nevertheless, it is possible to determine the exact abnormal movements possible after ligament division in an anatomical specimen, and a clinical diagnosis which does not correspond with such findings is incorrect.

An excellent study of amputation specimens was presented by Brantigan and Voshell in 1941 in which all the facts are laid out.[1] In addition they present a long list of contradictory statements that were commonly made 40 years ago. Unfortunately, such statements are still being made. A recent personal independent study of specimens confirms their findings.

In a completely extended knee joint both collateral and cruciate ligaments are taut, and in this position the condyles fit together. No rotatory movement is possible. The exact position of full extension (and by this is meant the full extension for that particular person) varies from person to person. It might be 5° less or more than the neutral position. When examining an abnormal knee a comparison with the normal uninjured one is necessary to determine the position of full extension for that individual. As the normal knee flexes, the tibia immediately rotates internally a few degrees, and this pattern is followed in its smooth course of further flexion. As soon as flexion starts it is possible to rotate the tibia on the femur. This freedom to rotate is essential for many physical functions. Although difficult to measure accurately, the range of rotation varies between 5° and 20°. External rotation is greater than internal rotation.

The axis of this normal rotatory movement is not central and this can be observed by palpating one's own knee at a flexion of 90°. One hand grasps each tibial condyle. As rotation occurs the lateral tibial condyle rotates predominantly; therefore, the pivotal point is to the medial side of the center. With this normal rotation there is no subluxation of the condyles.

Rotation of the flexed normal knee is possible largely because in flexion the lateral ligament is relaxed. The cruciate ligaments are less taut than in full extension but are still tight. Similarly, the medial ligament is less taut but is not relaxed in any position of flexion.

When the ligaments are divided, subluxation of condyles can be produced. With such subluxation the normal axis of rotation will shift.

MEDIAL LIGAMENT

The anatomy of the medial ligament is important. It consists of three portions—superficial, deep, and oblique. The superficial part is a vertical band with a distinct anterior edge extending from the medial femoral condyle distally and slightly forward in the extended knee (Fig. 21-1A). It is attached to the tibia about 2.5 cm distal to the joint line and then extends further down the tibia. It is separated from the deep part over the joint line, and as the knee is flexed it glides, to a slight extent posteriorly over the deep portion.

The deep part of the medial ligament is derived from the joint capsule deep to the superficial part. It is a thick strong structure attached to the femoral and tibial condyles just beyond the articular cartilage. The peripheral edge of the medial meniscus is firmly attached to it and runs into the oblique part of the ligament.

The oblique part of the ligament is a fan-shaped structure arising from the medial femoral condyle behind the attachment of the superficial part (Fig. 21-1B). It extends distally and spreads out to attach to the posterior half of the medial tibial condyle just distal to the joint line. The peripheral edge of the medial meniscus is attached to it. Anteriorly it blends completely with the superficial and deep parts. The posterior oblique edge blends with the posterior capsule, which covers the back of the medial femoral condyle. It may be difficult to distinguish these two structures in the extended joint, but in flexion the posterior capsule is very lax whereas the oblique part of the ligament is still tight though not taut.

DIVISION OF THE MEDIAL LIGAMENT

When the medial ligament is divided, a constant abnormal pattern of movement is produced. The extent of the abnormal movement is dependent on the extent of the division. Abnormal movement is constant, whatever the level of division between the proximal attachment on the femoral condyle to the distal attachment just distal to the articular cartilage of the tibia. However, if the ligament is completely divided down to bone at a distance of 2.5 cm or more from the tibial joint line, no abnormal movement is possible. If such a distal tear is found in an injured knee with instability, the instability is due to an associated more proximal lesion.

In full extension no abnormal movement is possible. With a few degrees of flexion an abnormal rotatory movement can be produced. This reaches a maximum at about 90° and then diminishes slightly with further flexion. When the tibia is strained forward, the medial tibial condyle rotates externally and marked forward subluxation occurs. In a specimen it

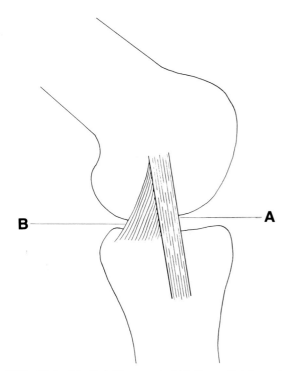

B ─────────────── **A**

FIG. 21-1. *Medial ligament.* **(A)** Superficial part. **(B)** Oblique part.

is obvious that the posterior horn of the medial meniscus restricts this abnormal rotatory movement somewhat. Abnormal movement will increase when the meniscus is removed. Rotation is an essential part of the subluxation. If external rotation is forcibly prevented as the tibia is pulled forward, subluxation of the medial tibial condyle is also prevented.

As the medial tibial condyle rotates in this way the anterior cruciate ligament touches and then is angulated over the lateral femoral condyle and finally may tear. This is the mechanism of the double lesion of torn medial and anterior cruciate ligaments.

When the medial ligament is divided a valgus stress will cause abnormal opening of the medial side of the joint. This, however, does not occur when the joint is fully extended, and even in flexion it is grossly diminished if external rotation is prevented. The joint opens because of a rotatory subluxation. The gap between the divided ends of the

ligament widens slightly in full extension and approximates in flexion if external tibial rotation is avoided. This ligament division produces the clinical instability termed anteromedial instability (Table 21-1).

ANTERIOR CRUCIATE LIGAMENT

The line of direction of the anterior cruciate ligament is a clue to the control it exerts on abnormal movement. It extends distally forward and medially from the back of the intercondylar surface of the lateral femoral condyle to the front of the intercondylar area of the tibia. It is taut in full extension and very full flexion and also in midflexion when the tibia is internally rotated, but it relaxes

TABLE 21-1. SUMMARY OF TYPES OF INSTABILITY

Name	Cause
Anteromedial instability	(a) Medial ligament (b) Medial ligament and anterior cruciate ligament
Anterolateral instability	Anterior cruciate ligament. It is increased by posterolateral capsular division.
Anterior instability	Combined lesion of medial and anterior cruciate ligaments
Posterior instability	Posterior cruciate ligament
Posteromedial instability	Posterior cruciate ligament and medial ligament
Posterolateral instability	Posterior cruciate and lateral ligaments
Opening with valgus strain (a) In flexion	
1. slight	Medial ligament
2. gross	Medial ligament with either anterior cruciate or posterior cruciate ligaments
(b) In extension	Medial ligament and both cruciate ligaments
Opening with varus strain (a) In flexion	
1. slight	Lateral ligament
2. gross	Lateral ligament and either anterior or posterior cruciate ligament
(b) In extension	Lateral ligament and both cruciate ligaments
Lateral slide subluxation	Medial ligament and both cruciate ligaments
Medial slide subluxation	Lateral ligament and both cruciate ligaments

slightly with external rotation. It follows, therefore, that this ligament is particularly stressed when the tibia is internally rotated and the knee is either forcibly flexed or fully extended. The anterior cruciate exerts a control on abnormal internal rotation of the tibia. When the ligament is divided in a specimen, the extent of abnormal movement produced varies but is of a constant pattern. The abnormal movement produced affects the internal rotation of the tibia with anterior subluxation of the lateral tibial condyle.

It has been customary to test for anterior cruciate ligament damage by examining the joint for forward subluxation at 90° of flexion. Because this test is not sensitive instability has commonly been missed. With an isolated division or clinical tear of this ligament abnormal anterior subluxation *should be tested for in 5° of flexion only*. In this position it is always positive, in strong contrast to examination made with the joint at a right angle. Recently, clinicians have come to appreciate this fact, and the abnormal physical sign has been termed Lachman's sign.

If the ligament division is associated with extensive division of the posterolateral capsule, abnormal forward rotatory movement of the lateral tibial condyle will be detectable at 90° because the instability is more marked.

It must be emphasized that the abnormal movement is not an anterior subluxation of the tibia but of the lateral tibial condyle alone. When seen clinically this has been termed anterolateral instability.

COMBINED DIVISION OF MEDIAL AND ANTERIOR CRUCIATE LIGAMENTS

The abnormal movement possible with combined division of the medial and anterior cruciate ligaments will be predictable from the previous observations. It must be the summation of anteromedial subluxation from medial ligament division and anterolateral subluxation caused by the anterior cruciate ligament lesion. In full extension abnormal movement is still not possible. As flexion commences, abnormal movement is possible immediately

and consists of both lateral and medial anterior rotatory subluxation of the tibia, and therefore of anterior subluxation. The rotation externally of the medial condyle is always greater than the rotation internally of the lateral condyle. The classic anterior draw sign at 90° used by clinicians is therefore produced by a combined lesion of the anterior cruciate and medial ligaments and not by one ligament division alone.

When a valgus stress is applied to a specimen with this combined lesion it is still not possible to open up the medial side of the joint in full extension. In flexion, however, the possible opening is greater than that obtained when the medial ligament alone is divided.

The same findings apply to a combined lesion of the medial and posterior cruciate ligaments. The joint is stable in full extension but can open widely in flexion.

The medial side of the joint will open with a valgus strain in full extension only when the medial ligament division is combined with that of both cruciate ligaments.

LATERAL STRUCTURES OF THE KNEE

The lateral side of the knee joint is passively protected by four main structures—the lateral ligament, the strong fascia lata, and the tendons of the popliteus and the biceps femoris. Any significant trauma to the lateral side will tear the lateral ligament together with any or all of the other structures.

It has been noted that the lateral ligament is taut in extension but that in flexion it is the most relaxed of the joint ligaments. This allows normal rotatory movement. At the extreme of normal rotatory movement in flexion the ligament becomes tight but not taut.

When the ligament is divided in isolation it is remarkable how little abnormal movement occurs. There is no increase in the normal range of rotatory movement. Abnormal internal rotation is prevented by the intact anterior cruciate ligament, and abnormal external rotation is prevented by the screwing up of the two cruciates on each other and also by the intact medial ligament.

When a varus strain is imposed on the extended knee the lateral joint line does not open. It will open to a slight extent with a strain in flexion. Divided ligament ends will separate obviously in full extension and will approximate in flexion of 30° or more.

If a lateral ligament division is combined with a division of either of the cruciates, the joint is still completely stable in full extension but opens widely in flexion. The joint will open with a varus strain in extension only when the lateral ligament division is combined with a division of both cruciate ligaments.

POSTERIOR CRUCIATE LIGAMENTS

The posterior cruciate ligament can be divided either from the posterior aspect of the joint after division of the posterior capsule or from the anterior aspect between the femoral condyles with preservation of the posterior capsule. It matters not which approach is employed. Division of the ligament allows a posterior subluxation of the tibia, the extent of which is variable in various specimens. This is the posterior draw sign. It is not detectable in full extension and is first obvious as the joint is flexed to about 10°, becoming maximal at 90°. Because the normal axis for rotatory knee movement is to the medial side of center, the lateral tibial condyle rotates backward slightly more than the medial condyle with this posterior subluxation.

POSTERIOR CRUCIATE AND LATERAL LIGAMENTS

The division of the posterior cruciate and lateral ligaments allows posterior tibial subluxation and particularly, posterior subluxation of the lateral tibial condyle. In a clinical situation this is called posterior and posterolateral instability (see Table 21-1).

POSTERIOR CRUCIATE AND MEDIAL LIGAMENTS

Division of the posterior cruciate and medial ligaments produces a complicated swinging rotatory instability, with gross lateral shifting of the normal axis point. The medial tibial condyle subluxes forward and backward, and in addition there is posterior subluxation. Clinically, this would be described as anteromedial, posteromedial, and posterior instability.

JOINT CAPSULE

The capsule surrounds the joint and varies in strength and thickness. On the medial and lateral sides it blends with the corresponding collateral ligaments. On the medial side it can be said to form a functional part of the ligament, and on the lateral side it binds together the four main structures named previously.

The anterior joint capsule is a thin structure extending from medial to lateral ligaments with the patellar tendon intervening. In specimens the anterior capsule cannot be seen to contribute to the passive stability of the joint. When it is completely excised, no abnormal movement is produced. It appears to function only with the extensor mechanism.

The posterior joint capsule extends from the posterior edge of the oblique part of the medial ligament around to the lateral ligament. Where it embraces the posterior condyles of the femur it can be strong or flimsy. It is completely relaxed in flexion and very taut in full extension. Centrally it is reinforced by an expansion from the semimembranous tendon. If the entire posterior capsule so described is excised without touching the collateral ligaments, no abnormal mobility can be produced.

REFERENCE

1. **Brantigan OC, Voshell AF:** Mechanics of ligaments and menisci of the knee joint. J Bone Joint Surg 23:43, 1941

CHAPTER 22
INJURIES OF THE CAPSULAR AND CRUCIATE LIGAMENTS

Arthur J. Helfet

The key to successful treatment of injuries to the ligaments of the knee is accurate diagnosis. Although sprains may be treated adequately by prompt and conscientious conservative means, ruptures of stabilizing ligaments invariably require surgical repair for recovery of perfect function.

D. H. O'Donoghue,[4] who writes from an exceptionally wide experience of severe injuries of the knee joint, considers that function of the ligament depends not only on its strength but also on its length, since a ligament that is elongated does not carry out its function of preventing abnormal motion of the joint. In addition, we should maintain that *the function of the capsular ligaments* is not only to prevent abnormal movement but also to give adequate purchase to the muscles that control normal movement. The function of a cruciate ligament is that of a guide rope and not a checkstrap. The objects of treatment remain identical. Both the integrity and the length of the capsular ligaments must be restored or the function of the ligament must be replaced by static or dynamic tendon transplant.

CLINICAL FEATURES OF THE ACUTE STAGE

Ligaments are injured at their junctions with tissues of different elasticity. For the collateral ligaments these junctions are the insertions to the femur, the tibia, and the meniscus on the medial side, and to the femur and the head of the fibula on the lateral side (Fig. 22-1). Sometimes a flake of bone comes away with the ligament, or it may snap transversely, in which case the torn ends, though ragged, are well defined. At other times interstitial fibers are pulled longitudinally and rupture at different levels within the substance of the ligament, when it will appear intact though elongated.

The variations in types of tear are many. A 17-year-old high-jump champion "sprained" his left patellar ligament. It was rested by splinting for 3 weeks, after which he started training again. The first time he tried to jump, the knee gave way. At operation it was obvious that the sprain was a coronal rupture of the ligament with complete detachment of the upper end of the posterior half from the pa-

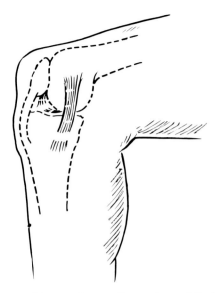

FIG. 22-1. Ligaments usually rupture at their bony attachments to the femur or the tibia.

tella. The fresh injury had avulsed the lower end of the ligament and its expansion from the tibial tubercle and the front of the tibia. At operation the site of fresh injury is denoted by hemorrhage and ecchymosis. At the time of accident, the patient feels immediate acute pain which may subside in a few minutes—in which case the joint stiffens up and is painful again a few hours later when local swelling becomes evident. More commonly, the knee remains painful, and movement and weight-bearing are difficult or intolerable. Synovial effusion always follows and is bloodstained; occasionally, a frank tense hemarthrosis develops, depending on the extent of damage to the synovium. The degree of pain and the rate of increase of effusion are proportional to the extent of the intra-articular bleeding. Severe bleeding causes severe pain.

The first distinction between sprain and rupture is the severity of the pain. Sprains are always painful and remain so on attempted movement. After rupture of a ligament, acute pain subsides and non-weight-bearing movement, though weak and unstable, is relatively painless. Locally, the point of sprain is more tender and sensitive, though there is more local swelling when the ligament has rup-

tured. This may be due to the dispersion of synovial effusion through the torn capsule, which prevents the painful distention of the knee seen in closed injuries. After a sprain the patient may be able to take weight, albeit very painfully, but after a severe rupture of the capsular ligaments the patient has a subjective fear for the stability of the knee and will not venture to put weight on it at all.

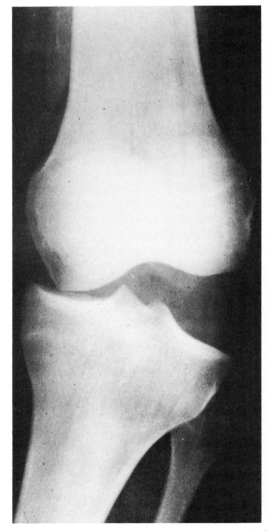

FIG. 22-2. Anteroposterior roentgenogram of the knee in forced adduction showing abnormal separation of femur and tibia. The lateral ligament has been wrenched off the head of the fibula with a flake of bone.

To test lateral instability the leg must be almost straight. The word "almost" is used deliberately, for when the leg is forced into the extreme of extension and lateral rotation, even if both cruciate and medial collateral ligament are ruptured, instability cannot always be determined—that is, in the so-called screwed home position, the knee is stable. Only after more extensive tears of the capsule can clinical instability be detected with the knee quite straight. The leg must be just off the straight when abduction and adduction strain are applied. Many knees in this position allow an impression of slight laxity, but there is no mistaking the "opening" of the side of the joint when the ligaments have ruptured. The palpating finger seems to slip between the femur and the tibia.

Doubt may arise when the capsule is strained or partially torn anterior or posterior to the ligament. In such a case attempted movement is painful, and abnormal abduction or adduction cannot be elicited with certainty. When any doubt exists, the knee should be examined under general or local anesthesia. For the latter, 10 ml to 15 ml of 1% procaine in saline is injected intra-articularly, and locally into the tender area.

Anteroposterior roentgenograms of the knee at the extremes of forced abduction or adduction confirm the abnormal separation of the femur and the tibia (Fig. 22-2). Arthrograms are useful in establishing the diagnosis. (See Fig. 22-3 and Chap. 9.)

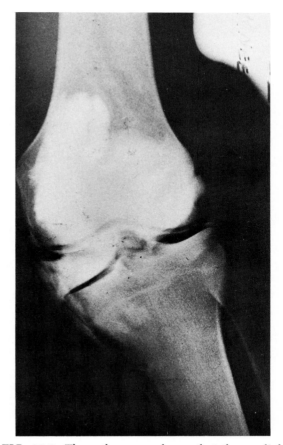

FIG. 22-3. The arthrogram shows that the medial capsule is ruptured. The medial meniscus has been separated from the tibia.

straightens completely. In such a case it is often possible to displace the meniscus again by straightening the knee while forcibly holding the tibia in internal rotation.

ASSOCIATED LESIONS OF THE SEMILUNAR CARTILAGES

By careful examination it is often possible to diagnose an associated derangement of a meniscus—usually retraction of the anterior horn of the medial meniscus. In this case, external rotation of the knee is restricted, and protrusion of the medial condyle of the femur and other rotation signs are present. The torn anterior end of the meniscus is tender. The diagnosis is confirmed if during examination the cartilage reduces and the knee suddenly

CHRONIC OR RECURRENT SPRAINS

Mild sprains may clear up completely even without treatment. Swelling and tenderness disappear and movement recovers. More severe sprains tend to leave a legacy of adhesions that manifest themselves by twinges or stabs of pain on certain movements. These stabs may be accompanied by a sensation of momentary weakness that simulates the giving way or buckling experienced in internal derangement of the knee. Occasionally these attacks are followed by swelling, stiffness, and local tenderness, and as the pain is felt in the same place, the history given by the patient suggests a torn meniscus. (Once the knee is examined, the differential diagnosis is easy, because extension is not limited and rotation is not blocked.) The patient feels the pain always in the same place on the same movement, and tenderness is localized to the ligamentous attachment.

Reference has already been made to the difficulty of diagnosing rotation sprains of the medial semilunar cartilage due to injury to the coronary ligaments (see Chapter 8). This applies also to sprains of the attachments of the semilunar cartilage to the deep part of the medial collateral ligament.

RUPTURES OF THE COLLATERAL LIGAMENTS

Because it has elastic components, ligament retracts after rupture or detachment from its insertion. The wrenched ends curl up and leave a gap. Rupture of a ligament is never an isolated lesion but is accompanied by damage of varying degree to adjacent capsular structures where similar changes occur. After complete rupture, therefore, it is unreasonable to expect the tissues to recover normal integrity and length merely by splinting the limb. The gap is crossed quickly enough by fibrous scar, but the structure as a whole is longer than previously, and the joint on that side remains lax.

The medial ligament and capsule are the important structures. The knee with a lax medial capsule is weak. The patient complains of weakness and of the knee giving way under strain or from sudden rotary movements. These symptoms are more severe when the cruciate ligaments also have ruptured. The attacks may be accompanied by pain and followed by swelling. The diagnosis is usually simpler than in the acute stage, for pain, swelling, and guarding muscle spasm are mild.

Rupture of the lateral ligament causes little

disability unless it is associated with disruption of the iliotibial band and further capsular damage, and rupture of the cruciate, when a particularly unstable knee results.

INJURIES OF THE CRUCIATE LIGAMENTS

Sprains of the cruciate ligaments are difficult to interpret clinically, except perhaps when they have been stretched by the medial condyle of the femur in a knee locked for some length of time by a bowstring or anterior horn tear of the cartilage (see Fig. 1-21). In this case not only the cruciate but also the capsule is stretched because laxity of the joint as a whole develops.

However, either cruciate may rupture from its femoral or tibial attachment. The cruciate may take with it part of a tibial spine, and quite often the anterior ligament tear includes rupture of its attachments to the anterior horn of the medial meniscus, which retracts. In other words, the distracting force tears both the anterior cruciate and the medial meniscus from their attachments to each other and to the tibia.

If the medial capsular structures remain intact, the clinical picture is that of the retracted meniscus with typical rotation signs, restriction of movement and site of tenderness. The torn cruciate is discovered only at the operation. The knee is not unstable, and repair of the cruciate is not important, although if the injury is recent the ligament should be sutured firmly to its soft tissue insertions.

Combinations of cruciate and capsular damage give rise to major disabilities of the knee. They are, of course, usually the result of gross injuries caused by lateral hinging or subluxation or actual dislocation of the joint. If the knee is examined soon after the accident, diagnosis of the wrenched unstable knee is obvious. The patient is in shock and in great pain. Swelling is rapid. Once the leg is splinted, pain may subside quickly.

Injuries of this type are always associated with tears of the synovium, often with displacements of semilunar cartilage, occasionally with tibial plateau fractures, and rarely with injuries to nerves. If the popliteal vessels are damaged, the vascular problem is predominant and demands immediate assessment and treatment. However, the management of blood vessel injuries is not within the compass of this monograph.

Broadly speaking, widespread damage treated conservatively results in either a stiff or an unstable knee. The patient presents for treatment months later with a knee that gives way or is restricted in movement or that suffers from both defects. Dense adhesions limit movement and cause pain if movement is forced. After undue strain the knee tends to swell and ache. Musculature is poor and difficult to improve.

With lesser damage, instability is the disabling symptom, though extremes of movement also may be restricted.

The patient complains that the knee gives way chiefly on slopes and stairs. It seems that the tibia does not remain on the helicoid track on the medial condyle of the femur but slides straight forward. The incidents are painful and may be followed by swelling, with muscle spasm and pain. On the other hand, for a while at a later stage the derangements may become relatively nonpainful, and the patient is able to carry on immediately after each episode.

With the patient either sitting or lying down with muscles relaxed, these abnormal movements may be elicited passively. The classic test is the demonstration of "anteroposterior glide." With the knee flexed, it is possible to slide the tibia forward and backward on the femur (Fig. 22-4). Sometimes the patient, while sitting with knee flexed, can actively subluxate and reduce the tibia on the femur. However, it should be appreciated that if the leg is extended fully with full outward rotation of the tibia, the knee is locked, and anteroposterior glide can no longer be demonstrated.

The patient may simulate this action to stabilize the knee when walking. The foot is fixed on the ground in external rotation, and

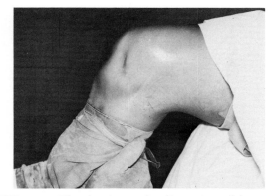

FIG. 22-4. The classic test for disruption of the cruciate ligaments is the demonstration of anteroposterior glide. With the knee flexed it is possible to slide the tibia forward and backward on the femur.

as the leg straightens, the femur is internally rotated on the tibia (see Fig. 6-34).

The articular cartilage of the unstable knee deteriorates after repeated derangements, and traumatic arthritis inevitably develops in untreated knees.

TREATMENT OF LIGAMENTOUS INJURIES

ACUTE SPRAINS

If acute sprains are untreated, traumatic exudate tends to organize by depositing fibrin, which is replaced by fibroblasts and then by fibrous tissue. These links of fibrous tissue, or adhesions, between components of varying elasticity lead to the troubles and the discomforts of chronic sprains. Therefore, treatment for the fresh injury should aim to relieve pain and to promote the absorption of exudate to prevent this organization of fibrous tissue. In the early stages pain is relieved fairly quickly by rest obtained through a compression bandage and, depending on the severity, by bed or splinting. Hot and cold compresses or local heat and light massage promote the rapid absorption of exudate, chiefly by stimulating local circulation. Deep massage is traumatic and at this stage aggravates the condition. The best agent of all is static muscle drill. The

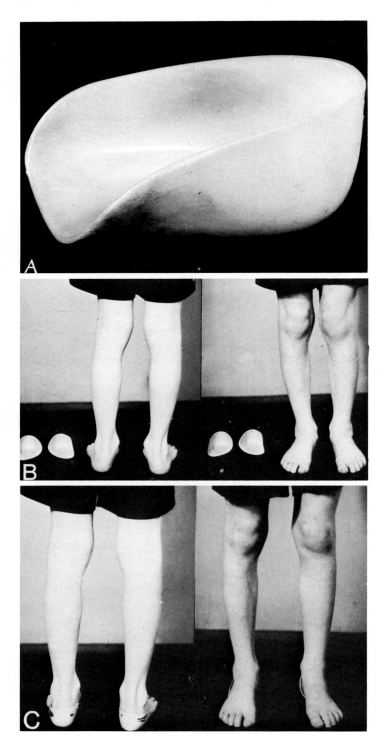

FIG. 22-5. (A) The heel seat molded of plastic. **(B)** The everted feet. **(C)** Complete correction in the heelseats. (Myron Medical Products Ltd. Maidenhead, Berks, England)

muscle is contracted fully, held in contraction for a second, and then relaxed. This is repeated 12 times at intervals of 1 hr. Exercise against gravity and against resistance follows. Faradization is of value, as an educational aid only, when the patient finds difficulty in actively contracting the thigh muscles.

Some 30 years ago, LeRiche advocated the treatment of sprains by the immediate local injection of procaine. He contended that the traumatic exudate contains metabolites that irritate the local sensory nerve endings; this initiates a reflex that causes further exudation of metabolites. A vicious circle is established, and the process is prolonged. The procaine breaks the reflex by anesthetizing the nerve endings, and the swelling resolves. The patient is allowed to bear weight immediately. Whether LeRiche's theory is right or not, the local injection of procaine in saline undoubtedly does relieve pain and accelerates recovery. After the injection a crepe or compression bandage is applied. If the injury is mild, the patient is allowed to walk with full weight-bearing; if the sprain is severe, he may walk on crutches. Tilting the medial side of the heel of the shoe on the injured side or wearing a heelseat inside the shoe is an aid to comfort and recovery, for it takes stress off the medial ligament. The heelseat is a device that holds the os calcis vertically. In this way, by preventing the heel's rolling over into eversion, it controls the arch.[6] The shape and the agility of the foot are preserved, and the heelseat is effective in correcting flatfoot, in relieving foot strain, and incidentally, therefore, in preventing strain on the medial side of the knee (Fig. 22-5).

CHRONIC AND RECURRING STRAINS

Once the symptoms and signs of chronic strain are established, the condition is treated by manipulation under either local or general anesthesia. By this time tenderness is localized, and the movements that cause pain are known. Manipulation under local anesthesia is more effective than that under general anes-

thesia when muscle strains are involved, for example the insertion of the quadriceps to the patella. It is also effective for minor strains. A solution of procaine is injected into the tender area. As soon as the anesthetic is effective, the patient performs the previously painful movements against resistance. If flexion is painful, sitting on the haunches will rupture the adhesions. For capsular and more extensive adhesions, manipulation under Pentothal anesthesia is advisable and effective.

Wasting of the thigh muscles and chronic or recurrent synovitis associated with chronic strain of the knee are treated by a regular and conscientious program of static and active exercises. There is no doubt that recovery of normal muscle power is the prime requisite in the restoration of stable function of the knee and its ability to withstand the demands of sustained effort.

RUPTURES OF CAPSULAR AND CRUCIATE LIGAMENTS

Capsular and cruciate ligament ruptures have been grouped under one heading, since injury is rarely confined to one ligament. Moreover, the broad principles of treatment are the same for all.

The object of treatment is recovery of function with full active movement, the most important movement being full extension of the knee with outward rotation of the tibia.

It is essential when ligaments are sutured that the femur and the tibia should be in their correct rotational alignment. This rule applies equally to splinting during conservative treatment and after operation.

I am convinced, as are other writers, that the *best results are obtained not by conservative treatment but by prompt and meticulous suture of ruptured ligaments.* Most patients who suffer disability later and require further treatment are those who have been treated by splinting without surgical repair.

One hears of isolated cases in which after complete rupture of the medial collateral ligament, the patient recovered a knee strong enough to stand up to the strain of violent games. These patients naturally do not seek further orthopaedic opinion. However, many knees, after excellent conservative treatment with an initial 8 to 12 weeks of splinting, break down under strain. Indeed, although I can report two patients who gained international rugby football caps and a number who play first class (major league) club football after suture of the medial ligament, I have not seen any patient stand up to the rigors of first class football after conservative treatment. O'Donoghue[4] and DePalma,[1] in reviews of their experience, record similar conclusions.

There is no doubt, also, that the main bastions of stability in the knee are the medial ligament and the medial capsule. Rupture of the lateral ligament in itself is not markedly disabling. However, when associated with cruciate plus iliotibial band and capsular damage, a particularly unstable knee is produced. The muscles probably cannot compensate for capsular weakness while bearing weight without the stabilizing effect that the lateral ligament and the biceps exercise on the leg through the fibula.

When the anatomical disturbances produced by the injury are considered, one is more convinced of the desirability of operative reconstruction of the capsular structures of the joint. The torn fibers of the ligaments tend to retract and curl up, and moreover, flaps of ligament and synovium may turn in between the joint surfaces. After conservative treatment, the probabilities are that the extra-articular ligamentous tears will be replaced by scar or fibrous tissue and that the intra-articular fringes will be absorbed or replaced by intra-articular fibrous adhesions. The result is instability or restriction of movement—the common sequelae.

Conservative Treatment

Mild sprains are easily distinguished from complete ruptures of ligament. Difficulties arise when the signs of complete rupture are cloaked by partial rupture and sprain of the adjacent capsule. When doubt exists, the knee must be examined under anesthesia. If skin

abrasion and infection preclude open operation, or if the age or the general condition of the patient contraindicates it, or when the extent of the rupture is small enough to warrant the gamble, conservative treatment is prescribed. If the skin heals cleanly within 2 or 3 weeks, suture of the ligament still should be considered. O'Donoghue is prepared to plan incisions that bypass clean abrasions because he considers early operation to be of urgent importance. My experience upholds this view.

Any displacement of the meniscus must be reduced by manipulation before the limb is splinted. The knee is held with the joint closed on the side of the rupture and with the femur and the tibia in correct rotational alignment. This means that the tibia is rotated outward; to hold it in this position the foot must be included in a plaster-of-Paris splint extending from the fold of the buttock. If manipulation is necessary, or after any severe injury, it is well to administer a general anesthetic. Tense synovial effusion or hemarthrosis is aspirated. The knee is maneuvered gently to ensure that movement is not restricted by a displaced meniscus or interposed soft tissues, and a compression bandage plus the plaster-of-Paris splint are applied with the knee in the corrected position.

Thigh muscle drill should be started next day, when the patient is up and walking on crutches. When swelling subsides it may be necessary to change the plaster splint. After 4 weeks the boot of the splint is removed, and the patient may take weight, protected by the back splint. In the treatment of a medial ligament injury, a heelseat is worn or the heel of the shoe is tilted on the inner side. The back splint should be removed at regular intervals for gentle non-weight-bearing flexion-extension exercises. If power and stability are adequate, the patient may indulge in slowly increasing unprotected weight-bearing after 8 to 12 weeks.

However, if the knee is still weak, a caliper with extension spring should be used to re-educate the thigh muscle and to add stability. If movement remains restricted by adhesions, these are broken down at the appropriate time by gentle manipulation under local or general anesthesia.

Surgical Repair

The presence of clean abrasions does not preclude early operation. After adequate preparation with medicated soap and hibitane or 2% iodine in 70% alcohol, the leg is toweled and the operative area coated with an aeroplastic self-sterilizing spray. Clean abrasions are excluded by the plastic skin that is formed, and the incision is planned to avoid the affected area. Of course, if the skin is infected, open operation is absolutely contraindicated. When abrasion is present, surgery must be planned and performed under an "umbrella" of chemotherapy or antibiotics.

The operation should be performed with the patient lying on his back with leg extended and a small sandbag behind the knee. Before starting, adduction, abduction, rotation, and anteroposterior movements of the tibia on the femur are tested. The incision will depend on the ligament or ligaments to be repaired. The medial collateral ligament and capsule are explored through a longitudinal incision in line with the anterior fibers of the ligament, extending from the upper border of the femoral condyle to some 3 in below the joint line. Points of maximum hemorrhage give a lead to the site of rupture, which varies in type and degree. The full extent of the lesion should be ascertained carefully before deciding on what sort of repair is necessary.

If the ligament with part of the capsule is completely ruptured, or if the ligament with the adjacent capsule is avulsed from the femur or the tibia, it is usually possible to examine the interior of the knee joint without further incision. If this is not possible and preoperative examination has suggested derangement of the medial meniscus, the knee joint should be opened by the usual anterior horizontal incision to explore the anteromedial compartment or a vertical incision in line with the posterior border of the tibia to expose the posterior horn of the cartilage. It is not always necessary to remove the cartilage. The decision depends on the type of damage. Transverse or longitudinal tears in the substance demand excision of the meniscus, as does complete detachment. If the anterior horn has been disrupted from the anterior cruciate, or if the anterior cruciate and the meniscus both have been detached cleanly from their tibial anchorage, repair may be feasible. Both ends may be sutured back to the stump of soft tissue or are attached to the tibia in the manner of O'Donoghue. Limited peripheral tears will also reunite to torn coronary ligament. Operations to remove or reattach the semilunar cartilage are performed with the knee flexed. When completed, the knee is straightened. If the cartilage has been retained, complete extention and lateral rotation of the tibia are tested. Only if these movements are free and unrestricted can the suture be considered satisfactory. If not, the knee should be flexed again and the meniscus removed. It is important during the operation to protect the fat pad from injury.

While the ligament and the capsule are repaired, the knee should be straight, with careful adjustment of the rotational alignment of the femur and the tibia. Various techniques for the repair of torn ligaments are available, and one or more of these may be necessary in a particular case. If a flake of bone has been avulsed with the ligament, it should be replaced carefully and held with a boatnail or staple. If the lower end has avulsed from the tibia, it also may be fastened to the roughened bone surface by these metal appliances or by suture to the surrounding periosteum and soft tissue with linen or fine wire. Or small drill holes in the tibia may be used to anchor the ligament with wire or linen sutures. Defined ruptures of ligament or capsule may be repaired by interrupted sutures with imbrication or by a modification of the Bunnell type of suture. If the ligament is lax through ill-defined interstitial ruptures of fibers, darning from one end to the other using catgut with enough tension to tighten it is a worthwhile procedure. The essential features are careful and complete repair of the damage so that tension and length of the capsule are finally as near normal as possible. If the damage has been so extensive or is of such ragged character that this cannot be achieved, immediate reinforcement by the semitendinosus tendon or of the lateral by half the biceps tendon should be added. The type of suture material is not really important. Fine chromic catgut or linen or Bunnell pullout wire sutures may be used. My own preference is for linen, except when the ligament needs shortening by darning, in which case catgut is used.

LATERAL LIGAMENT

Interstitial ruptures of the lateral ligament are extremely rare. Disruption occurs either from the femoral attachment or, more commonly, from the head of the fibula, when the insertion of the biceps tendon also is damaged. Avulsion with a flake of bone is fairly common, for the lateral ligament is compact and firmly attached to bone. More extensive injury involves the iliotibial band, where the tear may be ragged and irregular. The same principles of repair apply on the lateral as on the medial side. It is as important before deciding on the method of suture to examine each structure separately and to define the exact extent of injury but only after the popliteal nerve has been defined, isolated, and protected. The injury may have displaced the nerve from its normal track. Repair of each structure must be meticulous and separate because, as explained in Chapter 1, adherence of the lateral ligament to the popliteus tendon or to any point of the joint line, or malalignment between the lateral ligament and the iliotibial band acts as a brake to flexion.

CRUCIATE LIGAMENTS

The importance of the cruciates in stability of the knee joint in the presence of an intact capsule is not as great as is generally thought. When the integrity and the length of the capsular ligaments have been restored, patients are able to do arduous work demanding strength and stability in the knee joint and even to play football in spite of an unsutured cruciate ligament. This may not apply to the athlete who demands a knee capable also of the higher flights of speed. O'Donoghue, who has unrivaled experience in treating athletes, prescribes synchronous repair of these ligaments. From the present series, instances can be reported in which patients have returned to strenuous occupations after restoration of the capsular ligaments only, in the acute stage, or after replacement of function by extra-articular tendon transfer in the later phases. One patient had ruptured the upper end of the lateral ligament, the iliotibial band, and the anterior cruciate in an underground accident in a gold mine. In spite of a long period of conservative treatment, his knee was so unstable that he could walk only in a caliper. He had to give up his employment. After repair of the lateral ligament by biceps tendon transfer and imbrication of the iliotibial band and capsule, he was able to return to his work as a miner underground. Another, a bricklayer, young and powerful, tore all the medial capsular attachments and the anterior cruciate ligament. He reported for examination a year later, able to walk only in a caliper. After transfer of the tibial tubercle and transposition of the semitendinosus tendon, he was able to return to normal work, including carrying hods full of bricks up ladders.

If during the operation for the acute injury, the anterior cruciate is found to be detached from its inferior insertion, the opportunity of suturing it back to the bone ought to be taken. However, in the usual run of cases, except in most expert hands, I doubt the propriety of transarticular and intra-articular procedures for suture of the upper end of either cruciate. The lower end of the posterior cruciate is sutured only when an extensive tear necessitates exposure and also repair of the posterior capsule of the joint. Unless there is unhealed capsular damage, it is doubtful whether an isolated tear of the posterior cruciate disorganizes function materially.

Both O'Donoghue[4] and Smillie[5] have described a technique of practically extra-articular suture of the inferior end of the anterior cruciate ligament. Two drill holes pass through the tibial tubercle, being aligned to emerge in the joint at the site of attachment of the anterior cruciate ligament. The suture is passed up one track, is darned into the lower end of the ligament, and then emerges through the parallel track to be tied in front of the bone. O'Donoghue describes a similar simple suture for the lower end of the posterior cruciate. Two parallel holes are drilled from the front to the back of the tibia. The suture goes through one drill hole, emerges posteriorly, is plicated through the tibial stump of the posterior cruciate, and goes back out the other hole.

The length of time before the patient is allowed to bear weight on the limb after the operation depends on the extent of the injury. If it has been severe, crutches should be used for at least 6 weeks. After the operation, a compression bandage is applied with a plaster-of-Paris cylinder extending from buttock fold to toes with the foot at right angles. The knee is held just off the straight with full external rotation of the tibia. This position of splinting is always important, and its significance will be realized when we remember the effect of the locked knee on the normal cruciate ligament. If external rotation of the tibia is prevented, the cruciate is stretched by the medial condyle of the femur. After the plaster splint has set, it should be split anteriorly in case of swelling. If constriction threatens, the bandage also should be divided through the opening. After 2 weeks, the sutures are removed, and the splint is changed. While this is being done, the position of the knee should be maintained carefully by a trained assistant. The patient is allowed to walk with crutches. After another 4 weeks, the cylinder is replaced by a back splint without including the foot. At this time, the knee is clinically stable, and periodic gentle flexion exercises are prescribed with the proviso that each time the knee is flexed, it should be fully extended before the next knee bend. Thigh muscle drill is started from the first postoperative day, and the patient may graduate to straight-leg rais-

ing, first without and then with an added weight.

After 6 weeks the patient learns to take weight first with a backsplint and then, when strong enough, with a crepe bandage. He should not return to strenuous sport for 4 months.

Substitution Operations for the Cruciate Ligaments

Operations for anatomical intra-articular replacement of the cruciate ligaments have not been included in this volume. Since 1942, when extra-articular transposition of patellar and semitendinosus tendons was first used, intra-articular procedures have had no special indication or merit.

COMPLICATIONS

Such complications as ensue are controlled by careful and timely after-care. Effusion may require aspiration, and swelling, specific therapy. Slow recovery of movement is accelerated by intra-articular injections of procaine followed, while the joint is anesthetized, by active and gentle passive stretching. Occasionally, adhesions prevent certain movements or arcs of movement, and when these movements are attempted, pain results. In such cases, gentle manipulation under Pentothal anesthesia is helpful. Calcification of the injured ligament of painless or painful character (Pellegrini-Stieda) is relatively uncommon. Injections of procaine and hydrocortisone locally into the tender area usually relieve the symptoms. The development of late osteoarthritis depends on the damage caused to articular cartilage at the time of the accident.

Residual laxity of the capsule with weakness or instability of the knee joint is a possible sequel, the result of inadequate suture or faulty after-care. The regimen for untreated ruptures of ligaments discussed in the following paragraphs would then be applicable.

Treatment of Old Ruptures of the Cruciate and Collateral Ligaments

Over the years a variety of operations have been designed to correct the instability due to old ruptures of the collateral ligaments of the knee joint. Most of these have relied on grafts of fascia lata or tendon to substitute for the ruptured structures. A number of these reconstructive operations have permitted comfortable use of the knee over the years but only if it is not exposed to prolonged and undue strain. It is rare that the grafted tissues stand up both to time and stress without stretching of the capsule, which causes recurrence of laxity and weakness. More successful were McMurray, who used the semitendinosus as a fixed graft to replace the medial ligament, and Hauser, who pedicled the inner half of the patellar ligament as two cross strips to replace the medial ligament and capsule. DePalma describes an admirable operation in which the anterior half of the biceps tendon is pedicled from its lower attachment to replace the fibular collateral ligament. I use the semitendinosus and the biceps tendons as active ligaments respectively for medial and lateral repair in the manner to be described.

If we consider that the cruciate ligaments act as checkstraps that prevent anteroposterior movement of the tibia on the femur and that the resulting instability after rupture of these ligaments is due to absence of these checkstraps, then the only logical course of treatment is anatomical replacement of the checkstraps. On the other hand, if the cruciate ligaments are guide ropes that keep the tibia on its normal helicoid track on the medial condyle of the femur, it is possible to replace this function by extra-articular tendon transplants. This principle is applied in the following two ways:

by transfer of the tibial tubercle medially to ensure lateral rotation of the tibia while the knee is extending, and

by transposition of the semitendinosus tendon to preserve synchrony of excursion of the femur and the tibia during flexion of the knee.

In this way the guiding mechanism, of which the cruciates are a part, and the motor mechanism, represented by the thigh muscles, are both reinforced, and the muscles are given better purchase on the tibia.

A series of 40 patients who were successfully stabilized by these methods has convinced me of the advantages of replacing the function rather than the anatomy of these ligaments. In every case stability has been improved, and most patients recovered the ability and the confidence to undertake normal activities, even when strenuous. None of them has been permitted violent games such as football in which sudden abnormal, unexpected strains are probable. But strains that are foreseen and taken deliberately can be withstood after adequate retraining of the leg muscles. All the patients recovered confidence on rough ground. Two do work on ladders, and several ride horses without qualm. DePalma, who uses these methods, reports similar satisfaction with his results.

An interesting facet is that postoperatively the knee remains unstable when examined passively. When the muscles are relaxed, anteroposterior and lateral laxity still may be elicited. When the muscles are properly conditioned, active movements are stable.

Transposition of the Semitendinosus Tendon

T. P. McMurray originally described an operation in which he used the semitendinosus tendon to replace the anatomy of the medial collateral ligament.[3] He anchored the tendon by suture in two grooves cut in the line of the ligament in the femur and the tibia. The operation I use (Plates 22-1 and 22-2) also substitutes the tendon for the medial ligament, but by permitting the semitendinosus to run free in a groove in the femur, instability is prevented in abduction by active contraction of the muscle. In addition, the muscle helps to restore the function of the cruciate ligament because, by contracting when the knee flexes, it ensures synchrony of movement between the femur and the tibia. In other words, it prevents the tibia from running away from the femur. It has been my practice to transplant the tibial tubercle and to defer the operation for transposition of the semitendinosus to a second stage 4 weeks later. It is felt that although the transplanted tibial tubercle should be splinted for approximately 6 weeks, it is desirable to start active movements of the knee joint 3 weeks after the transposition of tendon. The stage of union reached by the tibial tubercle should be firm enough after 4 weeks to permit the gentle maneuvers and movements required during the operation for transposition of the semitendinosus tendon. On one occasion the semitendinosus was transposed first, and movement was initiated after 3 weeks. Six weeks from the time of the original operation the tibial tubercle was transplanted. The operation provided an opportunity to examine the semitendinosus. It was gliding smoothly in a well-lined groove. More recently, both operations are performed at the same time. After 3 weeks the splint is removed for gentle active movements but is reapplied for weight-bearing.

With the patient supine and almost straight the operation is performed through a long, slightly curved incision in line with the medial collateral ligament (Fig. 22-6). By sharp dissection the upper femoral condyle is gently cleared in line with the posterior border of the shaft of the femur and down to the reflection of the synovium of the joint. A gutter is cut, inclining posteromedially and wide enough to accept the tendon comfortably (Fig. 22-7). The maximum depth is approximately ½ in. The proximal and distal edges of the gutter must not be sharp. The semitendinosus, which runs most posteriorly of all the hamstrings, is identified. The tendon is freed down to its insertion and sufficiently far up the thigh to release enough length to bring it forward between the other hamstrings and slip it into the gutter. Gentle flexion of the knee and a dissector to lever or shorehorn the tendon into the groove facilitates this maneuver. Because of the inclination of the groove, the tendon, once settled, is quite stable and does not tend to slip out. The groove is converted into a

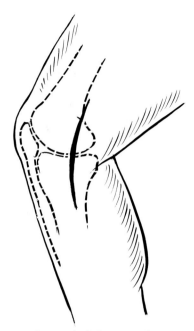

FIG. 22-6. A long, slightly curved incision in line with the medial collateral ligament.

tunnel by interrupted linen suture of periosteum and capsule. Postoperative conditioning of the hamstring muscles is an important feature of this operation. Thigh drill is started the day after the operation, and when movements are commenced 3 weeks later the patient is taught to contract the hamstrings consciously every time the knee is flexed. This should develop into a habit to give him permanent control of the knee.

In 1977 20 patients who had been treated for medial instability of the knee by transposition of the semitendinosis tendon were reviewed. All the operations had been performed at least 2 years previously. There were two interesting findings. Over the years stability had improved, for use of the knee, and exercise had strengthened and in some instances hypertrophied the muscle. This compares favorably with the long-term results of ligament replacement by strips of fascia or tendon. In time, all these static reconstructions stretch and to some extent weaken. Originally the procedure was designed to substi-

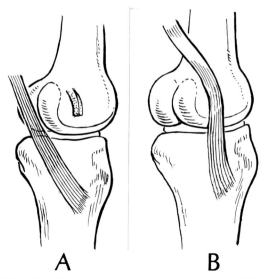

FIG. 22-7. Lively replacement of the medial ligament by transposition of the semitendinosus tendon. A groove **(A)** is made in the medial condyle into which the tendon is transplanted **(B)**.

tute for the collateral ligaments. But because of the new alignment the lively tendon also prevented anteroposterior instability. When the thigh muscles were relaxed, medial laxity and the drawer sign could still be elicited, but when the hamstrings were contracted the knee was stable. The postoperative training program conditioned the hamstrings to activate on all concerned movements, bringing practically normal stability. Most patients were enabled to resume suitable activities including sport.

Replacement of the Lateral Ligament of the Knee

The same principle may be used on the lateral side of the knee. At first the whole biceps tendon was transposed into a groove in the lateral condyle of the femur in the same way as the semitendinosus in the medial condyle, and this worked well. In another operation the biceps tendon was anchored in a groove on the femur by suture. In this way, satisfactory stability was also regained and retained. It is now found sufficient and preferable to use the anterior half of the biceps tendon (Fig. 22-8).

A longitudinal incision is made in the line of the biceps extending below the head of the fibula. The popliteal nerve is defined and retracted. The tendon is split longitudinally, leaving both ends attached. The outer surface of the lateral femoral condyle in line with the posterior border of the shaft is cleared as far down as the reflection of the synovium of the joint. A groove or "hook" is cut, directed medially and posteriorly in the same way as that on the medial side for the semitendinosus. The anterior half of the biceps is then slipped into this groove, which is converted into a tunnel by suturing periosteum and fascia. Care is taken to prevent injury to the capsule of the joint and the popliteus tendon. Adherence between the new ligament and these structures would cause restriction of flexion.

Since this description was recorded, instead of the biceps tendon it has been found as suitable and in most instances more convenient to replace the ligament with a middle slip of the iliotibial band. The slip is not detached from its insertion into the tibia because by its normal contractions it acts efficiently as a dynamic ligament.

The replacement of a torn ligament by an active tendon or "dynamic ligament" is particularly effective. It is more powerful and long-lasting than tenodesis.

I have used no other method since this one was devised during World War II. It is important to start isometric contractions soon after operation to prevent adherence in the bony groove. Postoperative stiffness of the knee has not been a significant problem. Very occasionally transient tenosynovitis of the semitendinosus has required a few days of splinting and an injection of a corticosteroid.

POSTOPERATIVE CARE

After each of these operations the wound is closed in layers. A compression bandage followed by a posterior gutter plaster splint is applied from midthigh to the lower third of the calf. After 2 weeks the sutures are removed, and the patient is allowed to walk on a back splint with crutches. Thigh drill is started on the second or the third day, increas-

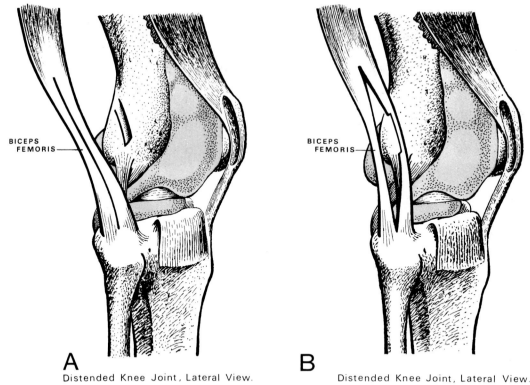

BICEPS
FEMORIS

A

Distended Knee Joint, Lateral View.

B

Distended Knee Joint, Lateral View.

FIG. 22-8. (A) The biceps tendon is split in its length, leaving both ends attached. A groove or hook is cut in the surface of the lateral condyle. **(B)** The anterior half of the split biceps tendon is hooked in the groove in the femur.

ing in frequency and in intensity as the weeks go by. Three weeks after semitendinosus transposition the splint is removed periodically for gentle active flexion exercises. After 6 weeks the patient may take weight, still wearing the back splint, which is not finally removed for another 2 weeks. After tibial tubercle transplant, a back splint is worn until the insertion of the patellar ligament is no longer tender. Normal activities should not be permitted until the thigh muscles have recovered normal power.

TREATMENT OF RECURRENT SUBLUXATION AND DISLOCATION OF THE TIBIOFIBULAR JOINT

Subperiosteal excision of the head of the fibula was an early operation for the unstable joint (Fig. 22-9). Patients lost their pain and functioned satisfactorily, but we were uncertain whether full power and stability would always be restored and would be retained. More recently, arthrodesis is preferred.

The joint is exposed through an incision curved anteriorly and extending some 2 in down the fibula. The peroneal nerve is isolated and retracted. The articular surfaces are exposed, denuded of cartilage, and apposed. A lag screw is inserted through the head of the fibula to hold it to the tibial surface. Usually tension of soft tissues resists firm apposition and may prevent sound ankylosis. Oblique osteotomy of the neck of the fibula releases these tensions, and by the time the arthrodesis is sound the osteotomy site has united (Fig. 22-10).

A long plaster cast is applied from midthigh to toes. After 4 weeks the patient may discard

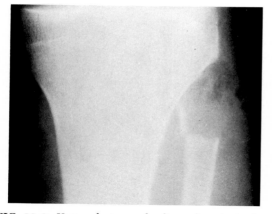

FIG. 22-9. X-ray photograph after subperiosteal excision of the head of the fibula and suture of soft tissues.

crutches and take weight on a rubber heel. The cast should be worn till fusion is sound, usually in 8 weeks.

INJURIES OF THE PATELLAR LIGAMENT

Contusions and sprains are discussed in Chapter 26. Rupture or avulsion of the ligament has been an infrequent injury in the ex-

perience of this practice. Clinically, whereas after contusion or sprain attempted extension of the leg on the thigh against resistance is painful, after complete rupture it is not possible, and the attempt is relatively painless. Early active or passive flexion is also painless but may become uncomfortable as the range increases. The gap in the patellar ligament may be felt, especially when the quadriceps are contracted.

Precise diagnosis may be established by measurements (Fig. 22-11) of the increased distance between the patella and the tibial tubercle in the injured compared with the normal knee. These measurements are useful also at operation to determine exact tension when pulling the patella down for suture. After suture, the patient should walk with a back splint and crutches for the first 3 weeks and a back splint alone for 3 more.

ACUTE TRAUMATIC DISLOCATION OF THE PATELLA

It has been customary to treat acute dislocation conservatively. While the patella is displaced—always laterally—the knee is slightly

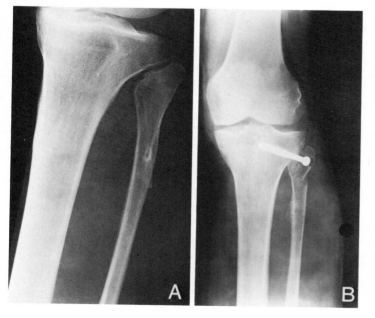

FIG. 22-10. (A, B) Pre- and postoperative roentgenograms, showing excision of the joint and apposition of the head of fibula to the tibia by means of a lag screw. Oblique osteotomy of the neck of the fibula has been performed.

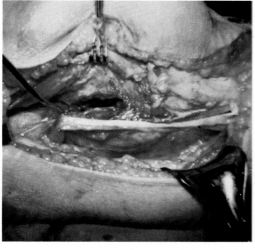

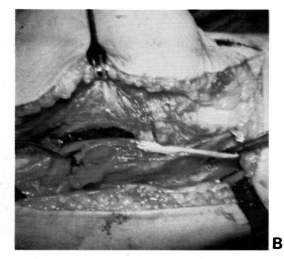

A

B

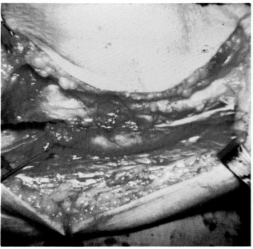

PLATE 22-1. (A) The semitendinosus tendon has been mobilized and a groove has been cut in the medial femoral condyle. (B) The tendon has been hooked into the groove. (C) The groove is converted into a tunnel by suturing the periosteum and deep fascia.

PLATE 22-2. (A) The normal configuration of the femoral condyles can be seen in this cadaveric knee. The trochlear walls are equal in depth, but the lateral condyle is longer than the medial. (B) In a patient with habitual dislocation of the patella, the trochlear groove is of adequate depth, but the lateral condyle is short—in this instance, shorter than the medial.

C

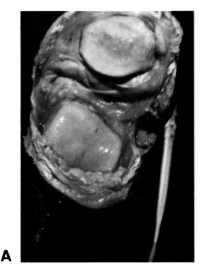

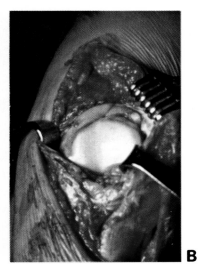

A

B

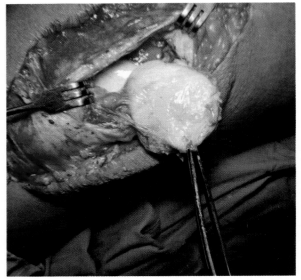

PLATE 22-3. Erosion on the medial articular facet of the patella.

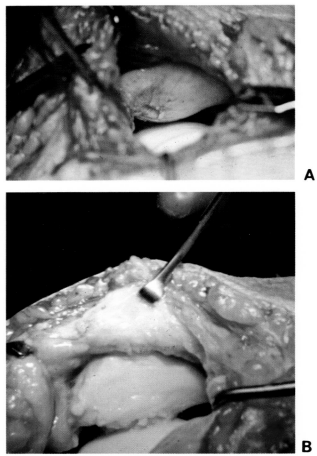

A

B

PLATE 22-4. Abrasions and disruptions of the articular cartilage of the patella should be trimmed.

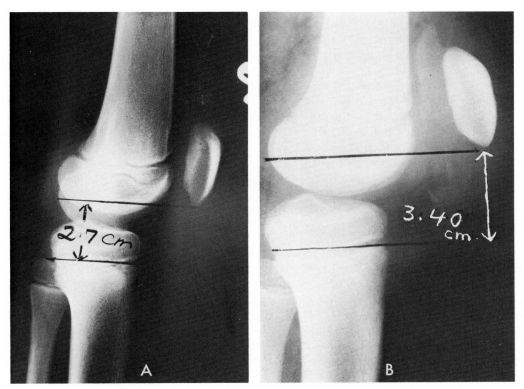

FIG. 22-11. (A) The distance from the epiphyseal line of the tibia to the lower pole of the patella in the normal knee is 2.7 cm. **(B)** In the injured knee with ruptured patellar ligament, the distance is 3.4 cm, an increase of 0.7 cm. Both roentgenograms are taken with the quadriceps contracted.

flexed, and is usually reduced as the muscles relax merely by straightening the leg. Anesthesia is rarely required. A compression bandage and back splint give comfort and permit weight-bearing. Aspiration of the point is seldom necessary. Thigh muscle drill is initiated. The splint should be worn for 4 weeks, after which movement and function return rapidly.

RECURRING TRAUMATIC DISLOCATION OF THE PATELLA

PREVENTION

Recurrence of the acute dislocation may follow if the capsule heals with loss of integrity and increased width, or it may follow ill-planned and poorly repaired long medial parapatellar incisions or inflammatory or infective processes that have distended the joint.

Realization of the true pathology leads to the conviction that *immediate repair of the split synovium and capsule is necessary in all cases of acute dislocation of the patella.* It is as important as immediate repair of ruptures of the medial collateral or the patellar ligaments.

TREATMENT

In contradistinction to habitual dislocation, traumatic dislocation invariably occurs in adolescent or adult patients. The resulting transverse weakness of the medial capsule of the knee joint is the basic fault to be repaired. Only surgery can effect a cure. The precise operation depends on the presence or absence of coincident anatomical or biomechanical weaknesses. Poor results are usually the consequences not of poor technique but of poor choice of operation.

An essential factor in successful long-term surgery is the appreciation in the particular patient of the track followed by the patella in its excursion from full flexion to full extension. The patella follows a sinuous path (see Chap. 1), and any interference, for example, when meniscal injuries lock rotation of the tibia on the femur, or when there is malalignment through medial transfer of the tibial tubercle and patellar ligament, leads inevitably to articular surface damage.

For high-riding patella the medial capsule must be tightened both longitudinally and transversely. (Invariably the lateral capsule is tight and should, as an initial stage, be released by longitudinal parapatellar division.) The transfer of the tibial tubercle medially with imbrication of the medial capsule, a frequent practice, carries dangers because, more often than not, the medial slope of the articular surface of the patella is tensed against the adjacent medial femoral condyle and leads to slow erosion and retropatellar pain. Moving the tibial tubercle lower as well as more medially (Hauser) to correct high-riding has a poor prognosis. In our experience it invariably leads to an eroded patella and retropatellar arthritis, and we no longer use this method. Besides disturbing the excursion of the patella, it often actually produces a twist on the tendon and patella.

The effect is not the same when the operation is performed as advocated for rupture of the cruciates with medial ligament laxity. Then it takes up capsular slack and ensures lateral rotation of the tibia, the normal func-

tion of the anterior cruciate ligament during active extension of the knee, and a necessary safeguard when a lax medial ligament threatens to produce weakness and instability. The additional rotation provided just aligns the patella so that in full extension it reaches its normal position in the trochlear groove.

On the other hand, if there is no transverse weakness of the capsule, medial transfer of the tibial tubercle may prevent the patella from reaching its position of comfort in the trochlear groove in full extension. Tension between the patella and the medial trochlear slope would result, leading to traumatic erosion of articular cartilage, a frequent cause of long-term disability after this operation. Medial transfer of the whole tibial tubercle should be performed only if longitudinal laxity of the capsule with or without a high-riding patella is a complicating factor.

The high-riding patella, lying as it does in the upper part or above the trochlear groove, is in its most vulnerable position for lateral dislocation. The operation described in Chapter 23, Fig. 23-10 is advised instead of the transfer of the tibial tubercle distally.

REFERENCES

1. **DePalma AF:** Diseases of the Knee. Philadelphia, JB Lippincott, 1954
2. **Helfet AJ:** A new way of treating flat feet in children. Lancet 270:1, 262, 1956
3. **McMurray TP:** The operative treatment of ruptured internal lateral ligament of the knee. Br J Surg 6:377, 1918
4. **O'Donoghue DH:** Surgical treatment of injuries to the knee. Clin Orthop 18:11, 1960
5. **Smillie IS:** Injuries of the Knee Joint. Baltimore, Williams & Wilkins, 1962
6. **Helfet AJ:** A new way of treating flat feet in children. Lancet, 270:1, 262, 1956

CHAPTER 23
DISLOCATIONS OF THE PATELLA

Arthur J. Helfet
A. W. Brookes Heywood

Although acute traumatic dislocation of the patella has a different etiological background and pathology from the more common recurrent dislocation of the patella, both conditions, because of their superficial anatomical similarity, will be considered in this chapter.

ACUTE DISLOCATION OF THE PATELLA

It is difficult to visualize the mechanism of traumatic dislocation of the patella in the normally formed and normally functioning knee when it occurs without disruption of the medial ligament. Personal experience and the histories of patients suggest that it results from severe abduction-flexion force on the fully extended knee while the foot is fixed and the quadriceps are fully contracted (e.g., the force exerted by a tackle obliquely from behind on the rigid knee while in the act of kicking a football with the other leg—see Fig. 23-1). In another instance, a forward's leg was

fully extended in the scrimmage when another player dived into his knee from the side and slightly behind. In both cases the quadriceps were powerfully contracted and the knee held straight when struck by a violent force into abduction and flexion. The patella in such a case nearly always dislocates laterally, tearing the medial capsule (Fig 23-2).

George Dommisse, of the Pretoria General Hospital, and one of us (A.J.H.) operated on the knee of a football player who had suffered traumatic dislocation 2 days previously. Under the anesthetic, with the muscles relaxed, the patella was lax enough to be subluxated to the outer side. The lesions in the fibrous capsule included a long vertical split immediately anterior to the medial ligament and a shorter split near the patella (Fig. 23-2, Plate 23-1). The synovium reproduced these lesions by a longitudinal parapatellar split as long as the patella and a much longer vertical tear just anterior to the synovial reflection, halfway back in the joint. As soon as the synovium was sutured, the patella was harnessed

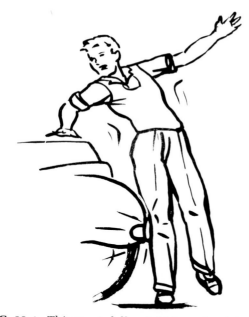

FIG. 23-1. This man's full weight is on the right leg with quadriceps braced. A pure abduction force would rupture the medial ligament. If he rotates his body and right thigh away from the car, he may dislocate the patella.

and could no longer be moved out of the trochlear groove. Suture of the capsule reinforced the stability. In another case a 16-year-old girl suffered an abduction and rotation strain on the weight-bearing fully extended leg. The foot was fixed by weight-bearing, and the femur rotated fiercely medially on the tibia. Again at operation a vertical split in both the synovium and the capsule was found, in this case only one. Before the synovium and capsule were sutured the patella was easily displaced, but repair brought complete stability.

When the quadriceps are contracted, the patella is at the limit of its upward excursion at a level where the trochlear surface of the femur is shallowest. The vertical splits in the capsule permit the lateral shift of the patella.

TREATMENT

Reduction is easy once the muscles relax and the knee is extended. Anesthesia is rarely re-

quired. Realization of the true pathology leads to the conviction that immediate repair of the split synovium and capsule is necessary in all cases of acute dislocation of the patella in adults. It is as important as immediate repair of ruptures of the medial collateral or patellar ligaments. Failure to effect immediate repair may result in recurrent dislocation of the patella.

RECURRENT DISLOCATION OF THE PATELLA

Only a minority of patients with habitual or recurrent dislocation of the patella can relate their condition to an acute traumatic dislocation; congenital factors are usually at fault. Recurrent dislocation of the patella is a common condition, especially in girls at the time of puberty, and the diagnosis is frequently missed. If the patella fails to find the normal condylar track in flexion it dislocates, usually laterally.

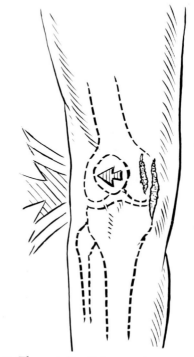

FIG. 23-2. The patella dislocates because of vertical splits in the synovium and the medial capsule.

GRADES OF PATELLAR INSTABILITY

Habitual dislocation. The patella is permanently and painlessly dislocated in all degrees of flexion of the knee.

Congenital dislocation. Habitual dislocation is present from birth.

Recurrent dislocations. The patella is usually centrally located but has occasional episodes of painful dislocation, almost always in a lateral direction.

Recurrent subluxation. The patella frequently starts to track laterally as flexion commences but is soon pulled medially into its normal groove, impinging on the lateral condyle as it does so.

THE MECHANICS OF INSTABILITY

The physiologic valgus of the knee creates an angle, convex medially, between the central quadriceps pull and the ligamentum patellae—this is the Q angle (Fig. 23-3). Quadriceps contraction therefore pulls the patella not only upward but also slightly outward, so that a permanent, normal, dynamic, lateral dislocating force exists. This force is countered chiefly by the immensely important vastus medialis, whose fibers pull directly medially on the patella and are supported by the epicondylopatellar ligament of Kaplan, which is a thickening of the medial capsule. A subsidiary buttress against lateral subluxation is the lateral condylar eminence. The balance between central location and dislocation is a delicate one. For dislocation to occur, the lateral dislocating force (Q angle, tight lateral structures) must overcome the restraining forces (medial quadriceps, medial capsule). In the normal knee, the patella lies slightly laterally in full extension. In a knee prone to recurrent subluxation of the patella, an episode is triggered by the leg being caught in external rotation as flexion commences with weight-bearing. Quadriceps contraction with the increased Q angle forces the high-riding patella

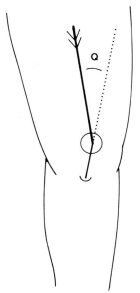

FIG. 23-3. The Q Angle

laterally as it descends, and it finds the lateral face of the lateral femoral condyle instead of the intercondylar groove. The tension of the medial capsule increases at 20° to 30° of flexion, either forcing the patella to jump the condyle to regain the groove or keeping it painfully trapped lateral to the condyle until tension is released by reflex inhibition and subsequent extension of the knee, which raises and disimpacts the patella.

ETIOLOGY

Congenital Diathesis

Women with this condition outnumber men 5:1. The majority of patients with dislocating patellae have a congenital laxity of the medial and posterior capsule, sometimes confined to the knees but more often manifest in multiple joints.[12] More serious lax-jointed disorders such as Ehlers-Danlos syndrome, arachnodactyly, and muscular hypotonia not infrequently involve unstable patellae. Recurring dislocation of the patella has been attributed to genu valgum, flattening of the lateral femoral condyle, laxity of the medial joint capsule, posterior ligamentous laxity causing hyperexten-

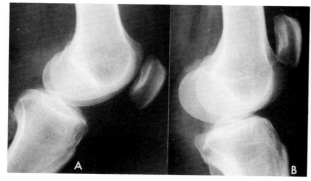
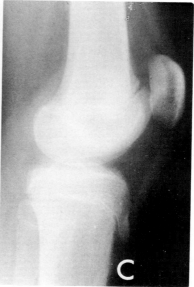

FIG. 23-4. In a normal knee the patella rests against the medial condyle of the femur when the knee is flexed **(A)**; when the knee is extended with the quadriceps contracted, the patella reaches the apex of the trochlear fossa **(B)**; and with the knee straight and the quadriceps relaxed, it rests comfortably in the trochlear groove **(C)**.

sion, excessive length of the patellar ligament, high-riding patella, abnormal lateral insertion of the patellar ligament of the tibia, and muscular hypotonia. In addition, the lateral capsule is usually abnormally tight.

The importance of joint laxity, aplasia of the lateral condyle, and the high-riding patella in the genesis of patellofemoral instability has been emphasized also by McNab[14] and by one of us (A.W.B.H.),[12] who, in evaluating 76 patients, was able to define trauma as the sole significant factor in only 5%.

Hyperextension or genu recurvatum is also present in a good proportion of cases with high-riding patella. With Alaia one of us compared eight consecutive cases of recurring dislocation with eight clinically and radiographically normal knees. Whereas the normal knee had a 5° average of hyperextension, in the dislocating group the mean angle of recurvatum was just over 9°.

Most initial dislocations occurred when a relatively trivial injury was superimposed on a congenital defect. In our practices the most common anatomical abnormalities have been laxity of the medial, with tightness of the lateral capsule, the high-riding patella, and a short rather than a flat lateral condyle (Figs. 23-4 and 23-5, Plate 23-2).

The lateral condyle normally acts as a buttress for the patella against lateral slip when the quadriceps are fully contracted. Both a short condyle and genu recurvatum allow the contracting extensors to pull the patella out of this groove at a lower level. The patella becomes high-riding and vulnerable.

This may be determined by lateral radiographs taken with the knee extended as far as possible and the quadriceps fully contracted (Figs. 23-4, 23-5).

Contraction Bands

Occasionally a tight vastus lateralis resulting either from scarring caused by intramuscular injections or from congenital contracture may cause habitual (permanent) dislocation.[4,8]

Injury

In approximately 5% of patients, congenital diathesis is absent, and a clear history of major trauma is obtained. In such patients the first dislocation usually occurs after puberty.

As described earlier in this chapter, the initial injury involves a violent external rotation and valgus strain in semiflexion with concurrent strong quadriceps contraction. Healing of the medial capsule in a stretched position results in lateral instability of the patella.

Below-Knee Amputation

Many years of walking with a below-knee prosthesis can cause late recurrent dislocation of the patella.[12]

EFFECTS ON THE PATELLA

Each time the patella dislocates or subluxates it jumps the edge of the lateral femoral condyle and is then dragged back again to regain its central position. On its way back across the condyle its medial facet is forced against the lateral edge of the lateral condyle, eventually resulting in chondromalacia patellae (Plate 23-3, Fig. 23-6).

Occasionally, osteochondritis dissecans results, in which an osteochondral fragment separates to leave a crater. Damage to the lateral femoral condyle also occurs. An occasional result of a major episode is an osteochondral avulsion fracture on the medial margin of the patella. Finally, generalized osteoarthrosis of the knee may be found in patients whose patellae have been dislocating unchecked for many years.

SYMPTOMS

The rare patients, usually children, with habitual (permanent) dislocation seldom have complaints. More common recurrent dislocations occur during adolescence or early adult life, most frequently in girls. Recurrent episodes of painful giving way of the knee are usually precipitated by a minor twist while running or while walking on uneven ground. Pain is felt medially owing to stretching of the capsule. The patient might be aware that the patella has moved but usually assumes it has

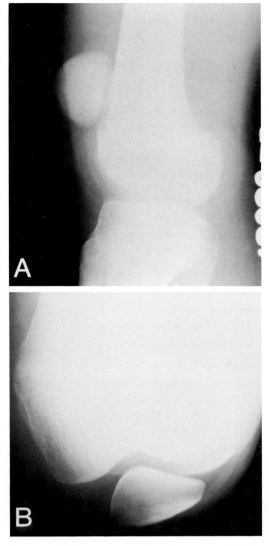

FIG. 23-5. This patient suffered recurrent dislocation at age 16, the first two incidents having occurred only a few months previously. **(A)** Note that in extension the patella lies above the trochlear ridge, which is short. The quadriceps is fully contracted. **(B)** In the tangential view it can be seen that the lateral ridge is not shallow. The patella dislocates because it is short.

displaced medially because of the painful prominence of the medial condyle. Most patients fail to relate their symptoms to the patella, saying only that the knee gave way with medial pain. Early episodes are usually followed by swelling; later ones frequently are not. Later, retropatellar pain and grating due to the onset of chondromalacia may be noticed by the patient, especially when sitting or descending stairs.

A family history of joint laxity, with or without instability of the joints, is frequently encountered.

PHYSICAL FINDINGS

Generalized ligamentous laxity occurs in about 25% of patients. On local examination, a medial meniscectomy scar may bear testimony to an earlier incorrect diagnosis. Hyperextensibility beyond 5° is common. The patella itself is frequently high and small, and its anterior surface may slope laterally. It is usually hypermobile in all directions, especially laterally, and a gentle lateral push on the patella may cause a start of apprehension from the patient, who recognizes this as being similar to the painful episodes (apprehension test). If the test is negative in full extension, hold the patella laterally with the knee fully relaxed. Now slowly flex the knee passively while still pushing the patella laterally; this should subluxate the patella, causing a start of apprehension. Sitting on the edge of the couch with the knee held extended, the patella is sometimes seen to lie laterally. On starting slow active flexion, the patella may drift off laterally and then jerk to the midline as flexion proceeds past 30°. Some or all of these signs are usually present bilaterally but are more prominent in the affected knee. Ten-

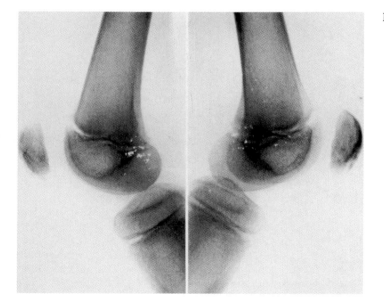

FIG. 23-6. Note thinning of the articular surface in these roentgenographic views of chondromalacia of the patella.

derness medial to the patella is common and is caused by stretching of the capsule early and by chondromalacia of the patella after some years.

RADIOLOGIC FEATURES

The lateral radiograph must be taken routinely in 30° of flexion to take up the slack of the ligamentum patellae. If the vertical height of the lower end of the articular surface of the patella above the tibial plateau is greater than the length of the patellar articular surface, the patella is abnormally high[4] (patella alta) and is prone to subluxations (Fig. 23-4, Fig. 23-7).

The axial view of the patella is taken with

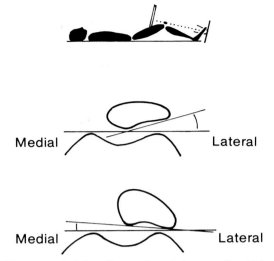

FIG. 23-8. Axial radiography of the patella. (After Laurin) **(A)** Axial view of patella. **(B)** When Laurin angle is open laterally, patella is stable. **(C)** When Laurin angle is open medially, patella is unstable.

the patient supine, both knees flexed to 20°, and the tube between the feet with the plate held vertical to the rays in front of the thighs (Fig. 23-8). This view gives the cross-sectional shape of the patella, the slope of the lateral condyle, and the geometric relationships between the two. At this critical point in the range of motion any lateral instability of the patella is most manifest. The patella that is prone to subluxation tends to be thick and narrow with a vertical medial facet. On the x-ray film, a line AA is drawn across the crests of the tibial condyles, and a second line BB is drawn along the lateral patellar condyle. If the angle subtended by these two lines is open laterally, the patella is stable. If the lines are parallel or make an angle open medially, the patella is unstable.[13]

MANAGEMENT

PREVENTION

Recurrence following acute traumatic dislocation may be prevented by early surgical repair of the medial capsule.

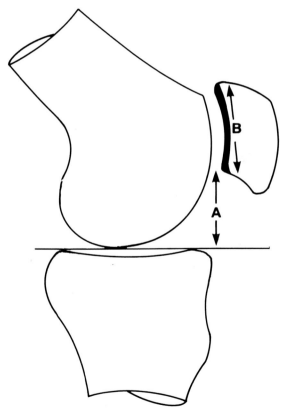

FIG. 23-7. *Patellar height* (Blackburne). Knee flexed 30°. If A is greater than B, the result is called patella alta.

CONSERVATIVE MANAGEMENT

Approximately 20% of adolescents with recurrent subluxation due to congenital diathesis may be successfully treated with intensive static quadriceps exercises only. The vastus medialis, which is crucial to the stability of the patella, is active only in full extension, and therefore resisted straight leg quadriceps exercises must be done at hourly intervals. A patellar stabilizing brace that consists essentially of an elastic sleeve with a check pad lateral to the patella and two straps embracing the knee, one just above and one below the patella, help to prevent acute episodes.

After an acute dislocation, a period of 3 to 6 months without sports is advisable. Sporadic subluxations occurring years apart are probably best treated without surgery. A conserva-

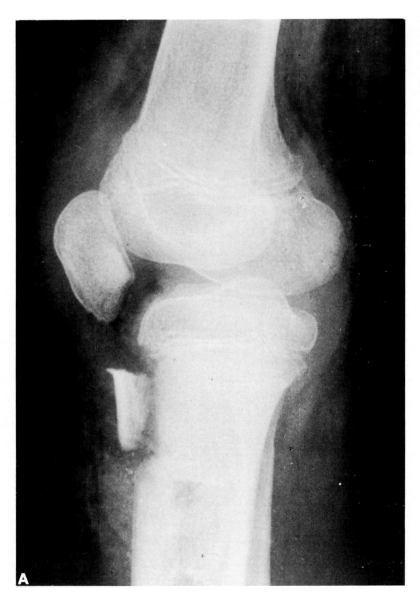

A

FIG. 23-9. (A) Two pitfalls in tibial tubercle transfer. The operation should not have been done before epiphyseal closure, and the tubercle has been moved too far inferiorly. Note the situation of the patella. (*Continued on opposite page.*)

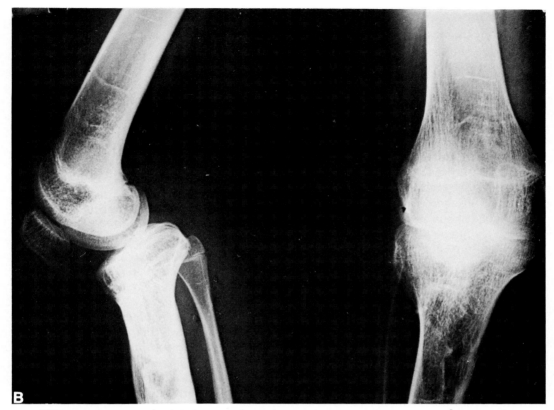

FIG. 23-9 (*continued*). **(B)** One year later the resulting anterolateral epiphyseodesis has sloped the tibial table forward and laterally, resulting in recurvatum and valgus deformity.

tive approach is especially important for recurrent dislocations that occur before closure of the epiphyses.

SURGICAL MANAGEMENT

Surgery is indicated if dislocations continue frequently. Surgical repair is not uniformly successful; many more methods have been devised than are in use today.

Two principles must be fulfilled: the contracted lateral parapatellar structures must be released, and the forces acting on the patella must be realigned. There is disagreement on the preferable and precise technique of realignment. Management varies with age. In choosing the operation, careful attention must be paid to the customary track used by the patella from flexion to extension. In the very

young, rerouting may be successful because the pliable adaptive growing articular structures may mold a new channel. In the adolescent or adult this is not always possible. Moreover, excessive surgical realignment may leave the knee worse off than before, and painful, irreparable osteoarthritis may become inevitable.

Small Children

For the rare instances in small children of habitual or congenital dislocation due to fibrous contracture of the vastus lateralis or other structure, early and radical surgical release is necessary.[2,3] Some cases discovered late in which there is good function are best left alone.

Older Children

The dislocating diathesis may lead to recurrent dislocations any time after the age of 8 years. Until the epiphyses are closed, to obviate anterior epiphyseodesis and subsequent recurvatum deformity (Fig. 23-9), the tibial tubercle must not be touched, and only soft tissue surgery is permitted. A narrow tourniquet is placed high on the thigh to permit full excursion of the quadriceps muscle. Surgical realignment should be performed through a lateral parapatellar incision curving downward and medially across the tibial tubercle. The lateral quadriceps expansion is released from well above the patella to the tibial tubercle without opening the synovium.

For patients in whom the high-riding patella is the salient mechanical derangement, the patellar ligament must be shortened (Fig. 23-10). A proximal central tongue of the patellar ligament is freed and buttonholed into the distal part. The amount of shortening required is small, a centimeter at most. Overshortening is a common error. The knee should be flexed on the table to ensure that the ligament has not been pulled too low, thereby causing the patella to impact in the intercondylar notch before full flexion is reached. Aftercare consists of a plaster-of-Paris backsplint for 6 weeks, which is removed for nonweight-bearing movements during the last 2 weeks.

An alternative technique is that described by Handelsman.* Two temporary sutures are placed as markers side by side, one in the ligament and one in the lateral expansion next to it. The ligament is now dissected free medially and then lifted carefully from its bony attachment in continuity with a distal prolongation of 3 cm of periosteum. The periosteum is then lifted medially and distally on the tibia to allow the ligament and its prolongation to be sewn under it a maximum of 1 cm medial and 1 cm distal to its original location. The marker sutures inserted previously facilitate the judgment of the exact distance, which will vary with the size of the limb, the degree of patella alta, and the severity of the dislocating diathesis. The marker sutures are removed, and two sutures are placed through drill holes in the bone below the epiphysis of the tibial tubercle. The knee must now be flexed to determine that the patella tracks normally and is not so low that it impacts between the femoral condyles before flexion is complete.

* Handelsman JE: Personal communication

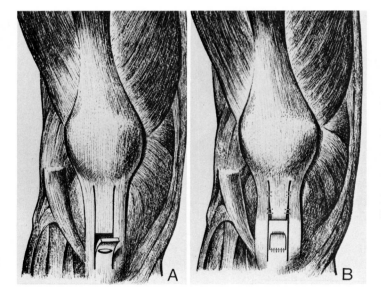

FIG. 23-10. Shortening the patellar tendon for patella alta. **(A)** The patellar tendon is exposed through a lateral parapatellar incision and division of the sheath. A guard is placed behind the tendon. Parallel incisions in the tendon release a central tongue, which is divided at the junction of the middle and distal thirds. The proximal portion is buttonholed into the distal part and fixed with sutures. **(B)** The amount of shortening need rarely be more than 1 cm. After the repair is completed the knee should be tested for an adequate range of flexion.

After Closure of the Epiphyses

In patients over the age of 14 years, when the danger of growth disturbance is over, the tibial tubercle may be involved in the surgical realignment. Most commonly the tibial tubercle or part of it is moved distally to lower the patella and medially to reduce the Q angle. Four alternative procedures will be described.

1. *The Hauser procedure (tibial tubercle transfer).* Despite criticism, this operation remains popular. After application of a high tourniquet, a lateral parapatellar incision is made, and the lateral quadriceps expansion is released from well above the patella to below the tibial tubercle (Fig. 23-11). When dislocations have been frequent and when painful retropatellar crepitus has been detected clinically, the joint is entered and the patella inverted for thorough inspection of its undersurface.[14] Plates 23-3 and 23-4 show the type of erosion that may be encountered on the medial facet. An area of fibrillated cartilage may be shaved down to bone. A deep ulcer with eburnated bone on its floor should be removed complete with the underlying bone by semipatellectomy as described by Sacks.[15]

    The tibial tubercle with the ligamentum patellae attached is now transplanted downward and medially. Several methods have been described. One of us (A. J. H.) described a "slot" method in 1948 (Fig. 23-12). A patient in this series developed a complication that necessitated a minor modification. The patellar tendon had been over-tautened, and consequently full flexion was not recovered; years later retropatellar arthritis developed. Unfortunately, in a way, the limitation of flexion of some 15° remained painless so that the excessive tightness of the quadriceps mechanism was not relieved. The technique has been modified by cutting the medial groove slightly upward instead of transversely. This maintains normal tension in the quadriceps mechanism in its new alignment. The patellar tendon has a more medial pur-

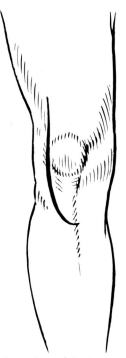

FIG. 23-11. A long lateral incision curving across the tibial crest below the level of the tibial tubercle.

chase on the tibia and so ensures earlier and increased lateral rotation of the tibia during extension.

The flap of skin and deep fascia is reflected to expose the patellar ligament and the tibial tubercle. Lateral and medial incisions free the patellar tendon. Care must be taken that this is complete on the lateral side. A block of bone of the same width as and including the insertion of the tendon plus 1/3 in proximally and distally beyond the insertion is removed, using small sharp osteotomes (Fig. 23-12). Care must be taken not to injure the fat pad with its synovial protection that lies between the ligament and the tibia. A groove the same width as the insertion of the tendon and at the exact level of the insertion is cut medially and slightly upward on the medial surface of the tibia (Fig. 23-12, *top, left*), extending approximately 1/2 in. The direction should be that of the circumference of a circle of which the patellar tendon forms the radius.

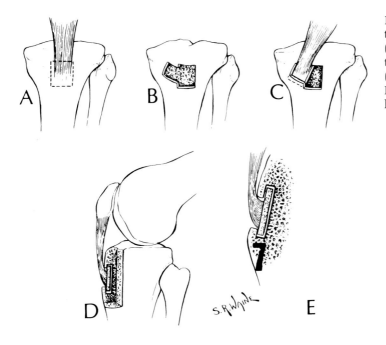

FIG. 23-12. Stages in transplantation of the tibial tubercle by the slot method. **(A)** The tubercle is removed. **(B)** A gutter is prepared to receive the tubercle. **(C)** The tubercle is transplanted. **(D, E)** Lateral views of the tubercle slotted home.

The cortical block of bone is kept for use as a plug to prevent the insertion from slipping out of the slot at the end of the operation. A sharp curette or gauge is used to scoop out cancellous bone from beneath the cortex both proximally and distally until enough room is cleared beneath it to slide in the oblong of bone to which the insertion is attached (Fig. 23-12, *top, right*). Once this is tapped home, it is held securely, and contraction of the quadriceps can only lock it more firmly. To prevent any medial slip, the block of bone removed from the slot is packed into the donor site at the tibial tubercle. The medial capsule is now sutured to the medial edge of the patellar ligament, and fascia is sutured over the raw bone surfaces (Fig. 23-12, *bottom, left and right*).

One of us (A. W. B. H.) prefers a modification of this technique that many find equally successful (see Fig. 23-13). A 1 cm width of tibial tubercle is demarcated by undercutting the ligament insertion medially and then is removed with an oscillating saw or small sharp osteotome, includ-

ing a 1-mm to 2-mm projection of cortex above the top of the ligament insertion. A second, shorter slot 1 cm wide is carefully cut 2 mm medial to the original bed, its upper margin 0 to 10 mm below the upper margin of the original bed, depending on how far the patella is to be displaced downward. Downward and medial displacement must be minimal (Fig. 23-14). The cancellous bone is removed from under the second slot, its upper and lower cortical lips being undercut to accept the tibial tubercle, which is now pushed in under the

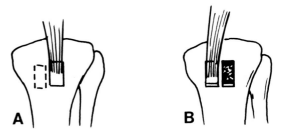

FIG. 23-13. Alternative Heywood method (see text).

FIG. 23-14. If the lateral capsule is not released, the patella may remain tensed against the lateral trochlear slope.

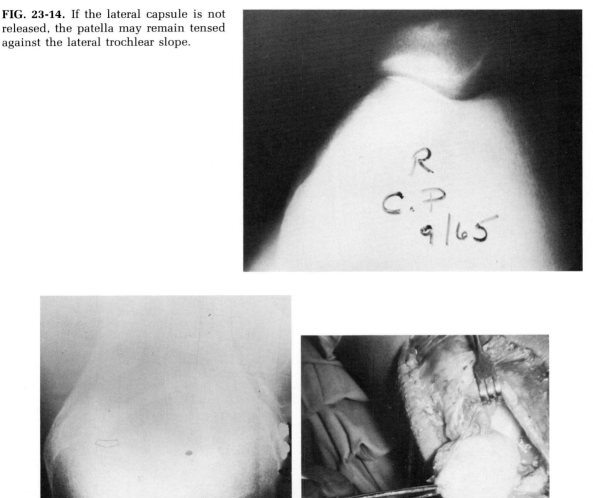

FIG. 23-15. (A) Tangential view of the patella after Hauser tibial tubercle transplant shows the patella to be twisted as well as displaced medially. **(B)** There is marked erosion on the medial articular facet of the patella. (See Plate 22-3 for color photo.)

lower lip and then pulled upward to impact it under the upper lip. Before suture, the knee is flexed fully to make sure that the tubercle has not been moved too far distally, thus causing impaction of the patella before full flexion (Figs. 23-14, 23-15).

After the operation, the limb is splinted in a plaster cylinder for 6 weeks.

2. *The Roux-Goldthwait operation.* When only transverse laxity of the medial capsule is at fault, the Roux-Goldthwait operation,

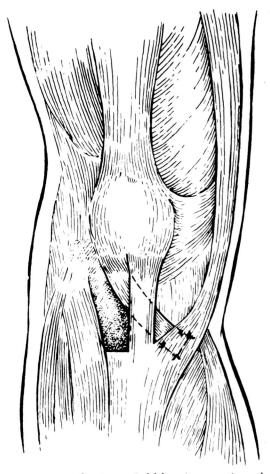

FIG. 23-16. In the Roux-Goldthwait operation, the patella and the patellar ligament are freed from the lateral capsule. The lateral half of the patellar tendon, with half of the tibial tubercle, is then mobilized, passed behind the inner half of the tendon, and slotted into the medial surface of the tibia with fair tension.

which prevents abnormal lateral excursion of the patella without altering the mechanics, is suitable. In addition, the relaxed capsule should be reefed or imbricated longitudinally. The Campbell procedure, a simple operation, should be used as an alternative or in addition to imbrication for gross medial capsular laxity.

As illustrated in Figure 23-16, the lateral quadriceps expansion is released longitudinally to allow the patella to return to its central position. The lateral half of the patellar tendon is then transferred medially without undue tension with its bony attachment.

The result is demonstrated by the roentgenograms of a 17-year-old boy shown in Fig. 23-5. The unstable patella was treated by this operation. Figure 23-17 shows the level of the patella after the operation. The lateral half of the tibial tubercle has slotted into the medial surface of the tibia. The patella lies in the trochlear groove with normal tension, and the patient is comfortable. Aftercare is the same as that described for the Hauser operation. Both the Hauser and the Roux-Goldthwait operations have been criticized, the former because it can disturb

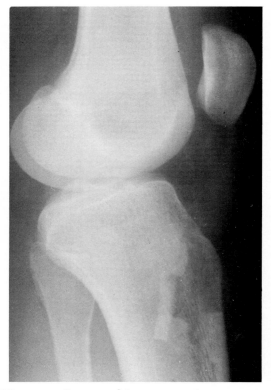

FIG. 23-17. Compare this postoperative roentgenogram with those of the patient's knee before the Roux-Goldthwait operation (Fig. 23-5). The knee is extended and the quadriceps contracted.

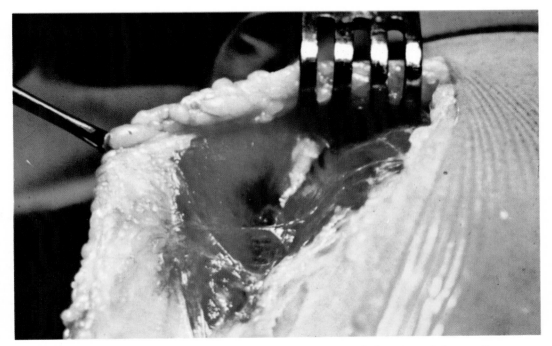

PLATE 23-1. Vertical tear of the medial capsule in acute dislocation of the patella.

FIG. 23-18. The Campbell operation. Beginning at a level with the articular surface of the tibia, a strip of capsule 5 inches long and ½ to 1 inch wide is dissected, leaving the base attached proximally. The cut margins of the capsule are closed, thus taking up transverse slack. Through two slits on either side of the quadriceps tendon the strap is passed around the tendon and sutured to the soft tissues in the region of the adductor tubercle.

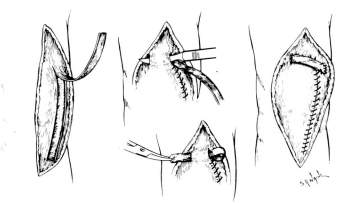

the patellar mechanism excessively and cause retropatellar arthritis* (Fig. 23-15*A*, *B*), and the latter because it may fail to realign the forces sufficiently.[13] Either criticism is valid if the operation is done inexpertly (see Fig. 23-15).

The success of either procedure requires meticulous surgical techniques matched with a sound appreciation of the biomechanical principles involved, and excessive displacement must be avoided.

3. *Patellectomy.* When retropatellar arthritis is caused by recurrent dislocation, patellectomy alone will not solve the problem. Rerouting of the quadriceps mechanism is necessary also; otherwise recurrent dislocation of the regenerated central tendon is likely. In patients in whom rerouting has stopped the dislocation but late painful retropatellar osteoarthritis has supervened, patellectomy usually cures the symptoms at the cost of a slight extensor weakness. When patellectomy is done, it should be a simple "shelling out" by sharp periosteal dissection with a knife, without formal repair of the quadriceps mechanism. Prolonged postoperative immobilization is unnecessary after such patellectomy.

4. *Soft Tissue Realignment.* Soft tissue realignment of the patella has obvious advantages before epiphyseal closure. Even after maturity, the dangers inherent in

overdoing correction by tibial tubercle transfer incline some authors* to favor soft tissue correction. Others[1] have found a high incidence of failure unless soft tissue procedures are accompanied by tibial tubercle transfer. Various methods in use today include those of Campbell,[11] Galeazzi,[7,13] and Wagner.[14,*]

5. *The Campbell operation* (Fig. 23-18) provides a medial checkstrap to lateral mobility of the quadriceps tendon. Beginning at a level with the articular surface of the tibia, a strip of medial capsule 5 in long and ½ in to 1 in wide is dissected, leaving the base attached proximally. The cut margins of the capsule are closed, thus taking up transverse slack. Through two slits on either side of the quadriceps tendon the strap is passed around the tendon and sutured to the soft tissues in the region of the adductor tubercle.[12] In addition, longitudinal release of a tight lateral capsule may be necessary. The operation has the virtues both of taking up transverse slack and of stabilizing the patellar mechanism.

Complications

Complications may result from injury, poor technique, or choice of the wrong operation.

When recurrence is due solely to the effects of the longitudinal tear of the medial capsule,

---

* Handelsman JE: Personal communication

* Handelsman JE: Personal communication

the edges tend to retract and, when treated conservatively, may heal with a gap and consequent weakness and further dislocation.

Arthrotomy should be used to detect osteochondral fractures or damage with fragmentation of the articular surface of the patella or femur. A lateral parapatellar approach is needed to release the lateral capsule. At the same time, the synovium is opened. Condylar fragments are removed, and the articular abrasions are trimmed (Plate 23-4). Associated ruptures of the menisci should be determined by careful preoperative diagnosis, including arthroscopy.

Two errors in technique are failure to release the lateral capsule, which may lead to recurrent subluxation or even dislocation, and second, pulling the patella and the patellar ligament too far distally or medially (Fig. 23-15*A, B*). This leads to restriction of flexion and compression of the patella in the trochlear groove and so to retropatellar arthritis, a frequent sequel of the Hauser operation.

Unfortunately, only in the relatively inactive is the long-term prognosis after patellectomy satisfactory. A fibrous or fibrocartilaginous pseudopatella may form and in time develop its own painful relationships with the articular surface of the femur unless it in its turn is realigned.

REFERENCES

1. **Alaia L, Helfet AJ:** Short Trochlear Groove in Recurrent Dislocation of the Knee. Report of N.Y. Academy of Orthopaedic Surgery, April, 1963

2. **Baker RH, Carroll N, Dewar FP et al:** The semitendinosus tenodesis for recurrent dislocation of the patella. J Bone and Joint Surg 54B:103–109, 1972

3. **Blackburne JS, Peel TE:** A new method of measuring patella height. J Bone and Joint Surg 59B:241–242, 1977

4. **Bose K, Chong KC:** The clinical manifestations and pathomechanics of contracture of the extensor mechanism of the knee. J Bone Joint Surg 58B:478–484, 1976

5. **Bowker JH, Thompson EB:** Surgical treatment of recurrent dislocation of the patella. J Bone Joint Surg 46A:1451, 1964

6. **Crosby EB, Insall J:** Recurrent dislocation of the patella. J Bone Joint Surg 58A:9–13

7. **Galeazzi R:** Nuove Applicazione del Trapionto Muscolare e Tendineo. (XII Congress Soceita Italiana di Ortopedia) Arch Ortoped 1922:38, 1921

8. **Green JP, Waugh W:** Congenital lateral dislocation of the patella. J Bone Joint Surg 50B:285–289, 1968

9. **Goldthwait JE:** Slipping or recurrent dislocation of the patella. Boston Med Surg J 150:169, 1904

10. **Hauser EDW:** Total tendon transplant for slipping patella. Surg Gynecol Obstet 66:199–214, 1938

11. **Helfet AJ:** Function of the cruciate ligaments of the knee joint. Lancet May 665, 1948

12. **Heywood AWB:** Recurrent dislocation of the patella. A study of pathology and treatment in 106 knees. J Bone Joint Surg 43B:508–517, 1961

13. **Laurin CA, Levesque HP, Dussault R et al:** The abnormal lateral patellofemoral angle. J Bone Joint Surg 60A:55–60

14. **McNab I:** Recurrent dislocation of the patella. J Bone Joint Surg, 1952

15. **Sacks S:** Semipatellectomy. S Afr Med J 36:518–520, 1962

16. **Speed JS, Knight RA:** Campbell's Operative Orthopaedics, 3rd ed. St. Louis, CV Mosby, 1956

17. **Wagner LC:** A plastic operation for recurrent slippings and dislocation of the patella. J Bone Joint Surg 14:332–334, 1932

CHAPTER 24
KNEE INJURIES IN NONCONTACT SPORTS

Daniel N. Kulund

In the past, those major knee injuries commonly encountered in contact sports have tended to monopolize the therapeutic and academic interests of orthopaedic surgeons to the exclusion of injuries occurring in noncontact sports. But with the recent upsurge of public interest in noncontact sports such as jogging, running, tennis, squash, and racketball, there is an increasing interest in injuries that are neither major nor caused by direct trauma, nor are they adequately described in much of the orthopaedic literature. In this chapter attention will be paid to aspects of the more common knee injuries encountered in noncontact sports.

INJURIES TO THE ANTERIOR ASPECT OF THE KNEE

RUNNER'S KNEE PERIPATELLAR PAIN IN RUNNERS

Virtually any injury causing knee pain in runners has in the past been labeled "runner's knee," but we prefer to restrict this term to injuries with characteristic symptoms occurring most commonly but not exclusively in recreational joggers and long-distance runners.

The athlete with runner's knee usually complains of anterior knee pain or discomfort, most often localized to the patella, after a predictable running or jogging distance. The discomfort becomes worse when running is continued, and when running is continued after a stop of a few minutes, there may be a grating or catching sensation in the affected knee. These symptoms typically develop gradually over a period of weeks without a history of direct trauma. The discomfort is reproduced by walking up or down stairs. A classic symptom of this condition is the so-called movie sign—discomfort that occurs after sitting with a flexed knee for a protracted period and that is relieved by fully extending the knee. Therefore, at the movies the athlete chooses an aisle seat to be able periodically to extend his knee fully.

There is considerable interest in the tissue origin of the discomfort in runner's knee. Although some feel that this syndrome is due to chondromalacia of the patella, others argue that the discomfort arises from the soft tissues surrounding the patella, particularly the anteromedial and anterolateral capsule.[18] James and his colleagues[16] believe that chondromalacia of the patella should be diagnosed in runners only if there is retropatellar crepitation and definite patella facet tenderness; this distinction is not mentioned by others. In most cases of runner's knee, deep palpation of the peripatellar structures alone is sufficient to reproduce the symptoms, and Mayfield[28] points out that, in contrast to the prolonged disability caused by true chondromalacia patellae, peripatellar pain in runners is usually a transient phenomenon that resolves rapidly when the correct treatment is prescribed. Others have used the term "patella compression syndrome"[18,35] to describe patella-related pain in the absence of chondromalacia.

There is now general agreement that runner's knee results from abnormal lower limb biomechanical function during running.[16,24,40] Specifically, it is held that prolonged, excessive subtalar joint pronation occurring for more than 75% of the stance phase of running causes abnormal transverse plane rotation at the knee. It is abnormal movement that is believed to cause the soft tissue trauma that results in runner's knee.

Prolonged subtalar joint pronation is usually the compensatory mechanism for one or more of the following anatomical factors[13]: tibia varum, functional equinus due to tightness in the gastrocnemius–soleus muscle group, subtalar varus, forefoot supination, and Morton's foot. Other factors contributing to runner's knee are leg-length discrepancies, hip anteversion, patella alta, and "squinting" patellae with increased Q angle.* [16]

A clue to the diagnosis and treatment of runner's knee is the presence of any static anatomical abnormality etiologically linked to

---

* Lines drawn from the anterior superior iliac spine to the midpoint of the patella and from the tibial tubercle through the same point form the Q angle. When anatomical variations increase the Q angle, the result is "squinting" patellae.

the condition. Overall alignment of the lower limb should be checked, particularly limb-length discrepancies, anteversion of the hips, genu varum or valgum, patella alta, excessive Q angle, tibia vara, leg-heel alignment, heel-forefoot alignment, foot type, and the flexibility of the posterior calf muscles. Observation of the running gait assists in assessment of the functional significance of these static abnormalities. More sophisticated analyses of running gait and subtalar joint function are possible but are not yet sufficiently specific to have clinical relevance for individual athletes.

Once the lower limb has been examined for the presence of anatomical abnormalities, local treatment can be given. Ice should be applied to the sore area both before and after running. Ultrasound and drug medication (aspirin 600 mg to 900 mg four times daily) may also be prescribed. If there is associated vastus medialis wasting, the strength of this muscle should be increased by isometric, isotonic, or isokinetic exercises; in the latter two exercises, resistance should be applied only through the last 15° of knee extension because only through this arc of movement is the vastus medialis maximally active.

For the definitive treatment of seriously symptomatic runner's knee, a foot orthotic device that will compensate for any abnormal lower limb anatomical factors by controlling the prolonged excessive subtalar joint pronation should be prescribed.[2] This mode of therapy, first popularized empirically, effectively reduces both the symptoms of runner's knee and the extent and duration of subtalar joint pronation.[2]

CHONDROMALACIA PATELLA

The symptoms of chondromalacia are essentially identical to those in runner's knee except that they are usually more debilitating and more resistant to therapy.

Much of the confusion that arises in differentiating between true chondromalacia patellae and the peripatellar pain of runner's knee can be attributed to the belief that Clarke's test is specific for chondromalacia patellae. In Clarke's test, the examiner holds the patella firmly in a distal position with the knee fully extended. The patient then contracts the quadriceps muscle firmly. Pain or discomfort sufficiently severe to prevent a sustained muscular contraction is believed to be diagnostic of chondromalacia patellae. However, sensitive synovia may also be pinched by this maneuver, thereby producing a false-positive result in a normal knee. For a more specific test, flex the knee 30° and place the thumb on the lateral side of the patella. Medially directed pressure that pushes the patella into the patella groove, which is innocuous in the normal knee, reproduces the symptoms of chondromalacia. As previously stated, the diagnosis of chondromalacia patellae should not be made unless there is definite retropatellar crepitation and facet tenderness.

The treatment for chondromalacia patellae follows the same principles as those described for runner's knee. Foot orthotic devices are prescribed to prevent excessive subtalar joint pronation. If the patient is a runner, he is advised to avoid cambered roads and downhill running because cambered roads cause excessive ankle pronation in the uppermost leg and running downhill increases the forces exerted between the patella and the femur, possibly adding discomfort.

Inflexibility in the hamstrings is another factor that adds to patellofemoral contact. Tight posterior calf muscles increase subtalar joint pronation, particularly running downhill, which requires greater ankle dorsiflexion. Therefore, a carefully prescribed program of calf and hamstring stretching exercises is an important therapeutic adjuvant. Medication in the form of aspirin or, in more severe cases, phenylbutazone may also be prescribed. Aspirin inhibits the enzyme cathepsin and has been shown to arrest cartilage degradation.[37]

DeHaven and his colleagues have described a four-stage approach to the rehabilitation of athletes suffering from chondromalacia patellae.[9] In phase 1, symptomatic control is gained by reducing all activities even to the point of using crutches. Salicylates are given routinely in this phase. The second phase is a progressive exercise program using only isometric exercise for the quadriceps muscles but isotonic or isokinetic exercises for the hamstring and other muscles. Phase 3 begins when symptoms are controlled and the athlete is able to sustain an isometric contraction against a predetermined weight, calculated from the size of the athlete and the demands of his particular sport. In this phase the athlete begins a graduated straight-ahead running program. As the strength of his quadriceps increases, faster running is allowed until the prescribed goals are achieved, at which time cuts, hard stops and starts, jumps, and figures-of-eight are introduced. The fourth phase is a maintenance program of unrestricted activities and resistance exercises performed two or three days a week.

A recent therapeutic introduction for this condition is a knee brace similar to the counterforce brace used for the treatment of tennis elbow.[21] This brace incorporates an infrapatellar strap that displaces the patella superiorly and slightly anteriorly. When worn below the popliteal crease, it compresses the patellar tendon and alters the patellofemoral relationship without impeding patellar mobility. Interestingly, it was discovered by a physician who observed his tennis partner wearing a knee sleeve or elastic knee guard below the patella. In reply to the doctor's recommendation that the sleeve should be worn over rather than below the knee, the partner replied that when worn in that position, the sleeve actually worsened the pain. Whether this new infrapatellar brace will prove universally effective has yet to be established.

In patients with chondromalacia patellae, surgery is indicated when pain and disability persist in spite of prolonged treatment. In these patients a causal defect in alignment usually exists and requires correction. The procedures are described in Chapter 14.

At operation to realign the extensor mechanism, changes are sometimes seen in the articular cartilage of the patella, the deep levels of which may undergo changes in the ground substance and collagen and separation—the

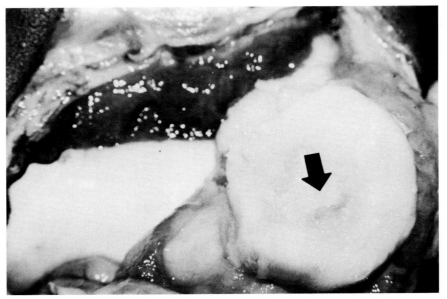

FIG. 24-1. Soft, fibrillated cartilage (*arrow*) behind the patella.

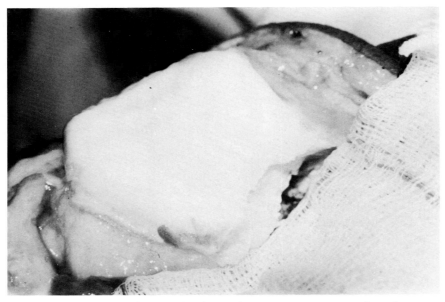

FIG. 24-2. Broad area of soft cartilage (Fig. 24-1) now shaved down to firmer cartilage.

so-called blister effect—though the cartilage surface itself may look smooth. These areas are not excised because they usually reconstitute after successful realignment of the knee extensor mechanism. In other cases the cartilage may have a soft, fissured, and fibrillated appearance. When this involves only a small area, excise the soft spots down to the subchondral bone, but for a larger area, shave down only to firmer cartilage (Figs. 24-1 and 24-2). Often only soft cartilage is found, in which case avoid deep shaving and remove only those pieces of cartilage that seem likely either to slough and irritate the synovium or to form loose bodies. The new alignment and the postoperative exercise program will reduce shearing forces on the patella, thereby allowing better nutrition to reconstitute firm cartilage. If there are small facets that are badly osteoarthritic and painful, consider local facetectomy because full function usually recovers after this small procedure. However, even if the patella is severely involved, facet resection is preferable to removal of the entire patella, because patellectomy leaves the extensor mechanism at a functional disadvantage. Total replacement of the patellar surface by high-density polyethylene material has not yet been applied to the treatment of chondromalacia in athletes.

JUMPER'S KNEE

Jumper's knee is the eponym used to describe patellar or quadriceps tendinitis. Typical symptoms occur after jumping, kicking, climbing, or running and consist of discomfort, tenderness, or pain either in the patellar tendon or at the superior or inferior poles of the patella. This discomfort may commence after a single jump but more commonly only after repetitive activity.

Traction or overload leads to focal degeneration of the tendon with fraying of fibers near its patellar attachment. There are four phases of jumper's knee. In phase 1, pain appears only after activity and without undue functional impairment. In the second phase pain lasts during and after the activity, but performance is still at a satisfactory level. In phase 3 pain comes on during and is prolonged after the activity. The athlete can no longer perform at his accustomed level. There is point tenderness near the patella and pain on extension of the knee against resistance. If heavy stress is applied during this period the soreness may presage rupture of the extensor mechanism, which is the fourth stage of the injury.

Occasionally there may be localized swelling over the patellar tendon insertion. Although x-ray films are usually normal, at times they reveal a lucency at the inferior pole of the patella or prolongation of the inferior patellar pole. An avulsion fracture or other irregularity in the inferior pole may be noted, as may the presence of calcium within the patellar tendon.

The pathology of jumper's knee includes focal tendon degeneration with fraying of fibers near its patellar attachment. This is not a benign, self-limiting condition because some continuity of fibers is lost, leading to development of a mucoid degeneration, fibrinoid necrosis, and scarred nodules.

Blazina and colleagues[5] believe that there may be three mechanisms contributing to jumper's knee—traction overload, circumscribed circulatory impairment similar to that causing supraspinatus tendinitis or biceps tendon ischemia in swimmers, and an aberrant immunologic or metabolic response to injury. Others[13,16] feel that prolonged subtalar joint pronation of the type believed to cause runner's knee is also a factor in jumper's knee.

Treatment of jumper's knee includes immersion before exercise in a warm whirlpool or treatment with warm packs. After exercise ice massage, an ice towel, or an ice whirlpool is used on the tender area. Attention should also be given to any anatomical abnormalities. If an anti-inflammatory drug is given, knee extension against resistance should be prohibited because of the risk of tendon rupture. Although local steroid injections reduce inflammation and pain, they may be dangerous because they tend to cause further degeneration. They should be used only with the informed consent of the injured athlete. Steroid injections may also mask symptoms, thereby leading to continued overuse and potentiating complete rupture of the tendon.[15] In phase 3 the athlete must rest his knee for a prolonged period and consider either giving up his sport or submitting to surgery. The treatment of phase 4 (complete tendon rupture) is, of course, surgery.

Surgery for jumper's knee is often curative.[38] Granulation tissue, when present in a hole in the distal pole of the patella, is removed. This deposit of damaged, degenerated tissue is similar to that found in the extensor carpi radialis brevis in "tennis elbow" or in the Achilles tendon of runners with chronic Achilles tendinitis. This material is scraped out through a longitudinal tendon slit that does not otherwise disrupt the tendon. The precise tender spot can be located more easily under local anesthesia, but general anesthesia is usually preferred.

PATELLAR TENDON RUPTURE

As mentioned in the previous section, quadriceps or patellar tendon soreness sometimes precedes a complete tendon rupture in which the patellar tendon is pulled from its origin at the inferior pole of the patella. Only rarely does the tendon rupture in its midportion.

In complete tendon rupture, operate early to allow anatomical repair before the tissues swell and weaken. Freshen the distal pole of the patella and reattach the tendon through drill holes. When the rupture is old and some tissue scarring has occurred, place a pin through the tibia, attach a wire to the pin, and loop it around the patella. This prevents separation of the anastomosis.

Postsurgical rehabilitation demands great skill because most sportsmen who develop these injuries are involved in activities in which deep knee flexion is of the utmost importance and they must regain full flexion.

Because patellar tendon rupture is associated with prolonged rehabilitation and the risk of never again reaching peak performance, prevention of these injuries is vitally important. Athletes should be encouraged to stretch the quadriceps muscles adequately. Furthermore, heavy training should be avoided whenever patellar tendon pain is being treated with anti-inflammatory drugs.

TRAUMATIC TIBIAL EPIPHYSITIS (OSGOOD-SCHLATTER'S SYNDROME)

Pain at the tibial tubercle and the development of a "knee knob" is noted in many youngsters active in athletics. The diagnosis of tibial epiphysitis can be made if localized tenderness is elicited by pressure over the tibial tubercle and if pain is produced when the knee is extended against resistance.

Tibial epiphysitis is a traction epiphysitis that results when the powerful quadriceps complex that inserts into a small area of tibial tubercle exerts a contraction sufficiently powerful to cause tubercle avulsion and separation in an area of developing bone formation.

Mital has described the four stages of change that occur in the proximal tibial epiphysis during adolescence.[31] The initial cartilage stage is followed by the apophyseal stage, during which ossification centers form within Henke's disk, a cartilage plate projecting downward in front of the tibia. This is followed by the third or epiphyseal stage, during which these ossification centers fuse to the rest of the epiphysis. Stage 4 refers to closure of the growth plate. Because all of these stages occur during adolescent development, disruption of the epiphysis usually occurs between the ages of 8 and 13 years in girls and between 10 and 15 years in boys. In the past, the injury has been more common in boys than in girls, but as more girls participate in sports, the incidence of this injury will increase in girls.

In the athlete with tibial epiphysitis, the x-ray picture depends on the developmental stage of the epiphysis. The best radiologic view is achieved with the knee rotated slightly inward so that a true lateral view of the tubercle is obtained. In the early stages of tubercle development, there may be no apparent radiologic changes other than swelling. Sometimes a separate fragment may be seen a few weeks after injury. During the apophyseal or epiphyseal stage, small or large avulsed fragments may be apparent; if so, it is important to compare the two knees because the nonsymptomatic epiphysis may look equally disrupted. Occasionally the epiphysis with the worst radiologic appearance may be totally asymptomatic. Therefore, the radiologic findings should not be the main criterion for either diagnosis or treatment. Their importance lies in excluding other more serious conditions such as osteomyelitis, arteriovenous malformations, and osteosarcoma, which may cause pain, tenderness, and swelling in this area.[8]

Tibial epiphysitis is a self-limited condition that resolves spontaneously with closure of the proximal tibial epiphyseal plate. Therefore, conservative treatment of this condition is advised. Reduced athletic activity encourages healing, and, as soon as the soreness abates, a quadriceps stretching program should begin. Many adolescents have extremely inflexible quadriceps muscles, so that quadriceps stretching should be part of all preliminary warm-ups in adolescent games, training, and contests. Steroid injections are unnecessary because of the natural history of the condition and should be avoided because of the dangers previously described. An avulsed piece of bone noted either radiologically or on palpation can be removed. It is possible to remove a portion of the tubercle at surgery without adversely affecting the quadriceps mechanism.

Occasionally, tibial tubercle fractures may follow a traumatic tibial epiphysitis. These fractures occur when a kick is interrupted in striking an opponent or when the cleats catch, both resulting in sudden overpull on the tendon insertion. Watson-Jones classified three injury types.[42] The first is an avulsion of a piece of the tubercle, which may then be pulled up to the level of the joint. The second is an epiphyseal fracture in which the tubercle is hinged upward but has not entered the knee joint. Type 3 is a progression of the type 2 fracture that has extended into the knee joint or has been displaced proximal to the tibia. When a tibial tubercle fracture occurs during the cartilage stage, the only radiologic sign of the condition may be patella alta. In this condition the radiolucent cartilage lies at knee joint level, blocking extension of the knee. In type 3 fractures, reattachment of the displaced piece is required.

Consider the possibility of a stress fracture of the tibial tubercle when a youngster has pain and swelling about the proximal tibia. Such stress fractures of the proximal tibial epiphysis have been mistaken for malignancies.[8]

QUADRICEPS TENDON RUPTURE

Rupture through the substance of the quadriceps tendon or avulsion of a portion of the proximal patella by the quadriceps is often preceded by a prodromal period of soreness. This soreness persists for days and follows any unaccustomed heavy activity. The injury is most often encountered in older athletes with degenerated tendons. It may also follow steroid injections into the tendon or the use of anti-inflammatory drugs.[4,15]

The mechanism of quadriceps tendon rupture is usually an abnormal stress produced by an eccentric quadriceps contraction as the athlete inadvertently slips into forced flexion while attempting vigorously to extend the knee. A good example is the tennis player who reflexly attempts to extend his knee while slipping on a sandy, unswept court. The rupture usually occurs when the knee is at about 90° of flexion, at which angle the force on the extensor mechanism is immense. Quadriceps tendon rupture has also been reported in weightlifters during splits with marked knee flexion.[12,19]

On clinical examination, a gap is felt above the patella, and the patient is unable to extend the knee actively. Lateral radiographs show a low patella with sometimes a fragment of bone avulsed from the superior pole.

For immediate treatment, the knee should be wrapped in a compression bandage, and the patient should be allowed to walk only on crutches. In most instances prompt surgery is advised, during which the tendon is reattached by suture to the patella through drill holes. If there is a large fragment this is replaced and sutured along with the tendon. A small fragment may, however, be excised before the tendon is repaired. In recurrent or old quadriceps tendon ruptures, it may be necessary to reflect some proximal tendon and incorporate this into the repair.

After surgery a *careful* rehabilitation program must be instituted to restore full knee flexion without endangering the repair. This is especially important in collegiate football players, wrestlers, rodeo steer wrestlers, and hockey defensemen who must frequently drop their knees into acute flexion.

An effective method for restoring quadriceps flexibility is the contraction-relaxation method, in which the quadriceps is contracted against resistance, then relaxed and further flexed by passive stretch.

In most athletes who are involved in explosive sports (springing, football, weightlifting, and so on), the quadriceps are overdeveloped and not stretched as frequently nor as adequately as the hamstrings. To avoid injury, this inflexibility should be rectified with an adequate stretching program, particularly in the prodromal phase of tendon soreness, when the levels of activity should also be reduced. Individuals on anti-inflammatory drugs should probably not participate in strenuous training or competition during this phase, and steroid injections should be avoided.

SUBLUXATION OF THE PATELLA

In the past it has been thought that lateral dislocation of the kneecap out of the femoral groove occurs only in women. It is now known that male athletes also develop subluxation of the patella due either to weakness or to malalignment of the knee extensor mechanism.[14] These injuries are more likely to occur when there is a valgus force at the knee, as in the "cutting" maneuver in football. It should be noted that unnecessary meniscectomies have been performed when the diagnosis of recurrent patellar subluxation has been missed.

Although a valgus force at the knee is the common mechanism, a number of factors predispose to patellar subluxation (see also Chapter 22). These include the larger pelvis of the female, anteversion of the hips, external rotation of the leg, a shallow or short femoral groove or flat patella, and knee recurvatum from ligamentous laxity.

Q angles of more than 15° increase the propensity to subluxation. However, an increased Q angle is not diagnostic of patellar subluxation, since many Q angles of more than 20° are not associated with this condition. In men the higher lateral condyle, a deeper intercondylar groove, and the wedge-shaped patella tend to prevent lateral subluxation. However, hard cuts may overcome these protections, especially if the quadriceps is weak and the pes anserinus does not give support during internal rotation.

The symptoms of a repeatedly subluxing patella include catching, giving way, and medial knee pain resembling a medial meniscal lesion. Catching occurs when the patella pops back into the groove as the knee begins to extend from a flexed position. Tugging on and tearing of the medial capsular structures as the kneecap slides laterally produces the medial knee pain.

On clinical examination it may be noted that in the sitting position the subluxing patellae sometimes point laterally like grasshopper eyes. Such patellae are generally more mobile and sometimes lie higher than is normal.

A number of radiographic methods are available to identify patella alta, the abnormally high-lying patella.[14,29] In one method the knee is bent to 90° and the patella's location is noted. If a horizontal line parallel to the anterior surface of the femoral shaft passes across rather than above the patella, patella alta exists. A high patella lies proximal to the femoral groove and tends to slide to the side more easily. The intercondylar sulcus skyline radiographic view shows the depth of the femoral groove and the patellar shape and also reveals patellar tilt (Fig. 24-3). A tangential view of the knee flexed to 30° should also be included because this is the angle of bend at which subluxation is most likely to occur. In another approach, the knee is bent with the patient in the prone position, and a tangential radiographic view is taken from the foot area.

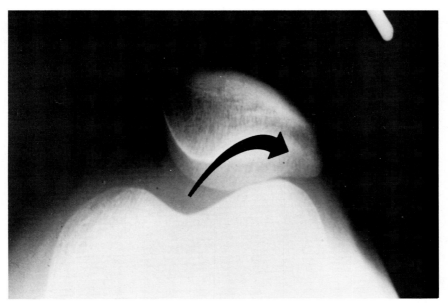

FIG. 24-3. Skyline view shows patellar tilt.

This technique is less satisfactory because it jams the patella into the patellar groove.

ACUTE DISLOCATION OF THE PATELLA

During a sidestep cut or when swinging a baseball bat, quadriceps contraction plus valgus and rotation stress at the knee can produce patellar dislocation. The diagnosis is readily apparent because in acute lateral patellar dislocation the knee is locked in flexion and the patella is displaced laterally.

The immediate treatment is flexion of the hip to relax the quadriceps; the knee is then extended to effect a gentle reduction, thereby reducing the danger of either bone chipping or articular cartilage damage. Because dislocation or reduction may cause chipping of a piece of lateral femoral condyle or a facet of the medial patella, it is imperative to perform radiographs immediately after reduction.

The treatment of choice is immediate operative reapproximation of the capsular structures to reduce future laxity without prolonging the recovery period. Bony damage such as lateral buttress or articular fragment frac-tures should be repaired with pins or small screws. After surgery the knee should be put in a plaster cast for 5 weeks. If treatment is nonoperative, the joint is aspirated to prevent any swelling that may cause further ligamentous laxity. As with operative treatment, the knee is placed in a plaster cast for 5 weeks.

In patients with recurrent dislocation, the "panic sign" or "apprehension sign" may be elicited (Fig. 24-4). When the patella is pressed laterally the athlete becomes apprehensive as he senses imminent redislocation. Recurrent dislocation is an indication for one of the knee reconstructive procedures discussed in Chapter 22.

QUADRICEPS MECHANISM INSTABILITY

For problems caused by instability of the knee extensor mechanism, the treatment options range from exercise and bracing to surgical reconstruction. Adolescent instability often disappears as bones mature because a steeper sulcus angle and improved patellar shape evolve with growth. Therefore, youth is an indication for conservative treatment. The exer-

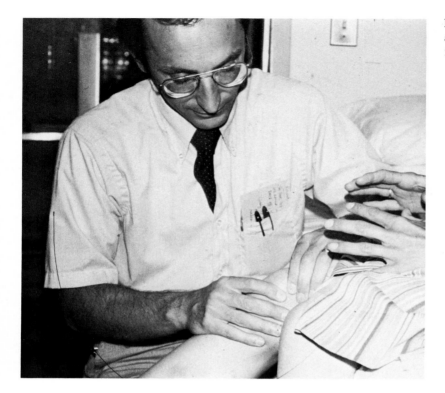

FIG. 24-4. Athlete becomes apprehensive as she senses imminent redislocation.

cise program is designed to strengthen and balance the quadriceps and hamstrings and to stretch the major muscle groups. The oblique vastus medialis must be strengthened because it acts to stabilize the patella in its groove.[23]

Bracing procedures may be tried in persons with knee recurvatum, a condition in which the buttressing action of the lateral femoral condyle is reduced. A felt "horseshoe" pad provides an external buttress (Fig. 24-5). Because the pad may slide in an elastic bandage, a knee sleeve containing a felt horseshoe is preferable (Fig. 24-6).

Examination of the feet is important in evaluating any extensor mechanism problem. Excessive subtalar joint pronation during the stance phase of running allows horizontal shift of the patella. Orthotics inserted into the sports shoe reduce the pronation and diminish valgus knee stress and horizontal patellar translation. These lightweight orthotic devices supplement the treatment program for patellar subluxation.

Should painful subluxation recur unduly, a surgical approach is indicated. The lateral patellofemoral ligament and the patellotibial ligament tether the patella laterally. Their release, combined with a strengthening and stretching program, results in improved patellar stability. No matter how much the quadriceps are strengthened, the lateral tethering ligaments always limit the position the kneecap can assume in the groove. After lateral ligament release, the patella will relax into the groove.

For gross malalignment of the extensor mechanism or ineffective lateral release, a more formal medial reconstruction is performed. A number of these reconstructive procedures are described in Chapter 22. Each has had its measure of success in vigorous athletes. A combination designed by McCue (Fig.

24-7) and labeled the "fix-it" operation includes a lateral release, examination of the joint interior, vastus medialis advancement, medial reefing, and, importantly, a pes anserinus transfer into the medial side of the patellar tendon. A procedure on the dynamic knee mechanisms must be meticulous. A vastus medialis transferred too far laterally may produce chondromalacia, whereas if the insertion is placed too far distally, the patella may rotate. For sportsmen requiring agile cutting ability, the pes anserinus transfer affords special benefit by adding to rotational stability. When the muscles inserting into the pes anserinus have been retrained either isometrically or with a pes strap or on a pes board, the internal rotation of the tibia during these cuts reduces the Q angle and diminishes the risk of lateral subluxation.

For the 5 weeks during which the leg is in a plaster cast after a lateral release or a medial reconstruction, the athlete builds his upper body strength and, with the good leg clipped on to an exercycle, maintains cardiovascular and muscular endurance through one-legged cycling. The complete rehabilitation program is described at the end of this chapter.

PREPATELLAR BURSITIS

Any acute knee injury, such as a blow from a lacrosse stick, or repetitive trauma, such as that caused by rubbing the knee on the mat in collegiate or freestyle wrestling or surfing with the old-style longer boards, may cause prepatellar bursitis (Fig. 24-8). Playing surfaces made of artificial turf also increase the incidence of this condition.

Puffiness or swelling in the prepatellar bursa usually does not affect motion, except for slight limitation of flexion as the skin becomes tense over the tender, swollen bursa. An abrasion with cellulitis may be difficult to differentiate from an abrasion over a reddened, inflamed prepatellar bursa. But this distinction is critical because needle aspiration in the presence of cellulitis may introduce an infection.

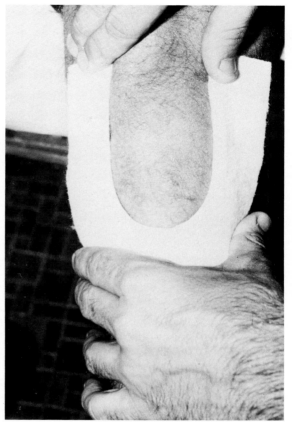

FIG. 24-5. Felt horseshoe pad provides an external buttress.

To prevent this condition in sports such as wrestling, protective kneepads should be worn that are large enough to cover the entire knee. The most commonly used pad is a flat piece of Ensolite that fits into the front knee pocket of the pants. In basketball, an elastic knee sleeve with an Ensolite inset may be used. Proper leg length and waist size of pants are important, and they should be tight enough to prevent the pads from sliding.[20] Athletes often choose pants of the new stretch materials that are too tight and too short. Hence, the patellar area is exposed and may be subject to bruising. When the kneepads ride over the knee, the pants become too tight in the popliteal region, so athletes cut the pants, further compromising the protective effective-

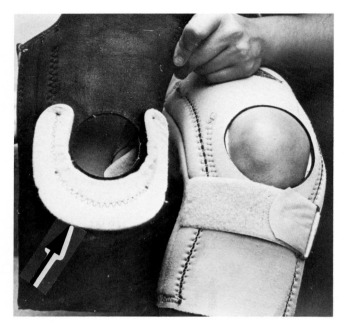

FIG. 24-6. Knee sleeve containing a felt horse-shoe pad (*arrow*).

ness of the kneepads. Kneepads are, of course, especially important in tackle football, where forces on the knee are increased, particularly by the weight of other players landing on top of the tackled athlete. Skateboard enthusiasts should also wear kneepads as protection from contact with cement (Fig. 24-9).

BIPARTITE PATELLA

Bipartite patella is a condition in which there are two ossification centers in the patella. The accessory ossification center usually appears radiologically in the superolateral segment of the patella as viewed anteroposteriorly and is bordered by a lucent line consisting of fibrocartilage (Fig. 24-10). Additional ossification centers may be lateral or distal, but the majority are superolateral. The incidence of bipartite patella is some 3%, and in about 40% of these cases the condition is bilateral.

Bipartite patella can cause knee pain, the onset of which may be gradual or may follow injury.[43] Kneeling induces pain, and there may also be catching during movements. The area of secondary ossification is tender to palpation, and the diagnosis is confirmed by the typical radiologic features described above.

The quadriceps is attached to the separate fragment, which may show malacic or arthritic changes and may possibly cause abnormal patellar movement. An unsound synchondrosis of a bipartite patella can follow injury, and this condition is difficult to distinguish radiologically from a patellar fracture. If the condition is bilateral or if the pain is recurrent, resection of the tender segment should be considered.

INJURIES TO THE MEDIAL SIDE OF THE KNEE

MEDIAL COLLATERAL LIGAMENT SPRAINS

Mild and moderate medial collateral ligament sprains follow sidestep cuts or occur when the knee is struck from the lateral side. They occur most commonly, but not exclusively, in contact sports.

A grade I medial collateral ligament sprain is defined as tears of microscopic fibers that do not produce gross ligamentous laxity. This is the most common injury in downhill skiing and occurs when the inside edge of the ski catches, leaving the trailing leg externally ro-then isotonic exercises and functional activities follow in sequence.

A grade II sprain is diagnosed when there is disruption and loss of ligament integrity. The damaged ligament lengthens enough to allow moderate instability, with 5° to 15° more lateral movement in the injured knee than in the sound knee. A grade II tear may be differentiated from a complete or grade III tear when, with the knee flexed to 20°, there is no endpoint resistance to extreme valgus stress. Alternatively, if there is resistance, it is "mushy" and not well defined.

Before any treatment commences, a firm diagnosis of the structures involved and the extent of the sprain must be determined. If necessary, this should include examination under general anesthesia.

The treatment of grade II injuries has been influenced by the finding that wearing a plas-

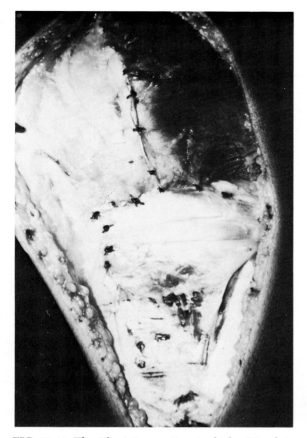

FIG. 24-7. The "fix-it" operation includes (1) a lateral release, (2) examination of the joint interior, (3) vastus medialis obliquus advancement, (4) medial capsular reefing, and (5) pes anserinus transfer into the medial side of the patellar tendon.

tated with the knee in valgus. The skier's momentum carries his body forward, increasing the stress on the medial knee structures.[26]

Examination reveals local tenderness and swelling with pain but no evidence of ligamentous instability when stressing the knee at 10° of flexion.[11] It should be noted that if guarding prevents an adequate assessment of ligamentous stability, examination should be repeated under anesthesia, general or local.

The treatment of grade I collateral ligament sprain consists in compression to reduce swelling followed by ice massage, an ice towel, or an iced whirlpool. Isometric exercises and

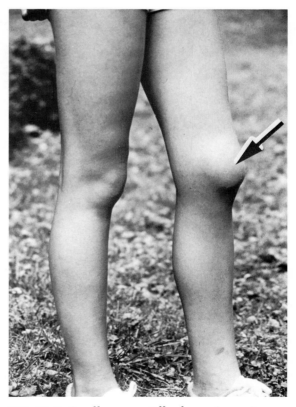

FIG. 24-8. Swollen prepatellar bursa (*arrow*).

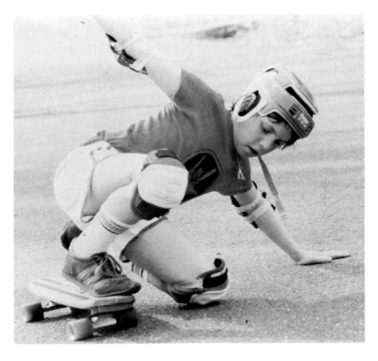

FIG. 24-9. Skateboarder wearing protective kneepads.

ter cast causes a dramatic deterioration in muscle function. Thus Tipton and co-workers found that the strength of intact or repaired medial collateral ligaments in dogs is influenced by the amount of exercise performed by the animal after injury.[41] The least strength was found in dogs whose knees were immobilized, whereas fiber bundles of larger diameter with significantly higher collagen content were formed in collateral ligaments of exercised dogs. Immobilization also led to significant weakening of ligaments in monkeys. Strength did not return to normal even after 20 weeks of resumed activity. Other studies have shown that rigid immobilization of the knee causes type I oxidative (endurance) muscle fibers to undergo significant reductions in their oxidative (endurance) potential but that a dynamic knee brace or a program of cycling prevents much of this weakening.[6,7] In view of these experimental findings, many grade II sprains are now treated by graded exercises rather than by cast immobilization.[10]

To accelerate recovery, Bergfeld and associates have outlined a functional approach.[3]

Based on the severity of the injury, grade II sprains are divided into two groups. After a day in a soft cast, the less severe injuries are placed in knee immobilizers while the more severely injured are fitted with lightweight hinged casts. Isometric exercises are begun in both groups. The knee immobilizers are removed three or four times a day to allow gentle flexion-extension movements, whereas those in hinged casts perform active movements. On the third or fourth day free isometric exercises advance to resisted isometrics and the patient uses one crutch in the hand opposite the injured knee. By the fifth to seventh day this crutch is discarded, and the patient concentrates on walking without a limp with heel-first weight-bearing. One week after injury, the knee is placed in a changing-axis brace, and, if the patient has no pain and the knee is not swollen, a program of isotonic exercises is prescribed. Once maximum isotonic contractions and pain-free motion is achieved, the athlete is advanced to isokinetic exercises on the appropriate apparatus.

Collateral ligament taping or a changing-axis knee brace, such as the Helfet helicoid brace (see Chapter 5), protects the knee during the rehabilitation program, lends added support to the knee, and accelerates return to practice and competition. This brace allows full movement in the normal range and restricts only abnormal deviations, thereby maintaining stability. The brace was devised to avoid the restrictions of mobility, speed, and performance caused by more cumbersome braces. It is a useful protective device for patients convalescing from injury when re-entering both contact and noncontact sports. It allows the normal muscles of the knee to control knee movements, which therefore remain in the normal pattern and are stable in any position of flexion and extension (see Chapter 5).

If taping is used, it should allow the patella to move freely and leave the popliteal fossa unencumbered.

BREAST STROKER'S KNEE

Ninety percent of competitive swimmers have symptoms in either the shoulder, knee, calf, or foot.[17] An important etiological factor in breast stroker's knee injury is the whip-kick. The kick causes a marked increase in tibial collateral ligament tension as the knee moves from flexion to extension, and this is accentuated by the valgus stress and external rotation of the tibia. The swimmer may have to use a flutter kick for a while until the knee soreness abates.

Ideally, breast stroke swimmers should have a few months of rest each year, when the knee is not subjected to these abnormal stresses. Happily, the number of swimming injuries has fallen significantly since the institution of complete and well-designed exercise and flexibility programs.

PES ANSERINE BURSITIS

The pes anserinus, or goose's foot, is the combined insertion of the sartorius, gracilis, and semitendinosus tendons in a row down the proximal anteromedial border of the tibia (Fig. 24-11). Although an aponeurotic connection exists between these tendons, they also

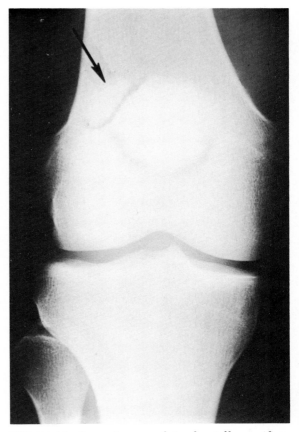

FIG. 24-10. Separate superolateral patellar ossification center (*arrow*).

operate individually in producing both knee flexion and internal rotation of the leg. The underlying tibial collateral ligament is separated from the pes anserinus by the pes bursa, which may itself sometimes become inflamed, causing a pes anserine bursitis. The signs of this condition are tenderness and swelling over the bursa.

The condition usually responds to local measures, including occasionally the injection of an aqueous steroid solution into the bursa. Compensation for any lower limb biomechanical abnormalities by a foot orthotic device may be required if the condition recurs.

A condition that may be difficult to distinguish from pes anserine bursitis results when prolonged ankle pronation causes repetitive contact between the medial gastrocnemius

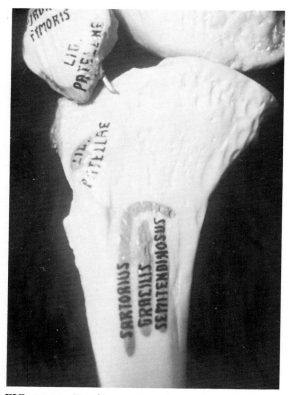

FIG. 24-11. Tendinous insertions of sartorius, gracilis, and semitendinosus into the tibia comprise the pes anserinus.

and the pes anserinus. The symptoms are similar to those of a pes anserine bursitis except that on palpation the tenderness is maximal between the tendon and the gastrocnemius, not over the bursa. For successful treatment, a foot orthotic device is necessary to prevent repetitive contact between these two structures.

HOFFA'S DISEASE—INFLAMMATION OF THE PATELLAR FAT PAD

Point tenderness over the anteromedial or anterolateral joint line without signs of a meniscal tear may be due to inflammation of the patellar fat pad (Hoffa's disease). Local therapies such as ice, aspirin, phenylbutazone, and even extra-articular injection with steroids about the fat pad should be tried. Arthroscopy may be needed to exclude the presence of a meniscal injury. On examination the tender puffy fat pad lies behind and bulges on each or one side of the patellar tendon.

INJURIES TO THE LATERAL SIDE OF THE KNEE

THE ILIOTIBIAL BAND FRICTION SYNDROME

This condition, which occurs almost exclusively in long-distance runners was first described by Nilsson and Staff.[33] The symptoms are characteristic. After a period of intensive hill or unaccustomed long-distance running, discomfort develops on the lateral aspect of the knee, particularly when running downhill. Symptoms usually progress rapidly, so that if training is continued the pain may become so excruciating that the athlete is unable to continue. A characteristic feature is the rapidity with which the pain disappears when walking or at rest; this is equalled only by the rapidity with which the pain recurs during exercise.

The symptoms that distinguish this condition from peripatellar knee pain in runners are the lateral location and the severity of the pain, the rapidity with which the symptoms occur during and regress after running, and the absence of the movie sign.[34]

The etiology of the iliotibial band friction syndrome is recurrent overriding of the prominent lateral epicondyle by the iliotibial band. This band, an extension of the fascia lata, inserts into the tibial tubercle of Gerdy. When the knee is extended the band lies anterior to the axis of knee flexion, but in flexion it passes posteriorly, crossing the lateral femoral epicondyle. For reasons that are unclear, in some runners this movement, when repeated sufficiently frequently over long distances, particularly when associated with the added strain of downhill running, produces an inflammatory response between the two structures.

On clinical examination the lateral femoral epicondyle is tender, and in advanced cases, when the knee is alternately flexed and extended, a creaking occurs that resembles the rubbing of a finger over a wet balloon. The specific diagnostic test is to apply thumb pressure over the lateral epicondyle with the knee in flexion. As the knee is extended and the posterior fibers of the iliotibial band cross over the epicondyle beneath the thumb, the pain is accurately reproduced.

Anatomical features frequently associated with the iliotibial band are genu varum, the cavus foot with a narrow range of subtalar joint movement, calcaneal varus, and forefoot valgus. In these conditions, the lower limb is unable to absorb the stresses generated during the stance phase of running, and these are therefore transmitted to the lateral aspect of the knee. Downhill running increases these stresses, whereas on a crowned road running causes jamming of the leg on the lower side and also increases lateral knee strain, particularly in the presence of the anatomical abnormalities described above.

Treatment includes attention to all factors that reduce the stress-absorbing capacity of the lower limb. Running shoes that provide maximum cushioning at the heel and forefoot should be used, and the flare on the shoe heel should be filed off on both its medial and lateral aspects. Running shoes with rigid heel counters and foot orthotic devices are usually contraindicated because most runners with this injury require more, not less, subtalar joint movement. Prescription of the Tules heel cup, which helps to dissipate the stress at heel strike, has been advocated by some authors.[18] The athlete is shown how to stretch the iliotibial band and is advised to do so for up to 20 min a day. He should initially run only on soft surfaces and avoid downhill running or running on roads that are excessively cambered. His training load should not cause him marked knee discomfort. Aspirin or phenylbutazone may be prescribed.

Local treatment for the injury includes regular ice treatment, physiotherapy, and hydrocortisone injections. In their initial study Nilsson and Staff reported that physiotherapy was less effective therapeutically than local hydrocortisone injection into the tender area.[33] An important practical point regarding cortisone injections is that the local area of tenderness is usually best defined immediately after the athlete has been running. Therefore, if it is de-

cided that an injection is required, a run to the point of pain should be made immediately before the injection, which should be followed by rest for 2 to 3 days before recommencing running. It must be emphasized that injection therapy is less likely to be effective if the athlete is not also advised about his running shoes, stretching needs, and choice of running surfaces.

POPLITEUS TENOSYNOVITIS

Pain at the lateral side of the kneecap can also be due to tenosynovitis of the popliteal tendon. Whereas the iliotibial band friction syndrome is initiated by uphill running, popliteus tenosynovitis starts with downhill work. This condition is common among backpackers who develop lateral knee pain and a "crunching" sound while descending from mountains.

The popliteus arises from the lateral femoral condyle as a pencil-sized, synovium-ensheathed tendon that passes deep to the fibular collateral ligament in a recess separating the lateral meniscus from the ligament. The tendon then has attachment to the lateral meniscus and the fibula, forming a conjoined tendon whose muscle belly inserts on the tibia.

The popliteus assists the posterior cruciate in retarding forward displacement of the femur on the relatively fixed tibia during stance phase, especially during downhill running.[25] By aiding and maintaining internal rotation of the tibia on the femur shortly before heel strike and for three-quarters of the stance phase, the popliteus prevents the lateral femoral condyle from rotating off the tibial plateau. The popliteus also retracts the posterior arch of the lateral meniscus.

Popliteus tenosynovitis causes soreness on the lateral aspect of the knee while weightbearing with the knee flexed to 30°. Pain is felt and may be accompanied by a crunching sound in sidestep cuts with the femur internally rotated. Rising from a crosslegged sitting position also elicits pain. In this position the fibular collateral ligament is prominent, and the popliteus may be palpated just anterior to the ligament.[27]

Popliteus tenosynovitis requires differentiation from lateral meniscal tears. Athletes with popliteus tenosynovitis usually do not report acute trauma, giving way, or locking. Tenderness is present just anterior to the fibular collateral ligament and superior to the joint, and often the peculiar crunching sound is heard.

Oral nonsteroidal anti-inflammatory drugs or local steroid injections in the bursa or about the tendon diminish inflammation. If the individual must run on hills, he should run up and ride down. Outward rotation of the foot in the stance phase alleviates some discomfort, as does a change to running on the other side of the road.

INJURIES TO THE BACK OF THE KNEE

ACUTE AND CHRONIC GASTROCNEMIUS STRAINS

Gastrocnemius muscle strains may produce knee pain that is usually localized to the posterior aspect of the knee. The acute gastrocnemius muscle tear frequently referred to as "tennis leg" has been well described and is usually easily recognized.[30] The injury is an acute one that occurs on excessive exercise in the middle-aged—for example, a vigorous game of tennis when unfit. The patient feels gastrocnemius pain, and the muscle is swollen and very tender at the attachment of the muscle fibers to the tendinous expansion.

Chronic gastrocnemius muscle strains that occur almost exclusively in runners and joggers are often overlooked. Symptoms are seldom acute, and the athlete usually presents with a history of one or more months of ill-defined, lower-limb discomfort but without real pain. The discomfort disappears rapidly with rest but typically recurs after running a predictable distance. Fast or uphill running usually produces more severe symptoms that come on more quickly than usual. Often the athlete can "run through" the discomfort and will usually seek medical advice only when he notices changes in his running pattern, usually a reduction in stride length or a feel-

ing of weak ankle "push off" on the affected side. Both these symptoms presumably result from protective spasm in the injured muscle.

Two other features are strongly suggestive of this condition. First, prolonged rest has no therapeutic influence, so that, in contrast to most other running injuries that do improve with a period of rest, chronic muscle strains show absolutely no improvement regardless of the duration of rest. Second, the runner with this injury will usually notice that after sitting for a prolonged period in the evening after running, he has difficulty fully extending the knee immediately after standing. This "stiffness" soon wears off with walking.

The diagnosis of chronic gastrocnemius muscle strain is confirmed by palpating an exquisitely tender "knot" in the muscle, usually in the region of the medial head of the gastrocnemius. Although the exact pathology of this knot is unknown, it presumably represents a chronic, low-grade inflammatory response to repetitive microtrauma, with the production of an overabundant mass of connective scar tissue. But regardless of the true nature of this injury, empirically the only effective therapy is vigorous manual cross-frictions to the injured area. Only when the local tenderness to palpation disappears and the firm knot has been manually dispersed will the athlete again be completely pain-free.

Other etiologic features are a short leg on the injured side and inflexibility of the calf muscles, both of which should be rectified by the appropriate advice. If the condition is recurrent despite adequate attention to all these factors, a foot orthotic device should be prescribed based on the empirical finding that this injury may be helped by the control of excessive prolonged subtalar joint pronation.

HIP INJURIES PRESENTING AS KNEE PAIN

SLIPPED CAPITAL FEMORAL EPIPHYSIS

In the young athlete with a normal knee, pain may be due to a slipped capital femoral epiphysis, the pain being referred to the knee via the obturator nerve. Lanky or heavy athletes are most often affected.

The diagnosis may be confirmed by radiographic examination of the hips in the frog position, which will show minor capital femoral slips. When this condition is diagnosed the femur should be pinned to prevent a large and potentially disastrous slip. If an acute slip should occur during activity, careful skillful moving is essential because awkwardness may produce a major displacement of the head of the femur.

INTERNAL DERANGEMENTS

THE SWOLLEN KNEE

Athletes develop swollen knees even after trivial trauma. A blow to the suprapatellar region might result in overnight swelling of the knee to melon size. To protect against suprapatellar pouch bruises baseball catchers now wear shin guards with suprapatellar extensions.

[In the management of internal derangements of the knee in sportsmen, Dr. Kulund reinforces the advice given in depth elsewhere in this volume. Traumatic synovitis requires urgent treatment—urgent precise diagnosis, aspiration, treatment of swelling, and early and adequate measures for rehabilitation. Loose bodies must be removed, and osteochondral fractures should either be removed or reduced with stable fixation. Surgery, when required, should be gentle and atraumatic and include careful repair of damaged structures.]

EDITOR

LOOSE JOINTS OR TIGHT JOINTS

Whether the athlete has loose or tight joints may have a bearing on injuries. Nicholas studied looseness and tightness of joints in professional football players.[32] His tests included supination of the hand with shoulder rotation, flexion of the spine, assumption of the lotus position, hip rotation, and knee recurvatum. He discovered an increased likelihood of knee sprains in loose-jointed athletes, whereas there were more muscle tears in the tight-jointed.

After screening, specific exercises were designed to increase the strength of players with loose joints and the flexibility of players with tight joints. It seemed that flexibility screening might offer a way to reduce knee injuries in contact sports and high-velocity athletics.

However, other surgeons, after systematic flexibility testing, have found no correlation between the frequency of knee and ankle injuries and the looseness of high school players' joints.[11]

Perhaps high school players are different from professional tackle football players. For example, as high school athletes mature, loose joints become tighter, and many loose-jointed sophomores become tight-jointed seniors. When joint flexibility was studied in 2,817 West Point cadets, no statistical relationship was found between flexibility and joint injuries sustained in general athletic competition.[20] Also, no relationship was found between subjective laxity tests and objective biomechanical knee ligament examination. Because there is no correlation between ligament laxity and type of injury, it may be a disservice to restrict high school athletes from participation in sports on the basis of ligament laxity testing.

Psychological as well as physical attributes probably determine injury rates and severity. Jackson found that personality factors do correlate with injury rates and severity.[20] He used Cattell's 16 personality-factor questionnaire (16 PF). Factor A contrasts reserved, detached, critical, and cool individuals to out-going, warm-hearted, easy-going, and participating persons. The "cool" athletes sustained the most severe injuries. Factor 1 contrasts gentle, dependent, over-protective, sensitive athletes to tough-minded, self-reliant, and no-nonsense ones. The gentle athletes were found to be more likely to be injured. So this test may have the potential to predict tackle football injuries.

Be sure that each athlete has the essential fourfold fitness base of strength, flexibility, endurance, and proper free gymnastic warm-up. Flexibility and psychological studies notwithstanding, a strong and flexible athlete has

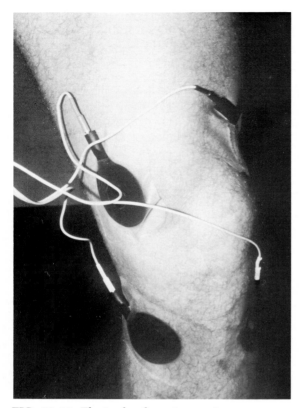

FIG. 24-12. Electrodes for a transcutaneous nerve stimulator placed around a painful knee.

a better chance of avoiding injury than a weaker and inflexible one.

THE POSTOPERATIVE KNEE EXERCISE PROGRAM

After knee operation, our goals are to restore muscular strength, power and endurance, flexibility, agility, and cardiovascular fitness. Toward these ends, therapeutic exercises are the most important modalities.[11]

Begin isometrics before the operation and reinstitute them in the recovery room to prevent dissociation of quadriceps function. Have the athlete initially perform 50% contractions for a few seconds and eventually advance to more forceful contractions to be held for 6 sec, 20 times an hour.

TRANSCUTANEOUS NERVE STIMULATOR

We have been able to reduce postoperative pain and soreness before, during, and after exercise by using transcutaneous nerve stimulators. The transcutaneous nerve stimulator (TNS) is a small, battery-powered device that produces a low-intensity electric current. Mild TNS currents stimulate large, fast, "A" touch or prick nerve fibers to close a "gate" in the substantia gelatinosa of the brain, blocking the burning pain signals transmitted by small "C" fibers. Perhaps TNS currents also induce the nervous system to release endorphins, which are endogenous, morphinelike painkillers.[39]

Place the electrodes over the site of pain or over the peripheral nerve serving the area (Fig. 24-12). Then attach the electrodes to the battery pack by a small cable. The athlete adjusts the electrical intensity, quality of sensation (pulse width), and repetition rate. He can leave the unit on for short periods or all day. Often, use of this device halves the need for postoperative analgesics.

STRAIGHT LEG RAISE

For active straight leg raising, the athlete places the sound leg under the ankle of the extremity operated upon. Using this technique, it is often possible to perform a straight leg raise independently on the day of the operation. Also, provide a sling to hold the leg up so that it can be lowered eccentrically with hip flexors. This lowering technique is usually easier than raising the leg and therefore allows more eccentric than concentric work to be performed.

WALKING

When a single leg lift is achieved, allow walking with two crutches. After 1 week, advance to a single crutch on the sound side for 2 or 3 more days. This aid is used until the athlete can walk unassisted without limping.

Never allow the athlete to limp. Even a minor limp results in a longer period of reha-

FIG. 24-13. "Scissor isometrics" exercise the quadriceps of the lower leg and hamstrings of the upper one.

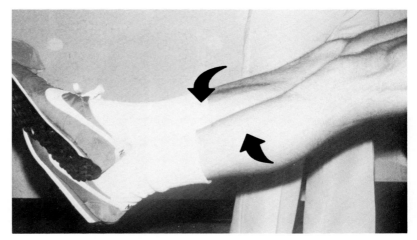

bilitation. When using the cane or single crutch, weight should be borne as much as possible with pressure on the hand grips to prevent a limp. The knee is kept straight and locked when walking, with concentration on heel strike rather than flat-footed walking with the knee bent. Also, ensure that a limp does not develop as a running program is reached. If limping occurs, activity is reduced.

Pillows under the knees are not permitted, and as soon as possible the knee is to be kept straight while reclining. For active hip extension, the sound foot is placed on the floor while the upper body is rested chest down on the training table. The hip is then extended on the operated side. Also, ankle flexion and extension and circles are repeated to provide a beneficial calf-pumping action.

ISOMETRICS

We use an isometric right-over-left and left-over-right method for early strengthening of the quadriceps and hamstrings. One leg is placed over the other in scissor fashion, and the legs are then contracted against each other (Fig. 24-13). Thus the hamstrings of the upper leg and the quadriceps of the lower leg contract. Hold the contraction for 6 sec and repeat 20 times. Then switch legs and repeat.

Since isometric strength gains are restricted to a small segment in the arc of motion, these contractions are performed at full extension, 45°, and 90° of knee flexion. Also abduct and then adduct the hips isometrically against hand resistance or a leather ball (Fig. 24-14). Isometrics provide some strength gains and serve as groundwork for advancing to isotonics.

Remove the sutures at 2 weeks. Then, when the knee is asymptomatic, is not significantly swollen, and has 90° of flexion, swimming pool work, isotonic weight-lifting, and stationary bicycle riding are commenced.

THE SWIMMING POOL

Underwater work serves as an early means of regaining both muscular strength and endurance.[36] The water reduces the effect of gravity, and the athlete is able to perform exercises without the pain that would be present without the buoyant properties of the water. Moreover, the pressure of the water helps return blood and lymph from the athlete's legs to his heart.

The athlete controls resistance in the water by altering his speed and the depth of the water and by goose-step walking first in water up to his armpits and then in shallow water. Hip abduction, flexion, and extension while holding onto the poolside are excellent conditioning exercises. Treading water is also a

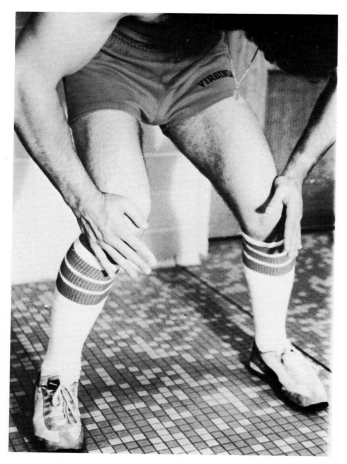

FIG. 24-14. Isometric abduction against hand resistance.

good exercise but is not used in early rehabilitation because the kicks might injure the knee.

ISOTONICS

Because isometrics build strength only at the angles used, isotonics are instituted to fill the gaps. Be sure to exercise the whole limb. For example, an isotonic hip flexion program strengthens the thigh muscles, as does work against a weight resting on or against a rubber tube held across the thigh. Ankle weights are avoided because they distract the knee, which normally functions in compression.

Begin the isotonic knee program by determining the athlete's maximum lift (ML). The ML is the maximum amount of weight that can be lifted once to full extension on the isotonic knee table. Repetitions start at 50% of the ML. This weight should be held at full extension for 3 sec each time, and the patient should try to increase to 10 repetitions (Fig. 24-15). When this goal is reached, add 1 or 2 more pounds. The hamstrings are exercised at 50% of the quadriceps working weight (25% of the quadriceps ML). The exercises are done slowly to prevent assistance from momentum. At first strength is gained from a daily workout. When strength gains peak, weight training is reduced to three sets of repetitions every other day.

As strength is gained on the isotonic program, power work can begin. Power is equal to force times velocity. If the knee table is used for power work, exercise is done three times a week with three sets of the maximum number of repetitions that can be accomplished with one-half of the RM in 30 sec. The

FIG. 24-15. Isotonic knee table work follows isometrics.

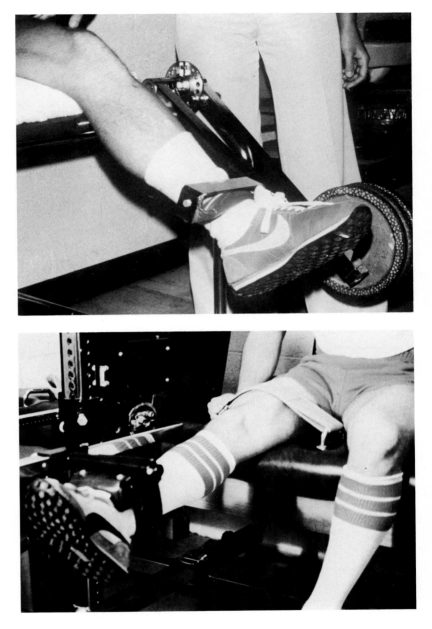

FIG. 24-16. Knee works rapidly against hydraulic isokinetic device to develop power.

exercises are performed as forcibly as possible using proper technique, and a rest of 20 sec between bouts is allowed.

ISOKINETICS

Isokinetic devices provide the best means for power rehabilitation because the knee can be exercised on them at fast speeds (Fig. 24-16).

We use isokinetic exercise for later rehabilitation. The advantages of isokinetic exercise include accommodation for fatigue or soreness, the ability to train at fast speeds, elimination of inertia and a read-out of peak torque, endurance, and total work.

However, early isokinetic exercise of weakened structures may produce edema and soreness and delay recovery if the athlete exerts

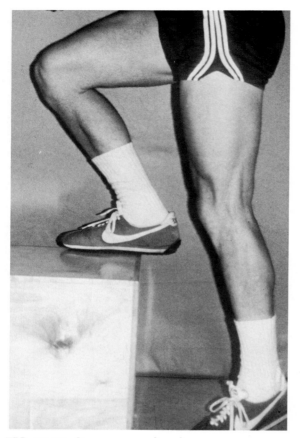

FIG. 24-17. Step-ups on a bench.

sitting, the leg is supported at the ankle so that flexion contracture is avoided.

THE VASTUS MEDIALIS

Because the oblique part of the vastus medialis rapidly atrophies after operation or immobilization, this part of the quadriceps was formerly considered solely responsible for the last 15° of knee extension. Lieb and Perry dispelled this notion by showing that this limitation of knee extension is related to total quadriceps strength and is not an indication of selective weakness of the vastus medialis obliguus.[23]

In truth, the vastus medialis obliquus is not the key motor for knee extension and power but instead serves a patella-centering function.[21] Consider, for example, that in amputated limbs a solitary vastus medialis obliquus will not extend the knee, whereas all of the long components of the quadriceps—vastus lateralis, vastus intermedius, vastus medialis longus, and rectus femoris—effect full extension. Normally, the last 15° of knee extension require 60% more force than is needed for extension up to the 15° position. However, when a weight is attached to the vastus medialis obliquus to keep the patella centered in the femoral groove, the force needed by the vastus lateralis to extend the knee decreases by 13%.

THE FUNCTIONAL KNEE PROGRAM

The injured athlete begins a functional knee rehabilitation program when performing advanced isotonics, riding the bicycle, and starting isokinetic exercises. The graduated functional program leads to the activities necessary in competition.

Athletes begin by walking about 2 miles, advancing without limp or pain to 1-mile jogs, and then proceeding to stair walking and jogging up stairs. This leads to step-ups for 5 min per day on an ordinary stair, advancing gradually to step-ups on an 18-in bench (Fig. 24-17). Next are sprints straight ahead for 40

too great a force. Also, the devices do not provide resistance, which would provide a stimulus for strength gains in terminal motion once the joint is "locked out." As full knee extension is achieved, the knee slows down, and consequently outside stimulus is least where it is needed most. In addition, the machines do not provide negative resistance for eccentric contraction.

Full knee extension is important because it is a stable position; if it is not achieved, walking is difficult and dangerous. It is reached by a limited arc technique with a bolster under the knee. However, if full active extension is lacking, the rest of the program proceeds while terminal extension is developed. When

FIG. 24-18. Isodynamic running is safer than jumping rope and provides proper body lean.

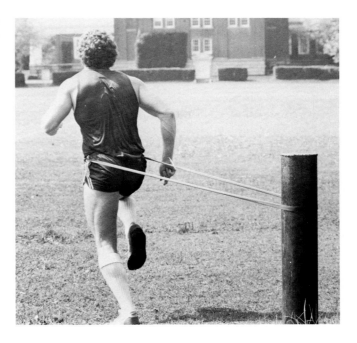

FIG. 24-19. An isokinetic machine prints out a strength and power analysis that precedes the athlete's return to practice.

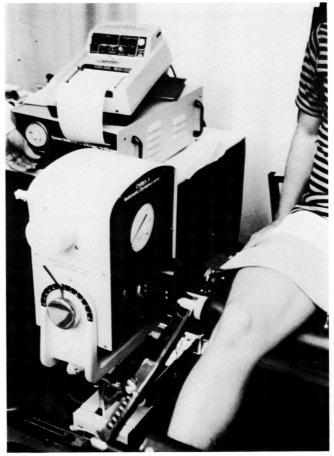

yards and 100 yards. At this time, 5-min bouts of rope skipping or isodynamic running (Fig. 24-18) may be started.

In the final phase, the athlete works in non-cleated shoes on starts, stops, jumps, rounded side-step cuts, and crossover cuts, advancing to hard 90° cuts, and running tighter and tighter figures-of-eight. Defensive backs run sideways and backward and perform carioca (crossover) steps. The athlete is now ready to demonstrate the 40-yard dash speed. Finally, this entire phase is repeated in cleats. When the functional tests are regarded as normal for this particular athlete, isokinetic strength and power is analyzed, and practice is resumed. (Fig. 24-19)

THE BICYCLE IN KNEE REHABILITATION

The exercise bicycle and lightweight touring bike are important parts of our knee rehabilitation program. Cycling restores muscular strength and knee flexibility and preserves muscular and cardiovascular endurance.[22]

Cycling strengthens both the quadriceps and the hamstrings. Be certain that the shoe is clipped onto the pedal so that the athlete can pull as well as push. A low saddle promotes greater knee flexibility, but, athletes who are unaccustomed to cycling sometimes have knee pain when seated too low, and the seat has to be raised.

Inactivity diminishes the oxidative enzymes in slow twitch muscle fibers. Cycling stimulates and restores these myochondrial enzyme systems.[6,7] Cycling can also provide a good training effect. Early in the rehabilitation program have the athlete clip in one foot and cycle one-legged; later, both feet can be clipped in. Later still, when the athlete pedals with his operated side, an isokinetic exercise bike is preferable to an isotonic bike. Although inertia makes an isotonic bicycle easy to pedal, if knee pain occurs, inertia keeps the crank spinning, and injury might result. On the isokinetic bike, resistance accommodates to the force applied, obviating injuries due to inertia. Bicycle touring affords a pleasant means of restoring strength, flexibility, and muscular and cardiovascular endurance (Fig. 24-20). The bike ride should be split into three 20-min segments, or it may be one unbroken ride for 1 hour each day.

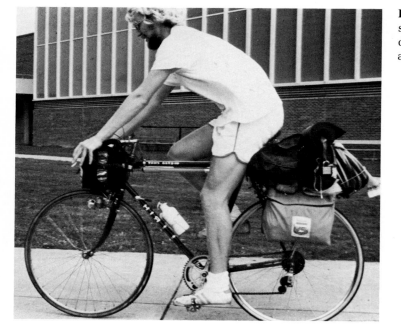

FIG. 24-20. Bicycle touring restores strength, flexibility, muscular endurance, and cardiovascular endurance.

SUMMARY

Knee injuries in athletics are second in frequency only to ankle injuries. An injured knee can distract, disable, or retire an athlete. To prevent ruined knees a precise diagnosis is essential, and treatment must be comprehensive. The athlete's physician needs a broad understanding of knee pathomechanics and a working knowledge of rehabilitation techniques. The ability to establish and supervise individual rehabilitation programs is important in the care of athletes.

REFERENCES

1. **Basmajian JV, Lovejoy JF Jr:** Functions of the popliteus muscle in man. J Bone Joint Surg 53A:557–562, 1971
2. **Bates BT et al:** Foot orthotic devices to modify selected aspects of lower extremity mechanics. Am J Sports Med 7:338–342, 1979
3. **Bergfeld J:** First, second and third-degree sprains. Am J Sports Med 7, No. 3:207–209, 1979
4. **Black HM et al:** Use of phenylbutazone in sports medicine: Understanding the risks. Am J Sports Med 8, No. 4:270–273, 1980
5. **Blazina ME et al:** Jumper's knee. Orthop Clin North Am 4:665–678, 1973
6. **Cooper DL, Fair J:** Trainer's Corner: Stationary cycling for post-op fitness. Phys Sportsmed 4, No. 6:129, June 1976
7. **Costill DL et al:** Muscle rehabilitation after knee surgery. Phys Sportsmed 5, No. 9:71–74, Sept 1977
8. **D'Ambrosia RD, MacDonald GL:** Pitfalls in the diagnosis of Osgood–Schlatters disease. Clin Orthop 110:206–209, 1975
9. **DeHaven KE et al:** Chondromalacia patellae in athletes: Clinical presentation and conservative management. Am J Sports Med 7:5–11, 1978
10. **Ellsasser et al:** Early mobilization of moderate knee ligament injury. Knee Symposium, Clancy, WG Jr, ed. Am J Sports Med 7, No. 3:206–213, 1979
11. **Eriksson E:** Sports injuries of the knee ligaments: Their diagnosis, treatment, rehabilitation and prevention. Science in Sports 8:133–144, 1976
12. **Funk FJ Jr:** Injuries of the extensor mechanism of the knee. Athletic Training 10, No. 3:141–145, Sept 1975
13. **Hlavac HF:** The Foot Book: Advice for Athletes. Mountain View, California, World Publications, 1977
14. **Hughston JC:** Subluxation of the patella. J Bone Joint Surg 50A:1003–1026, 1968
15. **Ismail AM et al:** Rupture of patellar ligament after steroid infiltration: Report of a case. J Bone Joint Surg 51B, No. 3:503–505, Aug 1969
16. **James SL et al:** Injuries to runners. Am J Sports Med 6:40–49, 1978
17. **Kennedy JC et al:** Orthopaedic manifestations of swimming. J Sports Med 6, No. 6:309–322, 1978
18. **Krissoff WB, Ferris WD:** Runner's injuries. Phys Sportsmed 7, No. 12:53–64, Dec 1979
19. **Kulund DN et al:** Olympic weightlifting injuries. Phys Sportsmed 6:11, 1978
20. **Kulund DN:** The Injured Athlete. Philadelphia, JB Lippincott, 1982
21. **Levine J:** A new brace for chondromalacia patella and kindred conditions. Am J Sports Med 6, No. 3:137–140, 1978
22. **Lyons R:** Trainer's Corner: Bicycle ergometer for injured athletes. Phys Sportsmed 2, No. 8:218, Aug 1974
23. **Lieb FJ, Perry J:** Quadriceps function: Anatomical and mechanical study using amputated limbs. J Bone Joint Surg 50A:1535–1548, Dec 1968
24. **Lutter LD:** Foot-related knee problems in the long-distance runner. Foot and Ankle 1, No. 2:112–116, 1980
25. **Mann RA, Hagy JL:** The popliteus muscle. J Bone Joint Surg 59A(7):924–927, 1977
26. **Marshall JL, Johnson RJ:** Mechanisms of the most common ski injuries. Phys Sportsmed 5(12):49–54, Dec 1977
27. **Mayfield GW:** Popliteus tendon tenosynovitis. Am J Sports Med 5(1):31–35, 1977
28. **Mayfield GW:** Runner's knee. Medicine and Sport 12:136–139, 1978
29. **Merchant AC et al:** Roentgenographic analysis of congruence. J Bone Joint Surg 56A:1931, 1974
30. **Millar AP:** Strains of the posterior calf musculature ("tennis leg"). Am J Sports Med 5, No. 5:191–193, 1977
31. **Mital M:** Osgood–Schlatters disease: The painful puzzler. Phys Sportsmed 5:60–73, June 1977
32. **Nicholas JA:** Injuries to knee ligaments: Relationship to looseness and tightness in football players. JAMA 212:2236–2239, 1970
33. **Nilsson S, Staff PH:** Tendoperiostitis in the lateral femoral condyle in long-distance runners. Br J Sports Med 7:87–89, 1970
34. **Noble CA:** Iliotibial band friction syndrome in runners. Am J Sports Med 8, No. 4:232–234, July/Aug 1980
35. **Parks RM:** Injuries of the endurance athlete. Medicine and Sport, 12:140–145, 1978
36. **Pease RL, Flentje W:** Trainer's Corner: Rehabilitation through underwater exercise. Phys Sportsmed 4, No. 10:143, Oct 1976
37. **Roach JE et al:** Comparison of the effects of steroid aspirin and sodium salicylate on articular cartilage. Clin Orthop 106:350–356, 1975
38. **Roels J et al:** Patellar tendinitis (jumper's knee). Am J Sports Med 6:362–368, 1978

39. **Roeser WM et al:** The use of transcutaneous nerve stimulation for pain control in athletic medicine: A preliminary report. Am J Sports Med 4, No. 5:210–213, Sept/Oct 1976

40. **Subotnick SI:** A biomechanical approach to running injuries. Ann NY Acad Sci 301:888–899, 1977

41. **Tipton CM et al:** Influence of exercise on strength of medial collateral ligament of dogs. Am J Physiol 218, No. 3:894–902, Mar 1970

42. **Watson–Jones R:** Fractures and Other Bone and Joint Injuries, ed 2. Williams and Wilkins, 1941

43. **Weaver JK:** Bipartite patellae as a cause of disability in the athlete. Am J Sports Med 5, No. 4:137–143, 1977

CHAPTER 25
MAJOR KNEE INJURIES IN CONTACT SPORTS

James A. Nicholas
W. Norman Scott

Statistically, major knee injuries are more disabling to the athlete than most other injuries. In 1978, 23% of the major athletic injuries to football players in the National Football League were knee injuries. In the North American Soccer League the figure was 25%. An increasingly sports-minded population and the high number of knee injuries are spurs to all primary care physicians to be familiar with and to recognize the distinctive types of knee disorders.

Knee motion occurs through a changing instant center of rotation. Its arc of motion is dependent on all the anatomical structures about the knee. Femoral and tibial conformity, patellofemoral congruence, muscle groups, menisci, and the collateral, capsular, and cruciate ligaments all contribute to the triaxial motion characteristic of the knee. Disruption of any of these structures affects the normal function of the knee. Each structure differs in importance, and the resultant anatomical variations in knee injuries demonstrate this.

The loose-ligamented gymnast is, for instance, apt to sustain extension mechanism problems with relatively minor trauma. These anatomical considerations combined with the demands placed on the knee by specific sports are the major elements in predicting, determining, and preventing injuries.

Treatment depends not only on the type and extent of the injury but also on the expectations and goals of the patient. Because the professional athlete wants to return to his livelihood, it is often not acceptable to treat ligamentous or meniscal injuries nonoperatively owing to the demands that will be placed on these damaged structures.

KNEE ANATOMY

Although the anatomy of the knee has been dealt with in the previous chapters, it is important to reemphasize certain structures when discussing athletic injuries.

391

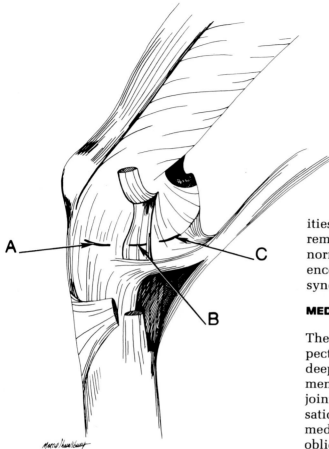

FIG. 25-1. Medial aspect of the knee. **(A)** Anterior capsular ligament. **(B)** Midcapsular ligament (deep medial [tibial] collateral ligament). **(C)** Posterior medial capsular ligament (posterior oblique ligament).

SYNOVIUM

The synovium, which lines the capsule, intracapsular ligaments, and tendons, has numerous ridges or recesses that are described as plicae. The three most commonly discussed synovial folds or plicae are (1) plicae synovialis suprapatellaris, a remnant of the complete septum of embryonic life that separates the suprapatellar bursa from the knee joint, (2) the shelf, which extends from the superior corner of the infrapatellar fat pad to the undersurface of the suprapatellar plicae, and (3) chordae obliquae synovialis, which are observed only in full extension when the retinaculum is under tension.[7] Some clinical entities, such as the medial synovial shelf syndrome, have been attributed to abnormal-

ities of these structures. It is important to remember that synovial folds or plicae are normal in up to 50% of knees, and their presence alone is not indicative of a pathologic syndrome.[5]

MEDIAL STRUCTURES

The ligamentous structures on the medial aspect of the knee include the superficial and deep components of the tibial collateral ligament, comprising the medial one-third of the joint. Anterior to this are the second condensations to the capsule described as the anteromedial capsular ligament, while the posterior oblique or posterior medial corner of the knee produces a cufflike posterior capsular ligament (Fig. 25-1). The medial retinaculum is an expansion of the vastus medialis obliquus aponeurosis and is of considerable importance, especially in patellar subluxation and dislocations. The common tendon of the sartorius, gracilis, and semitendinosus, the pes anserinus, inserts along the medial aspect of the tibia. This structure has often been used for extra-articular repairs of rotatory instabilities.[10]

LATERAL ASPECT

The lateral retinaculum or extension of the vastus lateralis, iliotibial tract, lateral collateral ligament, and the biceps and popliteal tendons represent the stabilizing structures on the lateral side of the knee (Fig. 25-2). The iliotibial tract, which inserts into the tubercle of Gerdy, is one of the strongest ligamentous

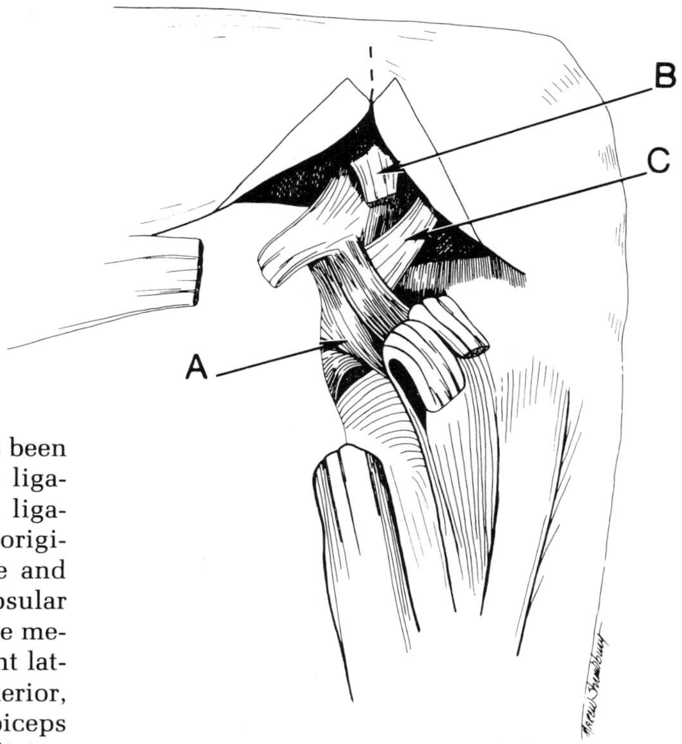

FIG. 25-2. Lateral aspect of the knee. **(A)** Arcuate ligament. **(B)** Lateral collateral ligament. **(C)** Popliteal tendon.

structures surrounding the knee and has been used for both intra- and extra-articular ligamentous repairs. The lateral collateral ligament, which is tight only in extension, originates on the lateral femoral epicondyle and inserts into the fibular head. The capsular condensations that were described on the medial side of the knee are not as prominent laterally but can also be divided into anterior, medial, and posterior segments. The biceps and popliteal tendon are the other stabilizing structures on the lateral side and reinforce the activities of the lateral collateral ligament, especially when it is lax in flexion.[10,13]

POSTERIOR STRUCTURES

The posterior capsule, divisions of the semimembranosus, oblique popliteal ligament, arcuate ligament, and popliteus muscles account for the stabilizing structures in the popliteal area of the knee (Fig. 25-3). The semimembranosus muscle has five distal expansions—the oblique popliteal ligament, the tendinous connection to the posterior horn of the medial meniscus, the anteromedial tendon, the direct head, and the distal portion of the fibrous expansion over the popliteus.[10] All these structures reinforce the posteromedial aspect of the knee. Contraction of the semimembranosus provides both static and dynamic stability to the posterior capsular ligament. The origin of the popliteus muscle has been described as a Y-shaped ligament that facilitates medial rotation of the tibia on the femur.[2] In addition to providing rotatory sta-

bility, it also pulls the posterior horn of the lateral meniscus posteriorly with knee flexion. The capsule becomes thick and in some areas fairly rigid and is characterized by the condensation that the senior author calls quadruple complexes.[13]

QUADRUPLE COMPLEXES

There are four structures on the medial side, four central structures, and four additional structures on the lateral side. The posteromedial corner is controlled by the semimembranosus tendon insertion, the pes tendons, the medial collateral ligament, and the oblique popliteal ligament. The central portion of the capsule is reinforced within the joint by the two cruciate ligaments as well as both menisci, which are attached to the capsule through the ligaments of Humphrey and Wrisberg. On the lateral side, the capsular reinforcement, as mentioned, is the biceps tendon, the iliotibial tract, the popliteal tendon, and the lateral ligament. These connect to

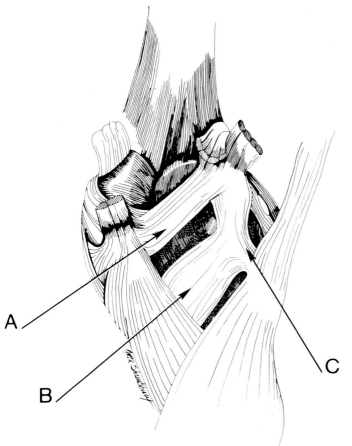

FIG. 25-3. Posterior aspect of the knee. **(A)** Oblique popliteal ligament. **(B)** Popliteus. **(C)** Arcuate ligament.

form the arcuate ligament (Fig. 25-4). Therefore, the posterior capsule controls a large part of the stability of the knee when it is forced into eccentric rotation (Fig. 25-5).[13] It plays little role in cadaver studies and is essentially activated *in vivo* by its muscular attachments. The dynamic component provides the stability.

DIAGNOSIS OF KNEE INJURIES

Medical students are constantly lectured on the importance of taking a good history. This cannot be overemphasized in diagnosing knee injuries. The position of the knee at the time of injury, mechanism of injury, amount of force, previous history of any knee injury, site of initial tenderness, audible sounds at the time of injury, and onset of swelling are im-

portant factors that make diagnosis easier for the clinician. Immediate swelling is usually indicative of a hemarthrosis and suspicious of capsular and ligamentous disruption. Delayed swelling, several hours after the injury, is indicative of synovial reaction and is seen more commonly with meniscal injuries. Inability to extend a locked knee may be associated with any intra-articular pathology, and the entire situation must be taken into account. Thus, a patient with a locked knee cannot always be considered to have a torn meniscus. Locking can be produced by anything that disrupts the normal biomechanical activity.[6] A valgus injury focuses attention on the medial aspect of the knee, whereas the mechanism of injury with a varus force usually disrupts the lateral complex. Since knee motion is triaxial, the resultant injuries often are three-dimensional

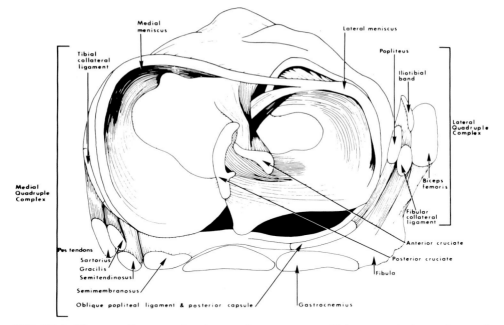

FIG. 25-4. There are three quadruple complexes—one medial, one posterior and central, and one lateral. They constitute the regulating function of the posterior capsule on knee stability. (Nicholas JA: J Bone Joint Surg 55A: 889, 1973)

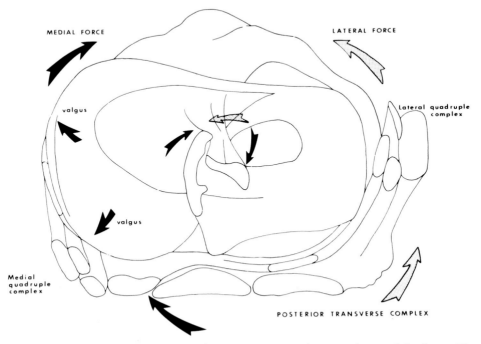

FIG. 25-5. The effect of rotation on the posterior capsular complexes of the knee. The medial quadruple complex resists external rotation and valgus. The lateral quadruple complex resists internal rotation and varus. (Nicholas JA: J Bone Joint Surg 55A: 899, 1973)

rather than straight compression-tension injuries. This makes diagnosis more difficult and again highlights the importance of an accurate history.

The diagnosis of ligament injuries has been discussed in previous chapters. The abundance of physical tests (Slocum, McIntosh, Losee "jerk," Helfet, Steinman, McMurray, Apley, Lachman, FRD, and so on) illustrates the existing confusion. Although some of the tests are quite accurate in describing specific knee derangements, they are not absolutely pathognomonic of isolated anatomical lesions. Thus, correct diagnosis of knee injuries requires an index of suspicion as determined by patient's body habitus, an accurate history, and physical findings. Attention to these details will lead to a correct diagnosis in a high percentage of cases.

Arthrography is well established as a diagnostic aid in determining meniscal lesions[15] (see Chap 9). It is accurate (95%) for medial meniscal tears but somewhat less reliable for lateral meniscal injuries (80%). This test, however, is no substitute for the clinical picture. It is an accessory screening procedure to a good examination. Asymtomatic meniscal tears are probably more prevalent than was previously thought. Arthroscopic procedures illustrate many clinically insignificant meniscal tears. Single contrast arthrography has recently been used to determine the status of cruciate ligaments. These results are encouraging to some but not to us because there is no dynamic display of cruciate ligament integrity. The clinician must rely on clinical or possibly an accurate stress machine examination.

Arthroscopic examination, which is often indicated in the acutely injured athlete, is more difficult than when done on an elective basis but will often allow a more exact diagnosis and possibly earlier return to athletic activities. As in many surgical procedures, however, arthroscopy is only as valuable as the experience of the surgeon performing it. Arthroscopic examination of the knee in acute injuries is more technically demanding and should be done only by the experienced arthroscopist.

The use of a stress-testing machine is becoming more popular and might possibly result in more accurate diagnoses in these complex knee injuries. Unfortunately, the parameters that must be considered in developing accurate machines are formidable obstacles. Hip rotation, abduction, adduction, tibial rotation, muscle relaxation, thigh and calf sizes, and manual resistance tests are only a few of the problems that must be sufficiently controlled to make stress machines accurate diagnostic tools. With increasing research and technology, these problems will undoubtedly be resolved, and the results should be helpful to the clinician and the patient.

KNEE INSTABILITY

The most serious major athletic injuries are those that involve stability. Forceful overrotation of the flexed knee with the leg fixed may disrupt many component parts. It is necessary to describe the resulting instabilities to understand both the mechanism and the rationale of management.[14]

SIMPLE STRAIGHT INSTABILITY

Simple instability denotes one-compartment involvement. For example, the medial complex structures such as the medial collateral ligament can be torn without involving the posterior capsule producing valgus deformity or one-plane laxity. This can result from a blow from the side or a fall from a height. Immediate pain, a feeling of weakness, and valgus laxity are the cardinal signs. The medial collateral ligament usually tears at its upper pole. Grading of these medial collateral ligament injuries is important to the treatment. A grade 3 or valgus opening of more than 1 cm in the highly competitive athlete may be sufficient reason for surgical repair. Grade I and grade II injuries can often be treated nonoperatively. After the correct diagnosis using the various methods as mentioned above, the specific activities of the patient must be considered before deciding on an operative or nonoperative approach.

When a nonoperative approach is used, we prefer immobilization in a plaster cast for up to 6 weeks. This should be followed by a Lenox Hill derotation brace for several months, night and day, depending on the extent of the injury. Active rehabilitation exercises are begun once the patient has progressed to the derotation brace.

In repairing medial collateral ligament injuries, the site of the tear determines the method of repair. Avulsions at the upper pole can usually be put back in place with a staple or screw. Inner substance tears, however, often require overlapping and imbrications of the collateral ligament or substitution, with pes plasty or posterior capsule advance. These tears are usually repaired with the leg flexed and internally rotated. Postoperatively, treatment is similar to that mentioned earlier. The integrity of the meniscus and posterior capsule must be determined prior to either operative or nonoperative treatment. The meniscus should not be removed if possible because it seems to enhance stability.

LATERAL INSTABILITY

Lateral instability of the simple type is primarily varus laxity. Pure lateral instability, however, is unusual. When present, the lateral ligament and usually the iliotibial band or the popliteal tendon are torn. In both instances, the patient feels the pop; the knee becomes quite unstable. Pain on flexion is localized to the upper end of the fibula and over the joint line. It should be noted that the lateral side of the knee is slightly lax in flexion because the lateral collateral ligament is relaxed in this position. If this is an isolated lesion, without any intra-articular cruciate ligament damage, several types of surgical procedures can be performed. They are primarily dependent on the nature of the injury at the time of surgery. The lateral edge of the arcuate ligament and posterior capsule can be advanced to the posterior aspect of the lateral ligament; the biceps tendon may be advanced either more proximally on the fibula or to the tibial condyle. The iliotibial band may also be used to reinforce the lateral collateral ligament when the remainder of the structures have been damaged. In general, a simple varus instability with no significant rotary laxity can usually be treated nonoperatively with immobilization for 4 to 6 weeks.

SIMPLE STRAIGHT ANTERIOR INSTABILITY

Simple anterior instability without medial or lateral compartment involvement is quite rare but has been described as a result of isolated anterior cruciate rupture.[4] Treatment of this injury remains controversial. Evidence in dogs suggests that disruption of the cruciate ligament may lead to early degenerative changes. There is no definitive evidence in humans to date, however. Indeed, we have seen athletes 10 to 15 years after untreated cruciate tears with no roentgenographic evidence of degenerative joint disease. For the professional athlete, acute repair is probably justified in view of the nature of his livelihood. Avulsion of the cruciate ligament with a fragment of bone is repaired by reattaching the fragment, using either wire or screw fixation. The question of how to treat substance tears, the most common type of cruciate ligament injuries, remains controversial. In our opinion, iliotibial band transfer should be considered in this instance. We have had good experience with this operation in patients with straight instability compared with the inconsistent results after static ligament transfers. Follow-up to date, after use of the iliotibial band for torn cruciate ligaments in old injuries, is encouraging. Follow-up, however, has been short, and further data are required.

Either a straight midline or a combination of medial and lateral parapatellar incisions can be used. The anterior one-third of the iliotibial band with a 1-cm × 1.5-cm piece of bone from the tubercle of Gerdy is dissected proximally to gain as much length as possible for passage "over the top." An incision is then made in the posterolateral capsule down to the periosteum. This allows easy access to the posterior aspect of the joint. With the use of special clamps or rubber tubing the bone block and part of the iliotibial band can then be transferred into the joint. An appropriate piece of bone is then removed, and, using a fixation screw, the transferred unit is countersunk with the leg in extension. Closure of the postero-lateral corner and medial parapatellar incision follows.

POSTERIOR INSTABILITY

Posterior instability from posterior cruciate ligament injury alone is also rare but may follow a blow at the front of the knee with the leg hyperextending so that the cruciate ligament is torn off the posterior aspect of the tibia. This is usually associated with a capsular tear as well. Except in athletes with moderate laxity, immediate surgical repair is recommended. An avulsion with a bone fragment, which may be reattached, has the best prognosis. Other methods for repairing torn posterior cruciate ligaments include gastrocnemius transfer,[8] popliteal tendon transfer,[1] semitendinosus,[9] transfer and the use of menisci. With substance tears of the posterior cruciate ligament this injury has a poor prognosis for highly competitive athletics, which are almost eliminated.

COMPLEX INSTABILITY

This type of instability is more common. Two or three axes of knee motion are affected. O'Donohue's triad is the classic type. It should be realized that anteromedial is not the only direction of instability. There are four types of complex instability that, if recognized and repaired early, lead to a satisfactory recovery.

Anteromedial Instability (Two-Plane Complex Anterorotary Instability)

The most common type results from anterior cruciate and medial collateral ligament rupture and often occurs with derangement of the medial meniscus. It is caused by violent external rotation and abduction, which cause the posterior medial tibial corner to rotate forward. The hamstrings and the posterior capsule restrain this movement, with the medial meniscus and collateral ligaments bearing the brunt anteriorly and medially. Marked laxity in flexion at about 15° results. Pain may not be very great; indeed, it may be possible to walk after the immediate symptoms are relieved. The patient often feels a pop. External rotation is increased, and valgus instability or anterior draw is often present.

Surgery is the preferred treatment for this injury. Many techniques are available, and the correct one depends on the type of ligamentous and meniscal disruption. Whenever possible, the medial meniscus is preserved, especially if there is a peripheral detachment that can be resutured. Repair of the cruciate ligament in the highly competitive athlete is recommended. Repair of the medial capsule depends on whether the residual medial collateral ligament is suitable and sufficient to anchor to the posteromedial corner and posteromedial complex.

An S-shaped incision is used. The pes anserinus tendons are exposed and turned up to see whether the medial ligament is torn underneath. Usually it is torn above the joint line. The intact part of the capsule posterior to the tear is identified. The knee is flexed, internally rotated, and displaced backward with varus stress. The posterior capsule is brought forward and distally to the side of the tear, and is fixed with a barb staple or sutures. It is of the utmost importance to insure firm fixation of the posterior and medial corner behind the tibia as well as the femur. Postoperatively, a long-leg plaster cast is applied for 6 weeks with the tibia internally rotated, adducted on the femur to produce a varus attitude, and displaced backward. The cast remains in place for a long rehabilitation period. A derotation brace is used after the casting immobilization. Ligamentous reconstruction needs a long period of after care that should not be compromised. Bracing and protection when participating in sports are mandatory until power is regained.

Anterior Lateral Instability

Anterolateral instability occurs when the leg is hit from the back or the side when the foot is planted with the tibia internally rotated and the strain placed on the lateral side. Some part of the lateral central quadruple complex or the anterior cruciate ligament, the lateral capsular ligaments, and the lateral meniscus tears. Internal-external rotation is increased, but an intact posterior cruciate ligament prevents backward tibial displacement. An anterior drawer sign and lateral laxity are present. The Ellison,[3] McIntosh, and Losee[11] are the most common extra-articular repairs used for this injury. If surgery is indicated, however, we feel that the anterior cruciate ligament should also be reconstructed late, whether by primary suture or by a secondary transfer, in addition to repairing the posterolateral capsule. A lateral approach is used to bring forward part of the posterolateral capsule behind the tear, along with the lateral head of the gastrocnemius. If a meniscectomy is done, the transferred capsule and advanced lateral ligament are stapled onto the posterior part of the lateral femoral condyle. The posterior capsule and the iliotibial band, if not used for a cruciate ligament reconstruction, are brought over the lateral ligament and popliteus and fixed to them. The operation is done with the tibia flexed, head backward with external rotation and backward displacement. Postoperative immobilization is imposed for 6 weeks with the tibia externally rotated and abducted on the femur. A reverse derotation brace is used after the casting. Again, a long period of rehabilitation, which varies in time depending upon progress in recovery of motion and stability, is observed. We do not wish a rapid return of motion earlier than 3 to 5 months postoperatively.

Posterolateral Laxity

Posterolateral laxity, a third form of rotary instability, results from rupture of the posterolateral compartment as well as impaired efficiency of the posterior cruciate ligament. It is caused by a forcable blow against the front of

the tibia with the leg externally rotated and planted in varus position. Instead of the posteromedial and medial compartments tearing, the posterolateral corner tears, usually somewhere along the course of the lateral ligament and popliteal tendon. Sometimes the biceps is avulsed. In such instances, because the posterior cruciate has been torn or is stretched, the lateral plateau of the tibia drops back with lateral posterior rotation and varus. In athletes, operative repair is mandatory to obtain a good result. Unfortunately, the importance of this injury is frequently neglected as a surgical emergency. The diagnosis is made from the presence of a posterior drawer sign, hyperextension, stress laxity in varus, and increased posterolateral rotation plus the local signs of tenderness. The medial compartment is quite stable.

Posterolateral repair is performed with the tibia internally rotated and displaced forward with the leg in valgus position. The posterior cruciate ligament should be repaired as previously described, or advanced if it is slack on the back of the tibia, thereby tightening it. The posterolateral corner is repaired as in anterolateral instability except that pes plasty is added to help check external tibial rotation.

Posteromedial Instability

Another type of instability that may be missed occurs in a posteromedial direction. It is rare but is seen occasionally, and can be seen early if a high index of suspicion exists. In this instance, a blow on the front of the leg, which is partially flexed and in external rotation, will tear the medial complex somewhere behind the medial collateral ligament above or below the joint line, often involving both menisci. The knee, having been driven backward, tears off the posterior cruciate ligament at its tibial attachment. Indeed, we have seen both ends of the ligament torn in such cases. A large saccular defect in the posterior compartment can be appreciated clinically under anesthesia by severe recurvatum as well as valgus laxity and increased internal rotation, the lateral compartment being uninvolved. Frequently, the patella's medial facet is also injured by a direct blow on the bone.

Surgical repair is very difficult. Restoration of the posterior cruciate ligament is essential. The tears in the posterior capsule are repaired, and we use the medial meniscus to anchor it. With the knee flexed, the entire capsule is mobilized forward to cover the medial ligament. The final position of the cast used in this situation is with the tibia displaced forward and the leg in varus in external rotation. It is possible, if one wishes, to transfer the biceps to the lateral side of the tibial crest. Results of this rare operation have sometimes been surprisingly good, but the key to success is to restore a stable posterior cruciate ligament and posterior medial support to allow the gastrocnemius to function.

Combined Complex Instability

When both medial and lateral or both anterior and posterior, as well as medial and lateral compartments are torn, combined complex instability exists. It is our opinion that transitory dislocation or at least subluxation is a preliminary. In many instances the peroneal nerve has been injured. The defects on both sides should be repaired in one stage through bilateral incisions. Operations for intra-articular transposition of the iliotibial band (i.e., Hey-Groves) or the semitendinosus have been disappointing. They should be considered a last alternative.

Rehabilitation, including a brace and an active exercise program, is stressed (as described in Chapter 24). Only those skilled in reconstruction surgery and conversant with the limitations should undertake these operations, which are primarily for patients with continuing instability despite restoration of power and the use of a brace.

KNEE DISLOCATION

Dislocation of the knee in athletes is infrequent but occurs in automobile or snowmobile racing, bobsledding, skiing, and motorcycle racing. It is a major injury requiring urgent hospitalization, immediate diagnosis, and reduction. Most dislocations are easily reduced and the sooner the better, sometimes even on a playing field. Careful examination to exclude popliteal artery laceration or peroneal nerve injury is imperative. Any question of vascular compromise requires immediate vascular consultation with the appropriate surgical procedures.

MANAGEMENT OF THE ACUTE DISLOCATION WITH NO ARTERIAL OR NERVE INJURY

In most cases, no lasting nerve, artery, or vein damage ensues after reduction. Instability is a problem. Unless the posterior cruciate ligament is intact, it is most unlikely that instability, treated conservatively with a cast, will be compatible with good athletic performance. Reconstruction will be necessary.

For this reason, ligamentous instability of the complexes in the mediolateral-anteroposterior compartments in dislocated knees should be operated upon at once. The prime purpose of surgery is repair of the posterior capsule, and its attachments to the medial and lateral tibial and femoral midaxial planes. The posterior cruciate demands top priority, and every attempt should be made to repair it. The anterior cruciate is usually so attenuated as to be irreparable.

Tears of the posterior cruciate ligament and posterior capsule are repaired at the same time. The medial and lateral capsules can be repaired at the same time or later, depending upon how much time is spent in surgery.

Neurolysis of the peroneal nerve, or transfer with enveloping fat away from the lateral complex tear, should be performed to avoid scarring of the nerve.

Dislocations of the knee are associated with so much ligamentous damage that one should try to repair the following structures (in order of importance):

1. Posterior cruciate ligament
2. Posterior capsule
3. Posterolateral corner

4. Posteromedial corner

5. Patelloquadriceps tendon tears

6. Anterior cruciate ligament

In all cases some loss of motion should be expected. Athletes can function with slight loss of motion but should be carefully rehabilitated to prevent contractures. After the cast is removed, bracing is necessary until power is restored.

DISLOCATION OF THE PROXIMAL TIBIOFIBULAR JOINT

Dislocation of the proximal tibiofibular joint is a rare injury produced by adduction of the lower leg with flexion of the knee. There are three types of dislocations, as described by Ogden.[13] Anterolateral subluxation is twice as common as posterior dislocation, which is usually associated with a peroneal nerve injury. The third type, superior dislocation, usually occurs with superior migration of the lateral malleolus.

Examination usually shows the fibular head to be somewhat more prominent than in the other knee. This, however, is not always reliable, and increased anteroposterior motion may be the only demonstrable sign. Roentgenographically, an acute dislocation becomes obvious when the fibular head is lying lateral to the tibial condyle in the anteroposterior view. The lateral view shows the fibular head sitting forward, overlapped by the tibia. Unfortunately, the roentgenographic diagnosis is often unreliable. Increased distance between the tibia and the fibula is often suggestive of the subluxation.*

In the acute dislocation, general anesthesia is often required to assure total muscle relaxation. The reductions are usually quite stable. Immobilization of almost any type usually works. Non-weight-bearing up to 2 weeks is usually advised. Return to full activity can be rather quick if there is no tenderness or pain. If an open reduction is required, several

---

* Turco V: Proximal tibiofibular subluxation, personal communication

methods can be used—arthrodesis, resection of the proximal fibula, fixation of the fibula to the tibia. We prefer Kirschner wire fixation.[17]

EXTENSOR MECHANISM INJURIES

Violent contraction of the quadriceps with the knee in a flexed position can lead to any one of four extensor injuries: quadriceps tendon rupture, fracture of the patella, patellar tendon rupture, and avulsion of the tibial tubercle. These depend on the age of the patient that is, quadriceps ruptures occur more commonly in the elderly patient whereas patellar tendon ruptures and tibial tubercle avulsions are usually found in the younger patient. Inability to extend the knee from a flexed position or to maintain quadriceps power against resistance are the usual physical findings with these injuries. In the athletic individual all four of these injuries should be treated surgically. The specific surgical techniques are described in detail elsewhere in this book.

DISLOCATION OF THE PATELLA

This injury usually results from some predisposing anatomical aberration such as increased Q angle, patella alta, dysplastic femoral condyle, vastus medialis dystrophy, or diffuse ligamentous laxity. Disruption of the medial retinaculum and osteochondral fractures are the usual pathologic findings.

The highly motivated athlete with no anatomical anomaly can usually be treated nonoperatively. A cylinder cast with the leg in full extension should usually be maintained for 6 weeks. Quadriceps exercises should be begun as soon as pain has subsided. A rehabilitation program as emphasized in a subsequent chapter is an integral part of this treatment.

In the professional athlete with either an increased Q angle or patella alta, surgical intervention is usually warranted. We prefer a proximal rather than a distal realignment. This is also coupled with a lateral release.

Recurrent subluxation of the patella without much disability at the time of the subluxation can be treated effectively in most patients with a prescribed exercise program.[18] Almost 80% of patients will respond favorably to this. If the patient does not respond favorably, surgical intervention is again warranted.

SUMMARY

The treatment of major athletic knee injuries is a growing and constantly changing field. With increasingly larger numbers of clinical investigators, new methods are constantly being tried. Athletes in all age groups will undoubtedly benefit from these advances.

REFERENCES

1. **Barfod B:** Posterior cruciate ligament reconstruction by transposition of the popliteal tendon. Acta Orthop Scand 42:438–439, 1971
2. **Basmajian JV, Lovejay JF:** Functions of the popliteus muscle in man. J Bone Joint Surg 53A:557–562, 1971
3. **Ellison AE:** Distal iliotibial band transfer for anterolateral rotatory instability of the knee. J Bone Joint Surg 61A:330–337, 1979
4. **Feagin JA, Abbott HG, Rokous JR:** The isolated tear of the anterior cruciate ligament. J Bone Joint Surg 54A:1340, 1972
5. **Fox JM, Blazina ME, Del Pizzo W et al:** Medial synovial shelft syndrome. Paper presented at the American Academy of Orthopaedic Surgeons, February 1979, San Francisco, California
6. **Frankel VH, Burstein AH, Brooks DB:** Biomechanics of internal derangement of the knee: Pathomechanics as determined by analysis of the instant centers of motion. J Bone Joint Surg 53A:945–962, 1971
7. **Gartz M:** Anatomy of the Knee: American Academy of Orthopaedic Surgeons Symposium on Arthros-
copy and Arthrography of the Knee, pp 44–53. St. Louis, CV Mosby, 1978
8. **Hohl M, Larson R:** Fractures and dislocations of the knee. In Rockwood CA, Green DP (eds): Fractures, Vol 2, pp 1131–1284. Philadelphia, JB Lippincott, 1975
9. **Hughston JC:** Posterior cruciate reconstruction. International Society of the Knee, First Congress, April 1979, Lyon, France
10. **Kennedy JC, Grainger RW:** The posterior cruciate ligament. J Trauma 7:367–377, 1967
11. **Losee RE, Ennis T, Johnson R, Southwick W:** Anterior subluxation of the lateral tibial plateau. J Bone Joint Surg 60A:1015–1030, 1979
12. **Nicholas JA:** Glossary of sports maneuvers in which the knee is immediately involved. Paper presented at the AAOS postgraduate course "The Injured Knee in Sports. Special Reference to the Surgical Knee," July 23–25, 1973, Eugene, Oregon
13. **Nicholas JA;** Injuries to knee ligaments. JAMA 212:2236–2239, 1970
14. **Nicholas JA:** The five–one reconstruction for anteromedial instability of the knee. J Bone Joint Surg 55A:899, 1973
15. **Nicholas JA, Freiberger RH, Killoran PS:** Double-contrast arthrography of the knee: Its value in the management of 225 knee derangements. J Bone Joint Surg 52A:203–220, 1970
16. **Ogden JA:** Subluxation and dislocation of the proximal tibiofibular joint. J Bone Joint Surg 56A:145–154, 1974
17. **Parkes JC II, Zelko RR:** Isolated acute dislocation of the proximal tibiofibular joint. J Bone Joint Surg 55A:177–180, 1973
18. **Schosheim P, Saraniti AJ, Bronson M et al:** The effects of a prescribed exercise program as treatment for subluxation or chondromalacia patella, submitted for publication
19. **Slocum DB, Larson RL, James SL:** Late reconstruction procedures used to stabilize the knee. Orthop Clin North Am 4:679–689, 1973
20. **Turco V:** Proximal tibiofibular subluxation, personal communication

CHAPTER 26
THE "DASHBOARD KNEE"

Arthur J. Helfet

A blow on the front of the bent knee is a frequent consequence of automobile and motorcycle collisions (Fig. 26-1). The sufferer is usually the passenger on the front seat, who is thrown forward and upward and strikes a knee against the dashboard. Fracture of the upper end of the tibia or of the patella, or backward dislocation of the tibia on the femur may result. But a lesion that might be called "the dashboard knee" merits discussion. It is less serious in its immediate consequence than frank fractures or dislocations but tends to cause protracted and troublesome disability unless the exact nature of the damage sustained is appreciated and adequately and specifically treated.

The site and the extent of the contusion depend on the position of the knee when struck —that is, if pointing forward or if the medial or the lateral side of the flexed knee receives the direct blow. The structures involved are the patellar ligament, the infrapatellar pad of fat, the anterior horns of the two semilunar cartilages, and the presenting articular surfaces of the femoral condyles.

The lesion is characterized by swelling and bruising of the tissues in front of the knee. There may be associated abrasions or skin wounds, and synovial effusion or hemarthrosis may develop. Unless the patella or the tibia has been involved, tenderness and pain in the early stages may not be severe. It is important to assess the exact extent of the injury and the tissues involved and to initiate treatment immediately. The formation of scar and adhesions should be prevented, for these are the main disabling factors when hemorrhage and swelling are given time to organize. A compression bandage, a back splint, no weight-bearing, heat, compresses—all these should be considered. The injury is a contusion that affects each tissue characteristically.

PATELLAR LIGAMENT

Oddly enough, patellar ligament injury does not cause the most trouble, although it is in the van of the accident. When it does, a scar has formed in the ensheathing tissues or in the substance of the tendon. Pain is felt whenever the ligament is tensed or strained, as in

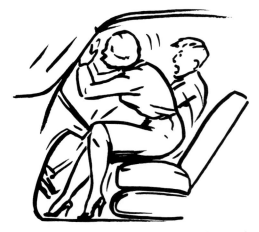

FIG. 26-1. As the passenger is thrown forward and upward, the knee strikes the dashboard.

climbing stairs or kicking a football. Kneeling on the tender knee is avoided. Active extension of the knee is painful, whereas passive extension is painless. Conversely, active flexion tends to be symptomless, whereas passive flexion may be uncomfortable. The injured part of the ligament is always tender on pressure. Injection of the tender area with procaine and hydrocortisone should be followed by "manipulation under local anesthetic." In other words, while the anesthetic effect of the procaine lasts, the patient is asked to do those movements that normally are painful. This would tend to break down the peritendinous and the intratendinous adhesions. Physiotherapy, including heat and deep massage or ultrasound, is useful in aiding resolution. Occasionally, manipulation under general anesthetic and even excision of the scar is necessary. The injury to the ligament is seldom isolated and is usually associated with damage to the infrapatellar pad of fat.

INFRAPATELLAR PAD OF FAT

Scar and adhesion formation in and around the fat pad not only interfere with function but cause disability through pain as well. The pad is a mobile structure, but following this injury it tends to become adherent to the tibia and to be tied by adhesions to the anterior horn of the nearest meniscus, most often, the medial meniscus (Fig. 26-2). The full range of functions of the fat pad are not clearly understood. It contains a high proportion of elastic fibers, and these, plus its synovial attachments, enable the mobile structure to adapt itself to and cushion the front of the knee joint as it opens and closes in reflexion and extension. It is also thought that it adjusts the intra-articular space in the knee joint to allow proper lubrication of the surfaces during movement. Adhesions at any point affect the mobility necessary for these functions.

In addition, when adhesions anchor the anterior horn of the meniscus, the rotator mechanism of the knee joint is affected. Extension and lateral rotation of the tibia are limited, with all the signs and symptoms of a retracted anterior horn.

Swelling of the fat pad as a whole simulates Hoffa's disease.[1] It is tender. The knee aches after activity and suffers recurring or persistent effusion. Forced extension is painful and aggravates the condition. When the semilunar cartilage is involved, rotation of the tibia is limited. There is specific tenderness over the anterior horn, and the patient may complain of pseudo-giving-way due to stabs of pain on certain movements.

Adequate physiotherapy is useful and important in the early stages. If the residual adhesions are mild, manipulation under general anesthetic is advisable. In those cases in which rotation is limited but painful when forced, manipulation may be dramatically successful because the adherent meniscus is mobilized. For the more heavily scarred fat pad, which does not respond to treatment by these methods, surgical excision of the scar and careful mobilization should be performed. It will be found that the fat pad is adherent above and anterior to the edge of the tibia. These adhesions must all be dissected carefully. Removal of the fat pad should be avoided. The knee without a fat pad is creaky and prone to strain on any exertion. Dissection of the scar must be meticulous. The fat pad is a vascular structure, and unnecessary trauma leads to new adhesions. Postoperative treatment to prevent further hemorrhage and

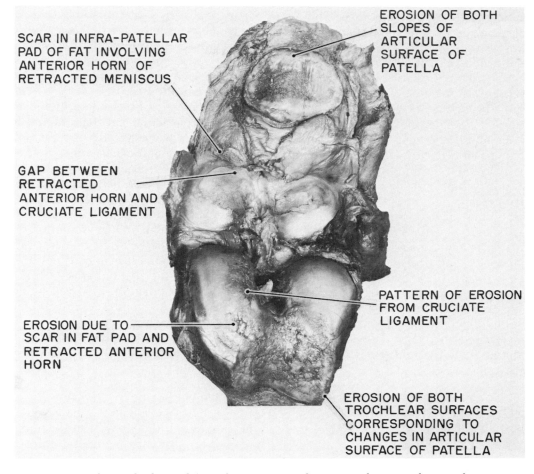

SCAR IN INFRA-PATELLAR PAD OF FAT INVOLVING ANTERIOR HORN OF RETRACTED MENISCUS

EROSION OF BOTH SLOPES OF ARTICULAR SURFACE OF PATELLA

GAP BETWEEN RETRACTED ANTERIOR HORN AND CRUCIATE LIGAMENT

EROSION DUE TO SCAR IN FAT PAD AND RETRACTED ANTERIOR HORN

PATTERN OF EROSION FROM CRUCIATE LIGAMENT

EROSION OF BOTH TROCHLEAR SURFACES CORRESPONDING TO CHANGES IN ARTICULAR SURFACE OF PATELLA

FIG. 26-2. Obviously this cadaveric knee was struck more on the inner than on the outer side. Though both surfaces of the patella are affected, the medial slope is much more so. There is a big hard scar in the medial side of the fat pad, and the scar involves the anterior horn of the medial meniscus, which has been detached from the cruciate ligament. The fat pad and the retracted anterior horn have caused a rounded pattern of erosion on the medial femoral condyle. (Royal College of Surgeons, England)

to promote absorption of reactionary swelling is vitally important. A Jones compression bandage for 10 days, followed by conscientious physiotherapy, is the course advised.

LESIONS OF THE ANTERIOR ENDS OF THE SEMILUNAR CARTILAGES

The medial or both anterior horns are commonly involved. The lateral semilunar carti-

lage seldom is injured by itself. The cartilage appears to be pushed back from its anterior attachments, and the anterior tip is embraced by the adjacent lobe of the fat pad in a bulky hard scar (Figs. 26-2; 27-4). If the lesion has been present for any length of time, a deep indentation is formed in the articular cartilage of the medial femoral condyle slightly more medially and anteriorly than the area of erosion from a retracted meniscus (Fig. 26-2). It may be possible to palpate the hard, tender lump in the anteromedial compartment of the knee. Rotation signs are present, and forced extension causes pain in this area. This is a troublesome knee that tends to become slowly but progressively worse—more so when the adjacent articular surface of the femoral condyle has shared in the contusion. Recurring or persistent effusion and wasting of the quadriceps are adverse factors.

Treatment by manipulation of the knee under an anesthetic may be attempted but now fails to relieve symptoms. Therefore, the lesion is explored through the usual horizontal incision, which may be extended slightly further medially and upward. The mass of scar involving the retracted anterior horn of the cartilage is usually adherent to the tibia. The meniscus and the scar in the fat are carefully dissected and excised. In these cases it may be difficult to remove the quite normal posterior horn of the meniscus in its entirety through the anterior incision. As long as the residual fragment is not injured surgically, it may be left without harm. However, it is always necessary to free and mobilize the entire fat pad.

CONTUSION OF THE ARTICULAR SURFACE OF THE FEMORAL CONDYLE

Again, it is usually the medial condyle that is involved. The blow falls on the anteromedial part of the articular surface of the condyle, or the damage may be secondary from pressure by the scar formed by the fat pad and the damaged anterior horn of the meniscus. The latter etches a progressive pattern of erosion that may be compared with that resulting from displacement of the semilunar cartilages. If the lesion lasts long enough, this knee follows a similar retrogressive course. Attacks of pain and swelling after activity increase in frequency and duration, the knee becomes more flexed, and eventually the patient feels he is walking on a stone in the knee. Excision of the cartilage and the scar and mobilization of the knee so that full extension is recovered may bring considerable relief. But on the whole these knees do not do as well after operation

as do their counterparts with traumatic arthritis due to a deranged meniscus. Convalescence is more protracted, and the recovery of comfort, power, and movement takes longer and is sometimes incomplete. There is no doubt that a badly damaged fat pad may be a lifelong hindrance.

This may also be the fate of the knee in which the articular cartilage of the femoral condyle has been directly and severely contused. The symptoms become progressively worse, as in chondromalacia or articular cartilage damage from other causes. At first the area is tender and the knee joint irritable. The products of the degenerating cartilage provoke effusion, discomfort, limitation of movement, wasting of the thigh muscles, and so on. It is wise in such a case to consider prolonged protection of the affected area, at first by rest in bed and bandaging, followed by crutches for walking until tenderness of the knee has disappeared. Aspiration of tense effusions or hemarthrosis using local anesthesia, repeated if necessary, and possibly Healon (see Chap. 4) accelerate recovery.

Quadriceps drill may be started early, with non—weight-bearing movements when swelling permits. At operation, the articular cartilage shows all the signs of degeneration. The area loses luster and compressibility, fibrillates, and appears slightly yellowish and more opaque. If protected for a sufficient length of time, the knee does tend to become symptomless, but it is unlikely that the long-term prognosis is satisfactory.

THE PATELLA

Contusion of the patella leads to gradual degeneration of articular cartilage, both of the patella and of the trochlear surface of the femur. The extent of cartilaginous erosion is usually more extensive than are the secondary effects of a displaced meniscus or recurring dislocation and depends on the severity of the original injury (Fig. 26-2). Symptoms, the assessment of disability, and treatment are discussed in Chapter 13.

It should be noted that although the dashboard may cause actual dislocation of the knee, a lesser injury may produce minor tears of capsule and ligament. These must be assessed carefully, for treatment for dashboard injury should never be delayed or casual in character. Every attempt must be made by conscientious therapy in the early days to prevent sequelae. As will be realized, disability from the four lesions described tends to become worse without, and lamentably, often in spite of, treatment.

REFERENCE

1. **Hoffa A:** The influence of the adipose tissue with regard to the pathology of the knee joint. JAMA 43:795, 1904

CHAPTER 27
THE STIFF KNEE

Arthur J. Helfet

In its broadest connotation, stiffness of the knee includes restriction of movement in one or more directions. It is a common sequel to injury of the knee joint itself, of the muscles of the thigh, or of fracture of the femur. It is an early symptom of arthritis, whether traumatic, rheumatoid, or infective in origin.

The knee joint is activated by flexion-extension and rotator mechanisms. However, when movement is limited, it is usual orthopaedic practice to place emphasis mainly on restrictions in the flexion-extension apparatus. Fixed limitations of movement are arbitrarily labeled as flexion or hyperextension deformities or "triple dislocation." But movement of the knee joint is a synchrony of flexion or extension with rotation, and, although one may be affected predominantly, limitation of range in any direction involves both. More often than not, the rotator mechanism is primarily at fault.

Treatment of the stiff knee without diagnosis and exact localization of the structure that is the brake to movement is difficult and unsatisfactory. To distinguish the different conditions is not often easy, for several structures may be involved at the same time. Adherence of the quadriceps to the site of fracture of the femur is not always the cause of limitation of flexion of the knee joint. Adhesions between the menisci or the fat pad and the tibia may be at fault. Attempts to increase flexion of the knee by hinging the joint under a general anesthetic or to correct flexion deformity by wedging a plaster cylinder posteriorly are unsatisfactory substitutes for removing obstacles to rotation of the menisci or to free movement of the fat pad.

ADHERENCE OF THE QUADRICEPS TO THE FEMUR

Stiffness after fractures of the shaft of the femur may be due to damage to and subsequent adherence of the quadriceps to the fractured area of the femur (Fig. 27-1). Charnley[4] has recorded evidence that this rarely happens when the fracture unites in reasonable time but is liable to occur when union is de-

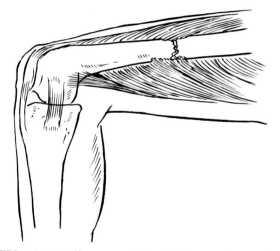

FIG. 27-1. Adherence of the thigh muscles to the shaft of the femur limits their excursion and therefore the range of movement of the knee joint.

layed. Similar restriction of movement occurs when the thigh muscles are damaged without fracture of the femur. They adhere to the bone or to each other. Injury to the hamstrings may result in flexion contractures, the deformity being combined with internal or external rotation of the tibia, depending on whether the medial or the lateral muscles are predominantly affected.

Involvement of the muscle alone may be inferred if rotation of the knee joint remains comparatively free. Unless the muscles have become fixed with the knee in complete extension, passive limitation of flexion is not associated with a proportionate loss of passive rotation. But this is a rare state of affairs, for fracture of the femur or damage to thigh muscles is often associated with coincidental sprain or contusion of the knee, or the prolonged splinting necessary in treatment may lead to stiffness, especially in old people.

The site of muscle adherence is tender to deep pressure, and the patient usually is able to localize the area from the sensation of local tension when passive movement is forced. Forced flexion does not produce pain in the knee joint unless tension between the patella and the femur or, if the patella is fixed, on the patellar ligament, becomes excessive. Often

the scar and the area of induration in the muscles are palpable.

The best preventive measure against adhesions after fracture of the femur is adequate reduction and splinting followed by conscientious quadriceps drill and hamstring drill, or what might more instructively be called "thigh drill," because exercise of the hamstrings is as important as exercise of the extensors. After 3 or 4 weeks, if induration persists and the patient has difficulty in properly contracting the thigh muscles, judicious injection of a mixture of procaine and hydrocortisone is helpful. Manipulation under a general anesthetic may be attempted after the fracture has united soundly and consolidated but will succeed only if the adhesions are few and minor. Massive adhesions will not yield to manipulation. At a late stage, when exercise, physiotherapy, stretching, and similar maneuvers, no longer bring further improvement, gentle freeing of the muscles, or quadricepsplasty as described by T. Campbell Thompson,[6] or recession of the quadriceps tendon as devised by Bennett,[2,3] all give good results. The interposition of a membrane of fascia, nylon, or metal between the muscles and the femur is seldom necessary.

Recent experiments[1] showed that hyaluronic acid implanted into a wound in a dog prevented intra-articular inflammation in a joint and a decrease in granulation tissue reaction and fibrous tissue formation in subcutaneous wounds (see Chap. 4). This holds promise that dehydrated membranes of pure hyaluronic acid may be most useful in preventing new scar formation in this and other operations on joints and muscles.

MALUNITED SUPRACONDYLAR FRACTURE OF THE FEMUR

The influence of malunion of these fractures on movement of the knee joint is not always appreciated. The femur may have united in perfect anteroposterior and lateral alignment, but if rotation has not been corrected, full extension or flexion may be mechanically blocked. It would seem that if the lower fragment is rotated laterally, the tibia reaches the limit of internal rotation before the knee is fully flexed. The opposite would hold if the lower fragment is in malalignment in internal rotation. Recovery of movement is possible only after corrective osteotomy.

ADHERENCE OF THE CAPSULE OF THE KNEE JOINT

Adhesions may form between fibrous and synovial capsules or between fibrous capsule, synovium, and bone, or they may bind synovium to synovium as in the suprapatellar pouch. The adhesions follow sprain or contusion (as in the dashboard knee), hemarthrosis, infected effusions or wounds, or ill-judged incisions.

In their formative or vascular stages these adhesions are acutely sensitive to movement and tender on pressure. When the adhesion is established as fibrous avascular tissue, tenderness, less marked, is present only on deep pressure, while movement is painful only when forced.

Adequate treatment in the early days after injury is necessary to prevent these sequelae. While the adhesions are vascular, treatment is conservative—physiotherapy and local injections of procaine, hyalase, and hydrocortisone. Manipulation at this stage is accompanied by the unpleasant sensation of tearing tissue and produces reactionary bleeding and exudate. Painful swelling and increased restriction of movement result. When the adhesion is formed and avascular, manipulation is accomplished with a sharp snap, and movement is immediately free. There is little or no reaction afterward.

The knee is ready for manipulation when tenderness is localized and present on deep pressure only. Extensive adhesions do not respond well to manipulation and are usually associated with damage to other structures, such as meniscus and fat pad, as well. In that event surgical mobilization is necessary.

Reference has been made to the limitation

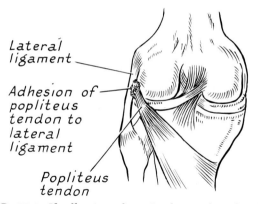

FIG. 27-2. If adhesions form in the tendon sheath of the popliteus or between the popliteus and the lateral ligament, movement of the knee joint is limited and painful.

of flexion that results from adhesions between the lateral ligament and the popliteus tendon or the lateral capsule (Fig. 27-2). Here, too, treatment to recover movement may require surgery.

ADHERENCE OF MENISCI AND FAT PAD TO THE TIBIA

Adherence of the menisci and fat pad to the tibia is responsible for stiffness of the knee joint after injuries associated with hemarthrosis (e.g., after rupture of the menisci from their vascular peripheral attachments) and after dashboard injuries. It is also a cause of stiffness after transient infection of the knee joint controlled by antibiotics. Adhesion of the menisci to the tibia is found in the knee in various stages of rheumatoid arthritis (Figs. 27-3 and 27-4).

This is true locking of the rotator mechanism. If the adhesions are firm and short, only hinge movement is possible. If the adhesions are lax, an arc of movement remains with synchrony of rotation approaching the normal. The condition is diagnosed either by the complete absence of passive rotation or by the relative restriction of rotation when compared with the extent of flexion or hinge movement

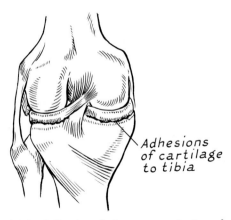

FIG. 27-3. Adhesion between menisci and tibia locks rotation and therefore limits flexion and extension.

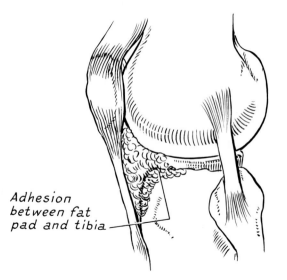

FIG. 27-4. The infrapatellar pad of fat is a mobile structure. If it becomes fixed to the tibia or the meniscus, movement of the knee joint is affected.

present. Pain on forced movement depends on the firmness of the ankylosis present. Early vascular adhesions produce sharp pain on movement, whereas more force is needed to give the same discomfort when the adhesions are dry and firm. Tenderness follows suit. The site of adherence is the site of maximum tenderness—usually the anterior horn of the meniscus or the fat pad or both. Because this con-

dition often follows hemarthrosis, adherence of the menisci and the fat pad may be associated with adhesions of the capsule to the femur and adhesions in the suprapatellar pouch. In this event, deep tenderness will be present over the femoral condyles, and thickening and tenderness may be palpable in the suprapatellar pouch.

The patient complains of limitation of movement with pain but usually adds a story of recurrent attacks of aching and effusion following undue activity of any kind. He may complain of illusory giving-way. On certain movements or on irregular ground a sharp twinge of pain gives the impression of momentary instability. He tends to guard the knee and walk with trepidation.

Attempts to recover movement by forced flexion or hinging are rarely successful. The arc of hinging may be increased, but the gain is at the expense of the capsule and in some instances includes stretching the cruciate ligament. The stretched capsule and cruciate ligaments are responsible for the anteroposterior laxity found in these otherwise stiff knees. However, this type of manipulation does sometimes free intracapsular adhesions. Recovery of rotation of the tibia on the femur is the maneuver to be practiced and is especially useful for mild adhesions between the fat pad and the anterior horn of the meniscus. The effect of regaining rotary movements may be demonstrated under general anesthesia. Without attempting flexion, gently manipulate the tibia on the femur in rotation. As rotation increases, flexion improves proportionately.

For mobilizing the really stiff knee, Sir Robert Jones described this method:

In breaking down adhesions of the knee, I teach that the knee should first of all be fully flexed and fully extended. It then should be fully flexed and slowly extended, and during the whole of the last act the knee should be rotated inwards and outwards at least ten or fifteen times.[5]

Sir Robert was especially skilled in manipulation. In my experience it is easier to regain flexion and extension as rotation is freed. Attempts to flex should be accompanied by forced medial rotation of the tibia and extension with lateral rotation.

Some adhesions give suddenly with a dramatic increase in the range of knee movement. In others, improvement is limited, and one feels an elastic block to further movement. Now, open operation is indicated and holds good promise.

At operation one finds the anterior horn or the anterior half of the meniscus adherent to the tibia. The semilunar cartilage may show the yellowish stain of old hemorrhage. The coronary ligament is impregnated with or replaced by fibrous adhesions, and the usual easy mobility of the anterior half of the meniscus has been lost. Unfortunately, too, one usually finds that the anterior horn has been detached from the cruciate ligament and is consequently retracted and thickened. When the meniscus has been tied down for some length of time it feels hard. It has lost pliability and resilience. If retracted or adherent it should be excised.

The common areas of fixation of the fat pad are to the anterior horn of the meniscus and to the anterior surface and the anterosuperior border of the tibia. The adhesions should be divided gently and the fat pad mobilized. In some instances, lobes of the fat pad are adherent to each other, and these fibrous bands also should be freed. Further damage to the fat pad with the prospect of hemorrhage and new adhesions must be avoided. As soon as the adhesions have been divided, rotation of the knee joint as a whole recovers. With the leg flexed over the end of the table this is easily tested. The leg then should be straightened to make certain that full extension with rotation has been recovered. Flexion is usually immediately possible well beyond the right angle.

Intracapsular adhesions are usually demonstrated between the femur and the capsule in the recess of the joint above the medial cartilage. They may be freed by gentle dissection or may be snapped by manipulation after the cartilage has been excised and the fat pad mobilized.

The timing of the manipulation or operation is important. If performed while the gran-ulation tissue and young adhesions are vascular, the resulting hemorrhage and exudate provide the basis for reformation. When they are avascular, there is little tendency to recurrence. Choosing the right time is a clinical decision, the main criteria being localization of swelling and tenderness and minimal reaction to limited activity or physical provocation.

After care is most important. Physical therapy and exercise after manipulation are designed to promote the absorption of any reactionary exudate and to maintain the range of movement gained. Excessive reaction denotes bad timing of the procedure. The knee should be rested and the manipulation repeated at a more suitable time. Postoperative care is the same as that after operation for the dashboard knee.

The following case reveals some of these features: A boy of 17 taking a broad jump landed on the outer side of the right foot and injured his knee. He suffered a painful internal derangement and was unable to take weight on the knee, which rapidly became distended. After admission to a hospital, the hemarthrosis was aspirated, but the surgeon was unable to reduce a "locked" knee. A few days later he performed an arthrotomy and reported a ruptured anterior cruciate ligament but no injury to the menisci. Postoperatively, full extension of the knee was not recovered. The patient suffered continuous disability with intermittent exacerbations, when aspiration and splinting with no weight-bearing were necessary.

A year after the original accident a severe and painful swelling necessitated admission to another hospital. The knee was severely distended and after aspiration still showed 10° limitation of extension. Flexion was possible through 50°, that is, from 170° to 120°, but both lateral and medial rotation were completely fixed. All the rotation signs were positive. The anterior half of the medial meniscus was tender.

At operation it was evident that both the anterior cruciate and the medial meniscus had been disrupted from their attachments to the tibia and to each other. The meniscus had retracted, leaving a gap of ½ in, and the anterior half had subsequently become adherent to the tibia. As soon as the meniscus was excised, full movement of the knee was possible. His convalescence was comfortable and benign, and he recovered a normally functioning knee.

This story illustrates dramatically the restriction of all movements when a point in the rotator mechanism of the knee is firmly tethered. As soon as the brake is released, both flexion and extension are recovered.

RHEUMATOID AND SEPTIC ARTHRITIS

All the components of the knee joint are involved in the inflammatory connective tissue reactions to rheumatoid and septic arthritis. As a consequence, the synovium is fibrotic, the menisci and the fat pad become fixed to the tibia, and adhesions form between the articular surfaces.

It was common practice when the articular surfaces are destroyed to arthrodese the knee. A comfortable rigid limb was the result. When the inactive phase of the disease is reached, because the joint is relatively insensitive, and if destruction of the joint surface is not gross, a more useful knee may be obtained by partial synovectomy, excision of both menisci, and freeing of the fat pad. Thirty to 60 degrees of comfortable movement has been recovered by this procedure. If the extremes of this range are not forced, the patient walks with short steps but with confidence, especially after an effort is made to recover muscle power. As long as movement is painless, this range, even though limited, has a distinct advantage over the arthrodesed joint and is especially worthwhile when the other knee is affected. It is easier to sit and dress, and the patients are content if able to walk to a car and to drive.

In recent years new techniques of arthroplasty have evolved, with increasing success. Following the progress in hip replacement, we have graduated from interposition of soft tissue and foreign materials through partial to total joint replacement. The special problems and difficulties that beset total replacement of the knee in its early stages have to a great extent been overcome. With the more advanced prosthesis in experienced hands, over 90° of painless and stable movement may be expected. Instead of the stiff knee, which in older patients is a serious handicap, there is promise of enough function "to carry, to comfort, and to supplicate," and hopefully eventually to "propel."

The perfect knee replacement device would have the following characteristics:

1. Replace normal movement or at least 120 degrees of flexion with approximately 13 degrees of synchronous rotation. It is not necessary to restore or replace the anatomy if a smaller and less cumbersome insert will reproduce normal function.
2. Have provision for joint stability inherent in its design and independent of the cruciate ligaments.
3. Be inserted with minimal removal of articular surface. This ensures that if it fails or loosens, it may be changed, or as a final resort the joint may be salvaged by arthrodesis.
4. Be of durable materials that articulate with minimal friction.
5. Be technically simple to insert.
6. Permit retention of the patella.

REFERENCES

1. **Balazs EA, Rydell NW:** Effect of hyaluronic acid on adhesion formation (in press)
2. **Bennett GE:** Preliminary report of lengthening of the quadriceps tendon. J Orthop Surg 1:530, 1919
3. **Bennett GE:** Lengthening of the quadriceps tendon. J Bone Joint Surg 4:279, 1922
4. **Charnley J:** The Closed Treatment of Common Fractures. London, Livingstone, 1957
5. **Jones Sir Robert:** Notes on Military Orthopaedics. London, Cassell, 1918
6. **Thompson TC:** Quadricepsplasty to improve knee function. J Bone Joint Surg 26:366, 1944

CHAPTER 28
OSTEOCHONDRAL FRACTURES OF THE ARTICULAR SURFACES OF THE KNEE

Joseph E. Milgram

Compared with meniscal derangements, osteochondral fractures occur relatively infrequently. However, they are by no means rare, and diagnosis is not particularly difficult. Early recognition permits prompt and often complete repair.

Osteochondral fractures of the knee result from direct application of external forces (impact, crush; impact shear) or indirect application of muscular and gravitational forces.

FRACTURE BY DIRECT INJURY

There are, to be sure, fractures of the articular surfaces that are sustained through direct injury, such as a violent blow striking the knee. Such fractures are often severe, for a whole condyle may be separated or crushed (Plate 28-1). The roentgenogram will point to the mechanism of injury—direct impact or extreme leverage.

They benefit in most instances from open accurate reposition and substantial metallic fixation (Plates 28-2, 28-3). Motion is subsequently commenced in bed with the limb suspended in a snugly fitted, hinged, long-leg plaster cast. This second plaster is applied 4 to 5 weeks after operation. Weight-bearing is delayed until the revascularization of bone underlying the articular surfaces is judged complete.

FRACTURE BY INDIRECT FORCES

Such forces expressed through excessive ligamentous tensions produced by motion, gravity, or muscular contraction are common in athletics.

INDIRECT FRACTURE BY AVULSION

A typical avulsion of the anterior **crucial** ligament may carry off with it a large osteochondral portion of the articular surface of the tibia, including the tibial spines. Such a segment, when fastened back securely into its tibial defect by a long screw or, better, by an encircling wire suture that passes through two drill channels from the anterior tibial cortex, and with the leg subsequently adequately immobilized in a plaster cast, usually heals well. The bony cortex unites, and the narrow clefts fill with fibrocartilage, restoring both articular and ligamentous function.

CONDYLE–TIBIAL SPINE CONTACT AFTER TIBIAL AVULSION

Yet in just such a lesion in a 10-year-old boy, after accurate replacement and securely retained screw fixation of the articular segment and tibial spines, there developed, with growth, a gradual local enlargement of both tibial spines. Seven years later it was found that the enlarged medial tibial spine was now

contacting the medial femoral condyle and had created a large condylar lesion containing a free body. Roentgenographic studies clearly revealed that the contact was made when the knee was in slight flexion and abduction of the leg or when the patient pivoted on the knee with the foot fixed on the ground (Plate 28-4). Normal adolescents may manifest surprising rotational ranges (Fig. 28-1).

In a normal cadaver's knee, experimentally produced contact between the tibial spine and the lateral surface of the medial femoral condyle was demonstrated by implantation of a series of electrical contacts flush with these two areas and rotating the femur inward in slight flexion and abduction. When rotated, the circuit was completed, and a light in the series circuit regularly flashed on contact (Fig. 28-2).

Condyle–spine contact is certainly the

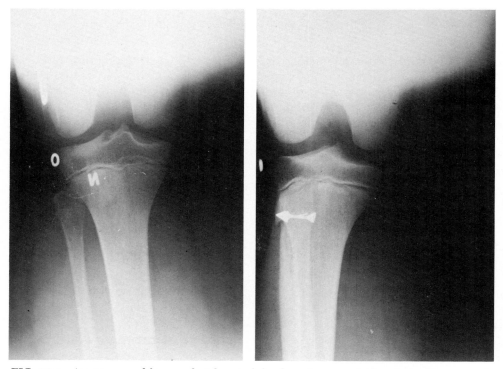

FIG. 28-1. An 11-year-old normal girl seated, leg hanging over table edge with a curved cardboard cassette underneath knee and leg: (*left*) anteroposterior view. (*Right*) On passive external rotation of the leg, fibular position measures the degree of rotation of the leg on the fixed femur.

cause of so-called osteochondritis dissecans in some patients. It has been blamed repeatedly by older authors, and correctly so in certain cases, such as the special example related above. In six other osteochondritis dissecans lesions occurring in our patients with no similar gross enlargement of the tibial spines, contact was suggested on x-ray studies during rotatory knee motions.

PATELLAR MARGINAL AVULSIONS, MUSCULAR OR TENDINOUS

Avulsion lesions of the cortical margins of the patella may require oblique and tangential roentgenograms of both knees for diagnosis and may need local excision if immobilization fails to relieve pain. Occasionally avulsion includes portions of the articular cartilage. Then bony reduction and open fixation may offer a desirable reattachment of quadriceps or ligamentum patellae.

OSTEOCHONDRAL FRACTURES BY PATELLAR IMPACT

Osteochondral fractures of the knee are not uncommon and as a rule are sustained by adolescents or young adults. They are almost invariably the consequence of indirect injury, of apparently excessive forces developed by a twist of the knee in either the erect or the flexed position during the course of violent athletics or energetic dancing. Most of the patients are limber and supple but otherwise normal. Rarely does a history of either previous knee disability or substantial injury exist.

Kroner, in 1904, reported the case of a 31-year-old woman who fell running and sustained a vertical frontal fracture of the patella.[5] The entire patella split into two frontal sections during a lateral dislocation. Subsequently, an "oyster shell fracture" was described by Villar in 1921.[14] "Verticofrontal fractures" were reported by Kleinberg[4] in 1923 and Lettloff in 1928.[6] Kleinberg suggested that a fall on the knee, forcing the patella downward against the femur, could

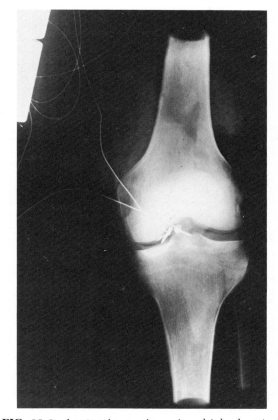

FIG. 28-2. Anatomic specimen in which electrical contacts, installed flush with the surface of the medial tibial spine and adjacent condyle, repeatedly demonstrated that electrical contact was completed when tibia rotated and abducted in the position of slight flexion of the knee.

shove or scrape off part of the articular surface, and later he described a lateral dislocation of the patella without fracture in which the medial border of the patella remained caught for 5 days on the femoral condyle.

The term tangential osteochondral fracture of the patella was introduced by Milgram[7] in 1943 to describe the nature of the forces involved in the mechanism of production of patellofemoral articular injuries.[8]

TANGENTIAL MECHANISM OF FRACTURE

As the knee is extended with the foot off the ground, the tibia rotates externally on the

VARIETIES OF INDIRECT OSTEOCHONDRAL FRACTURES OF THE KNEE

Fractures following spontaneous reduction of lateral dislocation of patella

1. Tangential osteochondral fracture of patella—acute.
2. Tangential chondral injury of patella and/or femoral groove for patella—recurrent.
3. Tangential osteochondral fracture of lateral femoral condyle—acute and recurrent.
4. Tangential compression fracture of lateral condylar wall—acute.

Fractures following tibiofemoral stresses

5. Cleft (or shell) osteochondral separation of femur (cartilage intact) initially—acute.
6. Osteochondral fracture (or erosion) (a) Following impingements of tibial spine, recurrent; some called "osteochondritis dissecans." (b) Meniscal lesion sequels.
7. Massive, pyramidal osteochondral fracture of medial femoral condyle—acute.
8. Posterior transcondylar fracture of medial femoral condyle—acute.
9. Posterior osteochondral fracture and irregular ossification of one or both femoral condyles.

Pathologic osteochondral fractures of known etiology

10. Osteochondral poststeroid fracture, medial femoral condyle.
11. Osteochondral poststeroid fracture, medial tibial condyle.
12. Osteochondral infraction, over subarticular area of cancellous weakening of many etiologies, local and general.

Pathologic osteochondral fractures of unknown etiology

13. Occasional varieties of osteochondritis dissecans in areas seemingly removed from likely trauma (cf. 6).

femur (see Chap. 1). If the foot is fixed on the ground, the tibia is fixed and the femur rotates. It rotates internally as the knee extends, bringing the lateral condyle anteriorly. If at this moment the quadriceps has contracted, it holds the patella while the lateral condyle glides internally beneath the patella. In relaxed knees the lateral condyle passes completely medial to the patella. As the quadriceps continues to tighten, the medial edge of the patellar articular surface engages the lateral articular edge of the lateral condyle of the femur. The patella is now momentarily fixed in the position of lateral dislocation. The exact area of engagement of the contiguous articular surfaces of the patella and the femoral condyle depends on the position of the knee in which the engagement has taken place.

As a rule, the accident occurs when the foot is fixed on the ground while the thigh twists or pivots medially on the fixed tibia. As the great quadriceps contracts, further extension of the knee is impeded by the fixed foot. Consequently, all of the quadriceps force is transformed into a medially directed force (tangential) that shoves the dislocated patella against the edge, the lateral wall, or the articular distal surface of the lateral condyle, depending on the degree of knee flexion.

The osteochondral separations result from this forcible impact of the dislocated patella on the lateral femoral condyle as the patella forcibly reduces itself from its lateral position. In other words, the patellar "hammer" may break in striking a glancing blow against the "anvil" of the lateral femoral condyle, thus creating a patellar osteochondral free body. In other cases the anvil is chipped or even crushed by the patellar hammer wielded by the powerful quadriceps.

Aside from these major and violent injuries, more subtle but also lasting damage may be inflicted on the patella and the lateral femoral condyle. The articular cartilage of the patella may be abraded, contused, split at the margins, or separated from its bony bed over a large area without becoming completely dislodged. Such loosened cartilaginous areas may not heal securely and later may undergo degeneration—so-called chondromalacia. Therefore, it may be difficult in later months or years to distinguish the changes that follow a single trauma from those of cumulative character due to innumerable traumas caused by imperfect kinesiologic construction, that is, the consequences of abnormal motion of the patella in congenital or recurrent subluxation and dislocation, or in back-knee, knock-knee, or ligamentous instability.

THE MANNER OF PRODUCTION OF OSTEOCHONDRAL FRACTURES OF THE PATELLA

The histories elicited from adolescents who have sustained osteochondral fracture of the patella indicate that dislocation and osteochondral fracture of the patella both occur in the phase of active extension of the knee—viz.:

1. A young female dancer doing a "split" slowly sank toward the floor with both knees in full extension when two "tears" took place, "a noise accompanying the second tearing pain." The knee swelled at once, and operation revealed both the typical medial inferior quadrant defect of the patella and the lateral condylar scrape.

2. A skater swinging into a turn on an extended knee slid the skate into a deep linear fissure in the ice and twisted on the fixed limb. Just before he fell, he felt a break and heard a loud breaking sound, with instant severe pain. Operation performed a few days later confirmed the osteochondral loss of the medial inferior quadrant of the patella and an abraded lateral condyle of the femur.

3. A boy trying to reach a shower wall-control above his head, while standing with legs spread widely, twisted and sustained instant disabling pain followed by immediate swelling. Still standing, he was assisted from the shower stall. Operation 2 days later confirmed similar lesions.

4. Another boy engaged in "Indian wrestling" with a comrade. As both stood with arms engaged, legs fully extended with feet

ACUTE LESIONS DUE TO PATELLOFEMORAL IMPACT

1. Tangential osteochondral fracture of patellar articular surface—free body comprising lower medial quadrant (Plate 28-5; Figs. 28-3, 28-4, 28-5, 28-6).

2. Chondral shredding (Fig. 28-5) or chondral separation from patella—small or giant blister (Fig. 28-5). "One-time" chondromalacia, Koenig. (See Fig. 28-18.)

3. Tangential osteochondral fracture of lateral femoral condyle

   A. Large, thin, curved free body or bodies, much cartilage, usually little bone (Figs. 28-7 to 28-14; Plate 28-6).

   B. Compression fracture of lateral condylar wall—depressed, extruding part of articular surface of the lateral condyle as a hinged osteochondral segment (see Figs. 28-15 to 28-20).

4. Reciprocal injuries to articular cartilage and opposing bone in the form of contusions, abrasions, and intracartilaginous hematomas (knee joint blood trapped between the peripheral tangential and the deeper columnar layers of cells of the articular cartilage) producing blood-stained cartilage that cannot be wiped clean at operation. It should be kept in mind that injuries to avascular articular cartilage that do not extend deeply enough to reach the vascular layer of the cortex simply do not repair themselves. Only the cartilage cleft that reaches blood will fill with clot that repairs by fibrocartilage that in time may resemble hyaline cartilage. Superficial cartilage abrasions and tabs will gradually break free, leaving damaged gliding surfaces. The most superficial layers of normal cartilage are tangentially disposed to facilitate gliding.

widely separated, the patient twisted his knee forcibly, with instant disabling pain. Still standing, the knee extended, he was helped to a couch. The knee swelled rapidly, and operation soon after revealed the typical patellar loss and the condylar contusion.

As a rule, patients who are suddenly stricken are flexible but not "double jointed" when surveyed later for evidence of joint hypermobility. Nor is there usually evidence of knock-knee or bowleg. Passive rotation of the flexed tibia on the femur seemed to be excessive in some patients but not in the majority.

OSTEOCHONDRAL FRACTURES IN RECURRENT DISLOCATION OF PATELLA

Most instances of osteochondral fracture of the patella occurred in patients who had not suffered previous dislocation of the knee. However, three of our patients recorded a history of numerous painless subluxations or dislocations in the past. With these exceptions, no knee with fresh osteochondral fractures revealed evidence of previous damage at operation.

After recurrent dislocation of the patella, the lateral condyle of the femur and considerable areas of the patella may undergo degenerative changes characterized by softening and shredding (see Figs. 28-9, 28-17).

Each of three adolescent females, after numerous lateral subluxations and dislocations during the course of many years, suddenly underwent a memorable episode in which very severe pain and a cracking sound accompanied the replacement of the dislocated patella. The knee at once distended with blood, and in two cases well-marked cutaneous linear hematomas that developed medial to the patella indicated medial capsule rupture. At the operations performed several months later, it was seen that osteochondral separation of the inferior quadrant of the medial surface of the patella had been sustained in each

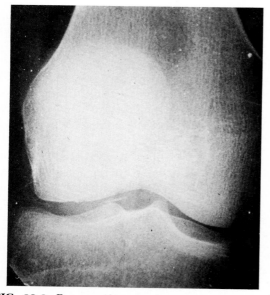

FIG. 28-3. Preoperative roentgenogram—a pencil line of fragment of cortex is visible at the tibial spine.

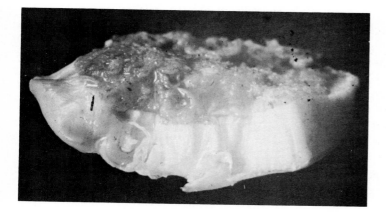

FIG. 28-4. A free body, avulsed from normal cartilage and bone, is characterized by the appearance of "palisading" (columnar lines of split cartilage). In addition, the appearance of the "chef's hat" (an adherent rim of the tangential layer avulsed from adjacent normal articular cartilage) is present early.

FIG. 28-5. Tangential forces have made glacial scratches in the body. The probe enters a cartilage blister.

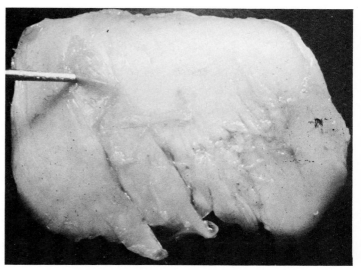

FIG. 28-6. Extensive acute tangential osteochondral fracture of the patella. Sole example in our series of a lesion so severe that it necessitates primary patellectomy.

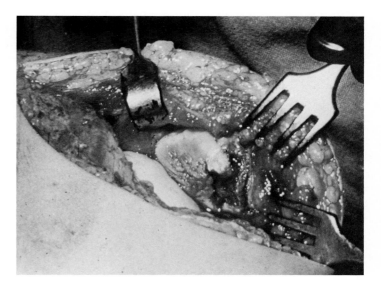

case. Also, the edge of the lateral femoral condyle was fissured and abraded, the gliding condylar surface was lusterless, and the lateral synovia was scarred. In each of the three the patellar loose body was removed. In two, medial capsular elongation of considerable degree was present. Subsequently, no pain or swelling was suffered, even though each patient resumed subluxation. Reparative reconstruction proferred later has not been accepted to date.

CASE HISTORIES OF TANGENTIAL OSTEOCHONDRAL FRACTURES OF THE LATERAL FEMORAL CONDYLE

Detailed histories of adolescents who sustained osteochondral fractures of the lateral femoral condyle indicate that possibly the patellar dislocation and certainly the femoral condylar fracture had occurred during the phase of considerable flexion of the knee, contrasting with the histories of fracture in exten-

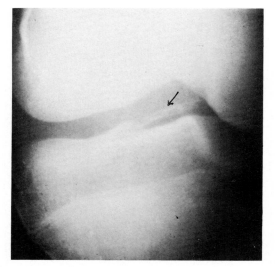

FIG. 28-7. This roentgenogram was made on admitting a patient with an osteochondral fracture of the lateral condyle made by impact of the patella. The double line of the fragment is visible on the anteroposterior view (*arrow*).

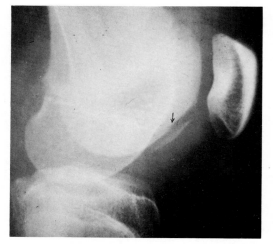

FIG. 28-8. Superficial defect is visible (*arrow*) on this lateral view of the lateral femoral condyle above a free fragment.

sion obtained in cases of patellar tangential osteochondral fracture—*viz.*:

1. A 16-year-old boy was crouching in a football game when he was tackled as he lunged forward. He twisted his bent knee, sustained instant knee pain and disability, and remained with the knee bent until he was carried off the field for medical attention. A large fresh segment of the weight-bearing surface of the lateral femoral condyle lay free in the joint. The patella was badly abraded, contused, and hemorrhagic.

2. An 18-year-old boy was squatting and leaning forward during a football game. As he projected himself forward forcibly, a player seized his ankle, fixing it to the ground. He twisted and felt instant "pain and tearing" in the knee. Disability was immediate. Operation 10 hours later revealed a fresh osteochondral fracture of the external femoral condyle. The patellar articular surface also was severely damaged, its cartilage having been loosened from its cortical bony attachment over a large area. The lateral condylar wall was the site of a depressed fracture (Figs. 28-14 to 28-20).

DIAGNOSIS IN FRESH CASES OF PATELLOFEMORAL INJURY

The history is suggestive, and as a rule diagnosis is not difficult. The knee is distended with blood, and the patient is usually unable to hold the knee actively extended or to activate the quadriceps strongly. The aspirated blood may contain fat droplets, particularly if an osteochondral body is visible on roentgenograms.

ROENTGENOGRAPHIC FINDINGS IN OSTEOCHONDRAL FRACTURES

Roentgenographic study is helpful in most cases. Usually only anteroposterior, posteroanterior, oblique and lateral views are possible, for the knee cannot be flexed without pain.

Patellar fragments, while occasionally based with a thick layer of bone (when they are easily seen on the lateral plate and when a corresponding defect is seen in the lower third of the patella in the lateral view), may be

FIG. 28-9. With the knee in extension, the condylar lesion is not exposed in tangential femoral lesions. Only the patella shows evidence of injurious contact.

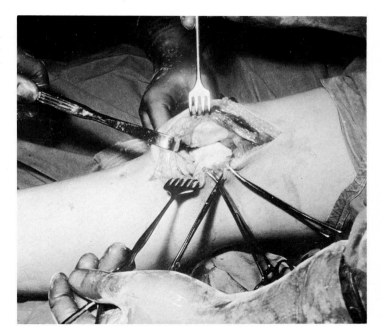

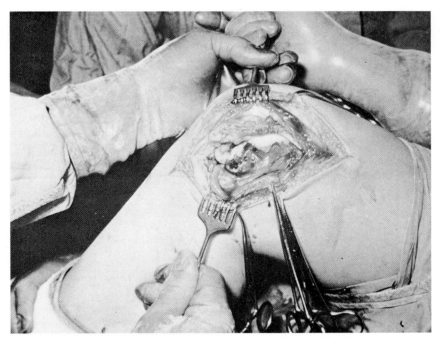

FIG. 28-10. With the knee flexed to 110° of extension, the condylar lesion is now visible (compare Fig. 28-9). Lateral condylar defect and free body lying anteriorly are seen. This indicates degree of flexion needed for patella to contact femoral condyle to produce distal lateral condylar articular surface avulsion.

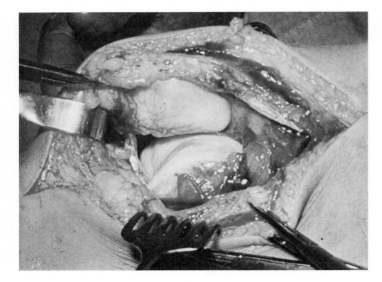

FIG. 28-11. A close-up view of the patella with the knee in extension reveals fresh, extensive loosening of normal cartilage from the bony bed. Hemorrhagic synovitis of the lateral condylar synovia is visible. The free body is seen tipped on edge at the left beneath the pole of the patella.

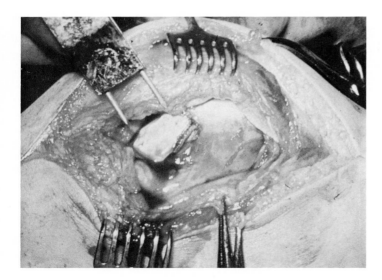

FIG. 28-12. A free fragment from a tangential osteochrondral fracture is replaced and is stapled into the defect on the lateral condyle. Knee is in flexion.

difficult to distinguish at first glance. However, if one studies the anteroposterior plate, one can usually see a pencil line of cortical bone ⅜ to ½ in long lying in the joint space between the condyles. Then, checking back on the patellar cortex in the lateral view, one can make out a marginal cortical irregularity of ½ in of the patellar articular surface matching the pencil line that marks the thick osteochondral body.

Femoral fragments are especially interesting because they usually arise from the curved distal end of the femur and consequently are curved and may include the groove for the lateral meniscus. The shadow of the body is projected as either a curved line (Fig. 28-21) or in the form of two lines with the ends overlapping (see Fig. 28-12). This type of shadow is pathognomonic of the lesion. Sometimes it is easier to distinguish the fragment on the an-

PLATE 28-1. Knee crushed by impact.

PLATE 28-2. Test of condylar replacement and matching of articular segments.

PLATE 28-3. Multiple screw fixation (clipped short for subsequent removal by threaded pin extractor).

PLATE 28-4. Condylar erosion and a free body arose from tibial spine—medial condyle contact.

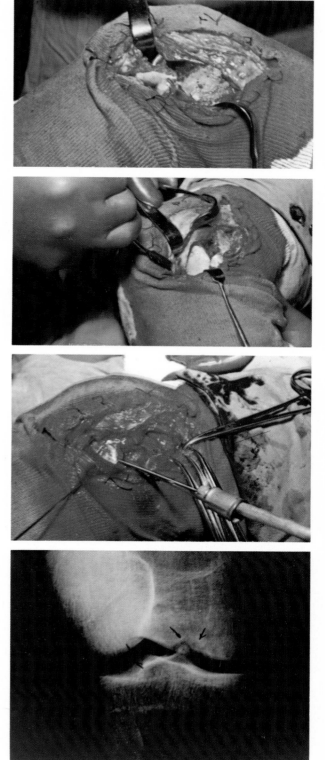

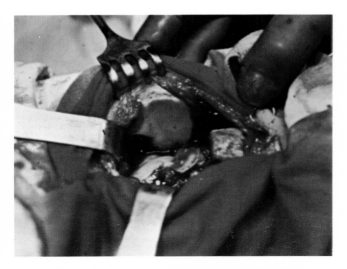

PLATE 28-5. In this view of a tangential osteochondral fracture of the patella an inferomedial quadrant defect is seen on the retracted patella. There is a free quadrangular body on the right. The external condyle is traumatized and hemorrhagic.

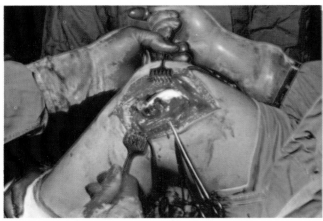

PLATE 28-6. With the knee flexed the femoral lesion is exposed. (Compare this with Fig. 28-9.) The patella is retracted, indicating degree of flexion necessary for patella to contact femoral condyle to produce tangential fracture of lateral condylar articular surface.

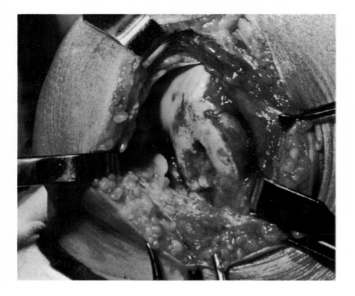

PLATE 28-7. Cortisone osteochondritis dissecans of femur. Typical appearance of ulceration of medial condyle. The cartilage lid lies partly visible to the left of the ulcer. Note ball-like contents. Woman, age 67. History of biweekly intra-articular injections of steroids over a 4-month period administered for calcification of the menisci. Fairly comfortable and surprisingly mobile at time of exploratory operation 3 months later.

FIG. 28-13. The knee was immobilized in a noncontact position of flexion until staple was removed 8 weeks later. Firm precise union was achieved, and the knee continued to be symptomless 2 years later.

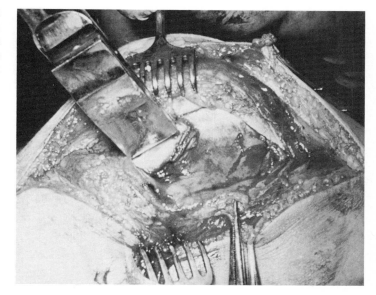

FIG. 28-14. Another variety of acute osteochondral fracture of the lateral femoral condyle is that in which the lateral subchondral table or wall of the condyle is compressed and hence depressed by patellar impact, bursting the articular surface. A clot fills the depression of the compressed condyle.

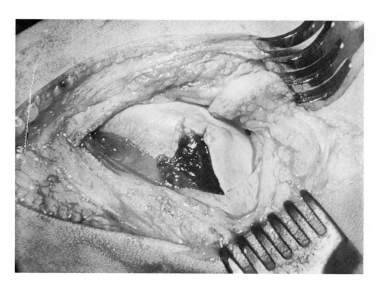

teroposterior than on the lateral view, although at times detection is impossible because of the minimal cortical avulsion that may accompany a thick cartilaginous fragment. When apparent, the defect in the cortical contour of the lateral femoral condyle also shows best on the anteroposterior view.

DEPRESSED FRACTURES OF LATERAL SURFACE OF LATERAL FEMORAL CONDYLE ASSOCIATED WITH OSTEOCHONDRAL FRACTURE OF ARTICULAR SURFACE

Depressed fractures of the lateral condylar wall from the "hammer of the patella" are easily discerned in the anteroposterior view as

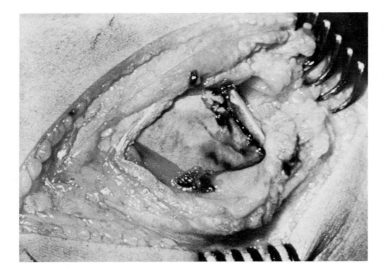

FIG. 28-15. After the clot has been removed, the depressed lateral condylar wall visibly displaces the articular surface forward out of line, necessitating its reduction and fixation.

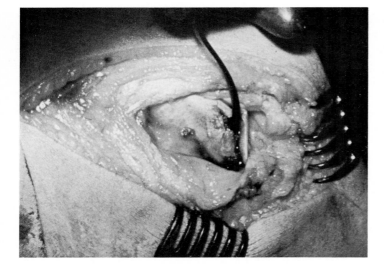

FIG. 28-16. Reduction of the articular surface—a skid levers out the depressed outer table of the femoral condyle to permit fitting the articular surface back in place.

depressions of the lateral wall of the condyle. The condylar articular surface may be undermined. Comparison with the normal knee makes the diagnosis clear. At operation the depressed segment needs to be elevated before the articular surface can be restored in contour. Delayed weight-bearing is desirable, since the cancellous structure must repair and consolidate if late flattening by such stressing is to be avoided (see Fig. 28-19).

EARLY TREATMENT OF OSTEOCHONDRAL FRACTURES DUE TO PATELLAR IMPACT

Early and ideal treatment is possible only if the diagnosis is made promptly after injury.

Patella

Usually the free body is small enough to discard without danger to the patellofemoral joint. The edges of the defect should be shaved slightly, and shreds should be trimmed if they threaten to become free

FIG. 28-17. Displaced articular segment is stapled back into accurate alignment. It is immobilized for 8 weeks thereafter, when staple is removed.

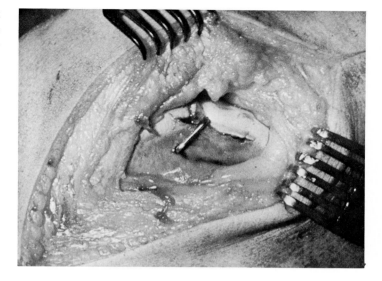

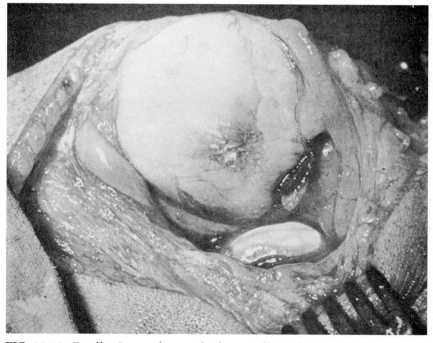

FIG. 28-18. Patella. Severe damage both centrally and at 5 o'clock position is visible. Centrally, articular cartilage has been loosened from its osseous attachment and otherwise traumatized.

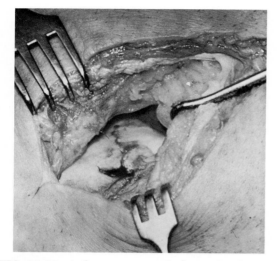

FIG. 28-19. Arthrotomy 8 weeks later. Staple is removed. Union of condylar fragments by fibrocartilage. A small subchondral defect persists—an indication to delay weight-bearing until condylar reconstitution is demonstrable on X-ray studies. Otherwise the condyle may flatten subsequently.

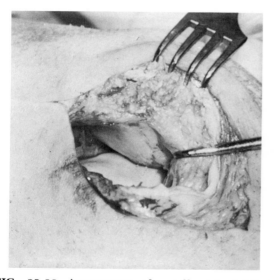

FIG. 28-20. Appearance of patella (at right) 8 weeks later. Cartilage irregularities still are visible at the lower pole of the patella.

bodies subsequently. Very rarely is patellectomy indicated, and then only in the case of virtually complete frontal plane decortication of the patella. Even then, in the young patient a trial of soft tissue flap covering might be considered. In an appropriate case the loose body, if not too thick to revascularize, may be fastened or stapled back into place. I have not replaced a patellar free body.

Femoral Condyle

A fairly large fresh osteochondral free body from the weight-bearing surface of the lateral femoral condyle carrying a layer of cortex should be replaced and secured in its original site. It should be protected for 3 months or more against contact or weight stresses by a cast applied in adequate flexion (checked by roentgenography if necessary). After union has been achieved, and any staple or nails removed, motion without weight-bearing is commenced. To prevent late flattening by compression of the condyle at the site of reimplantation, walking on this limb should be forbidden for 3 months after removal of the splint. To be sure, a stainless steel staple requires removal later, but it provides maximal fixation, and the second arthrotomy for its removal permits one to judge the repair achieved and to decide whether or not the patient may safely commence weight-bearing. The patella also may need minimal trimming of shreds arising from impact sites.

If the outer table of the femoral condyle is fractured and depressed, it must be levered out before the exploded hinged articular osteochondral segment can be pressed back into line with the rest of the articular surface (Figs. 28-14 to 28-20). A staple stabilizes the realigned table and the hinged articular segment while healing is progressing. The dead space beneath the once compressed and now elevated area must fill in before full weight-bearing on the area will be tolerated without late compression (Fig. 28-19).

LATE TREATMENT OF OSTEOCHONDRAL FRACTURES WITH SEPARATED BODIES

Fracture lesions of the patella or lateral condyle diagnosed months late (Figs. 28-22 and 28-23) are treated by removing the free body, because body and bed have undergone alteration and revascularization, and firm reattachment in good alignment is not likely. Furthermore, in fractures the site of the avulsed condylar segment is often surprisingly well repaired by slightly irregular fibrocartilaginous scar. Questionable lesions are those in which the area of loss is extensive, because the area usually corresponds to an area of condyle directly stressed in weight-bearing. I have no personal information on the results of late operative reimplantation of freshened old lateral femoral osteochondral grafts. Unfortunately, both cartilage cells and bone of specimens 6 weeks and 3 months after traumatic separation have at times been found to be nonviable despite their continuous immersion in joint fluid. Yet, if the cartilage appears to be relatively good, a thin layer of bone is present, and the site of projected implantation is as yet poorly covered, the experiment may be justified in special cases of fractures, particularly since freshening, drilling, and nail replacement have been successful in selected cases of osteochondritis dissecans of the medial condyle.[14]

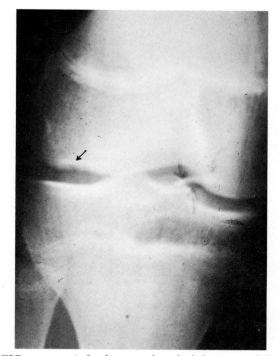

FIG. 28-21. A fresh osteochondral fracture of the lateral condyle. Curved free body (*arrows*). Defect origin is visible in the lateral femoral condyle (*small arrow*).

OSTEOCHONDRAL LESIONS OF MEDIAL AND FEMORAL CONDYLES DUE TO TIBIOFEMORAL CONTACT

Other condylar injuries, rarer and less well understood, follow forceful twists or violent pivoting of the femoral condyle on the contiguous tibia. These lesions affect the middle and the more posterior surfaces of the condyles well away from possible patellar contact. The medial femoral condyle with a longer excursion than the lateral seems to be particularly vulnerable.

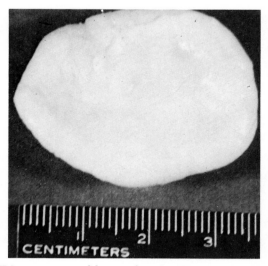

FIG. 28-22. An old osteochondral fracture (6 weeks) of the patellar body. Indistinguishable from osteochondritis dissecans of other than traumatic origin.

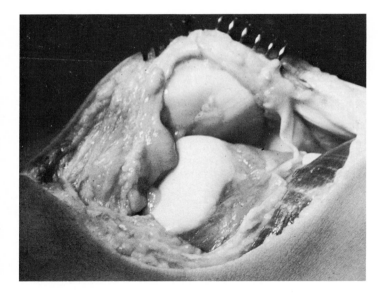

FIG. 28-23. A 9-month-old osteochondral fracture of the patella. Defect visible at site of origin on patella. "Osteochondritis dissecans" body lies above septum in opened suprapatellar pouch recess.

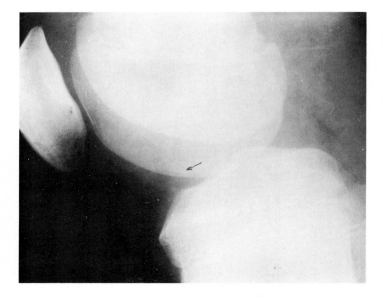

FIG. 28-24. Osteochondral cleft of the condyle was caused by sudden tibiofemoral crushing force of pivotal character (twist). Note the cleft (*arrow*) 10 hours after a dance injury (lateral view). Cleft must be sought. It is corroborated then on a flexion lateral view.

OSTEOCHONDRAL CLEFT IN THE MEDIAL FEMORAL CONDYLE

A singularly significant lesion—one that is probably of considerable clinical import and easily overlooked soon after injury—is the localized separation of the articular cartilage together with a thin, bony subchondral plate as the result of a single twist of the knee. It is followed by ache but not effusion. Only x-ray evidence of a pencil line that denotes a subcortical ½-in long cleft, with or without a tiny notch through the subchondral plate, enables the physician to recognize the site of a future osteochondral body (Figs. 28-24, 28-25).

The cleft is localized on two lateral films, one made with the knee extended and the other in flexion. Localization not only helps in reconstructing the probable position of the knee at the time of injury but suggests a position for immobilization in which further tibiofemoral contact may be avoided. This is the very time when immediate institution of complete rest and freedom from tibial contact will offer the femur the opportunity of rapid and full repair. The well-vascularized cancellous bone cleft will anchor the articular cartilage securely if it is immobilized for a sufficiently long period of time. In other words, incomplete fractures are denoted by a narrow bone cleft paralleling the condylar contour. A niche indicates that a cortical break may have occurred as well.

This traumatic lesion is undoubtedly one mechanism responsible for the subsequent production of shell-like osteochondritis dissecans. A careful search for this lesion may reveal that it is less rare than our present experience indicates. We have seen this lesion in three knees and in one ankle (lower tibia, bordering on upper surface of astragalus). In one knee a traumatic cleft lesion was not recognized, and the patient was treated with intra-articular steroids, whereupon a localized destructive lesion developed at the site, necessitating arthrotomy, which revealed a large, broken-down, ulcerated lesion of the femoral condyle.

OSTEOCHONDRAL CLEFT IN MEDIAL FEMORAL CONDYLE FOLLOWING A VIOLENT TWIST

A tall, rangy lad of 12 years dancing "the twist" in August 1962 crouched and twisted violently on the flexed knee when "something moved in the knee, and I think the kneecap jumped sideways. It hurt a lot but it did not swell much. I've been limping the past 10 days since then." Roentgenograms revealed a tiny notch or infraction of the cortex of the medial femoral condyle and a ½-in long subcortical cleft (Figs. 28-24, 28-25) indicative of incomplete localized avulsion of the cartilaginous surface of the condyle. The knee was placed in a plaster cast in considerable flexion, and he walked with crutches. The cleft filled with bone in 4 weeks, and clinically and roentgenologically the fragment reanchored. In 7 weeks the cancellous trabeculae regained

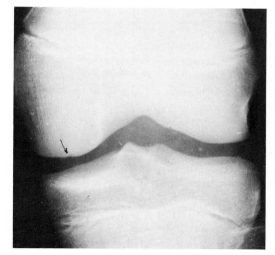

FIG. 28-25. Note notch in medial femoral condyle (*arrow*) (anteroposterior view).

normal configuration and retained this on follow-up roentgenograms.

An opportunity was afforded 11 years later to examine the site and appearance of the cleft healing in this patient when a bucket-handle fracture of the medial meniscus necessitated meniscectomy. The cleft site was oval, roughly ½ in long, and glistening. It was barely discernible, except for a slightly bluish tint in an otherwise glistening white medial femoral condyle.

TRAUMATIC MASSIVE OSTEOCHONDRAL FRACTURES OF THE POSTERIOR PORTION OF THE MEDIAL CONDYLES

We have seen two patients in whom large, thick pyramidal sections of the medial condyles separated after sudden severe trauma of the pivotal type. In one the sharply punched-out fragment of fresh bone and articular cartilage was ⅜ in thick, 1¼ in long, and ½ in wide. It is hard to understand the mechanism capable of producing a fracture fragment of this shape and relatively large size. Pivotal forces could conceivably be responsible, but no conclusive evidence has been obtained.

An even larger fragment separated in a 15-year-old girl. Her knee had been strapped into a reducing apparatus designed to produce automatic flexions and extensions of the knee by electrically stimulating the thigh muscles. Sudden excruciating knee pain occurred during a flexion motion, and when the repeatedly flexing knee was freed from the machine (and the patient revived) a large fresh fracture of almost the entire posterior portion of the medial femoral condyle was apparent. The fragment did not unite, and surgical removal of a body $1.25 \times 0.5 \times 0.7$ in has provided complete relief of pain. No signs of arthritis were present at follow-up 12 years after injury.

Kennedy[3] in 1966 reported the experimental production of several types of osteochondral fractures of each femoral condyle by combined rotation and compression forces in a "stress machine."

It seems reasonable to expect that if other, more complex motions of the knee could be simulated and tested on the cadaver under various excessive stresses, we would gain increased insight into the pathologic physiology that produces other clinical varieties encountered. Some of these lesions have not been recognized as traumatic in the past.

OSTEOCHONDRITIS DISSECANS

Osteochondritis dissecans is diagnosed when a segment of articular cartilage and underlying cortex of varying size and thickness separates from the host bone without apparent cause. Osteochondral fractures, particularly old ones, may be incorrectly so diagnosed, but as a rule the locality and the history differentiate the lesions. In others the history may implicate trauma (direct or indirect) but only occasionally conclusively—for example, when at operation tibial spine contact is demonstrable or a fragment from the medial femoral condyle is found attached to fibers of the posterior cruciate ligament. However, in most cases, traumatic etiology cannot be established. Infarction is a possible mechanism, but convincing proof is also lacking.

The lesion tends to occur in adolescents and is usually insidious. Discomfort may attract interest to the knee, or the first symptoms may be due to intermittent mechanical obstructions to motion due to a mobile free body. The patient may palpate "a bean" at times. During long intervals a loose body may remain lodged posteriorly or may come to lie anteriorly in a recess in the suprapatellar pouch separated from the joint by a valved septum (Figs. 28-23, 28-26).

Other cases may be diagnosed roentgenographically before separation has developed. In most instances these cases heal with prolonged noncontact and non–weight-bearing immobilization, and consequently, diagnosis in this stage is most desirable (Fig. 28-27; see also Chap. 8).

Not infrequently, the lesion is bilateral and often symmetrically located. Consequently, both knees should always be surveyed.

Roentgenograms should be taken in numer-

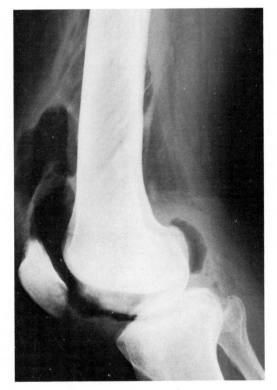

FIG. 28-26. Suprapatellar pouch, recess septum, and communication. Pneumoarthrogram.

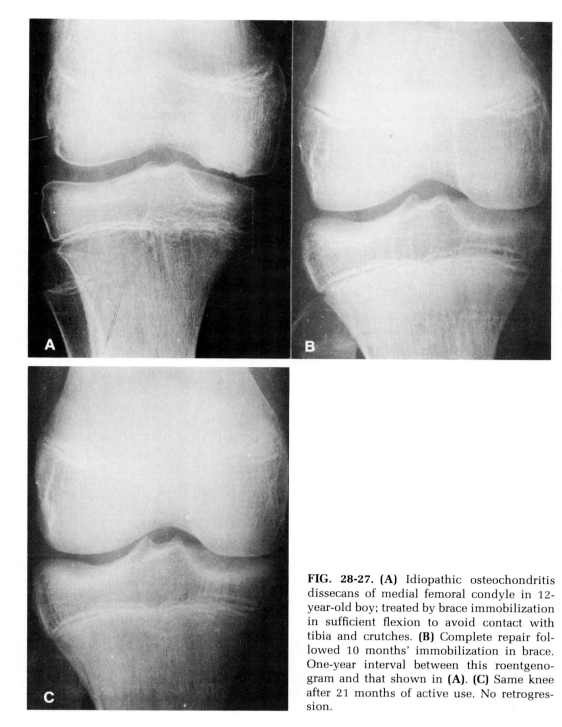

FIG. 28-27. (A) Idiopathic osteochondritis dissecans of medial femoral condyle in 12-year-old boy; treated by brace immobilization in sufficient flexion to avoid contact with tibia and crutches. **(B)** Complete repair followed 10 months' immobilization in brace. One-year interval between this roentgenogram and that shown in **(A)**. **(C)** Same knee after 21 months of active use. No retrogression.

ous positions. Not only should anteroposterior and lateral views be obtained, but posteroanterior and tangential views may reveal sites of pathology not otherwise visible.

Because tibiofemoral and patellofemoral impact trauma should be considered among possible causes for the symptoms, ligamentous stability of the knee joint should be tested carefully at rest and when stressed as back knee. Elbow and wrists are also surveyed for laxity.

The appearance of osteochondritis dissecans in young children may also be produced by localized disturbances in condylar ossification. These have been observed to clear up spontaneously at times without treatment.[12] In general, however, in the presence of roentgenographic evidence of localized condylar fragmentation, treatment should be instituted, particularly in children past 10 years of age.

Lesions of the posterior portions of the condyles, best seen on anteroposterior views, have been seen to heal in 6 to 12 months, often with use of braces that restrict area contact on these condylar sites.

Often roentgenographic findings indicative of femoral subcortical osseous separation are associated with operative findings of intact articular cartilage. Consequently, it is not desirable to excise the osseous lesion. Prolonged immobilization in a position evading contact with the tibia has been rewarded in many cases by disappearance of the lesion (Fig. 28-27). This advice by Green[2] and Banks[2] and others has been confirmed by us repeatedly.

Even when the bone of the fragment has apparently been completely separated and appreciably displaced by the defect it may incorporate and heal back into place; in two instances it left as a sequel a bony prominence on the condyle. In one of these cases (Fig. 28-28) the condylar prominence was seen to displace the patella sufficiently so that by contact with the edge of the femoral condyle as the knee flexed and extended a reciprocal furrow had been gouged longitudinally in the articular cartilage of the patella extending from its upper to its lower pole (Fig. 28-29).

Such persistent local prominence on healing is rather conclusive evidence that the lesion was indeed a true separation and not merely an anomaly of ossification. The fact that radiographic lesions, almost regardless of age and state of epiphyseal maturity, so often respond to 4 to 12 months of immobilization by incorporation into the bony structure of the

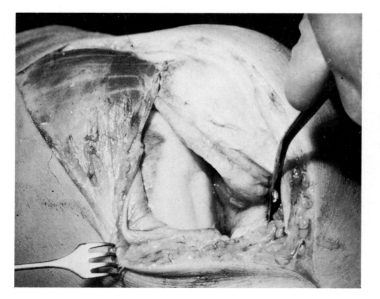

FIG. 28-28. Condylar prominence formed by displaced osteochondral fragment. Articular cartilage still intact. (See Fig. 28-29.) Knee joint was closed without surgical intervention, and knee was immobilized. The fragment healed, leaving a temporary condylar bony prominence that 2 years later had completely smoothed on X-ray. No functional or radiographic defect could be discerned.

FIG. 28-29. Reciprocal longitudinal groove in articular surface of patella produced by abnormal excursion of patella over edge of femoral condyle. (See Fig. 28-28.)

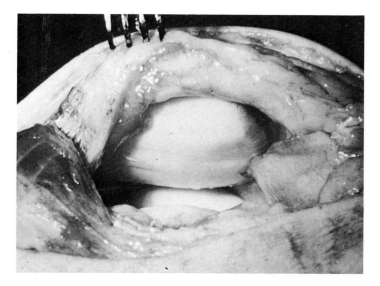

femoral condyles is further evidence that healing is a response to the therapeutic program involved.

A plaster cast or a rigid-knee long-leg brace with long-laced thigh and calf cuffs is provided in the position of flexion. The position of flexion is determined by roentgenograms showing that the lesion is not in contact with the opposite articular surfaces. Fixation and crutches for 4 to 11 months have been successful in healing even advanced lesions.

However, if one body has separated and its condition on inspection offers little hope of its incorporation by stapling back into a freshened bed, it is discarded. The cartilaginous edges of a defect may be shaved or trimmed conservatively, using a bent segment of a flexible razor blade. At times we have drilled the exposed femoral bone bed, using a fine jeweler's drill, so that the clot that forms might promote development of fibrocartilage to fill the defect. It is difficult to judge whether drilling materially aided repair. Centrally located sites of patellar osteochondritis dissecans also have been drilled. In the common case of localized dislodgment of the inferior medial quadrant of the patella in tangential osteochondral fracture, little subsequent disability is experienced after the loose fragment is discarded. We have not seen patellofemoral contact dis-

turbances follow such removal, but they have been reported by others.

In several cases of threatened separation of an osteochondritic fragment of the femoral condyle, we have drilled the bed from outside the joint under roentgenologic control. Preferably at open operation, the drill is passed through the medial wall of the medial condyle down to the bed of the lesion, care being taken not to perforate the articular cartilage. Unfortunately, only a few holes may be so drilled, but even so, it serves to stimulate vascularity for local repair. We have avoided drilling through intact cartilage from the joint side.

Patellectomy for indirect fractures or osteochondritis dissecans in childhood is rarely considered, and we have only once found it necessary in a complete tangential fracture.

Histologically, the loose bodies of osteochondritis dissecans are ultimately indistinguishable from fragments of old osteochondral fractures that have been in the joint long enough to show the effects of vascular separation from the host. A series of such loose bodies removed from patients at different and key intervals after injury reveal the progressive changes in the body that ultimately characterize specimens of osteochondritis dissecans. For obvious mechanical reasons, removal of all completely free bodies of whatever etiology is indicated, unless their recent origin and an adequate bone layer make the trial of reimplantation feasible.

The free body visible on roentgenograms may be difficult to find on opening the joint at operation. Occasionally it is posterior. It may also be found lodged in a compartment of the suprapatellar pouch. In some knees a complete septum with a semilunarlike valve is found, through which the free body at long intervals finds its way into parts of the joint where it may interfere with joint motion (see Fig. 28-23).

New bodies sometimes form and separate years after the initial arthrotomy for removal of a free osteochondritic loose body. Therefore, patients should be told before operation of the possibility of further operation if new areas separate at the margins of large condylar defects.

A not uncommon and rather unpleasant patellar lesion is osteochondritis dissecans of the middle third of the patella. It may be bilateral. Roentgenographic findings consist of subchondral cortical irregularity, or even crater formation. An arthrogram will at times be helpful. Pain on motion is not relieved by removal of one or more small bodies. Local curettage into bleeding bone and multiple drilling with a jeweler's drill followed by prolonged long-leg brace fixation in extension is advised. Patellectomy may ultimately be indicated. We have seen several unsuccessful metallic patellar implants.

Large condylar defects established in adolescence have produced evidence of degenerative changes in the third or the fourth decade, fortunately with few clinical complaints.

CORTISONE OSTEOCHONDRITIS DISSECANS

Since 1956 we have encountered the development of osteochondritis dissecans and cartilaginous free bodies in joints of patients who had been receiving steroid medication. Administration of the drug in a few earlier cases was oral, but in most patients the drug was instilled into the joint. No critical dose, particular steroid compound, or frequency of dosage could be ascertained. No age group was espe-

cially vulnerable, although most patients were 40 to 70 years old. Oral dosage was followed by multiple or bilateral joint lesions. Intra-articular cortisone, in our measured opinion, incited characteristic and severe lesions in the joint injected and that came to surgery. Injections were usually lateral in knees, but lesions were almost uniformly of the medial femoral condyle (Plate 28-7).

From 1956 to 1973 we have encountered 37 patients with 47 sites of joint destruction in which, after study, this diagnosis was reached. Of these, 29 knees of 26 patients had gross radiologic lesions. In all but two patients the lesion was located in the stressed prominence of the medial femoral condyle. In the two exceptions (who had taken oral steroids) medial tibial condyle areas were involved (Fig. 28-30).

The sequence of events in the knee joint appears to be as follows: Some months after commencing use of the drug, either intra-articularly or orally, the affected condyle presents an area of subchondral bone atrophy. Of particular interest are other deeper areas in the cancellous bone of both femoral and tibial condyles, where loss of trabeculation is discerned, often far removed from the later subchondral condylar lesion (Fig. 28-31).

Preceding the breakdown in the medial femoral condyle, bubblelike areas of absorption are apparent locally in the subcortical cancellous tissues. It is best seen in the early stage in the lateral view.

Next, the sclerotic cortical plate undergoes linear fracture or infarction and subsequently flattens. Separation of a cortical osteochondral body in the pivotal zone of the medial condyle follows. Pain is usually moderate, and motion is commonly surprisingly free for so severe a radiologic area of pathology.

At operation, cartilage necrosis and separation of cartilage from subcortical bone are exposed, often with deep dirty-appearing ulceration in the medial condyle (Plate 28-7). Loose, large cartilage fragments are often present. Cartilage destruction, subchondral defects, and aseptic necrosis of subchondral bone are confirmed at operation and are usually extensive.

In one instructive instance the steroid le-

FIG. 28-30. (A) Cortisone tibial osteochondritis dissecans in a woman, age 62. Anteroposterior view. Large fragment was separated from the medial condyle of the tibia, confirmed at operation. This followed 6 months of oral administration of cortisone. A decalcified lesion also appeared beneath the articular surface of the tibia in the ankle joint. **(B)** Lateral view of same knee.

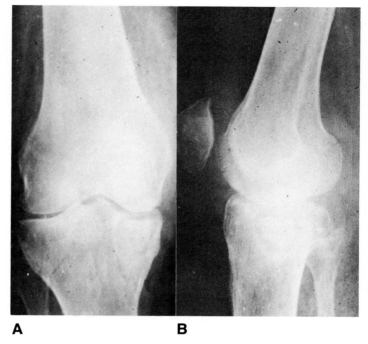

A   B

sion developed in the medial femoral condyle at the site of a previous purely traumatic subchondral cleft lesion in an active man. On elevation (at operation) of the cleft-pedicled flap, a nest of loose balls of necrotic, white-gray, poorly staining tissue was exposed, tightly packed in a deep medial condylar ulcer. The balls had been prevented from falling out into the joint by the persistence of one segment of the cartilage flap and were therefore visible in situ.

The mode of chemical action of the drug on articular cartilage has been intensively studied by Mankin.[7] To date there is no similar data available on the action of steroids on cortical and cancellous bone and marrow. It seems remarkable that following intra-articular injections such widespread, profound, deeply located lesions should develop.

The direct trauma of the concentrated stresses of weight-bearing, I believe, is the factor that fractures the locally atrophied subchondral cortex left unsupported by absorption of cancellous trabeculae, most often in this medial femoral zone. I believe that the chance distribution of atrophic zones is the reason it does not occur more frequently at the site of stress in the knee joint.

Three roentgenographically similar lesions have been seen in patients with osteoporosis who never received steroids. Two of these healed well with continued bracing and general measures aimed at improving the osteoporosis. As these knees were not opened, I am unable to report on their actual appearance.

I am not aware that similar major destructive and ulcerated lesions were reported prior to the introduction of steroids.

I distinctly do not believe that general use of steroids in knees is worth the unpredictable hazards instanced and have long dispensed with intra-articular administration.

The mechanism of action of the drug whereby these joint lesions are produced is not yet understood. Theories currently vary from loss of pain sensation and cessation of normal reparative processes in articular cartilage to vascular occlusions. It seems unlikely that direct trauma would involve normal subcondylar bone as deeply as the changes seen in these cases would postulate. My views are outlined above.

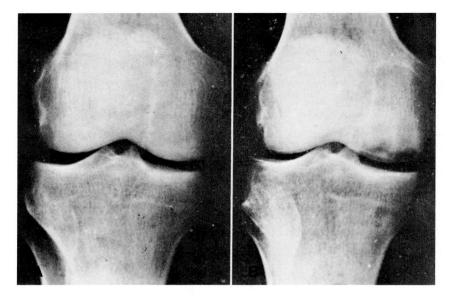

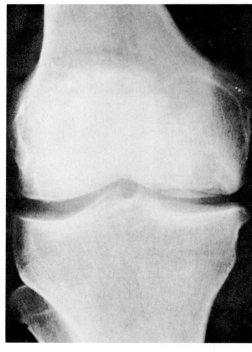

FIG. 28-31. (A) Cortisone femoral osteochondritis dissecans in 68-year-old man who had received 8 to 10 intra-articular injections of hydrocortisone over a period of 3 months. No oral medication. Initial roentgenogram. Normal medial femoral condyle. **(B)** Eight months later a large decalcified zone has appeared in the medial femoral condyle. **(C)** At 14 months collapse of decalcified zone with large, free osteochondral fragment is now visible beneath the medial femoral condyle.

Decalcified areas of cancellous bone are visible at 8 months deep in both femoral condyles, outlined faintly by scalloped sclerotic margins. Likewise, both tibial condyles contain subchondral cancellous areas of decalcification. Pivotal stress concentration produces the osteochondral fracture, exposing the "ulcer," which is the subchondral defect "with the lid off."

Ultimately, in the hip joint the progressive disintegration resembles the classic picture of a Charcot joint. Two cases have had both hips affected. In one young adult oral administration of moderate dosage for an atopic derma-titis of the forearm was followed after some months by hip disturbance that occasioned the discovery of the osteochondral lesions, which developed first in one hip and, after an interval of months, in the other. No critical dosage could be ascertained. Stopping cortisone therapy did not stop breakdown in the hips observed.

Spontaneous efforts at repair have been followed with interest in three severely unstable cases not subjected to surgical intervention. The knees in three patients treated by abstinence from steroids and continuous (day and night) use of a long-leg brace of the Goldenberg type, in which the axes of joint motion, including rotation, are controlled with special care, improved significantly in the course of a year. The area of destruction visible on roentgenographs compacted, regained contours, and then filled in, even if it did not return to normal. The associated instability of the joints was materially improved. The patients have continued with the brace in comfort for several years after the onset of conservative observation. Fusion was early refused by one particularly severely involved patient, and the alternative of a prosthesis was not tendered.

REFERENCES

1. **Freiberger R:** Aseptic necrosis of the femoral heads after high dosage. Corticosteroid therapy. NY State J Med 65:127, 1965
2. **Green WT, Banks HH:** Osteochondritis dissecans in children. J Bone Joint Surg 35A:26, 1953
3. **Kennedy JC:** Osteochondral fractures of the femoral condyles. J Bone Joint Surg 48B:436, 1966
4. **Kleinberg S:** Vertical fracture of the articular surface of the patella. JAMA, 81:1205, 1923
5. **Kroner M:** Ein fall von Flachenfractur und Luxation der Patella. Dsch Med Wochenschr 31:996, 1905
6. **Lettloff D:** Der verticofrontale Bruch der kniescheike, Austernschalenbruch. Arch Klin Chir 153:808, 1928
7. **Mankin HJ et al:** The acute effects of intra-articular hydrocortisone on articular cartilage. J Bone Joint Surg 48A:1083, 1966
8. **Milgram JE:** Tangential osteochondral fracture of the patella. J Bone Joint Surg 35:271, 1943
9. **Milgrim JE:** Osteochondral fractures of the knee joint. Mechanism of Production, pp 760–762. IX Congress Int. de. Chir. Orth. et da trauma. Transactions Bruxelles, 1964
10. **Milgrim JE:** Mechanism of production of patellar and femoral free bodies in the knee joint. J Bone Joint Surg 46B:787, 1964
11. **Milgrim JE:** Osteochondral lesions of the knee joint. Experimental tibial spine–femoral condyle contact. J Bone Joint Surg 48B:392, 1966
12. **Sledenstein H:** Osteochondritis dissecans of the knee with spontaneous healing in children. Bull Hosp Joint Dis 28:123, 1957
13. **Smillie IE:** Osteochondritis dissecans. Edinburgh, E & S Livingston, 1964
14. **Villar R:** Fracture vertico-frontale dite "en coquilles de Huitre de la Rotule." J Med Bordeaux 48:121, 1921

CHAPTER 29

THE PRINCIPLES AND PRACTICE OF STABLE INTERNAL FIXATION IN THE TREATMENT OF FRACTURES INVOLVING THE KNEE JOINT

M. E. Müller,
J. Goldsmith,
J. Schnatzker

Conservative treatment of fractures involving the knee joint has frequently led to unsatisfactory results with the knee joint remaining unstable, stiff, and painful. Open reduction and internal fixation in the past have similarly led to poor results. The choice between operative and conservative treatment of these fractures requires experience and judgment.

Since 1958, the AO group in Switzerland has devoted a great deal of time to the study of the many problems present in the treatment of fractures of the knee joint. From these studies have evolved techniques that are now standard. They permit anatomical reduction and rigid stable internal fixation so that plaster fixation can be abandoned and active painless mobilization of the joint and of the injured extremity can begin within a few days of surgery.

The best way to fix bony fragments accurately is by means of interfragmentary compression achieved with lag screws, tension band wire, or the so-called compression plate, or a combination of any of the three. The main principle of all these compression systems is to bring as large a fracture surface as possible under compression with the implant under tension. If the bony surfaces that are compressed are not large enough to permit rigid fixation, an autogenous cancellous bone graft must be employed.

The techniques that the Swiss AO Group found best will be discussed with particular regard to the type of fracture, operative exposures, biomechanical principles, and postoperative treatment.[4]

FRACTURES OF THE PATELLA

In fractures of the patella the following factors are important: mechanism of injury, number of fragments, damage to the articular cartilage, and rupture of the extensor apparatus.

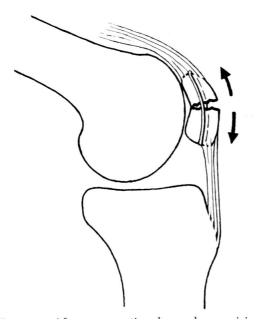

FIG. 29-1. After conventional cerclage wiring, with the wire running around the middle of the patella, the fragments invariably come apart on the anterior surface when the knee is flexed. Therefore, this procedure is not advisable.

Loss of the patella leads to degenerative changes in the femoral condyles and, on occasion, extensor lag of 10° to 15° may be present. Weakness during the last 10° to 15° of extension is the rule. For these reasons patellectomy will be exceptional. If the patella, as a result of direct trauma, is markedly comminuted, an accurate reduction is often impossible, and patellectomy is frequently indicated. If the extensor apparatus is intact, then only patellectomy is performed. If not, the quadriceps and patellar tendon are sutured together, and a triangular segment from the extensor apparatus is excised in order to shorten longitudinally the expansion of the retinaculae patellae.

In all other cases we make every attempt to maintain the integrity of the patella. If late degenerative changes do occur, a patellar prosthesis may be the best solution in preference to a late patellectomy.

In longitudinal fractures of the patella displacement of fragments usually does not occur. The extensor apparatus is intact, and no operative intervention is necessary. If the fragments separate, then stable fixation can be easily achieved after accurate reduction with one or two lag screws.

Transverse fractures or avulsions of the distal pole of the patella are usually the result of indirect trauma. These fractures are usually the result of a sudden powerful contraction of the quadriceps when the knee is flexed. This causes the patella to be forced against the femur, which then acts as a fulcrum. Separation of the fragments is the rule, and in most

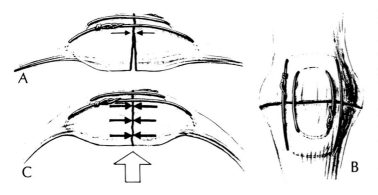

FIG. 29-2. The principle of tension band wiring of the patella. **(A, B)** The wire is passed around the insertion of the ligamentum patellae and the quadriceps in front of the patella. This wire is tightened until the fracture is slightly overcorrected. A second wire is passed more superficially. **(C)** As the knee is flexed and the quadriceps contracted, the pressure of the condyles against the patella compresses the bony fragments together.

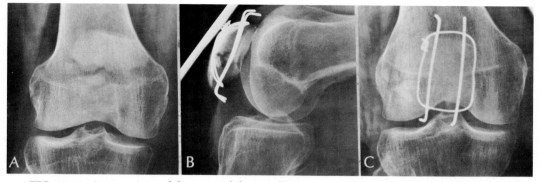

FIG. 29-3. A comminuted fracture of the patella (**A**) was managed by tension band wiring with Kirschner wires. (**B, C**) The Kirschner wires were first introduced longitudinally to stabilize the small fragments.

cases the lateral expansion of the quadriceps mechanism is ruptured.

TREATMENT OF SIMPLE TRANSVERSE FRACTURES

Wire fixation of simple transverse patellar fractures is not new. If circumferential wiring is employed, displacement of both fragments with a separation anteriorly is almost inevitable (Fig. 29-1). Pauwels has shown that if a circumferential wire is placed posterior to the center of axis of the patella, the fragments open anteriorly.[5] If, on the other hand, the wire is placed anterior to the center of axis, tensile stresses that previously caused the displacement and separation of fragments are converted into compressive forces and serve to maintain the reduction and apposition of fragments.

We expose such a fracture through a transverse incision centered over the patella and examine both femoral condyles. Prior to reduction the tendon fibers are scraped back from the fracture line for a distance of 2 mm to 3 mm. An accurate reduction is then obtained and maintained with two towel clips. Two wires are used to secure fixation. The first is placed deep to the insertion of the quadriceps and patellar tendon. The second wire is placed more superficially and passes through the Sharpey's fibers (Fig. 29-2). The fracture is

slightly overcorrected, and the wires are then tightened and tied. When the knee joint is flexed, the overcorrection vanishes, and the fracture surfaces are squeezed together with compression. The quadriceps expansion is then repaired, suction drains are inserted, and the wound is closed.

COMMINUTED FRACTURES

Comminuted fractures of the patella are exposed in the same manner as is a transverse fracture of the patella, but the fixation has to be supplemented with two longitudinal K-wires to stabilize the small fragments. The fixation is then completed with two tension band wires as illustrated in Figure 29-3.

AVULSION FRACTURES

Avulsion fractures of the lower pole of the patella cannot be stabilized with the tension band wire alone; the distal fragment tilts in toward the joint. A small distal fragment must therefore be stabilized with a small AO cancellous screw before the tension band wire is applied (Fig. 29-4). Only in the case of many small distal fragments that cannot be secured by means of screws is the excision of the lower pole the method of choice.

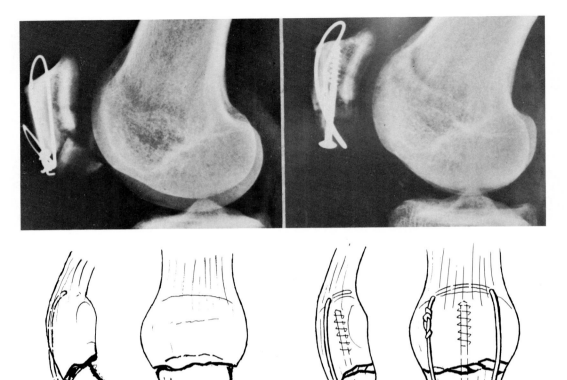

FIG. 29-4. (A) In avulsion fractures of the lower tip of the patella, tension band wiring alone tips the distal fragment. **(B)** The lower fragment must therefore be stabilized with a small cancellous screw before the tension band wire is applied.

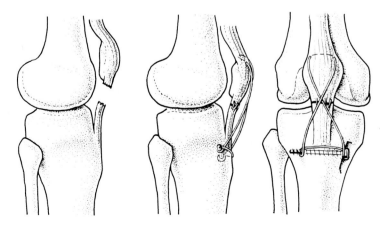

FIG. 29-5. Repair of a ruptured patellar tendon. The suture line is protected with a figure-of-eight tension band wire passed proximally around the quadriceps insertion and distally around the transverse screw inserted in the tibia just distal to the attachment of the patellar tendon. Immediate movement can begin without fear of disrupting the repair. The wire and screw are removed after 6 months.

FIG. 29-6. Postoperative positioning of patients with patellar or tibial fractures.

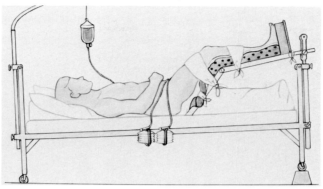

RUPTURE OF THE PATELLAR TENDON FROM THE PATELLA

In the case of rupture of the patellar tendon from the patella, the disruption of the tendon is repaired, but the suture line must be protected from tension. This is achieved by means of a figure-of-eight tension band wire placed proximally around the quadriceps tendon and distally around a cortical screw inserted transversely just distal to the tibial tubercle (Fig. 29-5). The wire and screw are removed after 6 months.

POSTOPERATIVE CARE

Postoperative splinting and positioning is extremely important. Fractures of the patella are immobilized in a compression bandage for 48 hours and protected during the postoperative period on a Braun frame, which maintains the knee in 45° of flexion. The foot is somewhat higher than the knee and the ankle is at 90° with the foot supported so it will not drift into equinus (Fig. 29-6). Quadriceps exercises are begun early with the help of a physiotherapist. Early flexion of the knee joint is most desirable because in extension the patella does not articulate with the femur. In flexion, on the other hand, the articular surface of the patella lies against the articular surface of the femur. Normally the patient with a fracture of the patella rigidly fixed will bend his knee joint approximately 70° to 90° after 1 week. It

is necessary to walk with two canes thereafter for an 8-week period.

FRACTURES OF THE LOWER FEMUR

Supracondylar and condylar fractures of the femur usually occur as the result of severe trauma because the distal femur is structurally very strong.

The reduction of these fractures and maintenance of the reduction by conservative means is difficult. It is important to note that in intercondylar fractures both the patellofemoral and the tibiofemoral joints must be reestablished to prevent posttraumatic arthritis. After conservative treatment a perfect functional result is the exception rather than the rule. Early motion is not possible in these cases, and stiffness of the knee joint ensues. Stiffness occurs because of incomplete reduction with shortening of the femur and formation of adhesions between the quadriceps and the fracture site, resulting in loss of the suprapatellar gliding mechanism.

In order to avoid these complications, an anatomical open reduction followed by rigid internal fixation is recommended. When severe bony comminution is present, autogenous cancellous bone grafting must be performed. Postoperatively the knee is maintained at 90° of flexion, and the active mobilization of the extremity begins on the day following surgery.

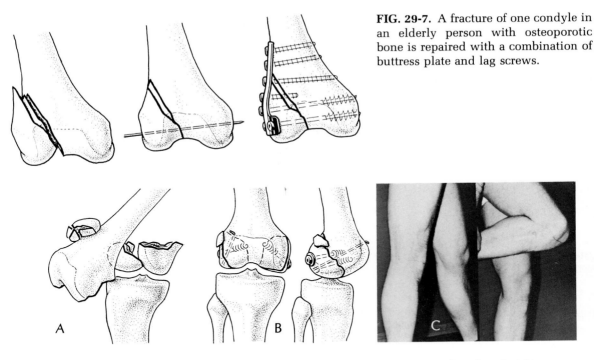

FIG. 29-7. A fracture of one condyle in an elderly person with osteoporotic bone is repaired with a combination of buttress plate and lag screws.

FIG. 29-8. A compound fracture of both femoral condyles (**A**) was reduced and stabilized with two cancellous lag screws. (**B**) Note that threads must not cross the fracture line. Movement was begun immediately. (**C**) Eight years after the operation the patient has full range of motion and no residual arthritis.

Fractures of one condyle have, as a rule, no ligamentous disruption associated with them because the ligament remains attached to the condyle. In a young person with strong cancellous bone such a fracture can be rigidly stabilized with one or two cancellous bone screws. These screws act as lag screws and therefore, as in all lag screws, the thread must not cross the fracture line (Fig. 29-7).

In compound fractures minimal internal fixation should be carried out. For young patients with compound fractures, débridement and simple screw fixation may be sufficient. Figure 29-8 illustrates a compound fracture of both condyles in a young patient with an excellent postoperative result.

Transverse supracondylar fractures are stabilized under axial compression by means of a tension band plate. If such a fracture is associated with bone loss medially, then this is filled primarily with autogenous cancellous bone at the time of the internal fixation. If such fractures are comminuted and have two, three, or four fragments, then reduction begins by reducing each fragment in turn and wherever possible securing interfragmentary compression by means of lag screws. Once the reduction is complete, the fractures are neutralized by a neutralization plate applied to the lateral cortex. For proximal supracondylar fractures a straight plate can be used that is slightly curved between the middle and the distal third of the femur. More distally, a condylar blade plate is used. Any bone defects are filled with autogenous cancellous bone.

Supra- and intracondylar fractures are stabilized by means of the AO 95° condylar blade plate. Fixation is again supplemented by autogenous cancellous bone whenever bone loss is present. In reduction and fixation of these fractures one always begins with the intra-articular fracture lines. Once the intracondylar

FIG. 29-9. (A) The standard condylar blade plate has two distal holes for cancellous screws and three holes for cortex screws. Condylar plates of longer shaft lengths for comminuted fractures are provided with seven, nine, or twelve holes. **(B)** The condylar plate guide is shaped like a mold for the shaft portion of the condylar plate. **(C)** The physiological axis of the tibia and femur showing the angles they form with the knee joint itself.

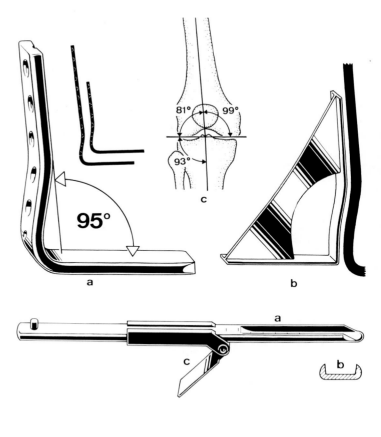

FIG. 29-10. This special seating chisel is made for inserting condylar blade plates. **(A)** To cut the channel for the blade it has a profile identical to that of the blade of the plate. During insertion it is held with the slotted hammer to prevent rotation. The hammer also serves as an extractor. **(B)** The standard U-section of the blade. **(C)** The chisel guide helps to establish the sagittal plane.

fracture is solidly fixed, the supracondylar component is dealt with. The condyles are rarely involved in comminution. But if such is present and results in bone loss, then again autogenous cancellous bone graft from the ilium must be employed. When the condylar blade plate is used, the axis of the frontal plane will remain physiologic as long as the blade of the plate is parallel to the articular surface of the knee.

The condylar blade plate as created by the Swiss AO in 1959 is a one-piece device with a fixed angle of 95°. The blade portion in profile is shaped like a U. The blade of this blade plate is always inserted parallel to the articular surface of the condyles, which subtends an angle of 81° with the anatomical axis of the femur (Fig. 29-9). As long as there are no anatomical abnormalities and the blade is inserted parallel to the articular surface, the plate portion will come to lie along the lateral cortex of the femur. Care must be taken, however, to direct the device properly in the sagittal plane because malposition such as recurvatum might ensue if the blade plate is improperly oriented. The standard condylar blade plate has two holes for cancellous screws of 6.5 mm diameter and three holes for cortical screws of 4.5 mm diameter.

The special feature of the AO angled plate is that the channel for the blade of the plate must be cut by means of a special seating chisel on which a guide for securing the orientation in the sagittal plane is adjustable (Fig. 29-10).

INTERNAL FIXATION OF INTRAARTICULAR FRACTURE OF THE DISTAL FEMUR

Surgical Exposure

The lateral approach is used. The skin and the investing fascia are incised, and the incision is carried to the level of the tibial tubercle. If the joint is to be widely exposed, the lateral

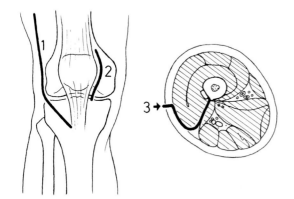

FIG. 29-11. (**1, 3**) The so-called mailbox approach for distal femoral fractures. Very sledom the knee joint must be inspected through a counter incision (**2**).

half of the infrapatellar tendon is reflected; a medial parapatellar incision is seldom necessary (Fig. 29-11). The vastus lateralis is retracted anteriorly and reflected from the intermuscular septum. The perforating vessels, wherever encountered, are ligated and cut. When complete, the exposure includes the lateral surface of the femur from the linea aspera forward, to and including the joint.

Technic

After the joint is exposed, the fracture lines are reduced under direct vision and temporarily stabilized by means of Kirschner wires (Fig. 29-12). Sometimes, especially in comminuted fractures of the condyles, the reduction is much easier if the knee joint is flexed 120° or more in order to relax all the flexors of the knee. The vertical component of the T- or Y-fracture should now be fixed under compression with one or more cancellous lag screws placed anteriorly and posteriorly to the projected position of the blade plate and 3 cm to 4 cm above the joint. Then the supracondylar fracture lines are reduced and tem-

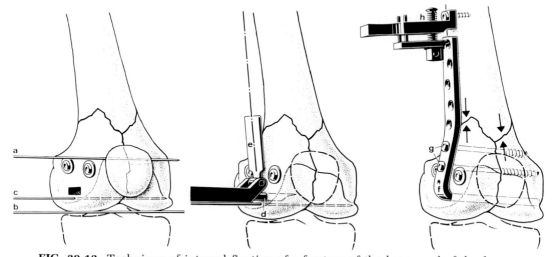

FIG. 29-12. Technique of internal fixation of a fracture of the lower end of the femur. One Kirschner wire is placed beneath the patella (**a**) and another in the joint parallel to the articular surface (**b**). The guide wire (**c**) is inserted into the bone 1 cm above the joint surface and parallel to the other Kirschner wires. The special seating chisel (**d**) is introduced parallel to the guide wire, and its aiming device (**e**) lies parallel to the femoral shaft. Two cancellous screws (**g**) are inserted into the distal fragment through the blade plate (**f**) before the tension device is attached proximally, (**h** and **i**).

FIG. 29-13. Postoperative positioning for fractures of mid- and distal femur.

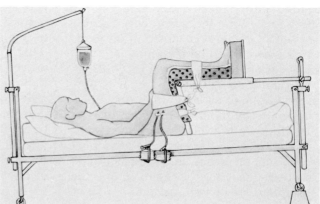

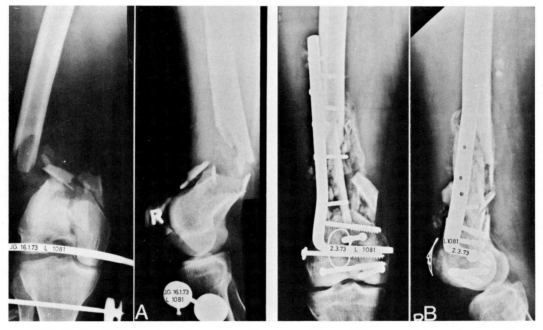

FIG. 29-14. **(A)** Comminuted compound fracture of the right femur with loss of 10 cm of bone. **(B)** After reduction of the joint surfaces and fixation of the fragments by means of four lag screws, the blade plate was inserted. The defect was filled with cancellous bone grafts, and a bone fragment was found in the patient's car after the accident. After 2 weeks the patient was able to walk with two crutches, and after 6 weeks he was able to bend his knee joint to 90°.

porarily fixed by means of bone clamps or Kirschner wires. One Kirschner wire is inserted transversely through the knee joint parallel to the articular surface of the femoral condyle. A second Kirschner wire is placed under the patella. The third Kirschner wire is inserted through the femoral condyle as low as possible—about 1 cm above the articular surface. It is inserted parallel to the first and second Kirschner wires respectively and serves then as the guide wire for the introduction of the seating chisel. The position of the third Kirschner wire, the guide wire, is now checked with the condylar positioning plate. The guide wire should be parallel to it.

The special seating chisel with its guide set parallel to the long axis of the femur is now hammered in, making sure that the chisel blade is parallel to the third or directional K-wire. This allows the blade plate to be correctly aligned in both the sagittal and coronal planes, no matter what the supracondylar comminution. The chisel is removed and the plate inserted. One or two cancellous screws are inserted not only in the distal part of the plate but also into the distal fragment of the fracture to increase the fixation of the blade plate. These cancellous screws, as they engage the medial cortex, increase the interfragmentary compression on the intracondylar fracture surfaces. The reduction of the supracondylar fracture is checked, and accurate axial compression is now obtained by securing the tension device to the femoral shaft and placing the plate portion under tension. Reduction should be perfect and the fixation rigid. If there is any loss of bony continuity medially, it must be reconstituted at the time of fixation with autogenous cancellous bone graft. The bone graft will serve in due time as a physiologic bone bar medially and will prevent bending forces from fatiguing the plate.

POSTOPERATIVE CARE

Once internal fixation is completed, the extremity is immobilized on a special splint with the hip and knee flexed to 90° (Fig. 29-13). Assisted active movements are begun in 48 hours. After 6 days the splint is discarded, and the patient is encouraged to sit with his leg over the edge of the bed and to begin active unassisted movements. With this postoperative regimen flexion has never been a problem. On the eighth postoperative day the patient is allowed out of bed. Full weight-bearing is not allowed for 2 to 3 months. In the interim partial weight-bearing not exceeding 10 kg to 15 kg (measured with the patient standing on a scale) is allowed. The patient uses two crutches. Plates are removed after 18 months. Before any metal is removed, however, the internal architecture of the cortex must have become homogeneous throughout as seen radiographically. The removal of these implants is necessary after bony union because these implants are rigid, provide too much stress protection, and prevent the bone from responding to normal physiological stimuli. There is also the possibility of metallic corrosion. Figure 29-14 gives an example of a severe femoral fracture treated by means of lag screws, condylar plate, and bone plasty.

FRACTURES OF THE TIBIAL PLATEAU

The metaphyseal portion of the tibia in its expanded cancellous proximal end is especially vulnerable to injury. The proximal tibia overhangs the shaft posteriorly and is not supported by diaphyseal cortical bone below. For these reasons fractures of the tibial plateau are more frequent than of the femoral condyles.

An associated medial ligamentous rupture may occur when the joint is mainly subjected to a valgus stress. If this stress is resisted by the lateral plateau, a tension build-up results in the medial ligament, causing its eventual rupture. If the plateau ruptures, no tension is generated medially, and the ligament remains intact. If further valgus force is applied, however, with further depression of the plateau, the medial part of the lateral femoral condyle may come into contact with the lateral tubercle of the intercondylar eminence and transfix it, shifting the fulcrum medially and thus causing further tension to be applied to the medial compartment. This tension, if great enough, will rupture the medial ligament. Thus, a medial ligament rupture may occur with an intact or a depressed tibial plateau.

We do not routinely explore the ligaments as does Courvoisier.[2] We rely on the clinical findings of medial discoloration, swelling, pain, instability, and stress ray films in order

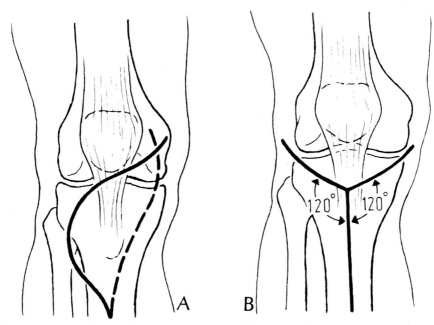

FIG. 29-15. (A) Incisions for the medial or lateral parts of the tibial plateau are centered over the medial or lateral condyle, respectively. **(B)** The arms of an incision to expose both parts of the tibial plateau must form 120° angles. This incision allows repair of both condyles and any associated ligamentous damage at the same time. If greater exposure is needed, the patellar tendon is elevated by Z-plasty.

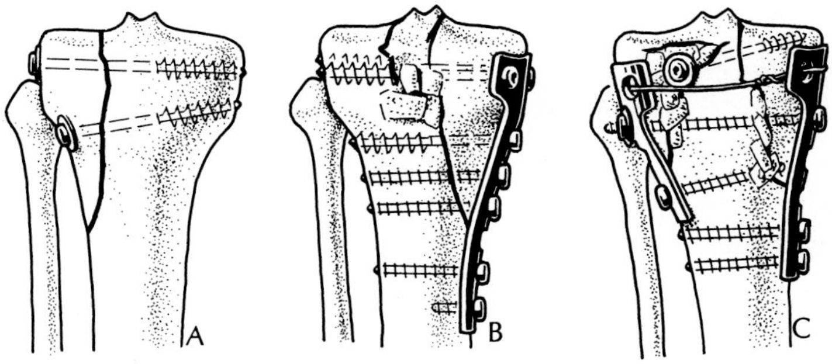

FIG. 29-16. The three classical tibial plateau fractures and their treatment. **(A)** Cleavage fracture. Two lag screws are sufficient only in young patients. **(B)** Depressed fracture. After elevation of the depression, a cancellous bone plasty is necessary. Fixation by means of lag screws and T-plate. **(C)** Comminuted fracture treated by means of a circumferential wire and two T-plates. Cancellous bone plasty is almost always necessary.

to establish our criteria for ligamentous exploration.

CHOICE OF TREATMENT

Böhler and others have shown that most of the tibial plateau fractures treated conservatively may achieve good to excellent results and that the only absolute indication for an open re-duction is an irreducible intra-articular fracture.[1] Before a conservative or a surgical course in undertaken, careful consideration must be given to all problems at hand, for a conservative approach may prejudice any subsequent surgery. Smillie has stated categorically that it is a mistake to attempt closed reduction using skeletal traction and powerful traction only to decide subsequently that the reduction is unsatisfactory.[6] The hazard of infection is greatly enhanced with the introduction of the Steinmann pin by the contusion of the underlying tissues and skin.

Surgical Approaches to the Head of the Tibia

An incision is chosen so that the final scar does not lie over the metal implant. Thus the position of the plate must be decided before the incision is made.

Surgical Approaches to Medial or Lateral Part of the Tibial Plateau

We employ either a medial parapatellar incision or a curvilinear incision centered on the lateral plateau (Fig. 29-15A). The joint is reduced under direct vision and provisionally stabilized with K-wires. Final fixation is carried out with lag screws or with lag screws in combination with a buttress plate.

Surgical Approach to Both Parts of the Tibial Plateau

A triradiate incision with 120° between its arcs gives good access to both medial and lateral parts of the tibial plateau simultaneously (Fig. 29-15B). The incisions meet not over the tibial tubercle but over the middle of the patellar tendon. To expose the articular surfaces the meniscotibial ligaments are incised and the menisci are elevated. To gain better exposure in very comminuted fractures it is necessary to elevate the patellar tendon. At the end of the procedure the meniscotibial ligaments are resutured. If a medial ligamentous disruption is also present, it can be repaired through the same incision.

OPERATIVE TECHNIQUES

We distinguish three types of tibial plateau fractures (Fig. 29-16):

Cleavage Fractures (Figs. 29-16A, 29-17)

Cancellous screws with washers alone are adequate only in young patients with strong cancellous bone and no osteoporosis. In all other patients a buttress plate is combined with the lag screws to prevent redisplacement.

Depressed Fractures

Depressed fractures should be elevated by upward pressure from below. It is sometimes desirable to drill a large hole 5 to 6 cm. below the joint line of the tibia and thus distal to the fracture. Then with a bone punch, introduced through the hole, elevate the depressed fracture. The fracture is overreduced slightly, and the resultant defect deep to the fracture is filled with autogenous cancellous bone. Fixation is then carried out as shown in Figures 29-16B and 29-18.

Comminuted Fractures (Figs. 29-16C, 29-19)

To repair a comminuted fracture it may be necessary to expose the whole plateau. For better visualization the meniscotibial ligaments may have to be divided as well as the patellar tendon. Sometimes reduction is only possible after a cerclage wire has been passed circumferentially around the upper tibia. Great caution is exercised so that the wire does not injure the posterior vessels and nerves. If a cerclage is used, fixation is supplemented with two T-plates. Extensive cancellous bone grafting is carried out to fill any ensuing defect, and wherever possible interfragmentary compression is achieved with lag screws. In these comminuted fractures we stress five points: (1) The joint under the meniscus must be restored. If the meniscus is torn in its substance, it is excised. If it is only peripherally detached, it should be resutured. (2) The reduction must be perfect. (3) Cancellous bone grafting must be employed.

(text continued on p. 456)

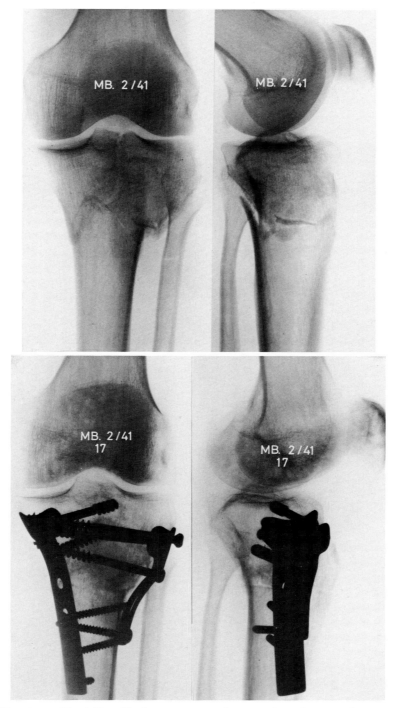

FIG. 29-17. (*Top*) Two T-plates were used to repair a cleavage fracture of both tibial plateaus. (*Bottom*) After 17 weeks there was no difference between the movements in the right and left knees, and the patient could bear full weight without pain.

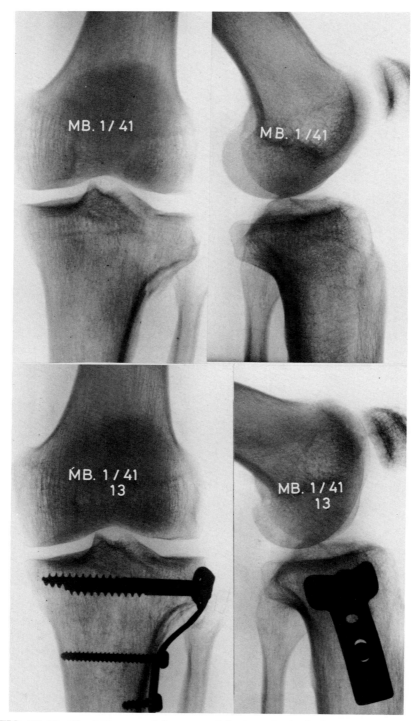

FIG. 29-18. (*Top*) Depressed fracture of the lateral tibial plateau treated by means of a T-plate and cancellous bone plasty. (*Bottom*) Result after 13 weeks. The patient was bearing full weight and had a normal range of movement.

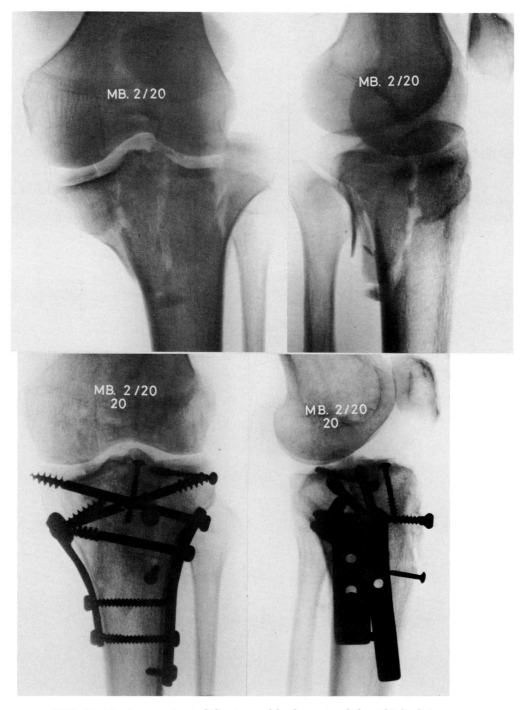

FIG. 29-19. A comminuted fracture of both parts of the tibial plateau required difficult internal fixation and rebuilding with cancellous bone. The tibial tuberosity was osteotomized during the operation to get an adequate view into the joint. The torn medial meniscus was excised. Twenty-two weeks after surgery the patient had 100° of flexion and could bear full weight.

(4) The fixation must be stable. (5) Associated ligamentous tears must be repaired.

Postoperative positioning as well as postoperative care is identical with that for fractures of the patella (Fig. 29-6).

SUMMARY

Fractures about the knee pose many technical, biomechanical, and biological problems. They are no longer unsolved problems, and the patient is no longer committed to life-long disability by the fracture. Full recovery is possible, but it requires careful preoperative assessment, meticulous surgery with no compromise in biological or biomechanical principles, and careful functional after care.

In conclusion, we can only reiterate the opening remarks of the AO Manual: "Open treatment of fractures is a valuable but difficult method which involves much responsibility. We cannot advise too strongly against internal fixation if it is carried out by an inadequately trained surgeon, and in the absence of full equipment and sterile operating room conditions. Using our method, enthusiasts who lack self criticism are much more dangerous than skeptics or outright opponents."

REFERENCES

1. **Böhler L:** Die Technik der Knochenbruchbehandlung. Wien, Maudrich, 1957
2. Courvoisier
3. **Müller ME:** Fractures basses du fémur. Acta Orthop Belg 36:566, 1970
4. **Müller ME, Allgöwer M, Willenegger H:** Manual of Internal Fixation. Technique recommended by the AO-Group- Berlin, Springer-Verlag 1970
5. **Pauwels F:** Gesammelte Abhandlungen zur funktionellen Anatomie des Bewegung-sapparates. Berlin, Springer-Verlag, 1965
6. **Smillie IS:** Injuries of the Knee Joint. Edinburgh E & S Livingstone, 1970

CHAPTER 30
EXTERNAL FIXATION
ABOUT THE KNEE

David L. Helfet
Andrew F. Brooker, Jr.

External fixation for treatment of difficult open fractures of the distal femur or proximal tibial plateau has played only a minor role during the past 30 years. As better engineered and more versatile frames have evolved, these devices have recently become more popular. Their easy, fairly atraumatic application and infinite adjustability throughout the healing period make them ideal for difficult clinical problems. The newer frames are more rigid than long-leg casts, yet wound débridement, skin grafting, and even burn care can be rendered to the soft tissues beneath them.

External fixation also enhances other, more established orthopaedic principles. Frames used to treat either distal femur or proximal tibial fractures generally permit early knee motion and do not require immobilization of the ankle or hip. The patients are permitted to get out of bed quickly and can walk and occasionally bear weight on the devices. In addition, simple amenities such as bathing or showering of the affected limb are generally permitted.

FRAMES

External fixation devices come in many types and sizes. For use about the knee, there are two principal configurations—the one-sided unit such as the Wagner, and those with transfixation pins with double uprights for stability (Fig. 30-1). We have abandoned the one-sided units for use in the knee area, preferring instead the transfixation device that is capable of adding additional planes of fixation to provide rigid support as required.

EXTERNAL FIXATION OF FRACTURES ABOUT THE KNEE

Open devitalized wounds in which débridement is essential and control of the fracture site desirable are a clear indication for external fixation. These injuries generally result from vehicular accidents, in which considerable energy is absorbed by the skeleton and overlying soft tissues; they are occasionally

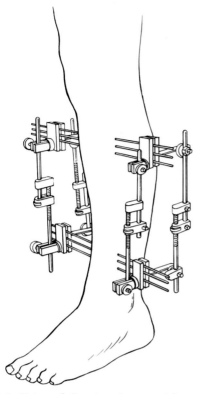

FIG. 30-1. External fixation frame with transfixation pins and double uprights.

grade I, but more commonly grade II or grade III compound fractures. The surgeon faces the difficult task of deciding on the viability of both overlying tissues and bony fragments. *Cast immobilization* is occlusive and restricts access to the wound. Traction gives good access but completely limits patient mobility, creating problems in treatment of associated injuries and complicating nursing care. Open reduction and internal fixation may be technically impossible or may require further dissection, devitalizing more bone and soft tissue in order to apply plates and screws.

External fixation, however, provides immediate stability with excellent wound access and does not preclude changing the treatment program to any of the above techniques at a later stage. Initial application is relatively easy, atraumatic, and provides a stable environment. If subsequent x-ray films reveal inadequate alignment, adjustments in all three planes and fine adjustment of limb length are easily carried out, often without the need for general anesthesia.

EXAMPLE 1

A 58-year-old man was crushed loading logs. He sustained bilateral femoral and proximal tibial fractures, of which both tibias and the left femur were open fractures with devitalized soft tissue. The injury resulted in bilateral "floating" knees (Fig. 30-2). He was treated initially with irrigation and débridement of the three compound fractures and stabilization of all of these with external frames (Fig. 30-3). One week later, he underwent open reduction and internal fixation of the right femoral fracture and final alignment of the external frames (Fig. 30-4). Two months after the injury, a concellous bone graft from the right iliac crest was placed on the right proximal tibia. The external fixation frames were removed 4 months after the injury, and the patient commenced range of motion exercises. Almost immediately he progressed to partial weight-bearing without problems. At his final follow-up visit, 8 months after injury, he was ambulating, bearing full weight with a cane (Fig. 30-5). His right knee range of motion was 0° to 110° and his left knee 0° to 90°.

EXAMPLE 2

A 48-year-old obese white man, a pedestrian, was struck by a car, which resulted in a bumper injury to the left leg. He sustained a closed proximal tibial fracture with an acute anterior compartment syndrome (Fig. 30-6A). Shortly after admission, he underwent complete fasciotomies of all four compartments through two incisions to relieve the pressure. The fracture was stabilized with an external fixation frame bridging the knee. Slight distraction was applied through the frame to reduce the fracture (ligamentotaxis) (Fig. 30-6B –E).

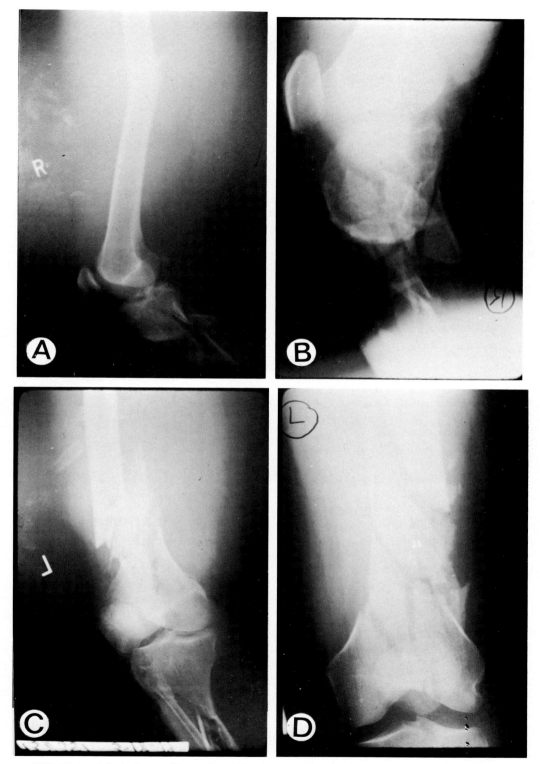

FIG. 30-2. Admission radiographs. **(A)** Fracture of right femur, closed. **(B)** Fracture of right tibia-fibula, open. **(C)** Fracture of left femur, open. **(D)** Fracture of left femur and tibia-fibular, open.

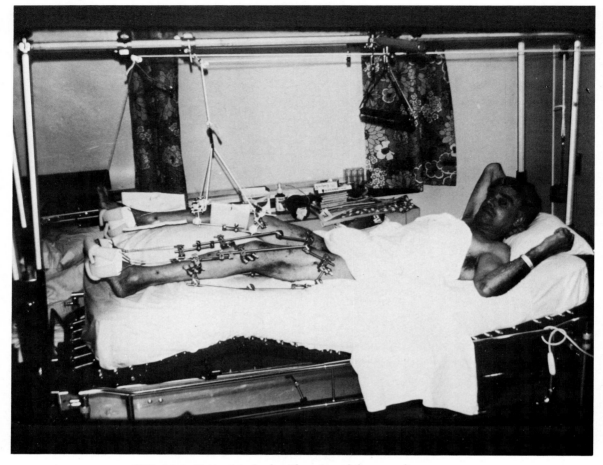

FIG. 30-3. Patient in bed with external frames after surgery.

EXTERNAL FIXATION OF LIGAMENT INJURIES

In current work at the Johns Hopkins Hospital, it has been shown that ligament repairs may suffer considerable stresses in a long-leg cast. Casting provides no resistance to anterior or posterior drawer type forces and frequently inadequate resistance to varus-valgus strains about the knee (Fig. 30-7). This fact has led, in some cases, to the use of external fixation frames to position and hold the knee following reconstructive surgery of the cruciate and collateral ligaments (Fig. 30-8). This concept is still in its infancy, but more rigid tibiofemoral fixation for knee ligament repairs and reconstructions may in the long run give more satisfactory results.

EXTERNAL FIXATION IN ELECTIVE SURGERY

Knee arthrodesis, either primarily or as a salvage procedure following failure of a total knee replacement, is ideally suited for external fixation. Open reduction and application of multiple plates can give rigid stability for primary knee fusion, but the procedure is large and quite traumatic to both bone and soft tissue. The concepts suggested originally by Charnley and refined by others have given satisfactory results in the most difficult circumstances. The external frame, applied in two planes, provides excellent rigid stability, eliminating the need for casting and allowing early ambulation or partial weight-bearing (Fig. 30-9A,B). This is appropriate because

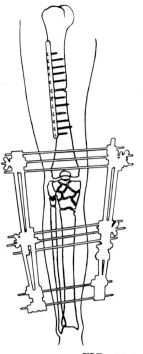 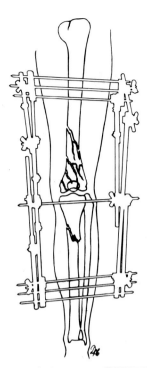

FIG. 30-4. Diagramatic representation of the management of femoral and tibial-fibular fractures.

many of these patients are either obese or debilitated and often have suspected subclinical infection. External fixation allows stability to be accomplished and the surgery performed without leaving implants in potentially contaminated areas. Furthermore, beyond removing the external fixator itself, subsequent removal of major hardware is eliminated. This obviates not only additional periods of protected weight-bearing but also the risk of further fracture following plate removal.

EXAMPLE 3

A 65-year-old obese white woman had previously undergone right total knee replacement for severe osteoarthritis. This became infected and was subsequently removed, and arthrodesis with internal fixation was attempted. She presented with an infected non-

(text continued on p. 464)

FIG. 30-5. Final result at 8 months shows full weight-bearing.

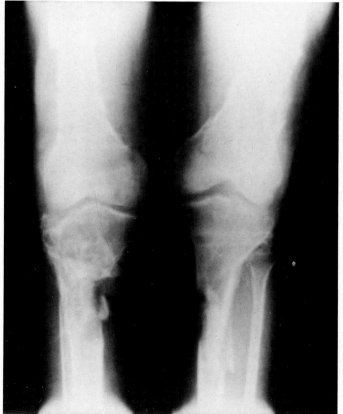

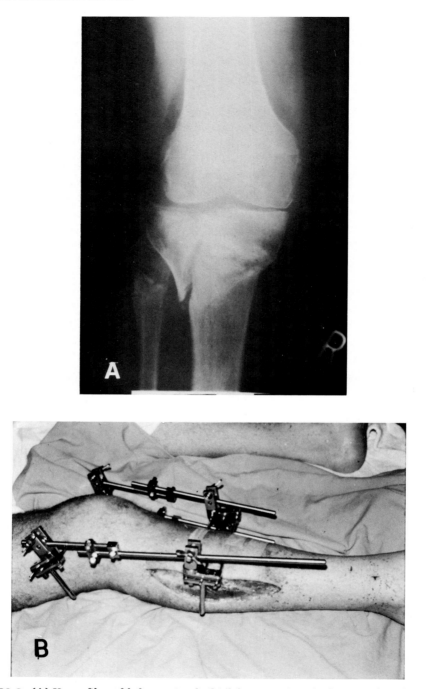

FIG. 30-6. **(A)** X-ray film of left proximal tibial fracture. **(B, C)** Photographs of patient after surgery in external frame. Note that frame gives excellent access to leg for wound care and compartment pressure monitoring. **(D)** X-ray film of left proximal tibial fracture reduced and stabilized in external frame. **(E)** Schematic representation of fracture of proximal tibia reduced and stabilized with external fixation, using ligamentotaxis (distraction across the joint using ligamentous pull for fracture reduction and stabilization).

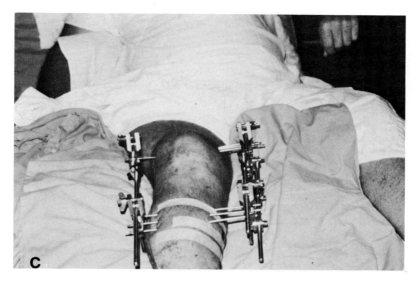

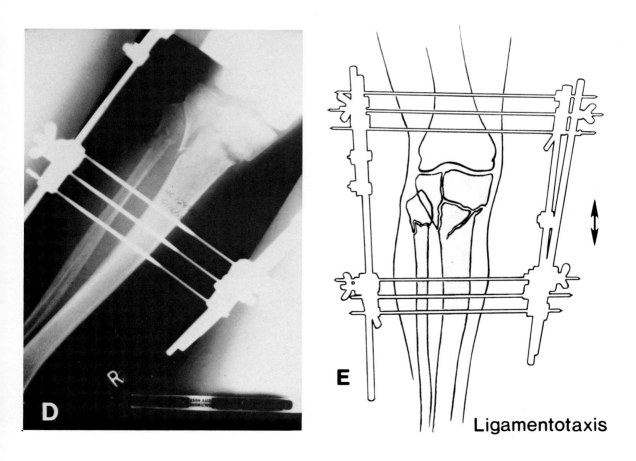

Ligamentotaxis

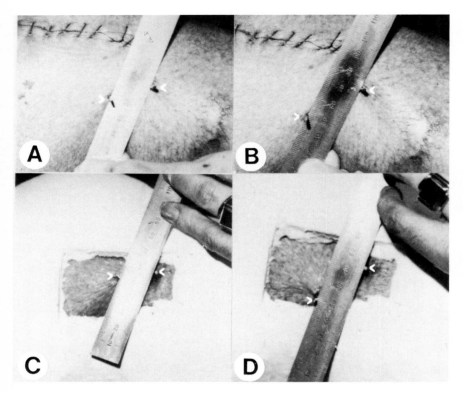

FIG. 30-7. A human autopsy knee specimen that had sustained medial lateral and anterior cruciate ligament transection. The markers represent Steinmann pins. **(A)** Resting position. **(B)** Anterior drawer stress position shows distraction of the pins.

The same leg was placed, with less than two layers of Sofrol, in a long leg cast with 45° flexion of the knee. **(C)** Resting in a cast. **(D)** Anterior drawer stress position in the cast. Note that same amount of movement is possible as with no cast. (Courtesy K. Krackow)

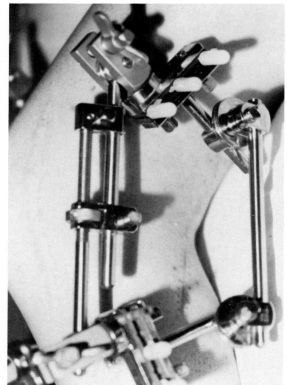

FIG. 30-8. Photograph of patient in external fixation after surgical reconstruction of the anterior cruciate and medial collateral ligaments of the knee. (Courtesy of K. Krackow)

union of the right knee (Fig. 30-10*A*). At surgery, the hardware was removed, and the nonunion débrided and stabilized with an external frame. After surgery, she was treated with continuous suction irrigation and the appropriate antibiotics. After removal of the drains, the external fixation device was compressed, and the compression across the nonunion was maintained for a full 12 weeks (Fig. 30-10*B*). A cylinder brace was applied after removal of the external fixation, for protection for a further 3 months, but she was bearing full weight during this time (Fig. 30-10*C*).

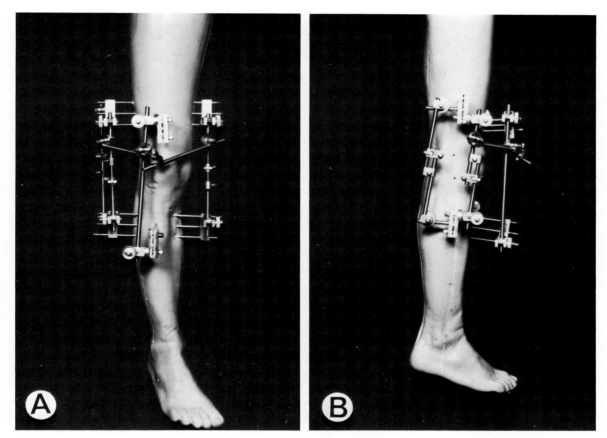

FIG. 30-9. (A, B) Frame configuration currently recommended for knee arthrodesis. Note two-plane stabilization.

HIGH TIBIAL OSTEOTOMY

Despite the success of total knee arthroplasty, proximal tibial osteotomy still has a major role in the treatment of knee arthrosis associated with varus or valgus deformity. Although the Coventry wedge osteotomy is the most commonly used procedure in the United States, elsewhere the high dome tibial osteotomy is more popular. In the latter procedure, external fixation is worthy of consideration. External fixation allows compression at the osteotomy site and at the same time allows early knee motion and weight-bearing. The major advantage of external fixation, however, is the ability to easily correct alignment of the osteotomy several days or weeks following surgery. This is important if the position is less then ideal or if there is slippage or motion of the original fixation (Fig. 30-11).

EXTERNAL FIXATION IN NONUNION

Two types of nonunion commonly occur about the knee. The first is failure of the tibial plateau fracture to unite. Such a problem is generally treated by open reduction and internal fixation. If infection is present, however, or if access is limited because of poor skin coverage, external fixation is a reasonable alternative. Unfortunately, a tibial plateau fracture usually does not provide adequate proximal bone to be gripped by the external frame and it is necessary to bridge across the knee.

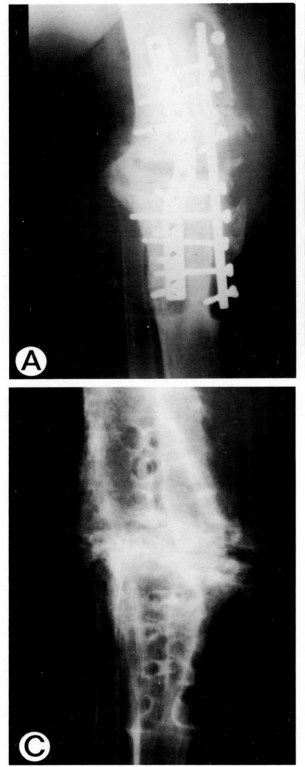

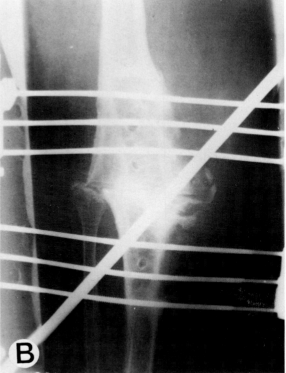

FIG. 30-10. (A) Infected nonunion of attempted right knee arthrodesis. **(B)** Compressed nonunion in external frame. **(C)** Final result at 6 months with union.

This prevents early knee motion and is a slight disadvantage.

The second and most frequently encountered type of nonunion about the knee is failure of the high tibial osteotomy. There is generally not sufficient bone stock between the nonunion site and the knee joint for adequate open reduction and internal fixation. The Hoffman frame, therefore, can be placed with pins parallel to the joint surface above the nonunion and perpendicular in the tibia below, permitting excellent access for débridement and bone grafting. It will also provide a method of compression of the nonunion site.

FIG. 30-11. X-ray film of frame for high tibial valgus osteotomy. Note that there are three pins placed horizontally through the proximal tibia and three pins placed vertically through the distal tibia.

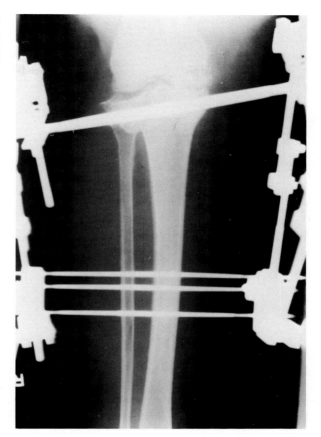

In this configuration, early knee motion can be undertaken, and healing of the nonunion can be expected.

EXAMPLE 4

A 22-year-old white man sustained a proximal tibial fracture that was treated closed with a cast. This progressed to a nonunion, for which a sliding bone graft was performed without success (Fig. 30-12A). The nonunion was explored and débrided, and an external fixation frame was applied with compression. This allowed full weight-bearing and mobility (Fig. 30-12B, C). The frame was removed at 10 weeks, and the patient was protected in a patella-bearing cast for a further 6 weeks (Fig. 30-12D).

SUMMARY

The development of stronger, more versatile external fixation devices has opened new areas for the use of external fixation around the knee. The Hoffman-Vidal type frame with double uprights and transfixation pins provides rigid fixation but allows mobility and change of alignment in all three planes and for length (compression or distraction) without the problems encountered in previous Roger-Anderson, Haynes, and Wagner type apparatus.

Today, periarticular knee fractures, compound fractures, burns, fractures with soft tissue injuries, nonunions, osteotomies, ligament repairs, and knee fusions are all amenable to external fixation.

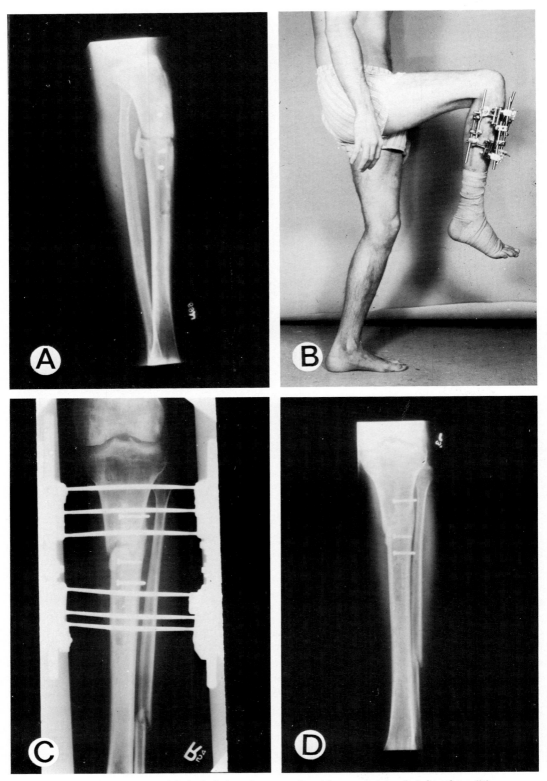

FIG. 30-12. **(A)** X-ray film of failed sliding bone graft with nonunion of right tibia. **(B)** Patient in external frame with full mobility. **(C)** X-ray film of compression of nonunion by external frame. **(D)** Final result with union of right tibia.

CHAPTER 31
REHABILITATION OF THE INJURED KNEE

James Nicholas,
Norman Scott,
A. J. Saraniti

Restoration of an injured knee to a high level of performance requires diligent work on the part of the patient and understanding of the muscle groups that require rehabilitation. Any operation is only as good as the patient's postoperative rehabilitation program. The orthopaedist cannot simply expect the patient to get better on his own.

To rehabilitate the knee, one should determine whether the defect is in motion, power, or stability, or in all three components. If there is loss of motion, it is important to ascertain whether it is intra- or extra-articular. Knees with intra-articular blocks to motion can be rehabilitated only by relieving contractures; such knees often require surgery. Extra-articular loss of movement results from contracture of the anterior quadriceps and thigh muscles, which limits patellar excursion, whereas lack of extension may be due to calf or hamstring contracture. The basic rehabilitative effort in

anterior or posterior thigh contracture is to stretch the muscles to increase excursion.

Lack of power is the most common result of knee injury and is often underestimated. Too frequently, only the quadriceps are considered, and the fact that other muscle groups in the proximal leg are subject to strength deficits is unrecognized. Dynamic control of the knee is a function of all muscle groups that **span** the hip and the ankle. For this reason, abductor and adductor power, particularly abductor power, is always lost after knee injury. Such loss of power can produce symptomatic synovitis.

Knee stability varies from patient to patient, depending on the body habitus. Loose-jointed individuals have a diffuse laxity of the ligaments. The ultimate goal in stability is not the same in these people as it is in tight-jointed persons. It is imperative to achieve maximum strength in an otherwise lax knee to increase

469

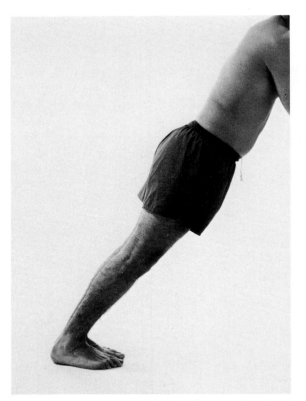

FIG. 31-1. Heel cord stretching helps to reduce heel cord and hamstring contracture.

the dynamic stability of the joint and to decrease the incidence of re-injury.

Power deficits can be tested manually with the patient seated by pushing down on the top of the thigh (just proximal to the patella). In the absence of pain, weakness in flexion is measured in terms of resistance compared with the opposite side. The average person can flex the hip 25 times against approximately 10% of body weight. Abductor power is tested with the patient lying on his side, abducting the leg against resistance. The hip and knee should be straight, and the weight is transmitted across the lower leg during this test. Knee extension power is tested with the leg at a 90° angle going to full extension, and flexion is tested with the leg in full extension bending against resistance for the latter.

Considering that for every step a person takes, a force of three to six times body weight passes through the tibiofemoral joint, any loss

of movement or power places a severe strain on the joint. The goal of rehabilitation is to attain equal power in both legs for all muscle groups. It can be achieved by a thorough understanding of the objective by the patient, careful measurement, and the use of active resistive exercises. Both legs should be strengthened to their maximum capacity.

RESTORATION OF MOTION

Loss of knee motion can occur from both intra- and extra-articular sources. It is often due to a combination of the two. For instance, a knee after hemarthrosis or injury to the patella heals, but contractures may develop in the quadriceps and upper thigh muscles. Because squatting is painful or not possible, the patient does not squat. However, if the hip and knee joints are normal, it is possible to obtain such movement by extending the hip, grasping the ankle, and bringing it toward the ceiling as one stands. This will stretch the anterior thigh musculature and produce increased excursion of the quadriceps.

Myostatic contracture of the hamstrings frequently causes limitation of extension of the knee and will produce tightening of the quadriceps mechanism along the patellofemoral ligaments. It is important to rid athletic persons of such contractures. An excellent exercise is wall stretching of the heel and calf muscles on an inclined plane (Fig. 31-1). The heel cord and calf muscles are stretched as the patient stands about 16 in from the wall with the heels placed square on the ground; the chest is moved to and against the wall while the knee remains extended.

To stretch the upper thigh, the foot is placed on a chair while the opposite knee is bent until the affected leg is parallel to the floor (Fig. 31-2). Usually this tends to flex the knee on the affected side. The patient forces the knee into extension as far as possible, keeping the foot dorsiflexed by bending the opposite knee. By these means, hamstring and calf muscles can be stretched to a considerable degree. If the spine is now flexed, all the muscles from spine to feet are stretched.

FIG. 31-2. A quadriceps stretching exercise in the standing position. This is an important test and treatment for anterior thigh contracture, which can limit knee movement.

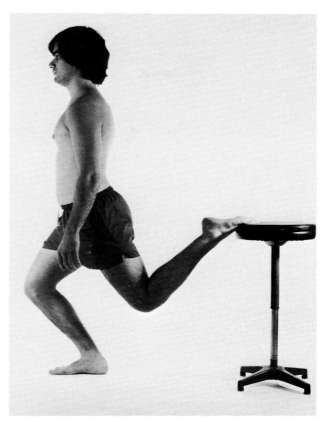

The abductors may be stretched in the manner described by Ober or by bending forward with the legs crossed, bending first to one side, then to the other. Lateral bending of the spine with the legs crossed while standing erect is another way to produce upper lateral thigh stretch.

It should be recognized that myostatic contracture entails loss of power and loss of adequate motion. Rehabilitation of the athlete's knee is not complete unless full power is recovered over the full range of motion.

ABDUCTION EXERCISES—
STRAIGHT LEG RAISING

The patient should lie on his side and lift sideways with weight over the ankle, beginning with ten repetitions if he can perform without pain. The weight the weakened leg can lift is actually very little and should not cause pain. The first target is the unaffected leg. When the two are equal, both legs should be strengthened. The weight the patient can lift sideways is in no way related to the amount he can lift while sitting.

After recovery of power and abduction and thigh flexion, knee extension exercises to obtain terminal vastus medialis power are performed, often with greater effect than with the conventional system described by DeLorme, whose system, if tolerated, is also used.

Once the maximum desired weight can be lifted, the exercises should not be discarded. Weight-lifting should be resumed every 3 or 4 months to see whether there has been a real decline in power. After injury there usually is, especially in hip flexion and abduction. The strength of the leg does vary, depending on the demands placed on it during specific seasons. In a nonathletic season the patient should be encouraged to retrain the leg. Such leg power is extremely important because even

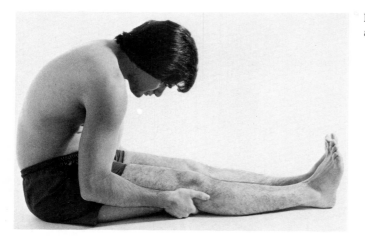

FIG. 31-3. Hamstring and calf exercise in a long seated position.

a slight loss will cause increased load on an already injured joint.

No weight-lifting should be done if it causes pain or swelling. Active resistive exercises of limited sets of perhaps 25 slide lifts and 10 knee extensions, repeated two or three times after a few minutes rest once a day, are usually adequate unless there are special weight-loading machines available.

POSTMENISCECTOMY REHABILITATION

After meniscectomy the first exercises are straight leg raising and quadriceps setting until motion gradually reaches 90° of flexion. At that point, rather than knee extension (from a flexed position), which may irritate the joint, hip flexion exercises are begun. This recommendation is based on the premise that the quadriceps muscle spans both the hip and the knee joints and is associated with the iliopsoas and lower abdominal muscles, which all contribute accessory power to the knee in athletic stress. In this way, power is developed in the quadriceps by transferring resistance to the upper end. In a seated position, the weight is suspended over the foot, and the knee is lifted off the table approximately 6 in. Two sets of 25 repetitions of this exercise are performed using the maximum amount of weight the patient can lift without pain. The opposite leg is tested to determine the maximum strength capacity of the legs. The aim is to develop equal power in both legs. Once this is accomplished, the patient is encouraged to achieve maximum power bilaterally. Many individuals can lift up to 40 or 50 pounds, after starting with as little as 5 pounds. This is extremely important in preventing re-injury. Knee extension against resistance, if not painful, is then instituted as well as active resistive abduction.

PERSISTENT STRETCHING

Continuous stretching during weight-lifting is important, especially in tight-muscled individuals. Tight-muscled athletes are usually unable to touch their toes with their hands and must do calf, hamstring (Figs. 31-3, 31-4, 31-5), and lower back stretching exercises if they are to participate in sports in which tight hamstrings endanger the knee. Loose-jointed people can easily put their palms to the floor, have recurvatum of the knee, and can often toe-out the entire extremity to 90°. In loose-jointed athletes, stretching exercises are useless because there is no contracture. Weight-lifting exercises are desirable for them because they may have considerable lack of power.

Many systems of rehabilitation are available after knee injuries and should be applied at all

FIG. 31-4. Hamstring and calf exercise in the standing position. This exercise should be performed with the leg held in a neutral position and in both internal and external rotation.

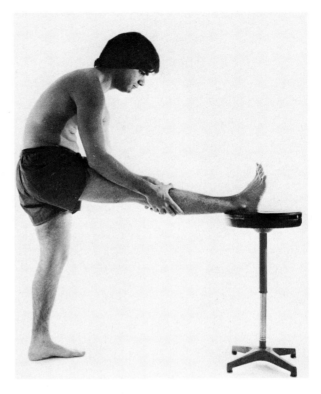

ages. Even a 70-year-old with a broken hip who recovers from the fracture and walks well may have residual thigh flexion and abductor weakness as well as contracture. Although the hamstrings and calf may be strong and have the ability to walk, there is usually contracture of these muscles, and the antigravity muscles are not strong. The system I have outlined has been valuable in recovering symmetrical strength, even in older people.

The use of a swimming pool is an excellent means for recovering thigh muscle power. Repetitive abductor exercises and walking in water with the level up to the groin will produce considerable upper thigh and abdominal abductor power. For good swimmers, treading water 200 to 300 times in the deep part of the pool is an effective way to develop upper thigh power. Goose stepping in the water with the knees fully extended is another way to strengthen the quadriceps. Flutter kicking in the water sometimes results in pain at the pa-

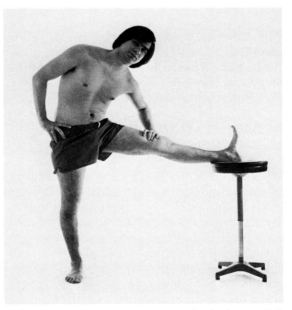

FIG. 31-5. Stretching exercise to both the medial hamstrings (semimembranosus and semitendinosus) and the hip adductors.

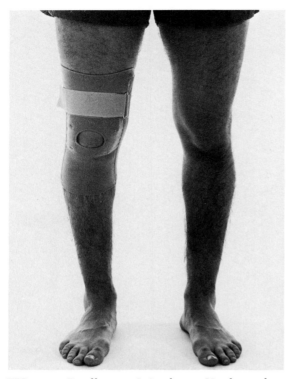

FIG. 31-6. Patella restraining brace. Used to reduce stress on the patellofemoral joint and to assist in proper tracking of the patella.

tella, a warning sign that exercises should be modified. Similarly, the butterfly and breast stroke should be avoided by patients with patellofemoral symptoms.

REHABILITATION OF EXTENSOR MECHANISM SYNDROMES

Rehabilitation of a weak knee with superimposed patellar pain is difficult. Whether the cause is subluxation, chondromalacia, or tendinitis, knee extension exercises often produce pain. Inability to perform exercises only aggravates the symptoms. Use of a patellar restraining brace (Fig. 31-6) can usually be prescribed as an adjunct to the exercises. The basic idea is to protect the patella from excessive movement and subsequent pain. Rehabilitation starts with sitting thigh flexion.

Such exercises as lifting the knee with the weight over the foot will cause no pain, whereas trying to extend the knee from a flexed position will aggravate symptoms. Instead of increasing the exercises, the patient can build up considerable power and then substitute more conventional quadriceps exercises. The second method is to see whether the patient can perform a straight leg raise in a sitting position without pain. If so, the patient, while sitting, can bend the knee from a raised straight leg position to the point where pain begins, usually about 30°. By flexing and extending the leg within this painless range, considerable power can develop before the leg ultimately reaches the full range of motion.

KNEE BRACES

Many supports are used in patients with symptomatic knees. Ace bandages and elastic wraps provide negligible stability and sometimes aggravate patellofemoral symptoms. Neoprene supports can be used after minor sprains but should not be used as a substitute for an exercise program.

Patellar restraining braces of many types have become popular. The basic idea is to protect the patella from excessive movement and contact with the trochlea. A hinged knee brace enveloped in a foam rubber support in the shape of a horseshoe has been used with success. This provides good protection for patients with patella alta. Cutout braces with relieving suprapatellar pads have also been successful in patients with extensor mechanism symptoms.

Braces for ligamentous instability require a more sophisticated approach. The Lenox Hill derotation brace and helicoid knee brace were developed specifically for ligamentous instabilities (Fig. 31-7; also, see Fig. 5-4). Rotational instability such as anteromedial, anterolateral, posteromedial and posterolateral, as previously discussed, can often be treated with these braces alone. The braces are used to supplement surgical procedures for these instabilities. Most ligamentous injuries, whether treated operatively or nonoperatively, are protected for up to a year with the use of these braces.

Many exercise modalities such as the Universal, Nautilus, and Cybex systems are commercially available for rehabilitation. In general, these machines can be of assistance to athletically minded patients. The overriding danger, however, is in allowing the patient to rely on the machines rather than on himself to do the work. Dedication and rehabilitation exercises done at home can be as effective as any mechanical aid.

The Universal machine offers a constant resistance throughout the entire range of joint motion. It can be applied in both upper and lower extremity exercises and is effective in building power and endurance. The disadvantage is that strength training is performed submaximally through a partial range of motion.

The Nautilus offers variable resistance through training. The resistive load is used to match an individual's force output. It allows for 16 exercises, which develop power and endurance in many muscle groups. From a practical point of view, this system can be used by 16 people at the same time. It is also one of the few units to apply head and neck exercises successfully. The difficulty with the Nautilus program is that a preset cam action does not provide for isotonic contraction throughout the entire range of motion.

The Cybex system offers accommodating re-

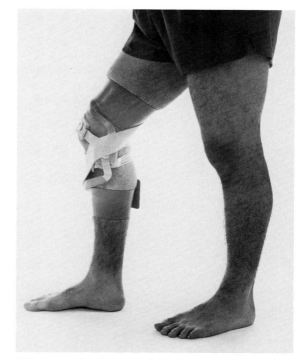

FIG. 31-7. The Lenox Hill derotation brace. Used to check simple and complex rotary instabilities.

sistive training with a preset velocity to resistance developed by the machine in response to the amount of muscle force exerted. Thus, this machine applies a maximal load throughout the range of motion. It can be used by only one person at a time, and this is somewhat of a disadvantage.

CHAPTER 32
TUMORS OF THE KNEE

Walid Mnaymneh

This chapter will deal with primary tumors and tumorlike conditions of the knee region, which includes the bones and soft tissues of the lower thigh and upper leg as well as the knee joint. This is a favored site of primary benign and malignant tumors, which do not differ basically from corresponding neoplasms in other parts of the body, whether they are primary in bone or in soft tissues. The general features of these tumors will be described briefly, with particular emphasis on diagnostic and therapeutic aspects specific to the knee region.

Tumorlike conditions consist of a group of lesions that are not true neoplasms but are the result of cellular proliferations of unknown cause that present as a "tumor," that is, a mass. These lesions present clinical, radiologic, and histologic features very similar to benign neoplasms but different in their biologic behavior and therapeutic management. They will, therefore, be considered with the benign tumors.

BENIGN TUMORS AND TUMORLIKE CONDITIONS

The common tumors that come to the attention of the orthopaedic surgeon are listed in Table 32-1, in decreasing order of frequency. They will be considered in four categories: (1) cartilaginous, (2) fibroblastic, (3) osteoblastic, and (4) giant cell tumor.

CARTILAGINOUS TUMORS

Osteochondroma (Osteocartilaginous Exostosis)

This is the most common benign bony growth in the knee region. Its pathogenesis is still controversial. The prevailing opinion is that it is not a true neoplasm but represents an aberrant growth of the epiphyseal plate[1,14] or an anomalous periosteal development with production of displaced nests of cartilage.[36] It arises at or near the epiphyseal plate of the distal

TABLE 32-1. BENIGN BONE TUMORS OF
THE KNEE (SURGICAL CASES)

Tumor	% of Benign Bone Tumors of the Knee
Osteochondroma	47
Benign giant cell tumor	28
Nonossifying fibroma	8
Enchondroma	4
Osteoid osteoma	4
Chondroblastoma	3
Chondromyxoid fibroma	2.5
Others	3.5

(Data taken from Dahlin, D. C.: Bone Tumors, 3rd ed. Springfield, Charles C Thomas, 1978.)

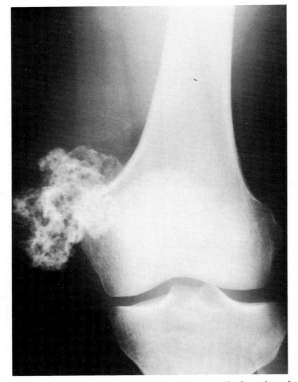

FIG. 32-1. Sessile osteochondroma of the distal
femur.

femur, proximal tibia, and proximal fibula, in
that order of decreasing frequency. The lesion
may be solitary, or multiple and hereditary. It
is more common in the second decade of life
and has a slight male predominance. Bony

protrusion is the usual presenting complaint,
followed by pain caused by pressure on
neighboring nerve structures. Occasionally,
the presenting manifestation is the result of a
fracture of the stalk of the tumor; very rarely,
pressure from the mass may result in the formation of a false popliteal aneurysm.[22] In the
multiple hereditary type, angular deformities
and shortening of the extremity are common.

Radiologically, the tumor appears as an osseous protuberance that may be either sessile
with a broad base (Fig. 32-1) or pedunculated
with a narrow stalk, tending to grow shaft-
ward. The exostosis is capped with a bluish
white layer of hyaline cartilage 2 mm to
5 mm in thickness. This cartilaginous cap acts
as the growth plate. By and large, the growth
of the tumor parallels that of the skeletal
growth of the patient. Hence, an enlarging
osteochondroma in a growing individual
should not raise much concern. In adulthood,
the cartilaginous cap becomes very thin or
nonexistent, and hypothetically, the growth
of the lesion ceases. If the tumor continues to
grow during adulthood, and especially if
there is irregularity and extensive calcification and thickening of the cartilaginous cap,
secondary chondrosarcoma should be suspected. This is not invariable; I have seen
cases in which lesions may show continued
growth and yet remain benign. About 1% of
the solitary and 20% of the multiple osteo-
chondromas undergo malignant transformation,[10,28] usually to a chondrosarcoma. Treatment is surgical excision; this is indicated
when the tumor produces pressure symptoms,
interferes with joint motion, or becomes
grossly unsightly. The tumor should be amputated at its base, flush with the cortex of the
bone, to ensure removal of the entire cartilaginous cap and circumferential periosteum.
Failure to do this may result in recurrence.

Enchondroma

An enchondroma in the knee region may be
either a solitary lesion or part of a multiple enchondromatosis. Solitary enchondroma is a
benign tumor of hyaline cartilage that devel-

ops within the medullary cavity of a single bone, whereas multiple enchondromas (Ollier's disease) are considered dysplastic lesions resulting from a developmental error in enchondral ossification.[10,28] In solitary tumors, neither sex nor age is a factor, and the lesions are often asymptomatic. Pain may result from fracture of an expanded, thin cortex curettage with bone grafting. Borderline tumors overlying a benign enchondroma. However, persistent pain without preceding trauma may indicate rapid growth and hence should arouse suspicion of malignancy. Radiologically, the tumor appears as a radiolucent lesion with spotty calcifications, a phenomenon shared by most cartilaginous tumors. Heavily calcified enchondroma may look like a bone infarct (Fig. 32-2). Ominous radiologic features include endosteal erosion, cortical penetration, and renewed growth of a previously stable enchondroma.[10,24] Microscopically, the differentiation between a benign enchondroma and a low-grade chondrosarcoma may be quite difficult, and a final verdict demands correlation of clinical, radiologic, and microscopic features.[10,14] Treatment consists of curettage with bone grafting. Borderline tumors should be adequately exercised and kept under long-term observation.[10] Occasionally, a solitary enchondroma may transform into a chondrosarcoma.[21] Malignant transformation is more common in multiple enchondromatosis, although the often quoted incidence of 50% appears to be too high.[28] Development of osteosarcoma has been reported both in solitary[56] and in multiple enchondromas.[3] When soft tissue hemangiomas are associated with multiple enchondromas, the condition is known as Maffucci's syndrome.[24]

Chondroblastoma

This is a benign cartilaginous tumor typically located in the epiphysis. It occurs predominantly in men in the second decade of life. The knee region is the most common site. Presenting complaints include pain, which may be of long duration, followed by tenderness

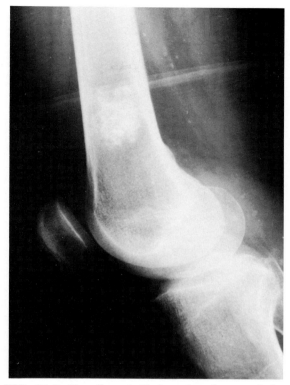

FIG. 32-2. Heavily calcified enchondroma of the distal femur.

and knee effusion. Radiologically, the tumor appears as an osteolytic lesion with or without mottled calcifications. The lesion is well defined with a thin sclerotic margin (Fig. 32-3). Chondroblastoma and giant cell tumor are the two primary bone tumors that characteristically involve the epiphysis of long bones. Microscopically, it consists of uniform round cells, the chondroblasts, and multinucleated giant cells, smaller in size and less abundant than those of the giant cell tumor. Occasional cases manifesting aggressive behavior are well documented in the literature, including local osseous and soft tissue recurrences[63] and pulmonary metastases.[12,26,55] Spontaneous or radiation-induced malignant transformation is also reported.[61,66] If feasible, *en bloc* resection of the tumor is preferable because curettage and bone grafting may result in recurrences in up to 25% of cases.[27]

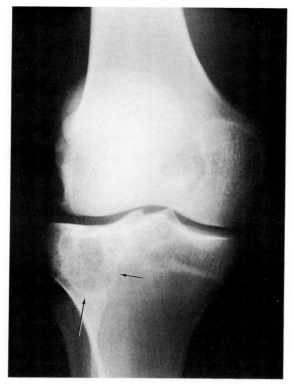

FIG. 32-3. Chondroblastoma of the lateral condyle of the tibia involving the epiphysis and adjacent metaphysis. There is a thin sclerotic margin surrounding the radiolucent lesion.

Chondromyxoid Fibroma

This is an uncommon, cartilaginous tumor with a metaphyseal, eccentric location. The proximal tibia is most commonly involved. It arises slightly more commonly in adolescent and young adult men. Pain is the usual presenting complaint. Radiologically, it presents characteristically as a sharply outlined, eccentric radiolucency with a thin rim of sclerosis. Occasionally, the overlying cortex is invisible (Fig. 32-4). Microscopically, the lesion is composed of lobules of cartilaginous tissue with myxoid and fibrous components. Treatment consists of either curettage or block excision. The latter is preferred because the recurrence rate after curettage is estimated to be 25%.[10] Bone grafting is often necessary. Well-docu-

mented cases of malignant transformation are extremely rare.[62]

FIBROBLASTIC TUMORS

Nonossifying Fibroma and Metaphyseal Fibrous Cortical Defect

Most authors agree that these fibrous lesions are not neoplastic. However, there is controversy about the histogenesis—that is, whether they result from failure of periosteum to lay down bone during the circumferential growth of the bone[14] or whether they are caused by a developmental aberration at the epiphyseal

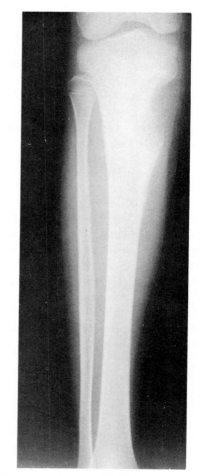

FIG. 32-4. Chondromyxoid fibroma of the proximal tibia. The cortex overlying the eccentric radiolucent lesion is missing.

plate.[9] Both lesions are identical histopathologically, and both arise in the metaphysis and migrate towards the diaphysis. They differ only in size. The fibrous cortical defect is small, usually less than 2 cm in size, intracortical, and asymptomatic. It is found in 35% of apparently normal children,[28] making it the most common lesion of the skeleton; it is often discovered incidentally on knee roentgenograms. Most of these lesions are self-healing; they either regress completely or become sclerotic. Nonossifying fibroma, on the other hand, is a large lesion that may produce pain and swelling. It may grow into the medullary cavity, weakening the bone and even producing a pathologic fracture. The majority of these lesions occur in childhood and adolescence. Both lesions occur more often in men. The radiologic appearance is quite characteristic and consists of an eccentrically located radiolucent defect, usually 2 cm to 5 cm in size (Fig. 32-5). It expands and thins out the overlying cortex. It is clearly demarcated with a thin sclerotic margin and may appear trabeculated. In the hands of the experienced, the x-ray appearance is so characteristic that biopsy is unnecessary. Treatment in the form of curettage and bone grafting is indicated only for large and symptomatic lesions. Unfortunately, this lesion is occasionally misdiagnosed radiologically and microscopically, leading to unwarranted and erroneously performed aggressive surgery.

OSTEOBLASTIC TUMORS

Osteoid Osteoma

Although the genesis of this lesion is not finally resolved, it is believed to be a neoplasm rather than an inflammatory or a reparative process by the majority of scholars on this subject.[10,24,68] It is a benign lesion characterized by a small central nidus, usually less than 1 cm in diameter, surrounded by a zone of dense reactive bone formation. It is more common in boys and young adult men. Pain, which may be present for any time from a few weeks to several years, is the most common

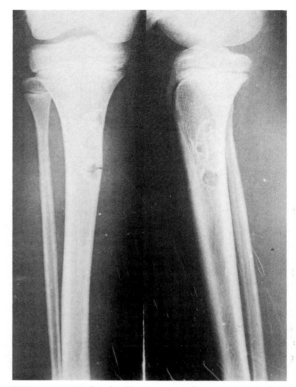

FIG. 32-5. Multiple fibromas of the proximal tibia. There is healing and sclerosis of the upper lesion, but a pathologic fracture is seen through the lower lesion.

complaint and is classically described as worse at night and responsive to aspirin. In a juxta-articular location, it may simulate arthritis. Radiologically, there is a central, radiolucent nidus surrounded by sclerotic bone. In cortical lesions, the sclerosis is so dense that tomography is required to demonstrate the nidus (Fig. 32-6). In cancellous lesions and in those arising near the end of a bone, there is usually little perifocal sclerosis. Technetium bone scanning shows a "hot" uptake. Angiography, especially if combined with magnification and subtraction techniques, reveals the hypervascular nidus, thus helping to localize the lesion; angiography may also be of value in differentiating it from osteomyelitis.[48] The ideal treatment is *en bloc* excision of the nidus with some of the surrounding sclerotic bone. Intraoperative roentgeno-

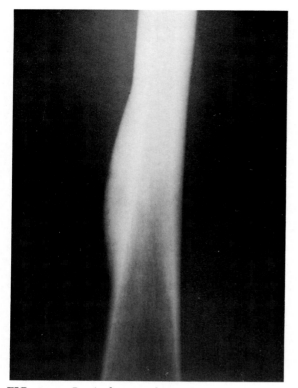

FIG. 32-6. Cortical osteoid osteoma of the lower femur showing the dense sclerosis surrounding the small radiolucent nidus.

graphic localization of the nidus is often needed. Recurrence is usually the result of incomplete removal of the nidus. Spontaneous healing is questionable because those cases that have been reported lack pathologic verification.

GIANT CELL TUMOR OF BONE

This lesion is still shrouded in controversy about whether it is a nonneoplastic or a neoplastic lesion, but it is increasingly accepted as a neoplasm. Recent ultrastructural and histochemical studies have demonstrated close similarity between the giant cells in giant cell tumor and normal osteoclasts. The knee region is the most common site of involvement. The peak age incidence occurs in the third decade, with a slight female preponderance. Painful swelling is the most common present-

ing complaint. Radiologically, the tumor appears as an expanded, radiolucent, often eccentrically placed epiphyseal lesion, frequently involving the adjacent metaphysis with absent or very little marginal sclerosis (Figs. 32-7B, 32-8A). Few instances have been reported in which the tumor is localized to the metaphysis prior to closure of the epiphyseal plate.[2] Microscopically, the character of the mononuclear stromal cells and the pattern of distribution of the giant cells are the two important clues in the histologic differentiation of this tumor from several other giant cell-containing lesions, such as aneurysmal bone cyst, nonossifying fibroma, brown tumor of hyperparathyroidism, and benign chondroblastoma.[28,44,45] Most giant cell tumors are histologically benign yet locally aggressive. Few undergo malignant transformation, particularly the irradiated ones, while few others are malignant from the outset.[10,45] Rarely, a benign giant cell tumor may metastasize to the lungs.[10]

Because of the high incidence of recurrence after curettage of the tumor and the potential of malignant transformation and metastases, giant cell tumors should be treated aggressively by means of *en bloc* resection. In young, active patients, resection-arthrodesis of the knee is indicated (Fig. 32-7).[17,45] Allograft hemiarthroplasty, which aims at preserving joint motion, is another surgical alternative (Fig. 32-8) that has not yet enjoyed wide acceptance, although preliminary studies suggest that allografts are well tolerated and often result in reasonably good function of the knee joint.[19,40] Proximal tibial allografts do better than distal femoral allografts.[19] Reconstruction following resection of a femoral condyle can be achieved by the use of an intramedullary bicondylar femoral prosthesis and bone grafts.[44] The use of customized total knee prostheses may be justified in older patients. Good results have been reported recently using cryosurgery after curettage of the tumor,[43] or just filling the curetted cavity with acrylic cement.[51] Further time and experience are needed to test the long-term results of these novel modalities of therapy. Radiotherapy has no place in the treatment of such tumors in the knee region.

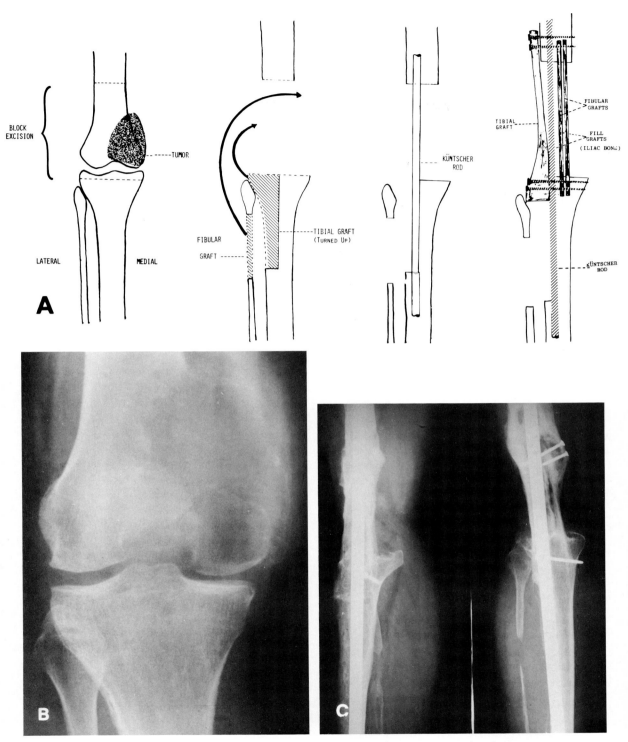

FIG. 32-7. (A) Diagram illustrating the surgical steps in the resection-arthrodesis procedure of giant cell tumor of the medial femoral condyle. **(B)** A large giant cell tumor of the medial femoral condyle with extension into the lateral condyle as well as the overlying soft tissues. **(C)** Two years after resection-arthrodesis procedure there is healing of the turned-up tibial and fibular grafts.

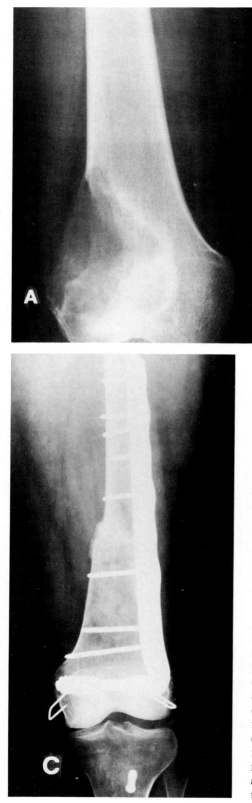

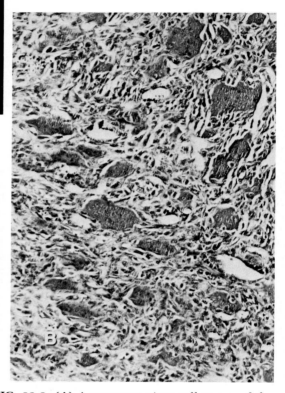

FIG. 32-8. **(A)** A recurrent giant cell tumor of the lateral femoral condyle showing the epiphyseal eccentric radiolucent lesion. **(B)** Microscopic appearance of the resected tumor. The mononuclear cells are polyhedral or round with a moderate amount of cytoplasm. This distinguishes giant cell tumors from the elongate and spindly cells of most other giant cell-containing lesions. The giant cells are uniformly scattered. (HE stain, original magnification ×1560) **(C)** One year after *en bloc* resection of the distal femur and massive hemi-joint allograft transplantation. There is good healing at the host–graft junction.

MALIGNANT BONE TUMORS

GENERAL CONSIDERATIONS

Not uncommonly, these tumors pose a difficult diagnostic puzzle and a major management problem. Hence, a multidisciplinary team approach is highly recommended. The time-honored cooperation between the orthopaedic surgeon, radiologist, and pathologist is essential to establish the correct diagnosis. In addition to ordinary x-ray films and tomography, newer diagnostic approaches are used, including ^{99m}Tc-labeled diphosphonate bone scanning to delineate intraosseous extension of the tumor and detect other unsuspected skeletal lesions, and biplane femoral arteriography to show tumor vascularity and to help delineate the extraosseous soft tissue mass as well as any encroachment on the popliteal vessels. Computerized tomography (CT) is helpful in demonstrating the axial extent of the tumor as well as its extraosseous extension. These diagnostic modalities are essential in determining the surgical feasibility of wide en bloc resection of the tumor, thus making the decision between en bloc resection and amputation. Lung tomography or CT scanning is performed to reveal any metastatic foci that are too small to be visible on plain x-ray films.

The biopsy is the final decisive diagnostic tool. The location of the biopsy is critical because the site must be removed en bloc with the tumor at the time of the definitive resection. Electron microscopy has enhanced the pathologic definition of some tumors, particularly the poorly differentiated small, round cell tumors.[47]

The management of malignant tumors demands team planning among the orthopaedic surgeon, chemotherapist, and radiotherapist. Recent advances in treatment have resulted in increasing survival rates and improvement in the quality of life of survivors. The present treatment plan is a two-pronged one, consisting in treatment of the primary tumor and control of subclinical occult metastasis.[29,59] Surgical ablation is usually undertaken for osteosarcoma, fibrosarcoma, chondrosarcoma, and malignant fibrous histiocytoma, whereas radiotherapy is recommended for Ewing's sar-

coma and non-Hodgkins lymphoma (reticulum cell sarcoma). Amputation is advised for the highly malignant tumors, while wide en bloc resection with skeletal reconstruction to preserve the lower extremity is recommended for low-grade malignant tumors such as parosteal sarcoma, low-grade chondrosarcoma and fibrosarcoma, and malignant fibrous histiocytoma. Reconstructive surgical techniques used in limb-saving procedures include bone grafting and arthrodesis,[17] customized prosthetic devices,[41,73] and allograft transplantation.[13,40] Adjuvant chemotherapy is used in highly malignant tumors in an effort to control subclinical micrometastases that are often present but unrecognized at the time of initial treatment. Unfortunately, the early optimism brought about by the use of chemotherapy seems to be losing some ground. Following the cessation of chemotherapy, relapses are being reported in increasing numbers, indicating that the drugs may be simply suppressing the inevitable appearance of metastasis.[15] Hematogenous spread to the lungs is the usual route of metastasis of malignant bone tumors. Wedge resection of pulmonary metastasis is recommended to improve the survival rate.[46]

The common malignant bone tumors of the knee region are listed in decreasing order of frequency in Table 32-2.

OSTEOSARCOMA

This is the most common malignant tumor of the knee region, where 55% of all osteosar-

TABLE 32-2. MALIGNANT BONE TUMORS

Tumors	% of Malignant Bone Tumors of the Knee
Osteosarcoma	65
Fibrosarcoma	7
Chondrosarcoma	6
Ewing's sarcoma	6
Non-Hodgkin's lymphoma*	5
Parosteal osteosarcoma	4
Malignant fibrous histiocytoma	2
Malignant giant cell tumors	2
Others	3

* Previously called reticulum cell sarcoma.
(Data taken from Dahlin, D. C.: Bone Tumors, 3rd ed. Springfield, Charles C Thomas, 1978.)

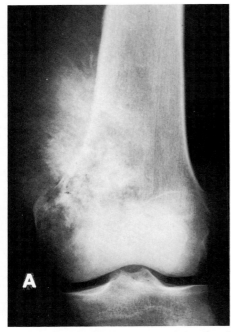

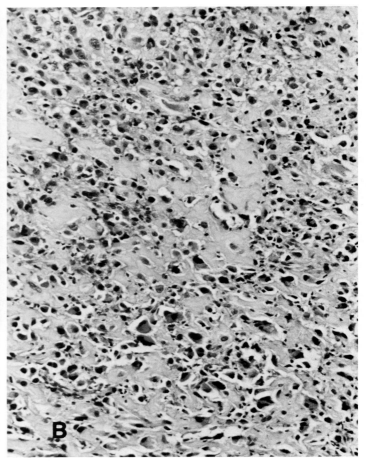

FIG. 32-9. **(A)** Osteosarcoma of the distal metaphysis of the femur showing the sunburst appearance. **(B)** Microscopic appearance of the tumor. The hallmark is the production of osteoid by the malignant cells. Osteoid is seen here as acellular material in the center, surrounding the tumor cells. (HE stain, original magnification ×1560)

comas occur. The highest incidence occurs in the second decade of life, with a gradual decrease thereafter. It occurs slightly more often in men. Pain and swelling are the usual presenting symptoms. Elevation of the serum alkaline phosphatase level is common. Radiologically, the tumor is metaphyseal in location and may appear as predominantly sclerotic, lytic, or a combination of both (Figs. 32-9, 32-10). Codman's triangle and a sunburst configuration of extraosseous ossification may be present. Telangiectatic osteosarcoma may mimic an aneurysmal bone cyst radiologically and grossly.[10,68] Contrary to the prevalent impression of the epiphyseal plate as a barrier to spread, a recent study has shown that the tumor often crosses the plate into the epiphysis.[64] This has been common in our experience also. Clinically undetectable intramedul-

lary foci of tumor that are separate from the primary lesion (so-called skip lesions) do exist[16] but are rare.

Owing to the use of recent, more informative diagnostic tools and the advent of adjuvant chemotherapy, management of osteosarcoma has undergone radical changes, resulting in improved survival rates.[13,30,59,73] Amputation is still the treatment of choice for the primary lesion. A midthigh amputation is recommended for proximal tibial tumors. For distal femoral tumors, there is still controversy about the level of amputation; a transmedullary thigh amputation is the preferred treatment by most authorities,[10] whereas hip disarticulation is recommended by those who believe that skip lesions are common.[16] Recent clinical studies, particularly those in which adjuvant chemotherapy was used, resulted in

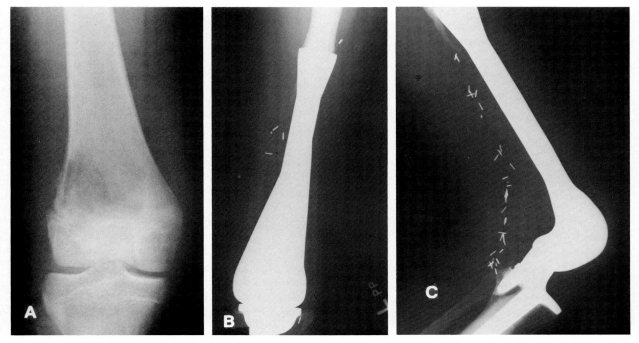

FIG. 32-10. (A) Predominantly osteolytic osteosarcoma of the distal femur in a 13-year-old girl. **(B)** Anteroposterior postoperative radiograph showing the customized prosthesis used in the limb-saving operation to restore skeletal integrity and knee-joint motion following radical *en bloc* resection of the distal femur and knee joint. **(C)** Lateral postoperative radiograph, showing the prostheses with the knee in flexion. (**A** courtesy Dr. H. Watts, Children's Hospital Medical Center, Boston, Mass.)

no difference in the local recurrence rate between the two levels of amputation.[13,73] By and large, I perform a high thigh amputation, 7 cm to 10 cm above the proximal edge of the tumor as seen on the bone scan (rather than on plain radiographs because the bone scan is more accurate in defining the tumor extent than plain x-ray films). A hip disarticulation is done instead if the proximal extension of the tumor does not allow this margin of normal tissue. Occasionally, if arteriography reveals no or only a small soft tissue mass with minimal or no encroachment on the popliteal vessels, and if the patient has reached full growth and his tumor is still mostly intraosseous, a limb-saving procedure is undertaken in the form of a radical *en bloc* resection, including a wide cuff of normal soft tissue and bone with the knee joint; skeletal reconstruc-

tion is achieved with prosthetic replacement[73] (Fig. 32-10) or allograft hemiarthroplasty.[13] The level of resection is determined in a manner similar to the determination of the amputation level. Multidrug adjuvant chemotherapy is given postoperatively, following either amputation or resection, to suppress any undetected pulmonary micrometastases or skip lesions and is continued for about 18 to 24 months. High-dose methotrexate and adriamycin are the commonly used drugs. Unfortunately, the early projection of a 70% 5-year survival rate has not materialized owing to late relapses. At present, an estimated 50% of patients attain a disease-free survival time of 3 to 4 years. Wedge resection of pulmonary metastases is recommended to further upgrade the survival rate.[46] Immunotherapy, although still in the experimental stage,[72] seems to hold

much promise, particularly adoptive immunotherapy[15,49] in the form of either interferon,
leukophoresis, or transfer factor.

PAROSTEAL (JUXTACORTICAL) OSTEOSARCOMA

Parosteal osteosarcoma is a peculiar type that
is much rarer and less malignant than the
usual intramedullary variety. Unlike ordinary
osteosarcoma, this type occurs in older people
and is much more common in women. Over
75% of tumors occur on the posterior aspect of
the distal femur.[47] Often the tumor is slow-
growing, and the patient presents with a
swelling of a few years' duration. The radiologic appearance is characteristic; the tumor
originates on the external surface, often encircling the shaft, and usually shows no medullary involvement and no Codman's triangle
(Fig. 32-11). The differential diagnosis includes
osteochondroma and myositis ossificans.
The recommended treatment for low-grade
tumors is wide *en bloc* resection-reconstruction with arthrodesis,[17] prosthetic replacement,[34,41,73] or allograft hemiarthroplasty.[13,40]
Recurrent high-grade tumors are best treated
by amputation. With early adequate treatment,
the 5-year survival rate is 80%.[10] The tumor
has a tendency to multiple local recurrences
if inadequately resected. Although there are
still no available clinical data on the use of
adjuvant chemotherapy, it is being recommended for high-grade tumors.[24]

FIBROSARCOMA OF BONE

This is a rare malignant tumor arising from
the fibrous element of the medullary cavity.
Fibrosarcoma may be primary or "secondary"[10] and develops after radiation therapy, in
a pre-existing giant cell tumor, or in Paget's

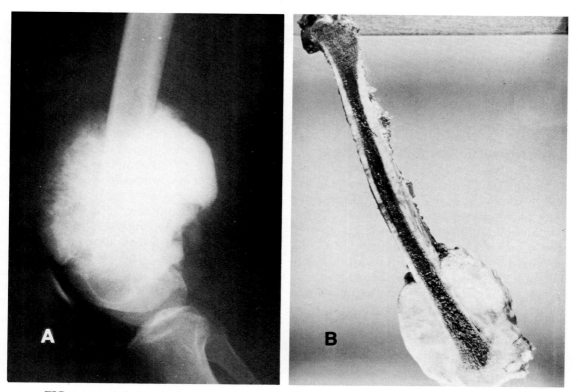

FIG. 32-11. (A) Parosteal osteosarcoma of the distal femur. **(B)** Sagittal section of the amputated femur showing the parosteal sarcoma encircling the shaft, with no medullary
involvement.

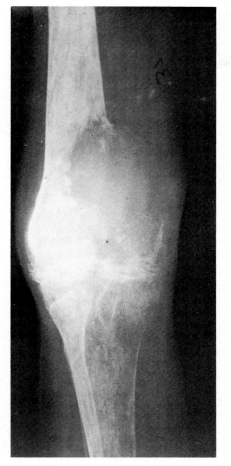

FIG. 32-12. Fibrosarcoma of the distal femur showing extensive osteolytic destruction of the medial condyle.

disease. It is evenly distributed from the second through the sixth decades of life and occurs as often in men as in women. It is usually metaphyseal in locatiion. Pain and swelling are the usual presenting symptoms. Radiologically, it appears as a permeative osteolytic lesion that may mimic osteolytic osteosarcoma (Fig. 32-12). Treatment usually consists of amputation;[54] however, the well-differentiated, low-grade fibrosarcoma has a better prognosis and can be adequately treated by wide *en bloc* resection-reconstruction techniques with preservation of the extremity.[10,40]

The reported overall 5-year survival rate is 35%.[25] The role of adjuvant chemotherapy has not yet been well established.

CHONDROSARCOMA

Compared to osteosarcoma, this is a relatively lower grade malignant tumor. It is more common in middle-aged men. It may be primary, arising *de novo* in a previously normal bone, or secondary, developing in a pre-existing, benign cartilaginous tumor. A rapidly enlarging osteochondroma or progressively painful enchondroma should alert the clinician to the probability of malignant transformation. Pain and hard swelling are the usual presenting complaints. Often the tumor has a slow clinical course. Metastases are rare and late in appearance. Radiologically, primary chondrosarcoma appears as a radiolucent lesion with stippled foci of calcification (Fig. 32-13). In osteochondroma undergoing malignant transformation, the surface becomes indistinct and fuzzy. To the pathologist, differentiation between low-grade chondrosarcoma and benign cartilaginous tumor can be very subtle and difficult.[10,14] However, nuclear pleomorphism and multinucleation differentiate this tumor from its benign counterpart. All parameters, including clinical course, x-ray films, bone scan, and arteriography should be carefully considered in the final assessment of borderline lesions. A symptomatic, vascular cartilaginous tumor in an adult with a "hot" uptake on the scan should be suspected of being malignant.[14]

Treatment of chondrosarcoma consists of either amputation or radical *en bloc* resection-reconstruction using bone grafts, allograft hemiarthroplasty, or a customized prosthesis. Local recurrence is the rule following inadequate excision. The average 5-year survival rate after adequate surgery is about 55%.[24] Chondrosarcoma is more resistant to chemotherapy than osteosarcoma. However, high-dose methotrexate is helpful in bringing about remission of this tumor.[59] Cryosurgery has been used in low- and medium-grade chondrosarcoma with seemingly encouraging preliminary results.[42]

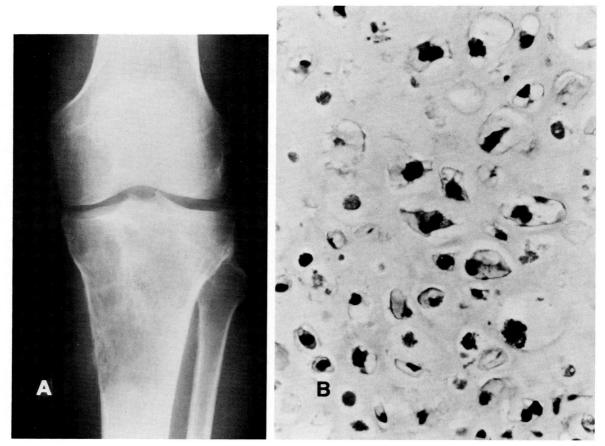

FIG. 32-13. (A) Primary chondrosarcoma of the proximal tibia, showing a radiolucent lesion. **(B)** Microscopic appearance of the tumor. The tumor cells show marked variation in nuclear size and shape, although they are still contained within lacunae. They are separated by a moderate amount of chondroid matrix. (HE stain, original magnification × 1560)

EWING'S SARCOMA

This is a highly malignant, small, round cell sarcoma that arises from the undifferentiated mesenchyme of the bone marrow. It is more common in men and occurs most commonly in the first two decades of life. Pain followed by tender swelling is the usual presenting complaint. Sometimes there is fever, leukocytosis, and elevated sedimentation rate suggestive of osteomyelitis. Radiologically, it appears as a mottled, destructive bone lesion, usually accompanied by an onion-skin pattern of periosteal new bone formation (Fig. 32-14). Osteomyelitis, eosinophilic granuloma,

malignant lymphoma, and osteosarcoma may mimic the tumor radiologically.[10] Bone scanning is helpful in determining the true intramedullary spread of the tumor, which is often more than that apparent from plain x-ray films. Microscopically, the demonstration of intracellular glycogen granules with PAS stain and electron microscopy help to differentiate this tumor from metastatic neuroblastoma and reticulum cell sarcoma.[10,68] The presently accepted treatment is radiotherapy to the whole bone to control the primary lesion plus multidrug chemotherapy (vincristine, Cytoxan, and adriamycin) to control micrometastases. In some centers where very aggressive chemotherapy regimens are given, a remarkable 5-year survival rate of 50% to 75% is reported.[50,57,58] Serious consideration, however, should be given to the possible ill-effects[35,71] of high-dose radiotherapy such as leg length discrepancy, joint contracture, muscle atrophy, and pathologic fracture as well as to the possible recurrent of the tumor and postradiation sarcoma. Moreover, recent reports have shown that surgical treatment of the primary lesion has actually given a better survival rate than radiation.[52,53] Hence, it is no longer considered unorthodox for the orthopaedic oncologist to advise amputation for Ewing's sarcoma of the knee region in the growing child when radiotherapy is expected to result in excessive shortening.

PRIMARY NON-HODGKIN'S LYMPHOMA

Non-Hodgkin's lymphoma was previously called reticulum cell sarcoma or lymphosarcoma. These tumors are found slightly more often in men and are common in adult life. A thorough search for signs of disseminated malignant lymphoma should be made, including bone marrow biopsy and lymphangiography. Radiologically, there is a nonmarginated, osteolytic, mottled permeative lesion (Fig. 32-15), which may be fairly extensive and frequently extends extraosseously. Sometimes marked irregular sclerosis of the lesion is seen. Treatment consists primarily of radiotherapy of the entire bone. Adjuvant chemotherapy is also given in some centers.[57] The reported 5-year survival is about 50%.[10] Primary lymphoma in bone has a better prognosis than disseminated disease involving bone. However, many of these primary bone lesions will develop lesions in other parts of the body. Pulmonary metastasis is relatively rare, in contrast to its high incidence in patients with Ewing's sarcoma.

MALIGNANT FIBROUS HISTIOCYTOMA

This is a new addition to malignant bone and soft tissue tumors and has a still unsettled histogenesis. It affects all ages but is more common in later life, with men slightly more affected. A painful swelling is the usual presenting complaint, often with a pathologic fracture. Radiologically, the lesion is usually metaphyseal in location and has a mottled, permeative lytic appearance with cortical destruction and without significant periosteal reaction (Fig. 32-16A). It may mimic fibrosarcoma, osteolytic osteosarcoma, or metastatic carcinoma. The lesion is composed of a bimorphic cell population, the histiocyte and the fibroblast, with a characteristic storiform pattern to the fibrous component (Fig. 32-16B). The current preferred therapy is similar to that for fibrosarcoma and osteosarcoma. Surgical ablation is the mainstay of the treatment, either amputation or radical en bloc resection with skeletal reconstruction and adjuvant chemotherapy. Available reports regarding survival and prognosis are scanty and conflicting. The 5-year survival ranges from 20% to 65%.[23,67] The usual sites of metastases are the lungs, other bones, and occasionally the regional lymph nodes.

TUMORS OF THE PATELLA

Primary tumors of the patella are very rare, with about 50 cases reported in the literature.[38,74] They are seldom considered in the differential diagnosis of patellar pain until radiologic bony changes become obvious. Most of these tumors are benign. The majority of the tumors in the reported cases are giant cell tumors. Other tumors include osteosarcoma, aneurysmal bone cyst, chondroblastoma, hemangioma, enchondroma, osteoblastoma, and reticulum cell sarcoma, in decreasing order of frequency. Patellectomy is generally curative except in osteosarcoma, for which more radical surgery is indicated.

SOFT TISSUE TUMORS OF THE KNEE

The differential diagnosis of a soft tissue mass in the knee region includes a long list of tumors, both benign and malignant, as well as

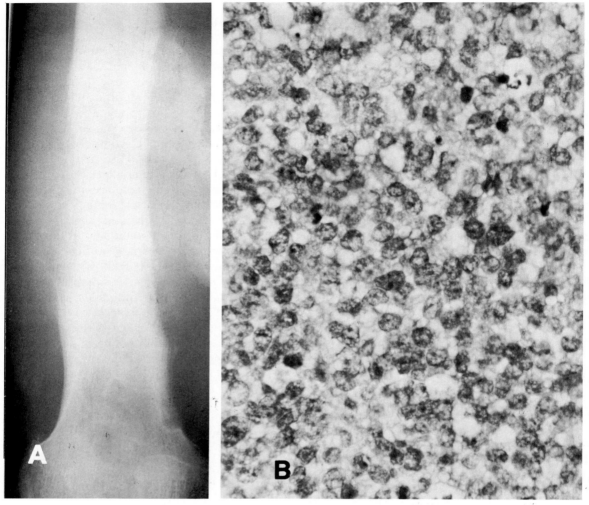

FIG. 32-14. (A) Ewing's sarcoma of the lower femur showing the onion-skin pattern of periosteal new bone formation. (B) High power microscopic appearance of the tumor. The tumor cells are small with ill-defined cytoplasm. The nuclei are round and vesicular with small nucleoli. (HE stain, original magnification × 2500)

nonneoplastic conditions such as traumatic, degenerative, inflammatory, circulatory, and metabolic disturbances and cysts. However, only soft tissue sarcomas will be discussed here.

About 40% of all soft tissue sarcomas occur in the lower extremities, and the great majority of those occur above the knee.[60] They can afflict any age group, the average age of incidence being 43 years, with an almost equal sex distribution. The soft tissue sarcomas of the lower extremity,[60] in decreasing order of frequency, are liposarcoma, fibrosarcoma, malignant fibrous histiocytoma, rhabdomyosarcoma, synovial sarcoma, leiomyosarcoma, malignant schwannoma, and angiosarcoma.

GENERAL CONSIDERATIONS

Soft tissue tumors have some features common to all of them. Their rate of local recurrence and metastasis is fairly similar. They have deceptively well-defined pushing borders, resulting in a pseudocapsule formed by fibrous and reactive connective tissue. This is not a true capsule, however, and tumor cells are found infiltrating the surrounding tissue. These tumors have a propensity to spread up and down musculoaponeurotic planes. Hematogenous spread is usually to the lungs. Spread to the regional lymph nodes is less frequent, especially in malignant fibrous histiocytoma, synovial sarcoma, and rhabdomyosarcoma. Clinically, the usual complaint is the presence of a lump. Attention should be directed principally toward the primary lesion, regional lymph nodes, and sites at risk for distant metastasis. Precise definition of the anatomical location and size of the tumor, fixation to deep structures, and invasion of bone and major vessels and nerves are feasible today through the use of bone scanning, gallium scanning, biplane arteriography, and CT scanning.

A staging system of soft tissue sarcomas has recently been outlined, and it appears to be more significant than the cell type and histogenesis[60,69] (Table 32-3). The parameters include histopathologic grading (G), tumor size (T), lymph node metastasis (N), and distant metastasis (M). Four stages are described, and 5-year survival rates have been shown to be inversely related to stage—75%, 56%, 26%, and 4% for stages I, II, III, and IV, respectively.

Surgery is the mainstay of treatment of these tumors. There is controversy about the choice of the surgical procedure and the adjuvant use of other treatment modalities. There are those who advise "radical local resection" or amputation if arteriography shows displacement of the popliteal vessels or if the femur or tibia are involved.[65] On the other hand, some workers advise "conservative" surgery followed by radiation therapy, which is presumably effective in eradicating any residual subclinical tumor tissue.[37,69,70] Proponents of the latter method of treatment claim results that are as good as those obtained by radical surgery or amputation while preserving the extremity. I subscribe to a middle-of-the-road approach in which a wide resection of the tumor, with an adequate surrounding

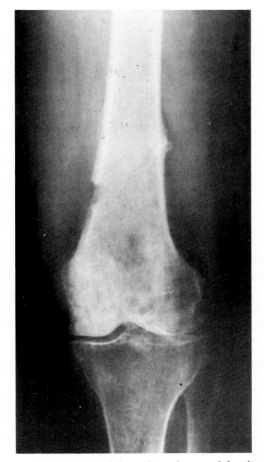

FIG. 32-15. Non-Hodgkin's lymphoma of the distal femur showing the mottled permeative osteolytic lesion.

margin of normal tissue at least 3 cm to 5 cm wide, is followed by radiotherapy (6000-rad tumor dose in 6 weeks). Occasionally, excision and simultaneous reconstruction of major blood vessels involved by the tumor is indicated to save the limb.[20]

A brief description of some of the special features of the common soft tissue sarcomas around the knee will be presented.

LIPOSARCOMA

Liposarcoma is a slowly growing, painless, deep-seated tumor. It is a much rarer tumor than lipoma. The average age of incidence is 52 years. Because of its relatively slow growth

TABLE 32-3. SOFT TISSUE SARCOMA STAGING SYSTEM

Parameter	Stage					5-yr Survival Rate (%)
G = Grade of malignancy (1, 2, or 3)	Stage	1A = G_1	T_1	N_0	M_0	76
		1B = G_1	T_2	N_0	M_0	
T = Tumor size	Stage	IIA = G_2	T_1	N_0	M_0	56
T_1 tumor < 5 cm in diameter		IIB = G_2	T_2	N_0	M_0	
T_2 tumor > 5 cm in diameter						
T_3 invasion of bone, major vessels, or nerves						
N = Lymph node involvement		IIIA = G_3	T_1	N_0	M_0	
N_0–No involvement	Stage	IIIB = G_3	T_2	N_0	M_0	26
N_1–Positive involvement		IIIC = Any G	T_{1-2}	N_1	M_0	
M = Distant metastasis		IVA = Any G	T_3	N_{0-1}	M_0	
M_0–No involvement	Stage	IVB = Any G	Any T	Any N	M_1	4
M_1–Positive involvement						

(Data taken from Rosen, G.: Past experiences and future considerations with T-2 chemotherapy in the treatment of Ewing's sarcoma. In Management of Primary and Soft Tissue Tumors, pp. 187–203. Chicago, Yearbook Publishers, 1977.)

rate, it may attain considerable size. The myxomatous liposarcoma is the most common type and has a better prognosis than the pleomorphic and round cell liposarcoma,[18] carrying a 53% local recurrence rate and a 77% 5-year survival rate.[31]

SYNOVIAL SARCOMA

Forty percent of synovial sarcomas occur near the knee (Fig. 32-17). They are most commonly found between the third and fifth decades of life. The tumor has an insidious slow growth with an average delay before diagnosis of 2½ years.[5] Although the lesion is located near the joint, it does not lie within or involve the joint except by secondary extension. About one-third of these tumors show calcific radiopacities, and 20% invade adjacent bone.[8,31] Metastasis is often to the lungs, and in 23% of cases there is spread to the regional lymph nodes.[31] Treatment today involves several modalities, but the commonly used protocols include wide local excision followed by radiotherapy and chemotherapy.[69,70]

FIBROSARCOMA

At present, many previously called fibrosarcomas are being diagnosed as malignant fibrous histiocytoma. Bona fide fibrosarcoma is more common in middle-aged men. The current treatment is wide en bloc excision plus radiotherapy. There is a 60% 5-year survival rate and a 50% recurrence rate.[54] Metastasis, which is usually to the lungs, occurs in 46% of cases.

RHABDOMYOSARCOMA

Rhabdomyosarcoma is a malignant tumor of skeletal muscles. Many of those tumors are being rediagnosed as malignant fibrous histiocytoma. The adult pleomorphic rhabdomyosarcoma usually develops in adult men, and 20% of the tumors in the extremities involve the knee region[39] (Fig. 32-18). The tendency of this tumor to extend along fascial planes and neurovascular bundles may account for the high recurrence rate (60%);[33] the 5-year survival rate is 25%.[39] The present mode of treatment is wide en bloc excision plus radiotherapy and chemotherapy.

MALIGNANT FIBROUS HISTIOCYTOMA

Malignant fibrous histiocytoma occurs more commonly in soft tissues than in bone. In fact, it is the most common soft tissue sarcoma in older people.[18] Many sarcomas that were formerly diagnosed as fibrosarcoma, liposarcoma, and rhabdomyosarcoma are now considered to be malignant fibrous histiocytomas. The most common site of this tumor is the thigh region (Fig. 32-19). The overall metastatic rate is 42%; metastases usually occur to the lungs, with about 28% to the regional lymph nodes.[18] Local recurrence rate is about 18%.[18] Treatment consists of en bloc excision plus irradiation and chemotherapy (Figure 32-19C).

FIG. 32-16. (A) Malignant fibrous histiocytoma of the distal femur showing the mottled permeative osteolytic appearance of the tumor. **(B)** Microscopic appearance of the tumor. The fascicles of spindle-shaped cells appear to radiate from a hypothetical point corresponding to the center of the field, imparting to it a storiform pattern. Notice the plump, polyhedral histiocytelike cells, as well as the few multinucleated giant cells.

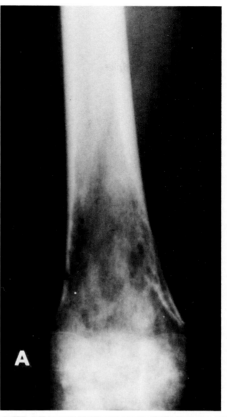

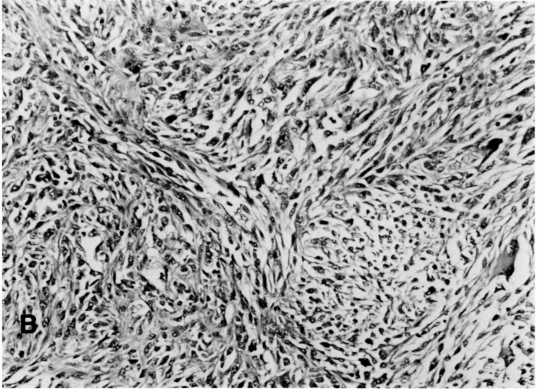

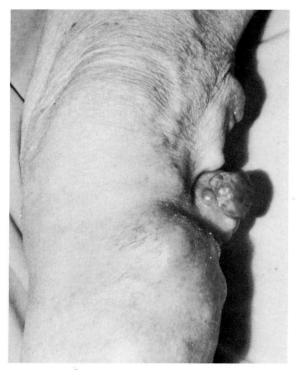

FIG. 32-17. Recurrent synovial sarcoma over the lateral aspect of the knee region. There were multiple recurrences of the tumor during the previous 8 years before this 75-year-old man agreed to an amputation. There was inguinal left node metastasis but no lung metastasis.

INTRA-ARTICULAR TUMORLIKE LESIONS

The two most common mass-producing lesions are pigmented villonodular synovitis and synovial chondromatosis.

PIGMENTED VILLONODULAR SYNOVITIS

Pigmented villonodular synovitis is a tumor-like proliferative lesion of unknown etiology, manifested by chronic, repeated painful swelling of the knee resulting from villous hyperplasia of the synovial tissue. The process can be localized and nodular or diffuse, in which case the whole lining of the joint looks reddish brown with grapelike masses protruding into the joint cavity (Fig. 32-20). The diffuse type is much more common.[32] The knee appears swollen, with a boggy synovium and frequently a bloody effusion. The lesion may invade bone and is then manifest radiologically as subcondylar osseous erosion and cystic destructive changes that may occasionally mimic a malignant process.

The ideal treatment is total synovectomy, which, technically speaking, can hardly be complete, thus explaining the high recurrence

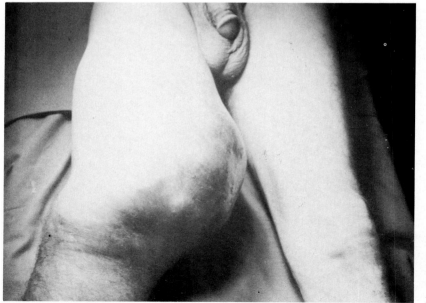

FIG. 32-18. A huge rhabdomyosarcoma of the soft tissue of the right lower thigh. Hip disarticulation was performed.

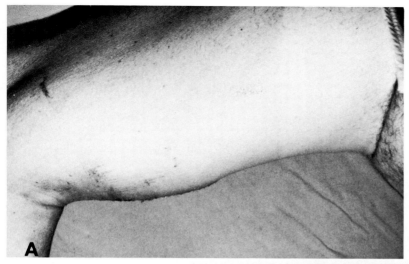

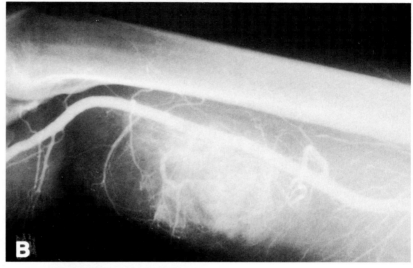

FIG. 32-19. (A) Malignant fibrous histiocytoma arising in the soft tissues of the posterior aspect of the distal thigh. **(B)** Arteriography showing the vascularity, size, and extent of the soft tissue tumor. **(C)** Gross appearance of the cut-open resected tumor. The patient was treated postoperatively with radiotherapy and chemotherapy.

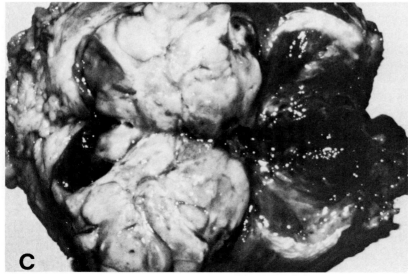

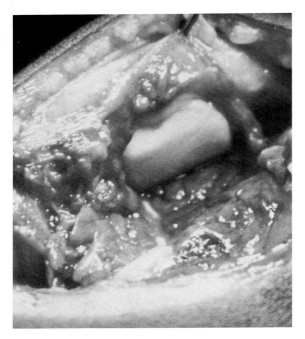

FIG. 32-20. Pigmented villonodular synovitis of the knee joint showing the hypertrophic villi of the synovium.

FIG. 32-21. Synovial chondromatosis of the knee joint showing numerous osteocartilaginous loose bodies.

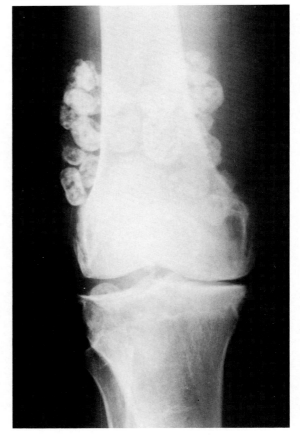

rate of 48%.[4] Moreover, extensive synovectomy often results in joint stiffness. Although radiotherapy may be beneficial, its neoplastic potential negates its use.

SYNOVIAL CHONDROMATOSIS

Synovial chondromatosis is produced by cartilaginous metaplasia of the synovial tissue of the joint, eventually resulting in the formation of many cartilaginous intra-articular loose bodies (Fig. 32-21). Some of these bodies undergo central calcification and ossification, imparting a radiologic appearance highly suggestive of the diagnosis. The knee is involved in two-thirds of the patients, and men are more commonly involved than women. The presenting complaints are usually pain, swelling, and locking, in that order.[7] The demonstration of chondromatous metaplasia in the synovial membrane, in addition to the calcified loose bodies, is essential for the diagnosis. The usual treatment is removal of loose bodies and excision of the involved synovium. Recurrences may occur, but chondrosarcomatous transformation is extremely rare.[34]

REFERENCES

1. **Aegerter E, Kirpatrick JA:** Orthopedic Diseases, 4th Ed, Philadelphia, WB Saunders, 1975

2. **Bogumille GP, Schultz MA, Johnson LC:** Giant cell tumor—A metaphyseal lesion. Proceedings of the American Academy of Orthopedic Surgeons, J Bone Joint Surg 54-A:1558, 1972

3. **Braddock GTF, Hadlow VD:** Osteosarcoma in enchondromatosis (Ollier's Disease). Report of a case. J Bone Joint Surg 48-B:145–149, 1966

4. **Byers PO et al:** Treatment of pigmented villonodular synovitis. J Bone Joint Surg 50-B:290–304, 1968

5. **Cadman NL, Soule EH, Kelly PJ:** Synovial sarcoma. Cancer 18:613–627, 1965

6. **Camblin JG, Enneking WF:** Immunotherapy in Osteosarcoma. In Jaffe N (ed); Bone Tumors in Children, pp. 215–233. Littleton, PSG Publisher, 1979

7. **Christensen JM, Poulsen JO:** Synovial chondromatosis. Acta Orthop Scand 46:919–925, 1975

8. **Craig RM, Pugh DG, Soule EH:** The roentgenologic manifestations of synovial sarcoma. Radiology 65:837, 1955

9. **Cunningham JB, Ackerman LV:** Metaphyseal cortical defect. J Bone Joint Surg 38-A:797–808, 1956

10. **Dahlin DC:** Bone Tumors, 3rd ed. Springfield, Charles C Thomas, 1978

11. **Dahlin DC, Coventry MD:** Osteogenic sarcoma: A study of 600 cases. J Bone Joint Surg 49-A:101–196, 1967

12. **Dahlin DC, Ivins JC:** Benign chondroblastoma: A study of 125 cases. Cancer 30:401–413, 1972

13. **Eilber FR:** En bloc resection and allograft replacement for osteosarcoma of the extremity. In Jaffe N (ed): Bone Tumors in Children, pp 159–167. Littleton, PSG Publisher , 1979

14. **Enneking WF:** Clinical Musculoskeletal Pathology. Gainesville, Stroten Printing Co, 1977

15. **Enneking WF:** Advances and treatment of primary bone tumors. J Fl Med Assoc 66(1):28–30, 1979

16. **Enneking WF, Kagan A:** Skip metastasis in osteosarcoma. Cancer 36:2192, 1975

17. **Enneking WF, Shirley PD:** Resection arthrodesis for malignant and potentially malignant lesions about the knee using intramedullary rod and local bone grafts. J Bone Joint Surg 49-A:223–236, 1977

18. **Enzinger FM:** Recent Developments in the Classification of Soft Tissue Tumors, pp 226–232. Chicago, Yearbook Publishers, 1977

19. **Faggard JM, Murray JA, de Santos LA et al:** Allograft hemi-joint arthroplasty for the treatment of locally aggressive primary bone tumors. Orthop Trans 3(1):207, 1978

20. **Fortner JG, Kim DK, Shiu MH:** Limb-preserving vascular surgery for malignant tumors of the lower extremity. Arch Surg 112:391–394, 1977

21. **Hamlin JA, Adler L, Greenbaum EI:** Central enchondroma—A precursor to chondrosarcoma? J Can Assoc Radiol 22:206–209, 1971

22. **Hershey SL, Lansden FT:** Osteochondroma as a cause of false popliteal aneurysms. Review of the literature and report of two cases. J Bone Joint Surg 54-A:1765–1768, 1972

23. **Huvos AG:** Primary malignant fibrous histiocytoma of bone. NY State J Med 76:552–559, 1976

24. **Huvos AG:** Bone Tumors. Philadelphia, WB Saunders, 1979

25. **Huvos AG, Higginbotham NL:** Primary fibrosarcoma of bone. Cancer 35:837–847, 1975

26. **Huvos AG et al:** Aggressive chondroblastoma. Review of the literature on aggressive behavior and metastasis with a report of one new case. Clin Orthop 126:266–272, 1977

27. **Huvos AG, Marcove RC:** Chondroblastoma of bone. A critical review. Clin Orthop 95:300–312, 1973

28. **Jaffe HL:** Tumors and Tumorous Conditions of the Bones and Joints. Philadelphia, Lea & Febiger, 1974

29. **Jaffe N:** Malignant Bone Tumors: Principles and Controversies in Treatment. In Bone Tumors in Children, pp 11–22. Littleton, PSG Publisher, 1979

30. **Jaffe N, Watts HG:** Multi-drug chemotherapy in primary treatment of osteosarcoma, an editorial comment. J Bone Joint Surg 58-A:634–635, 1976

31. **Johnston AD, Parisien MV:** Soft tissue tumors about the knee. Orthop Clin North Am 10:1 263–280, 1979

32. **Jones FE, Soule EH, Coventry MB:** Fibrous xanthoma of synovium, giant cell tumor of tendon sheath and Pigmented villonodular synovitis. J Bone Joint Surg 51-A:76–86, 1969

33. **Kehyani A, Booher RJ:** Pleomorphic rhabdomyosarcoma. Cancer 22:956–967, 1968

34. **King JW et al:** Synovial chondrosarcoma of the knee joint. J Bone Joint Surg 49-A:1389–1396, 1967

35. **Lewis RJ, Marcove RC, Rosen G:** Ewing's sarcoma: Functional effects of radiotherapy. J Bone Joint Surg 59-A:325–331, 1977

36. **Lichtenstein L:** Bone Tumors, 4th ed. St. Louis, CV Mosby, 1972

37. **Lindberg RD, Martin RG, Romsdahl MM et al:** Conservative surgery and radiation therapy of soft tissue sarcomas. In Management of Primary Bone and Soft Tissue Tumors, pp 289–293. Chicago, Yearbook Publisher, 1977

38. **Linscheid RL, Dahlin DC:** Unusual lesions of the patella. J Bone Joint Surg 48-A:1359–1365, 1966

39. **Linscheid RL, Soule EH, Henderson ED:** Pleomorphic rhabdomyosarcoma of the extremities and limb girdles. J Bone Joint Surg 47-A:715–726, 1965

40. **Mankin HJ et al:** Massive resection and allograft transplantation in the treatment of malignant bone tumors. N Engl J Med 294:1247–1255, 1976

41. **Marcove RC:** En bloc resection and prosthetic replacement in osteosarcoma. In Jaffe N (ed): Bone Tumors in Children, pp 143–158. Littleton, PSG Publisher, 1979

42. **Marcove RC et al:** The use of cryosurgery in the treatment of low and medium grade chondrosarcoma. Clin Orthop 122:147–156, 1977

43. **Marcove RC et al:** Cryosurgery in the treatment of giant cell tumor of bone. Orthop Trans 2(2):207, 1978

44. **Mnaymneh W, Dudley RH, Mnaymneh LG:** Giant cell tumor of bone—Clinicopathological study. J Bone Joint Surg 46-A:63–75, 1964

45. **Mnaymneh W, Mnaymneh LG:** Giant cell tumor of bone. J Cont Ed Orthop 19–31, 1978

46. **Mountain CF:** The role of surgery in the management of pulmonary metastasis. In Management of Primary Bone and Soft Tissue Tumors, pp 423–432. Chicago, Yearbook Publishers, 1977

47. **Murray JA, Finklestein JB, Spjut HJ:** Malignant bone-forming tumors. Inst Course Lect, Vol 27, pp 109–126. St. Louis, CV Mosby, 1978

48. **Murray JA, Thaggard A, Wallace S et al:** Artheriography of osteoid osteoma—An aid in differentiation and management. Orthopedics 2(4):359–365, 1979

49. **Neff JR, Enneking WF:** Adoptive immunotherapy in primary osteosarcoma. In Conflicts in Childhood Cancer, pp 289–296. N.Y., Alan R. Liss, 1975

50. **Pomeroy TC, Johnson RE:** Combined modality therapy of ewing's sarcoma. Cancer 35:36–47, 1975

51. **Presson BM, Woters HW:** Curettage and acrylic cementation in surgery of giant cell tumors of bone. Clin Orthop 120:125–133, 1976

52. **Pritchard DJ:** Surgical Experience in the Management of Ewing's Sarcoma. Presented at the Annual Meeting of the Musculoskeletal Oncology Society, Houston, April, 1979

53. **Pritchard DJ et al:** Ewing's sarcoma—A clinicopathological and statistical analysis of patients surviving five years or longer. J Bone Joint Surg 57-A:10–16, 1975

54. **Pritchard DJ, Soule EJ, Tayler WF et al:** Fibrosarcoma; A clinicopathological and statistical study of 199 tumors of the extremities and trunk. Cancer 33:888–897, 1974

55. **Riddell RJ, Louis CJ, Bromberger NA:** Pulmonary metastasis from chondroblastoma of the tibia—Report of a case. J Bone Joint Surg 55:848–853, 1973

56. **Rockwell MA, Enneking WF:** Osteosarcoma developing in a solitary enchondroma of the tibia. J Bone Joint Surg 53-A:341–344, 1977

57. **Rosen G:** Management of malignant bone tumors in children and adolescents. Pediatr Clin North Am 23:183–213, 1976

58. **Rosen G:** Past experiences and future considerations with T-2 chemotherapy in the treatment of Ewing's sarcoma. In Management of Primary and Soft Tissue Tumors, pp 187–203. Chicago, Yearbook Publishers, 1977

59. **Rosen G, Jaffe N:** Chemotherapy of malignant spindle cell sarcoma of bone. In Bone Tumors in Children, pp 109–121. Littleton, PSG Publisher, 1979

60. **Russell WO et al:** A clinical and pathological staging system for soft tissue sarcomas. Cancer 40:1562–1570, 1977

61. **Schijowicz F, Gallardo H:** Epiphyseal chondroblastoma of bone. A clinicopathological study of 69 cases. J Bone Joint Surg 52-B:205–226, 1970

62. **Sehayik S, Rosman MA:** Malignant degeneration of chondromyxoid fibroma in a child. Can J Surg 18:354–360, 1975

63. **Shoji H, Miller TR:** Benign chondroblastoma with soft tissue recurrence. NY State J Med 71:2786–2789, 1971

64. **Simon MA, Bos GD:** Epiphyseal extension of human osteosarcoma. Orthop Trans 3(2):235, 1979

65. **Simon MA, Enneking WF:** The management of soft tissue sarcoma of the extremities. J Bone Joint Surg 58-A:317–327, 1976

66. **Sirsat MV, Doctor VM:** Benign chondroblastoma of bone—Report of a case of malignant transformation. J Bone Joint Surg 52-B:741–745, 1970

67. **Spanier SS:** Malignant fibrous histiocytoma of bone. Orthop Clin North Am 8:947–961, 1977

68. **Spjut HJ et al:** Tumors of bone and cartilage, p 120. Armed Forces Inst Pathol Washington, D.C., 1971

69. **Suit HD:** Sarcoma of soft tissue. Cancer 28(5):1978

70. **Suit HD, Russell WO, Martin RG:** Management of patients with sarcoma of soft tissue in an extremity. Cancer 31:1247, 1973

71. **Tefft M et al:** Treatment of rhabdomyosarcoma and Ewing's sarcoma of childhood—Acute and late effects on normal tissue following combination therapy with emphasis on the role of irradiation combined with chemotherapy. Cancer 37:1201–1213, 1976

72. **Terry WD:** Present status and future directions for cancer immunotherapy. In Yamomura Y (ed); GANN Monograph on Cancer Research, pp 239–246. Raven Press, New York, 1978

73. **Watts HG:** Surgical management of malignant bone tumors in children. In Jaffe N (ed): Bone Tumors in Children, pp 131–142. Littleton, PSG Publisher, 1979

74. **Weinert CR, Jr, Wiss DA:** Unusual lesions of the patella. Orthopedics 2(4):378–383, 1979

Index